EDIBLE &
MEDICINAL
WILD PLANTS
of the
MIDWEST

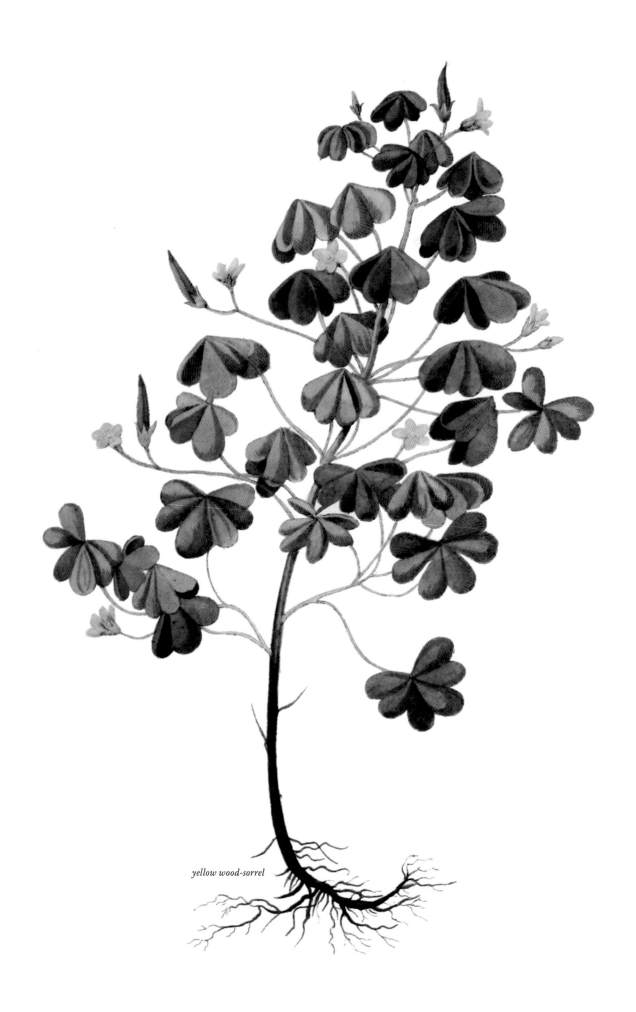

yellow wood-sorrel

EDIBLE &
MEDICINAL
WILD PLANTS
of the
MIDWEST

THIRD EDITION

Matthew Alfs

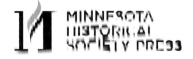
MINNESOTA
HISTORICAL
SOCIETY PRESS

mnhspress.org

The Minnesota Historical Society Press is a member of the Association of University Presses.

Manufactured in the United States of America

10 9 8 7 6 5 4

♾ The paper used in this publication meets the minimum requirements of the American National Standard for Information Sciences—Permanence for Printed Library Materials, ANSI Z39.48–1984.

International Standard Book Number

ISBN: 978-1-68134-175-0 (paper)

Library of Congress Cataloging-in-Publication Data available upon request.

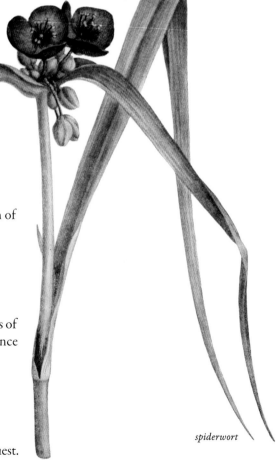

spiderwort

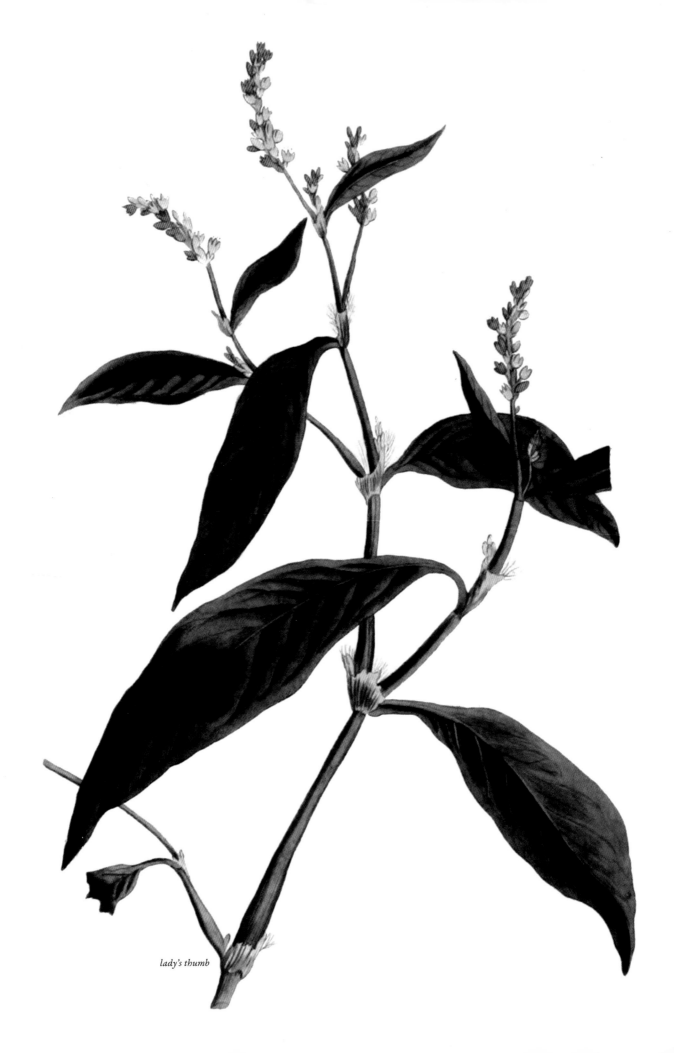

lady's thumb

Field Guide & Description of Plant Uses

Individual Plant Profiles Alphabetized by Common English Name

watercress

Acknowledgments

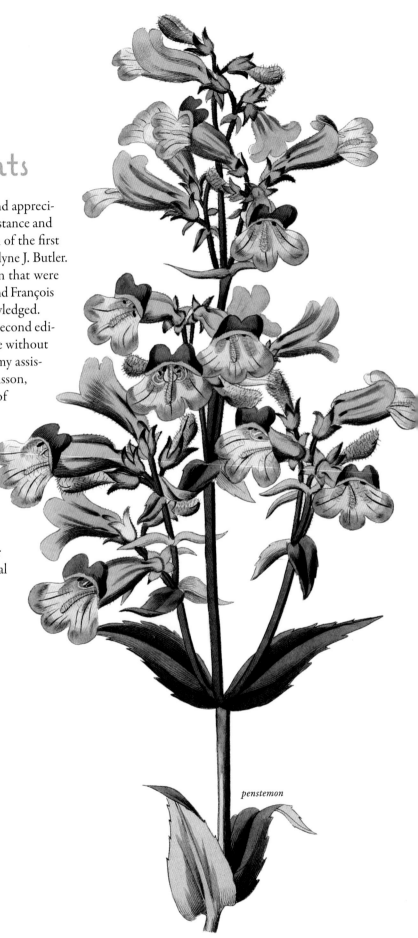

The author wishes to express his thanks and appreciation to the following people for their assistance and encouragement relative to the production of the first edition of this book: James Alfs and Carolyne J. Butler. Prepublication reviews of the first edition that were provided by Edelene Wood, James Duke, and François Couplan are also hereby gratefully acknowledged.

The timely and able production of the second edition in 2013 would not have been possible without the devoted and skillful aid provided by my assistants Deborah Garrido, Annika Christensson, Kara Carper, and Laurie Swadner, all of whom worked so diligently with me to prepare the text for publication.

This third edition, published by the Minnesota Historical Society Press, was accomplished with the able assistance of Josh Leventhal, Shannon Pennefeather, Madeleine Vasaly, Daniel Leary, and Susan Everson. I am deeply indebted to them for their sharp attention to detail and their additional efforts in producing this new edition.

penstemon

Preface

The bioregion encompassing the great states of the Upper Midwest (Minnesota, Wisconsin, Iowa, Michigan, and the Dakotas) has a varied landscape: coniferous forests in the north, prairie to the west and south, and deciduous woodlands and fields in the central portion. In view of this variety, one can surmise that a tremendous assortment of wild plants must flourish throughout this area. In fact, that is precisely the situation: even looking at simply the author's home state of Minnesota, more than two thousand species of vascular plants have been verified as carpeting its wild lands (Ownbey and Morley 1991: vii). Astoundingly, that is about one-tenth of all the known vascular species existing in North America (Moerman 1996).

A large number of our region's wild plants have been utilized for millennia as food and/or medicine by the local Indigenous peoples (see sidebar below). In the present day, in addition to traditionalists among these Native tribes, some non-Native wild-foods teachers and practitioners of indigenous herbalism enthusiastically perpetuate the hallowed tradition of a symbiotic interaction with the native flora in a culinary and/or healing context.

In view of our area's rich flora and of the protracted and colorful history of its utilization by some of its inhabitants as outlined above, it seems almost reprehensible that no significant study was published on the edible and medicinal uses of the wild plants growing in the Midwest prior to the twenty-first century. The present study is an attempt to remedy this deficiency. In doing so, it culls information from a variety of sources: phytochemical and therapeutic studies from the scholarly literature; historical and present-day uses by Native American tribes; the concerted uses of the plants undertaken by America's Physiomedicalist and Eclectic physicians of the nineteenth and early-twentieth centuries; clinical uses by herbalists of times past and present; and finally, my own utilization of our area's plants as both a wild-foods forager and a practicing herbalist.

When first published in 2001 as *Edible & Medicinal Wild Plants of Minnesota & Wisconsin*, this study charted a course that not only attempted to shed new light on the commoner plants but also focused on those plants which, while rich in medicinal and nutritional content, had been largely neglected. Thus, it "opened new doors" for those engaged in wild-plant studies by providing fresh and invigorating information. Twelve years later, I revised the book in a second edition with new and expanded information, and I amended the title to *Edible & Medicinal Wild Plants of the Midwest* to reflect the fact that the plants discussed flourish in a larger range than simply that encompassing Minnesota and Wisconsin—occurring also in Iowa, Michigan, the Dakotas, and other midwestern states.

I also added a section in each of the plant profiles summarizing my personal and/or clinical experience with that particular plant, entitling this section "Personal and Professional Use." This consistent, personal touch was evident in the first edition only in scattered spots in the text.

Several other features were added to this revised and expanded edition, including a history of herbalism in the United States and a chart comparing the

Wisconsin has been home to the Menomini (alternatively spelled "Menominee"), Winnebago (Ho-Chunk), Potawatomi, Oneida, Meskwaki (Fox), and Ojibwe (Chippewa) peoples. Minnesota has been home to the latter tribe (whose name in the Ojibwe language is "Anishinabe"), as well as to the Meskwaki, plus the Santee Dakota. Some of the aforementioned tribes spill over into Iowa, Michigan, and the eastern Dakotas as well: the Potawatomi to Michigan, the Meskwaki to Iowa, and the Dakota to the eastern Dakotas (even as the name of those states implies).

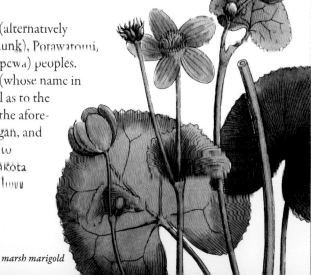

marsh marigold

nutritional content of wild foods to domestic vegetables (which evinces the nutritional superiority of the former over the latter! See page 13).

Now, here we are with the third edition of *Edible & Medicinal Wild Plants of the Midwest*. I have again updated the text based upon my further experience with the plants and upon newly published clinical trials and other scientific studies. In fact, this new research has been incorporated into more than half of the one hundred plant profiles featured in the book. The introductory material has also been updated and expanded, and new color photographs have been incorporated throughout the plant descriptions to allow for easy correlation between the text and the images.

In conclusion, my hope is that this third, revised and updated edition of *Edible & Medicinal Wild Plants of the Midwest* will continue to serve as a resource for those folks who hold a sincere appreciation for the remarkable flora of the upper midwestern states.

— Matthew Alfs

EDIBLE & MEDICINAL WILD PLANTS of the MIDWEST

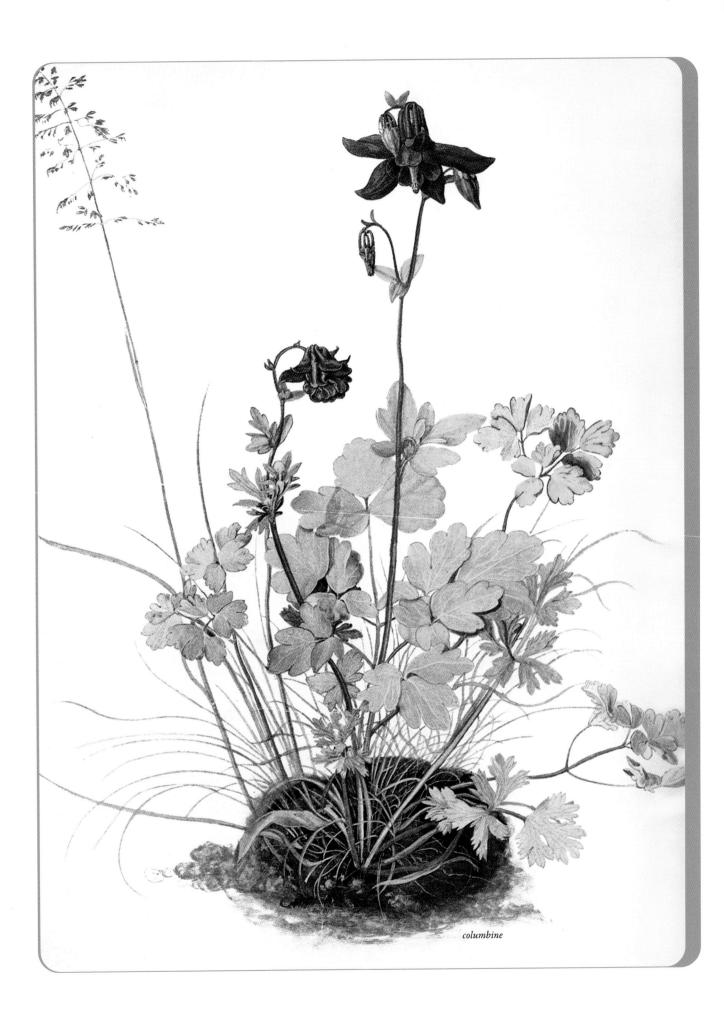

columbine

The Art of Wild-Plant Foraging

So many changes we have seen over the last century! My grandfather used to marvel that when he was born, people were still riding around in horse-drawn carriages, and yet when he reached his senior years, a rocket ship had carried men to the moon.

Yet, in serious contemplation, how many of the changes that we have witnessed have truly been for our good, as well as for that of the other creatures on this planet—not to mention the planet itself?

There is no doubt that baby boomers like me have, for most of our lives, dwelled in relative comfort—just a hop, skip, and jump away from the local supermarket, pharmacy, and haberdashery where our food, medicine, and clothing have all been easily obtained. Yet might we still be missing something on a deeper level that previous generations have experienced?

Here I remember that it was quite a revelation to me, as a lad in the early to mid-1960s, to learn that people of only a couple of generations ago—especially Native Americans and early settlers and pioneers—had subsisted largely off of nature's provisions for their food, medicine, and clothing, which they did through a symbiosis with the land that preserved both it and themselves. I couldn't help but wonder, even then as a young boy, whether we moderns had lost something—something, at least, of the spirit of adventure.

"Progress" powerfully changed the previous, self-sustaining way of life, my young self came to learn. Big cities, industry, and technology divorced us from the land as our provider so that we lost the feeling of kinship with it that we had once possessed. As a result, the wilderness become a terrifying monstrosity to many, with the general approach being "Tame that godforsaken 'wasteland.' Civilize it! Pave it over!"

Nevertheless, with the back-to-the-land movement initiated by Rachel Carson, Euell Gibbons, Bradford Angier, and others in the late 1960s and early 1970s, a sizable minority of the population began to adjust its attitude back to that possessed by its forebears. The wilderness, these people discovered, was not an enemy but the most intimate of friends. I think now it was inevitable that I, as I grew into my teens in the early 1970s, would stumble across the books of the aforementioned naturalists. As I did, I quickly found myself in harmony with the thoughts that they so clearly and logically presented. It was then that I realized something else: There was more than just *adventure* to this way of life. There was a sublime *spirituality* as well.

Here, though, my own sense of personal integrity compelled me to practice what I had now come to appreciate: that living in harmony with the land was the way to really

live. Gibbons's books, especially, imbued in me a burning desire to live an existence whereby nature's bounty would provide at least a portion of my food, medicine, and utility. So then, again almost inevitably, I, too, became a survivalist, a naturalist, and eventually an herbalist as well—spending long hours in the bush identifying, harvesting, and later preparing wild foods, medicines, and tools from hundreds of different wild plants.

In the present work, dear reader, I gladly pass on this accumulated knowledge and experience to you, admonishing you and entrusting you to use it wisely and with care as well as to closely observe the guidelines given in the way of both ecology and safety. Here my solemn wish is that you, too, can experience the oneness with nature that has so delighted my own soul over these past decades.

FORAGING RESPONSIBILITIES

First and foremost, it is important to understand that the path to a forager's nirvana requires some training in the art. And make no mistake about it: foraging for weeds is an acquired art. Not only must you learn where to look, but you must know something about botany, conservation, harvesting, gardening, meteorology, law, and the list goes on and on. I hope to make clear some of the specifics below, but the journey is really a matter of continual education—one in which firsthand experience becomes one of the most crucial factors.

So, then, let's see what I can do to get you prepared for your first forays into foraging ...

WHERE TO LOOK

Before I suggest where you might forage for wild edibles, I want to stress a very important point: *never collect plants from roadsides, no matter how tempting that may be.* Exhaust from autos, despite increasing antipollution measures, contains many harmful substances (including the toxic metal cadmium—also found in cigarette smoke—which collects in the body and causes great harm), and it settles on nearby vegetation like a noxious fog. Unfortunately, to further compound the problem, some edible and medicinal weeds actually act like natural magnets for such pollutants, possessing fine hairs or other characteristics that trap them. So, then, take the above-stated warning to heart. Your health is too precious to risk for a few scrumptious meals!

Having said this, we are left with the question, where does one look for edible and medicinal wild plants? Interestingly, the best foraging places are often the most overlooked. For example, the strip of land bordering each side of railroad tracks is often quite productive (as long as these areas haven't been sprayed to kill vegetation—many aren't, but some still are). Here you may stumble across plants not commonly found in the immediate vicinity—out-of-state plants may have become rooted in the area from windblown seeds that hitched a ride on railroad cars.

A variety of wonderful wild plants can be spotted on riverbanks and on the shores of lakes, which means that an activity such as canoeing or fishing could prove to be doubly rewarding (since fish and greens make a terrific combo).

How about that vacant lot you've noticed a few blocks down the road? Vacant lots are frequently quite rewarding for the forager in that they usually contain "the plants that follow the white man," as our Native friends used to describe the plants that seemed to sprout in the footsteps of the settlers. This highly nutritious and often easily recognized category of urban weeds includes such characters as lamb's quarters, yellow wood-sorrel, purslane, dandelion, chicory, and plantain.

Meadows are prime foraging locations, as are the borders of swamps and marshes. Open woods yield some interesting plants not found elsewhere, but woods in general are not as prime a location as the novice may imagine. On the other hand, the perimeters of woods can sometimes prove to be excellent natural pantries.

So-called "wasteland" is often quite ripe for foraging, although permission to forage on any such that may be privately owned should first be obtained. The same is true of the vacant lots mentioned above: for a small fee, you can usually check ownership of land in a plat book at the government office for the county in question. Nowadays, too, that information is often available online.

Even where public land is concerned, there are regulations that need to be considered. Numerous endangered species are protected by law; this is understandable and should be respected. Then, too, parks on all levels—national, state, regional, county, and city—usually prohibit the uprooting of plants, although some of them allow berry picking; in some cases, too, you may prove able to obtain a foraging permit from the park authorities to take some samples for "scientific or educational purposes." At any rate, should you be restricted in what you can collect, you can still use the parks for identifying plants and for studying them in their natural habitat. Here, a good camera with a macro lens for close-up photography becomes an invaluable tool.

It is a sad, but true, fact that so-called conservationists are pressing for firmer "look, but don't touch" regulations on other public lands as well. From my standpoint, these individuals would seem to lack an education in, and an appreciation for, genuine wilderness ecology. As well-known herbalist Michael Tierra has so well phrased it, "pseudo-ecologists ... make futile attempts to maintain natural environments as aesthetic monuments with no functional purpose, leaving signs saying 'do not touch,' 'do not pick the plants,' etc. The herbalist, along with the American Indian, appreciates nature not only for its beauty but also for the valuable resource of wild foods and medicines that grow in these all-giving bowers. Thus the herbalist views nature as a positive force, and as a provider and teacher" (Tierra 1998: xix–xx).

If well-meaning, but misguided, environmentalists such as these continue to get their way, one will encounter more rigid and far-reaching restrictions on foraging on public lands than there will be for the hunting of animals in these same areas—an incongruity that needs not be elaborated. (Of course, true conservation is vital for the forager, and this will be discussed below.)

Even worse than the misguided environmentalists, however, are the greedy land developers and politicians who are draining swamps, paving over wasteland, bulldozing woods, and spraying everything in sight with herbicides. Euell Gibbons said of this situation: "[A] real menace is the huge array of herbicides sprayed on roadsides, in fields, and over lawns. These are poisons and badly upset the balance of nature. They kill earthworms and wash into streams where they kill aquatic life. Another enemy is the engineering mentality that wants to bulldoze all the hills, fill all the marshes, pave over all open areas—never even knowing the names and natures of the billions of life forms they are destroying" (Gibbons 1973: 148).

That was decades ago, and the situation nowadays is considerably worse: natural resources are disappearing like the proverbial Cheshire cat! Sadly, unlike that fairy-tale feline, many of these natural wonders may never reappear.

SCOUTING PLANTS

As you study the field guide following this introductory material, you will see that certain plants favor particular locales, such as wasteland, meadows, moist woods, dry woods, hills, deserts, mountains, swamps, marshes, ponds, or other bodies of water. Study these habitats and you will be better prepared to scout out the particular species that may be appealing to you. For instance, if you come across boneset in a swampy region, you can—armed with knowledge of habitat—anticipate finding blue vervain or joe-pye weed growing along with it. You can also expect that wood-sorrel and lamb's quarters might be growing at the edges of clearings or paths, not to mention plantain, peppergrass, or shepherd's purse. Yes, you can become skilled enough that if you need a particular wild plant for a recipe or herbal formula, you will know just where to look for it out in the wilds. That not only is a time saver but also can be quite rewarding on a personal level.

Remember, too, that certain plants bloom only at particular times of the day (examples being spiderwort, chicory, and evening primrose) or in particular weather (the blossoms of chickweed and purslane open only on sunny days). Knowing this will help you plan your foraging so that you hunt for these plants when they are in bloom and thus easier to locate.

SAFE FORAGING

It might seem strange to think that you can encounter hazards when foraging, yet there definitely can be dangers. To begin with, the forager needs to be careful about where they are walking. You shouldn't be so intent on weed watching that you saunter into a hole, trip on a rock, or march into an overhanging branch that could poke an eye! This may seem laughable, but all of these things have happened either to me or to other foragers I have known.

A second caution has to do with insect pests. Mosquitoes and deer flies can ruin a foray into the wild if you are not prepared for their onslaught. Commercial sprays may contain substances that are damaging to the body's systems. Several studies have indicated DEET (N,N-diethyl-meta-toluamide)—the ingredient common to many sprays that, according to its sponsors and some independent studies, best repels mosquitoes—has the potential to cause serious problems. Since up to 15 percent of the chemical can be absorbed into the skin, allergic or toxic reactions may arise, and seizures have even been known to occur in children who have been doused with it (Silverstein 1990: 86).

Several commercial sprays coming on the market now reflect the increased awareness of the potential hazards posed by large concentrations of DEET. These largely herbal-based products may provide some protection without the damaging side effects of synthetic chemical sprays. Infusions made from chamomile, catnip, yarrow, or garlic, kept in a spray bottle in a pocket for repeated application, have proven helpful for some people (although those with allergies should be cautious in any use of the first two herbs). Essential oils of patchouli, eucalyptus, catnip, and/or pennyroyal have also been employed with success by many. Because essential oils are highly concentrated, a few drops are usually mixed with an innocuous base paste or oil or otherwise diluted and applied to pulse points (wrists, ankles, and neck). Most essential oils should never be applied full strength. Also, a bottle of pennyroyal essential oil should only be opened and applied when outdoors—never in a vehicle, as, in such a closed environment, it could potentially cause respiratory collapse. This is especially a hazard for infants or small children, but it can happen to adults, too!

Some sources have suggested that regular ingestion of vitamin B_1 (thiamine) for about a month prior to heading out into the mosquito-infested wilds may cut down on mosquito attacks, as it causes the skin to emit an unpleasant odor.

A more serious threat is that posed by ticks, especially the deer tick *(Ixodes scapularis)*, which can carry the debilitating Lyme disease. This tick, which used to be confined to small areas of the United States, is now spreading rapidly. In its early life as a larva, it often latches on to the white-footed mouse, picking up from it the spirochete that can cause Lyme disease in humans. It chooses a larger mammalian host (occasionally a human, but more often a deer) during its later nymphal and adult stages, sometimes transmitting to this host the infectious spirochete. Experts have found that, contrary to popular belief, the tick usually transmits spirochetes to humans during its nymphal stage (late spring and early summer) as opposed to its adult tick stage, although considerable transmission at this later stage is suspected as well. Compounding the risk is that both the adult tick and the nymph are very small and difficult to spot on one's body.

false Solomon's seal

How, then, can you protect yourself from the deer tick as well as from other ticks and similar parasites? While there are no surefire procedures, the tips listed in the box below may prove to be helpful.

In addition to these tips, there is this very important one: *all foragers with long hair should bunch up their hair underneath a hat.*

There are also some important cautions related to the particular act of harvesting wild plants. These will be discussed below.

HOW TO HARVEST

Foraging for plants is something to take seriously. You must be certain not only to identify the plant carefully (cross-referencing in several field guides is strongly recommended) but also to pick in a way that neighboring plants are not accidentally pulled with the desired one(s). One must also exercise caution so as to utilize only the particular parts of a plant that may be edible and to prepare these parts in a fashion that renders them safe and palatable. Also, individual allergies vary, so even wild plants that have been positively identified as edible must be sampled with caution. Some wild plants may even be related to domestic foods to which a person may be allergic.

In other words, we are dealing with a serious activity requiring an organized, teachable mind. Mistakes can be hazardous, even deadly. Contrariwise, care and enthusiasm can generate great rewards.

The serious forager, if anything, is well equipped. Never be without certain implements, all of which can be carried in one of those strap-on waist pouches designed for carrying small objects. For suggestions, see the box on the next page.

When gathering herbs to be dried for future use as a tea, be sure to collect them only on dry and sunny days, as the plants' essential oils are at their high point in this sort of weather. Then, too, leaves collected while wet tend to mold more easily when dried at home than do those collected during drier weather.

Plant parts should be collected when they are at their greatest point of utilization in the respective plant's growth cycle. Native Americans developed the following methodology in this regard, which modern herbalists have also adopted: *Roots* of annuals are collected in spring, prior to flowering; those of biennials are dug in the autumn of the first year; and those of perennials are gathered either in the fall or in the spring before the leaves start to grow. *Leaves* are usually collected only up to the time when the plant begins to blossom. *Flowers* are collected shortly after they began to

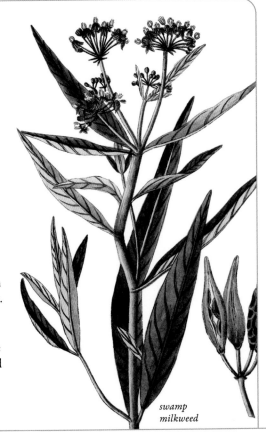

swamp milkweed

protect yourself

- ◊ Wear light-colored clothing.

- ◊ Wear long-sleeved shirts and long pants, tucking the latter into light-colored socks so as not to allow an entry point to the body.

- ◊ Ticks hate garlic! In view of this, some choose to make a garlic infusion and spray the contents onto their neck, wrists, and/or ankles (where the pulse points are located) or use an oil preparation in which the garlic has been heavily diluted by olive oil. Do not apply full-strength garlic to skin, as it may burn it! The skin of some people may even be too sensitive for dilutions. Some persons, if coming across the related wild onion (see page 269) while foraging, have elected to rub some of the crushed leaves or bulb onto the outer layer of their pant legs—again, not directly onto the skin.

- ◊ After returning home, take off all your clothes and put them in the dryer. Set on high, then tumble for at least twenty minutes.

- ◊ Visually inspect yourself in a full-length mirror for any ticks.

- ◊ Shower. This last tip may not be as helpful as the others; I have observed ticks clinging to my skin while under the shower, and they simply hunker down and bear it! The shower may knock off any wandering ticks, however.

appear. *Bark* is usually collected in the early spring, when it is most easily removed, with few exceptions.

When harvesting, be conservation minded. Do not take lone plants, but look for colonies. When these are located, take only a few plants at most—bearing in mind that wild animals often depend on such colonies for food. Native Americans cultivated this sort of fine attitude and even felt that if a lone plant was chanced upon, it could be supplicated to lead them to its plant brothers growing in a colony.

Consider, as well, what parts of a given plant you will really need before harvesting. Taking one or two leaves from a plant that has a half dozen or more will not hurt it, but bear in mind that taking more than that amount may kill the plant because leaves are needed so that it can produce enough food to survive through the winter. Harvesting a root will kill a plant for sure. If you feel a real need to take a root, break or cut off part of it, leaving the section that is attached to the stem, and then replant the herb. It may survive. (I have done this with certain plant species and have observed that it often works.)

Again, Native American tribes provide the proper example in wild-plant conservation. Typical of the attitude of contemporary tribes, those of the Missouri River region related these cherished instructions, inherited from their ancestors, to ethnobotanist Melvin Gilmore: "Do not needlessly destroy the flowers on the prairies or in the woods. If the flowers are plucked there will be no flower babies (seeds); and if there be no flower babies then in time there will be no people of the flower nations. ... Then the earth will be sad. ... The world would be incomplete and imperfect without them" (Gilmore 1977: 97–98).

CLEANING THE HARVEST

Nature's processes normally clean wild plants quite efficiently. Still, if you have serious doubts about possible recent contamination of harvested plants by dog urine, human spittle, or other pollution, you may elect to disinfect these plants before consumption. Boiling kills most harmful microorganisms, of course. Yet what if you wish to consume the plant raw—as a trail nibble or in a salad? Foraging guides often recommend soaking the plants or plant parts in a solution of 1 teaspoon to 1 tablespoon hydrogen peroxide to 1 gallon of water for at least ten minutes, afterward rinsing the plants thoroughly before consuming them.

Any plants gathered from fresh waters, as opposed to seawater—such as the rhizome of cattail (see page 72) or watercress (page 254)—*must* be cleaned if you intend to eat them raw, as such plants can harbor harmful water parasites. Cattail tastes fine when cooked, which usually kills any clinging parasites. Yet because watercress tastes best when eaten raw, such as in salads or on sandwiches, one would be wise to exercise great care in cleaning and disinfecting it should one elect to consume it in that manner. (At

inclination has been to bypass such an experience and to secure this healthful herb from commercial sources, where it is grown in protected beds.)

STORING THE HARVEST

If intending to dry and use all the aerial parts of an herb for a tea, it is best to hang the whole plant upside down in a cool, dry place out of direct sunlight. However, if only particular parts of a plant are needed, the method of choice involves the use of a drying rack. You can make a simple but efficient rack out of cheesecloth (not wire screen, which may impart a metallic taste) and some wood for frames. The important thing is to allow for air to circulate to all parts of the plant, as otherwise mold may set in. Not only is mold undesirable from the standpoint of taste and appearance, but certain molds can be quite dangerous (such as those developing in sweet clovers or in brambles).

When fully dried, break up—but do not fully crumble—the plant in your hand just enough to fit the pieces in a (preferably dark-colored) glass bottle or jar with a screw-on lid. Store in a cupboard or some other dry, dark place until ready to use. Check stock after a day or two (and periodically thereafter) for condensation or signs of mold. If the material is molded, throw it away. If you find no mold and see only condensation (indicating that the herb was not fully dried), the contents can often be removed, dried again, and bottled.

Herbs do deteriorate. Some are even hygroscopic—that is, they absorb moisture from the air, which reactivates their enzymes, precipitating deterioration. Typically, your stock should be stored for only a year (aromatic herbs) to a year and a half (other herbs), although certain herbs (e.g., shepherd's purse) should not be kept any longer than six months, as they can become worthless or perhaps even toxic if kept beyond that point.

Roots slated to be dried for decoctions should first be cleaned of all clinging dirt. If they are thick, slit them lengthwise one or two times before drying them.

be well-equipped

- Collecting bags (use cloth or paper; plastic induces specimens to mold)

- A small garden spade or a solid "digging stick"

- A clean pair of round-edged scissors (children's scissors)

- Small plastic containers for fragile specimens, such as berries

Fresh leaves, stems, flowers, berries, and roots can be stored in a refrigerator. Some keep for a long time, others for not so long. Trial and error will teach you which is which. Generally, roots and tubers will keep best, but some—such as Jerusalem artichokes—spoil in about a week and a half.

Berries, larger fruits, and vegetable shoots can often be canned for winter storage. Be sure to consult a post-1989 professional manual on this because improper canning procedures (some of which were not known to be risky when the older canning manuals were published) can result in production of the deadly botulism toxin.

Roots can often be kept fresh in a leaf-insulated pit in the ground, with a board placed over the pit and then more leaves and branches heaped thereon. The pit can be accessed by turning over the board, thus dumping the leaves.

Freezing is a fine form of preservation, but even here certain procedures and cautions should be understood. Fruits are the easiest to freeze. Berries and smaller fruits, such as wild plums, can simply be washed and frozen as is, although you may want to cut up larger fruits. Store them all in tightly sealed containers, allowing a bit of headspace for expansion.

Wild veggies, however, need a bit more work. Once washed and cut up, they should be blanched in boiling water, then cooled in ice water, then drained or patted dry, and finally sealed in plastic bags or containers for freezing. If you use containers for freezing, leave headspace in them for expansion; if you use plastic bags, squeeze out the air in them. For the blanching, use a wire basket (preferably nonaluminum) to dip the veggies into the boiling water, usually for two to three minutes, but see variations enumerated in the field guide under individual plant entries. Then, plunge the veggies into the ice water. Bear in mind that wild veggies, like domestic ones, must be used immediately upon thawing and cannot be refrozen for later use.

PREPARING THE HARVEST

As a health enthusiast, I believe that, when possible, fruits, vegetables, seeds, and nuts should be consumed raw. This allows one to benefit from the cleansing and invigorating power of the plant enzymes, which would be destroyed if the plant were cooked. Then, too, I believe that the solar energy trapped in the plant's cells can be utilized most efficiently by the body if the plant is consumed in its raw state. Raw foods also best provide the fiber necessary for colon health.

Still, light steaming usually preserves—at least to some degree—many of these benefits. Cooked food also requires fewer calories to digest, and this can be crucial in a survival situation. Then, too, of course, certain plants are only edible after being cooked. In fact, some of these must even be cooked in several changes of water or dried before being cooked. (These variations will be noted in the field guide.)

Here it should be stressed that plants purposed to be prepared as a potherb should almost never be immersed in cold water and then brought to a boil. Rather, in most cases, they should be placed directly in water that is already boiling, which is crucial to ensuring optimal flavor. Also, most plants that require short boiling periods should be put in very little

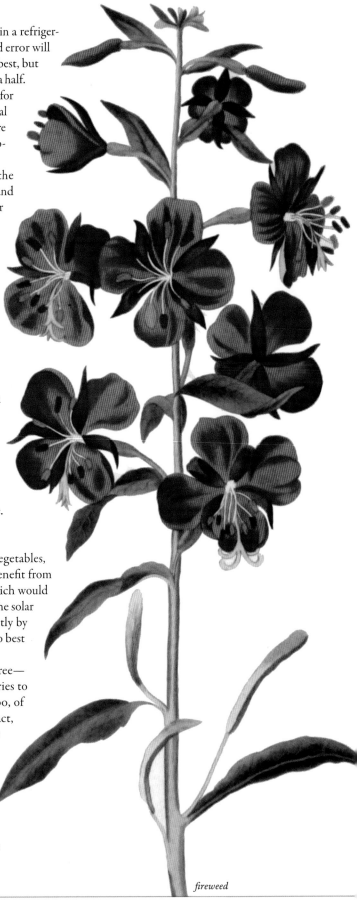

fireweed

water—generally, just enough to cover the plants, and sometimes even less. The less water you give the plant in which to disperse its natural flavors and oils, the better will be its taste upon its removal from the pot and the more bursting with nutrients it will be. Conversely, you will need a greater volume of water for those plants requiring longer boiling periods, such as cleavers (see page 86).

Although steaming is often preferable to boiling because it better preserves not only the taste but also the plant's beneficial nutrients, you should not steam any plants for which several changes of water are required. (These are noted in the field guide.) Many such plants are treated with this succession of water changes in the first place because they have poisonous or bitter principles that need to be boiled off into the earlier water, and steaming might not allow these principles to fully escape.

Most roots and tubers are best if baked. (I refer to a regular oven here, as I personally frown on the use of microwave ovens to cook food.) If instead boiled, however, they will need more water than other plant segments because they must be cooked for a longer period of time in order to reach the desired tenderness. Note that roots do not, as a rule, lend themselves well to being steamed.

Teas made from leaves or stems are prepared by infusion. This means that 6–8 ounces of water is heated until boiling, then combined with the appropriate herb and covered. (The amount of herb to use may vary from a level teaspoonful to a rounded tablespoonful—the weaker concentration for a mere culinary beverage and the higher concentration for a medicinal brew.) The mixture is then steeped for ten to twenty minutes or even longer in some cases. The longer you steep, the greater will be the flavor and the higher the potency of the herb, which is often beneficial if you are taking the tea for therapeutic purposes. See the appendix article "How to Make Herbal Preparations at Home" for more information on how to make herbal infusions. After steeping at least to the point that the tea is cool enough to drink, enjoy your beverage!

To me, herb teas are delicious, and I keep a cupboard stock of at least fifty different wildcrafted plants on hand at all times to allow for variety, as I am a voracious consumer.

Well, that's about it! I trust that you will find the preceding information helpful in maintaining your own joy of foraging. In conclusion, I leave you with this final wish: may you experience the wondrous way of weeds, not only during many daylight hours but also in your nighttime dreams, and that for many years to come! 🌿

Health, Medicine, & Weeds

Even as there are numerous benefits to health that can be gleaned from domestic vegetables, so this is true of wild plants, and sometimes even more so. Some such advantages present themselves on the most basic of levels. Take, for instance, our sense of sight. As to why we humans so often yearn to "get out in nature," especially when under great stress, it may be that the very color of wild vegetation, green, holds the key, for this color has been known to relax the mind, destress the eyes, lower blood pressure, and induce a reverence for the life that it represents (Wigmore 1985: passim).

Chlorophyll is the pigment that conveys this wondrous green tint to plants. This unique substance also appears to contribute substantially to human health when ingested, giving rise to an upswing in energy, improved overall health, and a heightened sense of well-being. Scientific studies have revealed, in addition, that chlorophyll can regenerate the blood, help heal some intestinal diseases, reenergize geriatric patients, and possibly help prevent cancer. Popular health writers such as Bernard Jensen and Ann Wigmore have done much to acquaint the public with the wonders of this powerful green vitalizer (Wigmore 1985: 120–21 and references), but knowledge of its benefits needs yet to be more ingrained in the minds of the public.

WILD-PLANT NUTRIENTS

Aside from chlorophyll, edible weeds contain numerous other components that provide health benefits. Euell Gibbons did much to bring this knowledge to the public by means of the many wild-plant analyses that he did and reported in his books (Gibbons 1971). Yet today, this information remains largely unknown. This is unfortunate in that wild fruits and vegetables are often far superior to their domestic counterparts in their nutrient content (not to mention their taste!) while lacking harmful preservatives, dyes, and waxes.

Take, for instance, lamb's quarters (see page 145), a sort of wild spinach, which outshines domestic spinach in its content of protein, vitamin C, and pro-vitamin A (Gibbons 1971: 161). That is quite an accomplishment, especially for pro-vitamin A, because spinach contains more of this vitamin than any other marketed green vegetable—approximately 8,100 imperial units per 100 grams, compared with 10,000–15,000 for lamb's quarters (Zennie and Ogzewalla 1977: 77). Many wild edibles, however, overflow with valuable nutrients in amounts that surpass most or all of our domestic veggies. Just staying with pro-vitamin A for now, several other common edible weeds surpass spinach in their content of this vitamin, including plantain (page 180), with 10,000 imperial units per 100 grams (Zennie and Ogzewalla 1977: 77); violet (page 248), with an incredible 15,000–20,000 imperial units per 100 grams (Zennie and Ogzewalla 1977: 77); and peppergrass (page 173), with 9,300 imperial units per 100 grams.

Another example of the ultrapotency of the wild is the stinging nettle (page 226), an edible plant (when properly prepared) that contains an incredible amount of protein—one source finds 42 percent by dry weight (Tull 1987: 16). That may be more than is contained in the leafy green portion of any other green plant, wild or domestic! But that is not all: nettle is also one of the richest sources of chlorophyll known in the plant world—so much so that it has been cultivated for commercial extraction of this substance. In fact, it is rich in a wide spectrum of nutrients, especially magnesium, calcium, chromium, zinc, and vitamin C. Its content of iron, although not particularly high, has proven to be quite bioavailable to humans because the large amount of vitamin C in the plant assures its absorption.

Arrowhead tubers (page 22), which have been a staple of many Native American tribes (whose knowledge saved the lives of the Lewis and Clark expedition, according to their own testimony), are an incredible source of energy, yielding up to 400 calories per serving and harboring a rich amount of potassium, phosphorus, and thiamine (vitamin B1).

The familiar chickweed plant (page 75), a staple of yards and gardens as well as available to the forager in various wild forms (especially in the Midwest as the delicious water chickweed, *Stellaria aquatica*), has one of the highest contents of vitamin C known in a green. It is also rich in copper, iron, magnesium, silicon, manganese, and zinc—a genuine nutritional powerhouse. As with stinging nettle, the high vitamin C content allows for good absorption of the plant's iron. Many foragers remark that more chickweed passes their lips than any other plant, and I confess to being among them.

Numerous other examples could be cited, but suffice it to say that edible weeds can be incomparably nutritious. In fact, the more than sufficient information available allows me to provide a chart of comparison between common edible weeds and the very best in marketed vegetables (see page 13).

As source material, I have used the US Department of Agriculture's nutrient databases (from the agency's periodically published book entitled *Composition of Foods* and its very useful website at www.nal.usda.gov/fnic/food-composition), James Duke's internet database, https://phytochem.nal.usda.gov/phytochem/search/list, and resources from my bibliography, listed on page 11.

OTHER PHYTOCHEMICALS

Aside from nutritional benefits, numerous wild plants contain one or more biologically active compounds that have made them popular in healing remedies, sometimes over centuries of use. In some cases, this is because certain amounts or combinations of these compounds have lent these plants to some very specific uses in human health. Thus, an individual plant may possess a combination of constituents that yields anti-inflammatory, antiseptic, antispasmodic, sedative, carminative (gas-expelling), or yet some other helpful effects.

Interestingly, many of the above-described effects on human health on the part of various plants have been known, and used, for hundreds—sometimes thousands—of years, although without detailed scientific knowledge of the mechanisms of efficacy. The wound-healing and blood-stemming (styptic) effects of the meadow-dwelling plant yarrow (page 282), for instance, were said to have been implemented by the warrior Achilles in tending to his injured compatriots during the Trojan War—over three millennia ago! Hippocrates and other ancient physicians were acquainted with many benefits from the plants and discussed them in their extant works. North America's Indigenous tribes have implemented over 3,650 vascular plants for medicinal or culinary benefits.

The discovery of the therapeutic properties in herbs is shrouded in mystery but probably was achieved variously by means of trial and error, by accident, by watching what other mammals (such as bears) ate when ill or lacking in some way, and perhaps by other means not known today. According to the ancient Jewish work known as the *Book of Jubilees* (composed during the first or second century BCE), faithful messengers of the Creator transmitted to Noah the knowledge of how to heal with the various plants; he, in turn, passed such knowledge on to his descendants (chapter 10, verses 11–12). At any rate, the accumulated knowledge was passed on to succeeding cultures. In fact, many North American

herbalists—even pharmacists—owe much of their plant healing knowledge to the Native Americans, already mentioned, who kindly shared their carefully cultivated storehouse of herbal knowledge with early settlers who found the labor of taming a new land to be compounded by various ills. This knowledge, in turn, was recorded in the various herbals and pharmacopeias to which later phytotherapists and pharmacists turned as the starting point for their own investigations.

In regard to the nuts-and-bolts specifics of the efficacy of herbal medicines, we are now living in a most exciting time, as only in this present age do we have the scientific tools necessary to adequately explain how plants heal by means of their chemical content—research that is being increasingly done in universities and other bases of scientific investigation (especially in Europe, Asia, Australasia, and Canada). All of these discoveries, coupled with an increasing frustration by the public with orthodox medicine (including the many thousands of deaths each year that have been established to be iatrogenic—that is, physician induced) have led to what, since the 1970s, has been called an "herbal renaissance." Botanical remedies now abound—not only in health-food stores but also, as they did at the turn of the previous century and earlier, in pharmacies. A recent study revealed that over one-fourth of the American public uses medicinal herbs (Rashrash et al. 2017). Books, magazine articles, and television commercials about herbal medicine are also commonplace. In short, herbal medicine has been mainstreamed.

To provide some insight into the medicinal usage of weeds, however, let's take a cursory look at how some of the plant compounds currently being investigated can make an impact on human health.

Alkaloids

Alkaloids occur in about 10–15 percent of vascular plants and are defined as generally toxic substances that affect the

resources

◊ Duke, James A., and Atchley, Alan A. 1986. *CRC Handbook of Proximate Analysis Tables of Higher Plants*. Boca Raton, FL: CRC Press. 389pp.

◊ Gibbons, Euell. 1971. *Stalking the Good Life: My Love Affair with Nature*. New York: David McKay Co. 247pp.

◊ Harris, Ben Charles. 1973. *Eat the Weeds*. New Canaan, CT: Keats Publishing Co. 253pp.

◊ Pedersen, Mark. 1998. *Nutritional Herbology: A Reference Guide to Herbs*. Rev. ed. Warsaw, IN: Wendell W. Whitman Co. 336pp.

◊ Zennie, TM, and Ogzewalla, CD. 1977. "Ascorbic Acid and Vitamin A Content of Edible Wild Plants of Ohio and Kentucky." *Economic Botany* 31(1): 76–79.

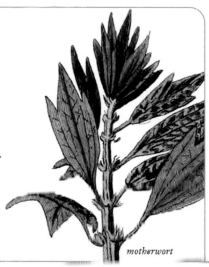

motherwort

central nervous system of living creatures. They contain heterocyclic nitrogen and are produced in plants from amino acids and related substances. Despite being generally toxic (they are often the substance that makes poisonous plants toxic—even deadly), a number of alkaloids have been put to use in small amounts, or in certain forms, as medicinal agents. In fact, alkaloids were among the first substances isolated from plants for medicinal purposes. Examples of commonly known alkaloids include quinine, codeine, ephedrine, morphine, nicotine, and caffeine (note the *-ine* endings). In the present work's main text, you will note various alkaloids referenced in conjunction with their therapeutic activities.

Glycosides

Glycosides are extremely abundant in the plant kingdom. They are defined as substances in which a sugar molecule is chemically bonded with a nonsugar molecule (called an *aglycone* or *genin*). In such a compound form, glycosides are often, although not always, inert, but when they are broken down into their basic components of aglycone and sugar—such as can occur via ingestion as well as by other means, including sometimes a mere picking or damaging of their plant source—the aglycone part is often rendered biologically active. Unfortunately, the nature of glycosides as just explained accounted for some of their unique and important antiviral properties being "masked" until the 1990s, when their aglycone components began to be more rigorously investigated (Hudson 1990: 119).

You will encounter many references to various glycosides scattered throughout the text of the field guide that follows. Note that certain of them, known as *cardiac glycosides* or *cardenolides*, are cardioactive—they affect the heart, either for good or for bad, depending on type and amount. References will be made as well to *anthraquinone glycosides*, which are laxative in small amounts and toxic in larger amounts. Various other types of glycosides will be referred to as well, including the following.

COUMARIN GLYCOSIDES

These are glycosides that are widely sprinkled among the many plant species, being characterized by an oxidized, phenolic sort of aglycone known as a *coumarin*. They display anticoagulant, antibacterial, anthelmintic, analgesic, estrogenic, and sedative activities (Farnsworth 1966: 165). Psoralen, a type of coumarin known as a *furanocoumarin* (wherein a coumarin has fused with a furan ring) and occurring in yarrow, has proven useful in the treatment of psoriasis (Fuller and McClintock 1986: 320). Furanocoumarins have also proven effective against many kinds of gram-positive bacteria, and it has been demonstrated that they possess the rare ability to bind DNA (Fuller and McClintock 1986: 320). A coumarin derivative known as scopoletin (technically known as a *hydroxycoumarin*) has

been found to be a powerful anti-inflammatory and antispasmodic agent useful in the treatment of allergies, menstrual cramps, and other troublesome conditions. This chemical is found in stinging nettle and in some other plants.

IRIDOID GLYCOSIDES

These are a group of bitter-tasting chemicals technically known as *monoterpenoid lactones*. They include aucubin, a powerful antibiotic compound found in plantain, mullein, and several other wild plants in sufficient amounts to make those plants useful as topical antiseptics for minor cuts, scrapes, bites, and other wounds. In addition, aucubin is anticatarrhal and increases the excretion of uric acid—which in excess amounts is connected with gout—by the kidneys.

Flavonoids

Flavonoids occur in all vascular plants—sometimes in free form, but often as the aglycone component of glycosides. Flavonoids that have been known to be biologically active have historically been designated as *bioflavonoids*. They are thought to play a vital role in restoring, if not also maintaining, human health (Middleton 1988). It has long been known, for instance, that bioflavonoids serve an important function in the maintenance of capillary walls (so much so that a common indicator of deficiency in bioflavonoids is frequent nosebleeds). In fact, initial enthusiasm on the part of a number of researchers had even designated them, collectively or sometimes individually, as a vitamin—vitamin P—though this designation was later shown to be technically inappropriate. Still, evidence accumulated to demonstrate that bioflavonoids do work synergistically with vitamin C in the body in an antioxidant-dependent, vitamin C–sparing way (Middleton 1988). Time has revealed that their role in human health is significant, contrary to what orthodox dietitians had once so confidently asserted.

Although flavonoids' role in maintaining human health has not yet been fully explicated, evidence for a role as therapeutic agents in the alleviation of health problems is strikingly impressive, and much research has focused on medical possibilities with these substances since the 1940s. In fact, two bioflavonoids—rutin and hesperidin—have been employed in orthodox medicine for several decades. Quercetin, found in many edible weeds, has captured the attention of biologists and other researchers, proving its worth in the restoration of human health in some very important respects. One of these, of great interest to those afflicted with hay fever and other kinds of allergies, is its not-too-long-ago-explicated role as an inhibitor of histamine-mediated allergic reactions (Middleton 1988). Also investigated have been the marked antiviral effects that this bioflavonoid has been shown to exert against some eleven kinds of "tough guy" viruses (Selway et al. 1986; Middleton 1988).

Comparison Chart of Wild vs. Domesticated Veggies

To interpret this chart, note the following: Figures given are for *100-gram servings* of foods in their *raw state* unless otherwise noted. Domesticated veggies are *italicized*. The four highest nutrient amounts for each category are put in bold. (Note that out of twenty-four winners here, wild plants nabbed twenty, while marketed vegetables secured only four!) "ND" = "no data available"

Vegetable	Protein (g)	Vitamin A (IU)	Vitamin C (mg)	Calcium (mg)	Iron (mg)	Potassium (mg)
Amaranth	**3.5**	6,100	80	**215**	3.9	50
Beet greens	2.2	6,100	20	ND	3.3	ND
Broccoli	3.4	1,542	93	48	0.9	325
Cabbage	1.4	133	33	47	0.6	246
Cattail shoots	1.8	ND	76	58	2.0	**639**
Cauliflower	2.0	19	46	22	0.4	303
Chickweed	1.2	ND	**350**	160	2.9	243
Chicory greens	1.7	4,000	24	109	0.9	430
Dandelion greens	2.7	**14,000**	35	**187**	3.1	397
Dock greens	2.0	**12,900**	**119**	44*	2.4	338
Fireweed greens	2.8	ND	68	186	2.7	382
Kale (cooked)	1.5	7,400	41	72	0.9	228
Lamb's quarters	**4.2**	11,600	80	309*	1.2	**684**
Parsley	Trace	5,200	**130**	140	**6.0**	550
Peppergrass	2.6	9,300	69	81	1.3	**606**
Plantain	2.5	**13,000**	8	184	1.2	277
Purslane	1.7	2,500	25	65*	3.5	494
Romaine lettuce	2.0	2,900	26	40	1.2	322
Sheep sorrel	2.1	**12,900**	54	66*	**5.0**	198
Shepherd's purse	**4.2**	1,554	36	**208**	4.8	395
Sow thistle	2.4	2,185	32	93	3.1	67
Spinach	3.3	6,715	27	99*	2.7	**557**
Stinging nettle	**6.9**	1,100	10	ND	**5.0**	20
Swiss chard	2.4	6,500	32	ND	3.2	ND
Turnip greens (cooked)	1.4	5,498	27	**197**	0.8	203
Violet	ND	**15,000**	**210**	ND	ND	ND
Watercress	ND	4,900	79	151	ND	ND
Wood-sorrel	0.1	2,800	ND	ND	ND	ND

* = Calcium available only or primarily in unusable oxalate form. ND: No data available.

Anthocyanins, a type of flavonoid that has been given a lot of press in the past few decades, are nitrogenous, water-soluble pigments responsible for the tints of flower petals in the red-violet-blue range and for certain autumnal colors occurring in leaves. Their contributions to human health were unappreciated until the 1960s but since then have been under intense study. Largely investigated in this regard have been the potent free-radical-scavenging abilities that anthocyanins have been shown to display. Then, too, like other flavonoids, anthocyanins strengthen blood vessels and have shown to be especially contributory to microcirculation in the eyes, where they also support the visual purple (rhodopsin) of the eye's cones, improving night vision and even myopia. Other research shows that they can favorably modulate how cholesterol functions in the body.

Partaken in their natural form in edible foods, both domestic and wild, most—if not all—flavonoids would appear to be safe, with any potentially harmful effects negated by other substances in the foods or by reactions occurring in the digestive processes.

Saponins

Then there are the highly interesting saponins, which possess a terpenoid aglycone (called a sapogenin). Although not as widespread in the plant kingdom as are flavonoids, they still occur in most flowering plants—the current state of phytochemical knowledge has isolated them in about six hundred plant species from almost one hundred different plant families. Curiously, saponins are quite a bit like soap particles, frothing greatly when mixed or shaken with water, although they are nonalkaline. (The term *saponin* is from the Latin word *sapo*, meaning "soap.") One common wild plant containing these compounds in abundance, bouncing bet (see page 50), is also known as soapwort because its leaves and stems can be crushed and rubbed on one's hands to produce a soapy froth to clean them—a feature that has been heartily implemented by both Native Americans and settlers of bygone times.

Because of the nature and amount of the saponins that saturate soapwort, however, this plant is potentially toxic if ingested (although, interestingly, several Native American tribes discovered preparative methodologies to offset this). Soapwort toxicity produces nausea, gastrointestinal irritation, and vomiting.

In the form and concentration in which they can be found in certain other wild plants, a number of saponins are thought to convey some health-restorative benefits upon ingestion of the plants in which they occur as constituents. For example, the saponin content in mullein helps to make an infusion of that plant a useful expectorant for those afflicted with colds, bronchitis, asthma, and similar complaints.

In their concentrations in certain other weeds, saponins appear to yield diuretic and laxative effects to their users. In yet others, such as chickweed (page 75), they produce a crude anti-inflammatory effect. (In fact, plant saponins have been implemented by pharmaceutical chemists to synthesize cortisone.) Saponins have also been shown to exert powerful antifungal and antibacterial effects (Hiller 1987).

Finally, research conducted since 1990 has found certain orally administered saponins to be immunomodulators, stimulating—in animal experiments—humoral and/or cell-mediated aspects of the immune system (Hudson 1990: 140–41).

Sesquiterpene Lactones

Sesquiterpene lactones are compounds occurring widely in several plant families, especially the Asteraceae (daisy) family. Aromatic and bitter in taste, they are usually concentrated in the leaves or flowers of plants and most particularly in the plant's glandular hairs (trichomes). They are being investigated with fervor owing to anticancer effects that have been elicited from them (Hausen 1992: 228). A number of sesquiterpene lactones also exert antifungal, anthelmintic, antibacterial, analgesic, and anti-inflammatory effects. Prominent in the latter respect are the *azulenes*, occurring in yarrow (see page 282) and in pineapple-weed (page 178), no doubt elucidating the traditional use of these herbs for gastritis.

Tannins

Tannins are phenolic substances occurring in many weeds and especially in shrubs and in tree bark. They occur in two forms: (1) *condensed tannins*, related to flavonoids, and (2) *hydrolyzable tannins*, derived from simple phenolic acids. Tannins possess the unusual ability to precipitate proteins. This property makes them useful in treating certain diseases or conditions, if used judicially. That last phrase is significant, for in large amounts—such as can be obtained through excessive consumption of black tea and even a number of herbal teas—tannins irritate intestinal mucosa. In small amounts, however, they serve the useful function of precipitating the protein contained in the mucosal cells, thus rendering these cells impermeable to any irritating substances that may be present. Likewise, they can inhibit infectious agents by disrupting their proteins and/or by starving them of their protein food source.

Not surprisingly, therefore, tannins are used to resolve diarrhea and to heal ulcers and various afflictions of mucous membranes throughout the body. Their well-documented use in aiding the healing of burns is also attributed to the aforementioned property. Virucidal abilities have also been discovered in these remarkable phytochemicals (Hudson 1990: 159–61).

Essential Oils

Essential (or volatile) oils are important constituents of some plants, especially aromatic ones. They can exert remarkable antibacterial and antifungal effects (Farnsworth 1966: 268). It is thought that the basis of their antiseptic action has partly to do with their ability to increase the flow of blood when coming in contact with mucosa. Likewise, they may aid a distressed digestive system by increasing the flow of gastric juices or by acting as a carminative. Species in the mint family (Lamiaceae or Labiatae) are renowned for their essential oils. Menthol, occurring in greater amounts in the essential oil of wild mint than in any other form known, including even the cultivated peppermint, is well known and appreciated for its decongestant and carminative effects but has also been found of late to be useful in the treatment of sports injuries with one study describing its efficacy as surpassing the more traditionally used salicylates (see wild mint, page 264). Thymol—which has been well known to orthodox medicine as a powerful antiseptic, anthelmintic, and antifungal—occurs in the most concentrated form known in the essential oil of horsemint, a wild meadow-loving herb characterized by its powerful, perfume-like scent.

Mucilage

Mucilage, the last individual plant component we will summarize, occurs in a number of wild plants, including in the common weed plantain (see page 180). When ingested, mucilage reacts with water present to form plastic-like masses that protect mucous membranes from irritants. Thus, it has proven popular in remedies for the relief of conditions involving irritated mucous membranes, such as sore throat and ulcers.

HOLISTIC MEDICINE

The study of the physical and chemical properties of plant- and animal-based crude drugs, including the plant components we have isolated above, is defined by the term *pharmacognosy*. It is a wonderful science, explaining a great deal relative to the healing powers of wild plants. But it does not explain *everything*, although unfortunately some of its advocates seem to think that it does. As heirs of the Cartesian philosophy that attempts to define everything by the sum of its components, many Western scientists have failed to grasp some important considerations that have not so readily eluded health researchers who have embraced a more holistic (wholistic) method of appraisal. *Holism* is a science that looks at things in their entirety and does not judge the whole solely by the sum of its parts. It also does not downplay the testimony of history as to how herbs have affected human health for hundreds—sometimes even thousands—of years.

On that latter point, let's get specific. The plant known as boneset (see page 44) was used by both Native Americans and early European settlers (as well as by enslaved people and, after the Civil War, emancipated black communities) to deal with colds, influenza, malaria, typhus, and dengue. Various health practitioners of the time, including many medical doctors, recorded in great detail the application and tremendous efficacy of this herb. With the advent of modern drugs, it fell out of use and has since been held by orthodox medicine to be practically worthless—devoid of significant biological or pharmacological activity. Starting in the 1970s, however, the herb attracted the attention of several phytochemists and other scientists who, in a number of skilled analyses and studies published in scientific journals, confirmed many of the herb's renowned medicinal abilities—especially immune-stimulating and fever-fighting activities. In the present century, additional scientific research has isolated the exact mechanism whereby boneset disallows viruses to take over body cells in order to replicate.

Here the question to be posed is this: how many years of potential benefit to users (without the harmful side effects often accompanying standard drugs) have been lost because orthodox medical practitioners and investigators employed a strictly reductionistic, and not a holistic, approach to evaluating this herb—dismissing it because it competed with drugs being hyped and because nobody cared enough to verify that it contained any of the "right stuff"? The tragedy of waste, not to mention the uncalled-for slurs on natural healers who had been employing these herbs all along, is assuredly a black mark on the record of orthodox medicine. Yet waste abounds still in the pharmacological field where researchers choose to experiment with extending the properties of existing drugs in preference to investigating the properties of the wide variety of crude drugs—plants—whose efficacy is already time-tested in various cultures. How many untapped powerhouses are thus being neglected remains anybody's guess.

Of course, the advances in phytochemistry are very helpful and much to be lauded. Even without this information, however, the herbal knowledge accumulated through centuries of use has refined the various applications of healing plants to an art. Hence, skilled herbal practitioners have, in our modern day, often helped persons abandoned as hopeless by the orthodox medical realm. In the hands of these skilled healers, the consistent results obtained—person after person, culture after culture, animal after animal—are the only testimony that herbs have ever truly needed.

In this regard, a brief history of the use of herbs by skilled herbal healers on American soil would no doubt prove to be of value, and so I will proceed with such below.

AMERICAN HERBALISM

Of course, the implementation of wild plants as food and as medicine in the United States began with its original inhabitants, the Native Americans, whose uses will be referred to time and again in the field guide to follow.

Herbal enthusiasts among the European settlers gleaned a great deal of knowledge about native plants from various tribes, amalgamating this new information with what they

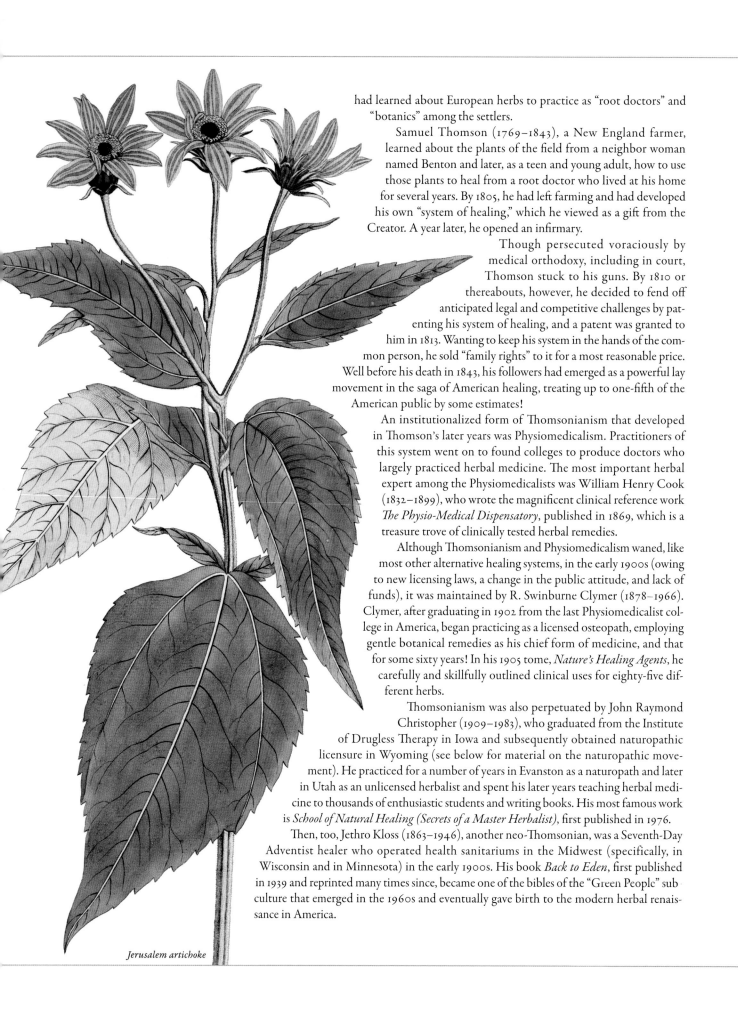

had learned about European herbs to practice as "root doctors" and "botanics" among the settlers.

Samuel Thomson (1769–1843), a New England farmer, learned about the plants of the field from a neighbor woman named Benton and later, as a teen and young adult, how to use those plants to heal from a root doctor who lived at his home for several years. By 1805, he had left farming and had developed his own "system of healing," which he viewed as a gift from the Creator. A year later, he opened an infirmary.

Though persecuted voraciously by medical orthodoxy, including in court, Thomson stuck to his guns. By 1810 or thereabouts, however, he decided to fend off anticipated legal and competitive challenges by patenting his system of healing, and a patent was granted to him in 1813. Wanting to keep his system in the hands of the common person, he sold "family rights" to it for a most reasonable price. Well before his death in 1843, his followers had emerged as a powerful lay movement in the saga of American healing, treating up to one-fifth of the American public by some estimates!

An institutionalized form of Thomsonianism that developed in Thomson's later years was Physiomedicalism. Practitioners of this system went on to found colleges to produce doctors who largely practiced herbal medicine. The most important herbal expert among the Physiomedicalists was William Henry Cook (1832–1899), who wrote the magnificent clinical reference work *The Physio-Medical Dispensatory*, published in 1869, which is a treasure trove of clinically tested herbal remedies.

Although Thomsonianism and Physiomedicalism waned, like most other alternative healing systems, in the early 1900s (owing to new licensing laws, a change in the public attitude, and lack of funds), it was maintained by R. Swinburne Clymer (1878–1966). Clymer, after graduating in 1902 from the last Physiomedicalist college in America, began practicing as a licensed osteopath, employing gentle botanical remedies as his chief form of medicine, and that for some sixty years! In his 1905 tome, *Nature's Healing Agents*, he carefully and skillfully outlined clinical uses for eighty-five different herbs.

Thomsonianism was also perpetuated by John Raymond Christopher (1909–1983), who graduated from the Institute of Drugless Therapy in Iowa and subsequently obtained naturopathic licensure in Wyoming (see below for material on the naturopathic movement). He practiced for a number of years in Evanston as a naturopath and later in Utah as an unlicensed herbalist and spent his later years teaching herbal medicine to thousands of enthusiastic students and writing books. His most famous work is *School of Natural Healing (Secrets of a Master Herbalist)*, first published in 1976.

Then, too, Jethro Kloss (1863–1946), another neo-Thomsonian, was a Seventh-Day Adventist healer who operated health sanitariums in the Midwest (specifically, in Wisconsin and in Minnesota) in the early 1900s. His book *Back to Eden*, first published in 1939 and reprinted many times since, became one of the bibles of the "Green People" subculture that emerged in the 1960s and eventually gave birth to the modern herbal renaissance in America.

Jerusalem artichoke

Eclecticism was a nineteenth-century movement in American medicine that came to influence almost one-sixth of the medical students in the United States. These aspiring physicians sought a medical practice of a more comprehensive, or "eclectic," nature than what was generally available—one inclusive of an education in alternative therapies such as herbalism and homeopathy Thus, Eclectic medical colleges arose to serve these venerable student goals, producing Eclectic physicians in the thousands.

Wooster Beach (1794–1868) founded the Eclectic movement in medicine in the late 1820s after having educated himself in an "eclectic" manner—combining an herbal education obtained from an old root doctor named Jacob Tidd with a regular medical education secured from a New York university. He launched a school—the Reformed Medical Academy—in 1829 and began writing and publishing books. Cofounders were said to include the eccentric botanist Constantine Rafinesque (1783–1850), who lived with Native Americans for a while in order to learn Native herbalism and was the author of an incredible tome on herbal medicine, *Medical Flora* (1828–30).

Other important Eclectic experts in herbalism were John King (1813–1893), who wrote the scholarly and influential *Eclectic Medical Dispensatory*, a standard herbal repertory among Eclectic physicians; John Scudder (1829–1894); Eli Jones (1850–1933); Finley Ellingwood (1852–1920); and John Uri Lloyd (1849–1936), a brilliant pharmacist and PhD who was co-reviser, with Harvey Wickes Felter (1865–1927), of King's *Dispensatory*. Lloyd also wrote an extremely valuable multivolume set on the medicinal plants of North America.

In the 1800s, as the pioneers moved westward, folk herbalism spread to the frontier and eventually to the Midwest, where it developed an enormous importance in view of the lack of trained physicians accompanying the westward surge. A big impetus here was the fact that many families moving west had purchased one or more of the "domestic medicine" manuals that were then being churned out in the east, consisting largely of Native American herbal remedies and authored by the root doctors or botanics. These include *The Indian Doctor's Dispensatory* by Peter Smith (1753–1816), first published in 1812, and *Domestic Medicine, or Poor Man's Friend* by John C. Gunn, first published in 1830.

Benedict Lust (1872–1945) was the founder of the American naturopathic movement, viewed by some as the heir to Eclecticism (which had largely migrated to England for the same reasons that the Physiomedicalists had ceased operations in America, as mentioned above). He opened a sanitarium and established the American School of Naturopathy. In the 1920s and 1930s, many German healers of a system known as Nature Cure immigrated to the United States, where they began cooperating with Lust's movement. One of these was Otto Mausert, a skilled herbalist who practiced in the San Francisco Bay area and who published the book *Herbs for Health* in 1932. Another important figure of the times was Thomas Deschauer, whose *Complete Course on Herbalism* was published in two volumes in 1940. In many ways, however, the most important book produced by this movement was *The Herb Book*, authored by Lust's nephew, John Lust, and originally published in hardcover by Benedict Lust Publications in 1974. This engaging work discussed some five hundred herbs in great detail. The popular American publisher Bantam Books made arrangements with Benedict Lust Publications to produce a mass-market paperback of *The Herb Book* later in that same year, paving the way for this valuable handbook to become extremely popular with the American public. It quickly became, in fact, one of the bibles of the Green People movement of the 1970s—which, as discussed just above, largely spawned the herbal renaissance in America, which brings us full circle back to the present!

Today, then, the Midwest boasts a number of practicing herbalists and various herb guilds where both practicing herbalists and lay enthusiasts can gather to hear lectures and experiences about herbs. Colleges also offer courses on herbal medicine conducted by herbal practitioners (including your author). ⋘

Field Guide & Description of Plant Uses

The field guide list plants in alphabetical order according to the plant's most oft-used common name. If you prefer, however, any plant can be located by its scientific name in the index appearing in the back of the book. At the beginning of each profile, a detailed physical description of the plant is provided, complemented by one or more color photographs of the plant. This descriptive material is followed by information on the plant's range and habitat and thereafter on its known major constituents.

In most profiles, information is given on how the particular plant may be consumed as food (i.e., whether raw or cooked or both), and instructions are usually given for cooking. Sometimes, too, skeleton recipes are provided.

Since the late 1960s, there has been a great resurgence of interest in herbal medication. In accord with this, a large and detailed section on the therapeutic benefits of the respective wild plants is provided. Here the reader will note that physiological functions of the plants are listed in lowercase italics (thus, *astringent*), while pathologies or other health conditions are listed in **bold** text (thus, **pneumonia**). Some readers, in consulting this information, may be surprised to learn that some of the most potent or multiuse herbal medicines are derived from the commonest of weeds. This simply underscores what Ralph Waldo Emerson said in his 1878 essay entitled "Fortune of the Republic": "What is a weed? A plant whose virtues have not yet been discovered." Nowadays, as noted in the previous section, a plethora of new information on the biological and pharmacological properties of these lowly weeds is being processed ever increasingly by scientists. Hence,

in referring to therapeutic uses old and new, I have made a special effort to reference published studies conducted by researchers that support the herbal uses that I have listed.

Here, however, an important point needs to be stressed: while specifics for herbal use are sometimes related, it should be understood that such material is included for informational purposes only and is not intended by way of prescription for maladies. Moreover, self-treatment, as well as self-diagnosis, can be risky. Overuse of a self-prescribed and self-administered herbal formulation may prove to be harmful, just as a weak formula—or an infrequent enough usage of a properly made formula—may prove to be ineffective. In such cases, precious time could be wasted while other methods of healing might have been implemented by professionals skilled in their use. Yet practitioners skilled in the use of medicinal herbs (chiefly clinical herbalists and naturopaths, but some pharmacists and medical doctors) are available in a number of states for consultations relative to the use of herbs to support health or healing in individual situations.

As to other features of the field guide: known cautions are provided at the end of profiles. One should pay special attention to these, as they are there to help offset potential problems. My only regret is that this material is not exhaustive: our present state of knowledge simply does not allow for certainties here, and therefore the cautions listed must be viewed as preliminary only and not by any means as comprehensive.

Referencing in the text is by author, year, and page, to be matched up in the references section at the rear of this volume. A glossary at the end of the field guide attempts to clarify the usage of certain technical terms that may at first bewilder the neophyte student of wild-plant ways. Another appendix section sets forth information on "How to Make Herbal Preparations at Home." The book rounds out, as mentioned earlier, with both a bibliography and a nearly comprehensive index.

I trust that conservationists will appreciate that I, a conservationist myself, have made a special effort to include in the following profiles only those plants that are commonly thought of as weeds or otherwise are common enough not to be threatened by judicious foraging. Thus, I have not included numerous endangered species sometimes listed in other foraging manuals, such as ginseng and goldenseal.

IMPORTANT NOTE

Prior to foraging or using plants for food or healing or even studying the field guide following, you are advised to read both the disclaimer on page v and the two introductions preceding, as such material contains some important cautions that will need to be observed.

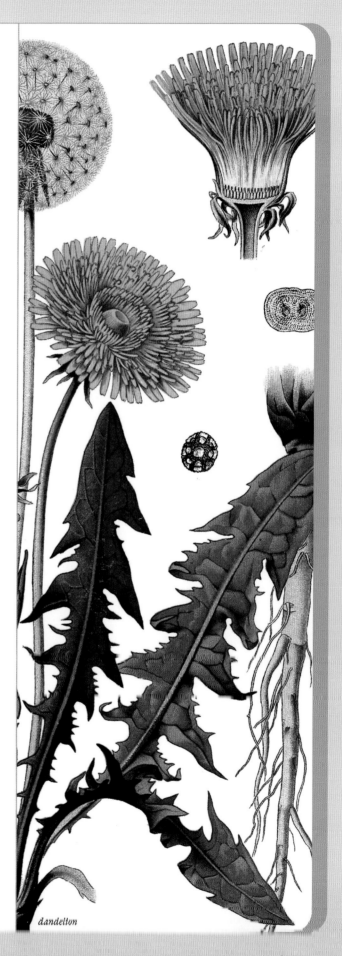

dandelion

FIELD GUIDE & DESCRIPTION of PLANT USES

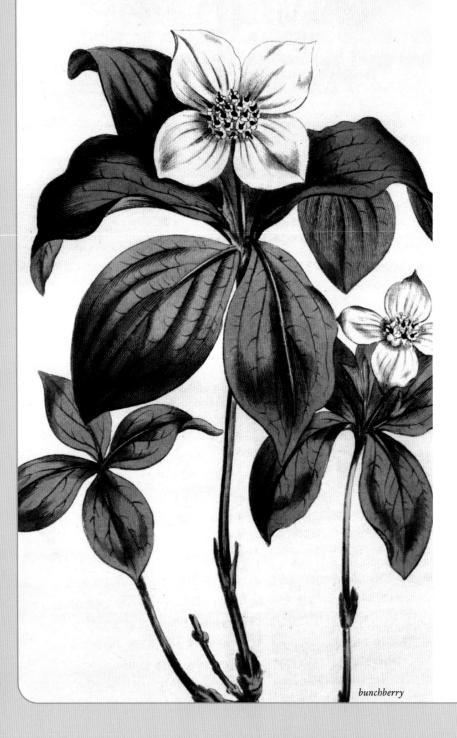

bunchberry

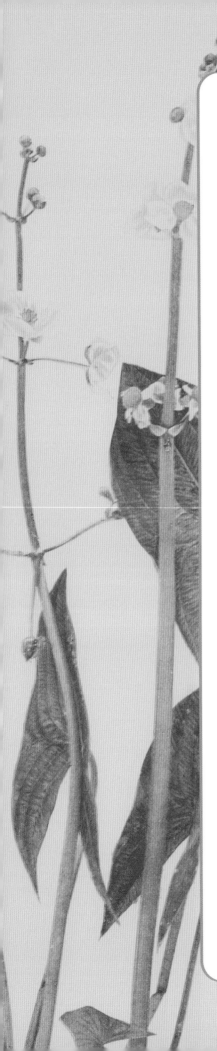

Arrowhead

WAPATO; DUCK POTATO

Sagittaria latifolia

DESCRIPTION

Arrowhead is an erect, perennial aquatic plant that grows 5–40 inches tall.

It is characterized by large, broad, dark-green, arrow-shaped leaves that are terminally situated on a basal leafstalk.

The plant's leafless flower stalk bears waxy, rounded, white, three-petaled flowers whorled in groups of three at spots along the stalk. Flowers can be either male (with a fuzzy yellow center) or female (possessing green mounds).

Long roots lie submerged beneath the mud, with the main one terminating (often at some distance from the main plant) in a tuber that is possessed of a milky juice.

RANGE AND HABITAT

Arrowhead can be found throughout the United States and southern Canada at the edges of freshwater ponds, slow streams, lakes, and marshes. It also thrives in ditches.

SEASONAL AVAILABILITY

Tubers are ripe for collection in October and November.

MAJOR CONSTITUENTS

Arrowhead contains diterpene ketones (trifoliones A, B, C, and D), diterpene glycosides (sagittariosides A and B), other diterpenes, and arabinothalictoside. Nutrients include phosphorus, potassium, and thiamine in significant amounts.

FOOD

If a quantity of the tubers can be gathered and cooked, they are a culinary delight. Raw tubers, while passably edible as a survival food, should not normally be consumed, as they contain a bitter, milky juice that can produce a stinging sensation in the throat. This principle is destroyed in the cooking process.

Arrowhead tubers can be prepared exactly as one would prepare potatoes. Once cooked, they can then be candied with thick maple syrup, if desired. (Delicious!)

The difficulty is in procuring the tubers in the first place. Reaching down for them with one's arm is often disappointing, not to mention messy. Native Americans who have used this food as a staple have waded into the water, barefooted, to dig up the tubers with their toes. Once thus released from the roots, the tubers float to the water's surface, facilitating easy collection. This has usually been done in the cold waters of autumn, when the tubers are at maximum growth, which is typically when the seed stock is left alone of the plant above the surface of the water or situated next to its shriveled remains.

Modern foraging manuals often recommend using a rake to do the same thing. That just doesn't set right with me, probably because it has the potential to inflict a lot of unnecessary damage to the colony. After all is said and done, I still think it best to employ the time-tested methods of the wilderness's original and most experienced students, the Native Americans. (Now, don't be timid—the water's just fine!)

HEALTH/MEDICINE

The Ojibwe have made a tea from the tubers for **indigestion** (Densmore 1974: 342). The Iroquois have esteemed this form of treatment for **constipation** (Herrick 1995: 239). The latter tribe has also implemented an infusion of the leaf for **rheumatism** (Herrick 1995: 239).

A Modern Herbal by M. Grieve states that arrowhead is *antiscorbutic* and *diuretic* (Grieve 1971: 1:57). The latter attribute was especially appreciated by early American healers, with contemporary medical botanist Constantine Rafinesque pointing out that the roots were viewed as being especially useful when "applied to feet or yaws and dropsical legs." He added that the leaves were also "applied to breast to dispel milk of nurses" (i.e., as an *antigalactic*) (Rafinesque 1828–30: 2:259).

A mid-1990s scientific investigation experimentally verified *antihistamine* properties for the diterpene constituents of the tubers (Yoshikawa et al. 1996).

PERSONAL AND PROFESSIONAL USE

I've enjoyed cooking and eating arrowhead tubers on a number of occasions. In my herbal practice, I have not had occasion to use this plant (which is not available on the herb market and must be wildcrafted) except on one occasion: I advised a client who was finished nursing and wanted to "dry up" her milk supply to try a topical application of the leaves, which grew in her area, because she did not like the taste of sage (*Salvia* spp.) tea, the usual recommendation of professional herbalists for this concern. She was not able to come for any follow-up visits but informed me over the phone that the arrowhead application "seemed to be working just fine."

CAUTIONS

Don't eat raw tubers, which can leave a sting in the throat.

Don't confuse arrowhead with the poisonous arrow arum (*Peltandra virginica*), the tubers of which are toxic unless treated in a long, involved fashion (including a thorough drying). Both plants grow at the edges of lakes and marshes and have, at first glance, a very similar appearance to their leaves. However, arrow arum's leaf veins all run diagonally from the midrib, while those of arrowhead run parallel to it, originating from a common point at the center of the leaf. Arrow arum's flower is also wrapped tightly in a spathe, unlike arrowhead's blossom.

Another plant that may be confused with arrowhead is the toxic wild calla, or water arum (*Calla palustris*), which has heart-shaped leaves that lack conspicuous lobes. When flowering, it possesses a large white blossom situated in a spathe. (As mentioned above, arrowhead's flowers are not set in a spathe.) ᕗᕗ

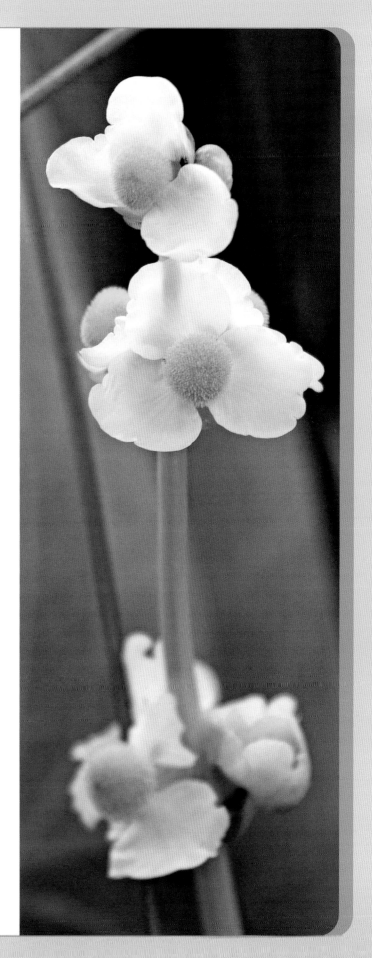

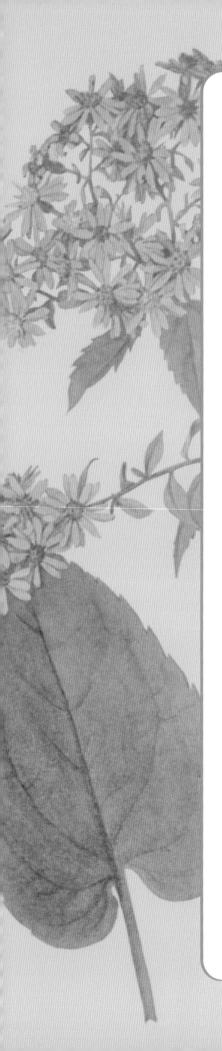

Aster

Aster spp.*; Symphyotrichum* spp.*; Eurybia* spp.*; Doellingeria* spp.

DESCRIPTION

There are over twenty-five species of aster in the Midwest. This member of the Asteraceae (or Compositae) family has flower heads composed of numerous ray flowers surrounding a central disk flower that is almost always yellow in color. The Midwest's major species include the following:

Symphyotrichum cordifolium (formerly *Aster cordifolius*) (heart-leaved aster, starwort) grows 1–5 feet high and is possessed of hairy, toothed, heart-shaped leaves that appear on very slender stalks. The ray flowers are violet-blue to pink-red in color. Dark-green tips adorn the flower bracts.

Symphyotrichum lanceolatum (formerly *A. lanceolatus*) (panicled aster) is tall and smooth stemmed. It has willow-like leaves that have few or no teeth and are conspicuously short stalked.

Eurybia macrophylla (formerly *A. macrophyllus*) (large-leaved aster, big-leaved aster) reaches a height of 1–4 feet and has large basal leaves that are thick and rough to the touch. The stem leaves are small, ovate, and sessile. The ray flowers are lavender colored, while the disk flowers possess a reddish tinge. The flower stalks are rough, possessing tiny glands.

Symphyotrichum novae-angliae (formerly *A. novae-angliae*) (large blue aster, New England aster) grows 2–7 feet high. It displays bristly, hairy, lanceolate leaves that clasp the stalk and are 1½–5 inches long. The ray flowers are a vibrant violet. The flower bracts are narrow, hairy, and sticky, as is the flower stalk.

Symphyotrichum puniceum (formerly *A. puniceus*) (purple-stemmed aster) can be anywhere in the range of 2–8 feet tall. Its stout stem is hairy and reddish in color. The leaves gradually taper down to their base, where they clasp the stalk. Here the ray flowers are also violet but sometimes quite pale.

Other species common to the Midwest include *Symphyotrichum boreale* (formerly *A. borealis*) (rush aster), *Symphyotrichum ciliolatum* (formerly *A. ciliolatus*) (Lindley's aster), *Symphyotrichum ericoides* (formerly *A. ericoides*) (heath aster), *Symphyotrichum laeve* (formerly *A. laevis*) (smooth aster), *Symphyotrichum lateriflorum* (formerly *A. lateriflorus*) (calico aster), *Symphyotrichum ontarionis* (formerly *A. ontarionis*) (Ontario aster), *Symphyotrichum oolentangiense* (formerly *A. oolentangiensis*) (azure aster), *Symphyotrichum sericeum* (formerly *A. sericeus*) (silky aster), *Doellingeria umbellata* (formerly *A. umbellatus*) (flat-top aster), and *Symphyotrichum lanceolatus var. hesperium* (formerly *A. hesperius*) (white panicled aster).

RANGE AND HABITAT

Aster is found throughout the Midwest in open, dry woods and in fields, thickets, clearings, damp meadows, and swamps.

SEASONAL AVAILABILITY

Asters become conspicuous in late summer when they begin to flower, being one of the last plants to do so in this area of the country.

MAJOR CONSTITUENTS

Aster is known to contain tannins but is otherwise largely uninvestigated.

FOOD

The heart-leaved aster (*Symphyotrichum cordifolium*), known in Maine as tongue, has long been used in that state as a green (Perkins 1929). Pillager Ojibwe have treasured the roots of large-leaved aster (*Eurybia macrophylla*), using them as stock for soups (Smith 1932: 398). The Algonquin of Quebec have preferred eating the leaves of this species, as have our own area's Ojibwe, who boil them with fish (Densmore 1974: 307; Black 1980: 108). The Flambeau Ojibwe have also consumed the young, tender leaves as food (Smith 1932: 398). Indeed, as the wild-foods authorities Merritt Lyndon Fernald and Alfred Kinsey pointed out, it is only the very young leaves that are edible because as they mature they become tough and leathery (Fernald and Kinsey 1958: 355).

HEALTH/MEDICINE

The heart-leaved aster (*Symphyotrichum cordifolium*) was used in nineteenth-century North Carolina as "an aromatic nervine in the form of a decoction and as an infusion for rheumatism and by old women, as *partus accelerandum*" (Jacobs and Burlage 1958). The early-nineteenth-century botanical investigator Constantine Rafinesque emphasized the nervine connection, suggesting that aster be tried in the place of valerian (*Valeriana* spp.) to deal with **epilepsy**, **spasms**, and **hysterics** (Rafinesque 1828–30: 2:198). The Physiomedicalist physician William Cook, after acknowledging indebtedness to Rafinesque for introducing the use of this plant to botanical practitioners, remarked that "experience has confirmed the brief account he gave of it. The root is relaxant ... acting slowly and rather permanently. Its principal power is expended upon the nervous system; and it is used in hysteria, nervous irritability, painful menstruation, rheumatism. ... [It is] in the class of the nervine tonics. It deserves more attention than it has received from the profession, and its abundance should secure for it a trial. It has been compared to valerian; but is less relaxing" (Cook 1985).

The Zuni have used panicled aster *(Symphyotrichum lanceolatum)* as an inhalant to stop **nosebleeds**: to accomplish this, several of the plants are crushed and then sprinkled onto live coals, whereupon the smoke produced is inhaled (Stevenson 1915). White panicled aster (*Symphyotrichum lanceolatus var. hesperium*) has been used in the same way by members of the tribe. They also have put this latter species to work to heal **wounds** from arrows or bullets, which they have done by soaking a cloth in a tea of the herb, lightly wringing it out, and proceeding to clean the wound with the compress. The wound is then washed a second time with more care and precision by using a twig wrapped with raw cotton that has been soaked in the tea (Youngken 1925: 165).

The young roots of the large-leaved aster (*Eurybia macrophylla*) have been made into a tea by the Flambeau Ojibwe to wash the head so as to relieve a **headache** (Smith 1932: 363). The Iroquois have made a tea from this species and from four other plants (including sweet cicely, page 237, and bloodroot, page 27) to treat **venereal disease** (Herrick 1995: 230).

Rafinesque tells of how he learned from a certain Dr. Lawrence of New Lebanon that a decoction of the tea was indicated in "many

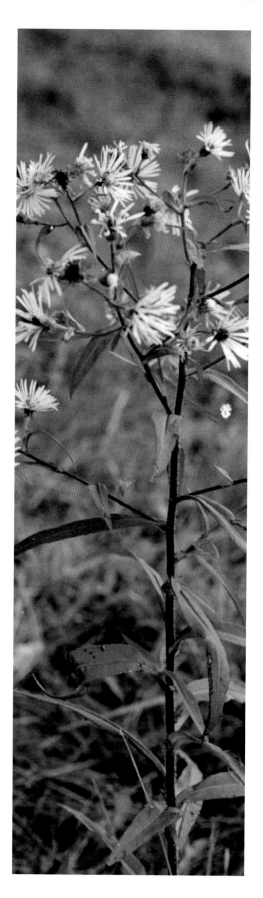

eruptive diseases of the skin" and that if applied externally to **poison ivy** and **poison sumac rashes**, it could even succeed in "removing the poisonous state of the skin" (Rafinesque 1828–30: 2:198).

The Cherokee have poulticed pulverized roots of large blue aster (*Symphyotrichum novae-angliae*) onto **painful areas** of the body (Hamel and Chiltoskey 1975: 24). They have also implemented a tea of the root to treat both **diarrhea** and **fever** (Hamel and Chiltoskey 1975: 24).

The Iroquois have likewise appreciated this species for the latter complaint, putting the roots and leaves from two plants into 6 quarts of water, boiling this combination down to 1 quart of fluid, and then drinking the tea frequently whenever the fever is pronounced (Herrick 1995: 230).

The purple-stemmed aster (*Symphyotrichum puniceum*) was listed in the twenty-first edition of the *United States Dispensatory* as an *astringent* and was also said to have been appreciated as a "stimulating diaphoretic in rheumatic and catarrhal affections" (Wood et al. 1926: 1213). The Woods Cree have similarly found that a root decoction serves ably as a *diaphoretic* to reduce **fever** (Leighton 1985: 31). The Iroquois have implemented it to the same end, infusing three or four roots in 2 quarts of water—taking it warm if the sufferer was chilly, but cooled if they were hot (Herrick 1995: 230). This species has also been used by the Woods Cree to alleviate illness that accompanies **teething** as well as to treat **amenorrhea**. Viewed also as a valuable *anodyne*, it has been chewed and placed onto an **aching tooth** to relieve the pain. It seems further to have been used in the treatment of **facial paralysis**, especially where a contortion or grimace is observed (similar to what occurs with Bell's palsy) (Leighton 1985: 31).

PERSONAL AND PROFESSIONAL USE

Although I always keep a tincture of one or two different local aster species on hand, I have not implemented this herb (either in my personal life or in my herbal practice) nearly as much as I probably should have relative to its wide availability in the Midwest and its strong historical testimony as a nervine, spasmolytic, and diaphoretic. This is probably because a number of other nervine or spasmolytic herbs (e.g., valerian, skunk cabbage, skullcap [page 212], and blue vervain [page 41]) have always been readily available to me, both in the wild and commercially from herbalist-run companies that I know and trust.

CAUTIONS

None reported, but this is undoubtedly because the herb is generally not available commercially. However, it is probably *best not to use it in pregnancy* owing to the fact that a number of other spasmolytic herbs have been shown to affect the uterus. ⋘

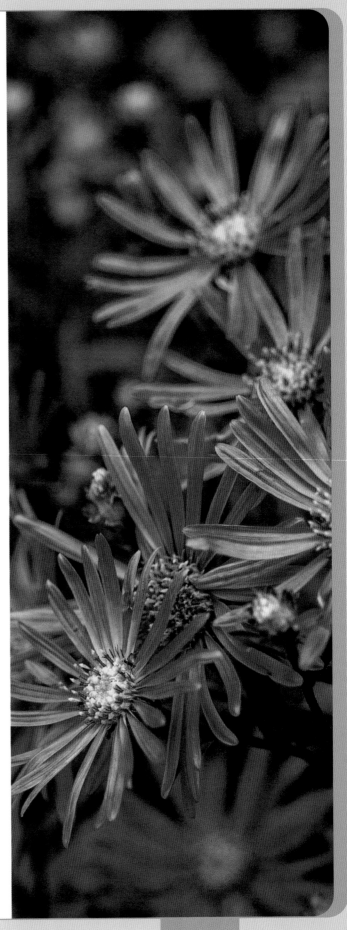

aster

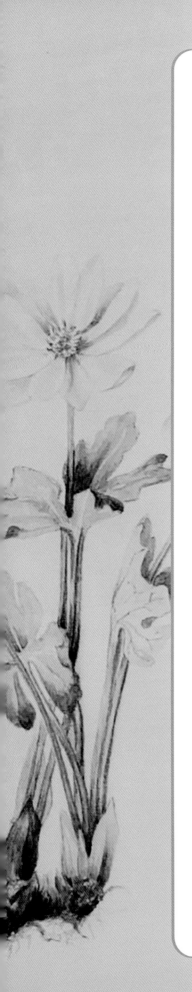

Bloodroot

RED PUCCOON

Sanguinaria canadensis

DESCRIPTION

Bloodroot is an odd-looking but most beautiful native plant that tops off at 6–12 inches.

The lone, large leaf (4–7 inches) is basal and palmate, with five to nine lobes. It is wrapped around the single flower bud as it emerges and then expands as the flower blooms. That blossom boasts eight to twelve oblong petals, is 1½ inches in diameter, and is situated at the end of the plant's leafless stem. Numerous golden stamens combine with its snow-white petals to give it a most lovely and striking appearance. Unfortunately, it opens only on sunny days and is relatively short-lived. However, as the flower appears early in the spring before many other plants open their blossoms, and as bloodroot tends to grow in colonies, this makes for quite a sight on an otherwise flowerless terrain during the muddy, lackluster days of late April and early May.

Bloodroot's rhizome and its flowering stem are filled with a reddish juice that exudes when damaged, thus illuminating the plant's common name.

RANGE AND HABITAT

Bloodroot thrives in colonies in rich woods throughout the Midwest, but it is getting harder to find as, sadly, nonnative species continue to replace our native plants.

MAJOR CONSTITUENTS

Bloodroot contains isoquinoline alkaloids (including sanguinarine, berberine, protopine, chelerythrine, chelidonine, sanguidimerine); organic acids (citric, malic); and resin.

HEALTH/MEDICINE

This is a plant with significant physiological activity, having been listed in the *United States Pharmacopeia* from 1820 to 1926 and in the *National Formulary* up until 1965. It possesses *drying* and *cooling* energies when used in small amounts and more *heating* energies when used in larger amounts.

Bloodroot has been a respected *vulnerary* in various cultures, especially among Native Americans. Modern herbalists use a bloodroot paste or vinegar extract of the fresh roots as a topical treatment for **scabies**, **ringworm**, **athlete's foot**, **tinea**, **warts**, and **eczema**, always being careful to apply it only to the diseased part of the skin (Gunn 1859–61: 756; Tierra 1988: 385). A 1907 study published in the *Journal of the American Medical Association* described the successful use of a bloodroot fluid extract in the treatment of papular and squamous eczema (Graber 1907: 705).

Probably bloodroot's most famous use has been as a salve for **surface cancers**, in which situations it functions as a powerful *escharotic*. This interesting treatment has accumulated a strong lay following (Naiman 1999). Previously, however, it was appreciated by physicians (Lewis and Elvin-Lewis 1977: 123), having been given prominence in orthodox circles due to the investigations of J. W. Fell, a nineteenth-century physician. Fell, having heard about how Native Americans living on the shores of Lake Superior had successfully applied it to cancer, had his curiosity aroused and ruminated about trying it on some of his "hopeless" patients with surface tumors. He eventually decided to try mixing a bloodroot extract with flour, water, and zinc chloride, then smearing the resultant paste on cotton or cloth and covering the tumors with this mixture, doing so on a daily basis. After some days, the tumors developed encrustation. As they did so, Fell made incisions approximately ½ inch apart in the hardened mass and then inserted the bloodroot paste into the cuts. In a mere two to four weeks, the cancer was reported to have been destroyed, with the mass falling out ten to fourteen days later and leaving a flat sore that healed rapidly.

Fell's technique was next tested in a controlled setting at Middlesex Hospital in London, where twenty-five cases (mainly involving breast cancer) were treated by his technique. Fascinatingly, remission occurred with each and every case. Three out of ten persons did eventually relapse and return for further treatment two years later, but this compared favorably to the eight out of ten also returning who had been treated by the standard medical procedures (Fell 1857). Judged in this light, the treatment appears to have been most successful.

Fell's procedures were abandoned not long after his death but were revived by several physicians in the 1960s, led by J. T. Phelan, who experienced dramatic results with a paste made of bloodroot and zinc chloride for carcinomas of the nose and the ear. These physicians reported that most of their patients were totally healed and that only a few experienced reoccurrences. Their results were widely published in respected surgical journals (Phelan et al. 1962; Phelan and Juardo 1963a; Phelan and Juardo 1963b). In 1972, the *American Journal of Surgery* even carried an article detailing the successful use of a similarly structured paste in the topical treatment of ulcerated breast lesions (grade III adenocarcinoma), which proved to be quite successful and concerning which a detailed follow-up found the subjects cancer free some eighteen months later (Sonneland 1972). Detailed analysis since has revealed that bloodroot's alkaloids are the active *antineoplastic* agents, which have been shown to produce therapeutic results on carcinomas and sarcomas in mice (Stickl 1929; Shear et al. 1960; Faddeeva and Beliaeva 1997).

Although bloodroot is most famous for its use in cancer, most herbalists no doubt have utilized the plant's root more often for afflictions of the respiratory tract, for which region it seems to possess a special affinity. Hence, the Pillager Ojibwe have implemented the root juice for **sore throat** (Smith 1932: 377), while the Forest Potawatomi have squeezed the juice onto maple sugar to use as a lozenge for same. They have also used an infusion of the root for **diphtheria**, which they recognized as a throat disease (Smith 1933: 68). Bloodroot has, however, been most predominantly viewed (including in the *United States Pharmacopeia* and *United States Dispensatory*) and implemented as a powerful *expectorant*, either by way of a tincture or as a decoction—the

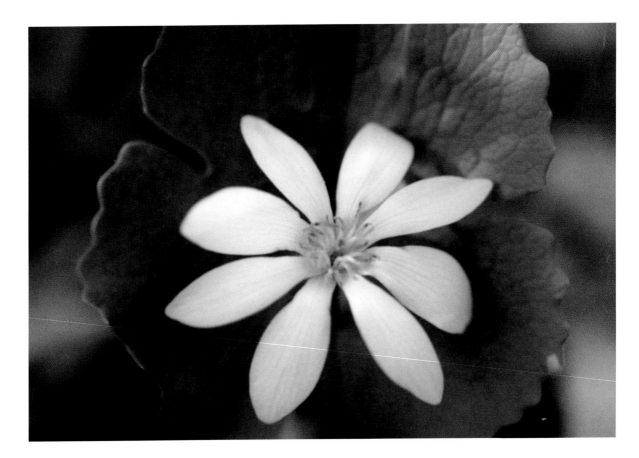

latter with 1 teaspoon of the root boiled in 1 pint of water and 1 teaspoon of this tea taken three to six times a day. This effect seems to be primarily due to the sanguinarine content, which constitutes some 50 percent of bloodroot's alkaloidal constituents (Karlowski 1991). The *US Dispensatory* recognized its use for "sub-acute and chronic bronchitis" through many of its editions. Eclectic physician John Scudder wrote in the 1870s that bloodroot was "valuable in bronchitis with increased secretion" and that "in minute doses [½–5 drops of the tincture, max] we employ it in cases of cough with dryness of the throat and air passages, feeling of constriction in the chest, difficult and asthmatic breathing, with sensation of pressure" (Scudder 1870: 208; cf. Ellingwood 1983: 242). Herbalist Peter Holmes, explicating the energetic principles involved in its indications, says that bloodroot is best used with what Traditional Chinese Medicine calls "lung phlegm cold," manifesting as a productive cough with sternal pain, but also with "lung phlegm dryness," displaying an unproductive and harsh cough that leaves a tickle in the throat (Holmes 1997–98: 1:232).

As for the "asthmatic breathing" mentioned by Scudder, Southwest American herbalist Michael Moore found bloodroot useful in treating **asthma** that is largely extrinsic and characterized by a dry, spastic cough (Moore 1994b: 4.2). California-based herbalist Michael Tierra finds it most helpful for asthma when there is cold and thick phlegm. Tierra also finds it invaluable for **pneumonia**, especially when dosed at 1 or 2 drops, repeated often during the day (Tierra 1988: 384). Early American physician Asahel Clapp wrote that he used it successfully for over thirty years for both spasmodic asthma and pneumonia as well as for **vesicular emphysema** and **tuberculosis** (Clapp 1852: 735). The Micmac have likewise used it for tuberculosis (Lacey 1993: 6). Of especial interest here is that an aqueous extract of the root was shown in 1954 to exert a powerful influence against a virulent human strain of tuberculosis, even in as high a dilution as 1:80! (Fitzpatrick 1954: 520)

The Cherokee have implemented small amounts of the root for **lung inflammation** (Hamel and Chiltoskey 1975: 26). Clapp had also found, over his thirty-year span of implementing the herb, that it "frequently cures or relieves pneumonic inflammation" (Clapp 1852: 735). Then, too, the leaves have been implemented by the Micmac to treat **rheumatism** (Lacey 1993: 6), and an infusion of the root has been used for the same purpose by several other tribes (Chamberlain 1888: 156; Vogel 1970: 355; Lewis and Elvin-Lewis 1977: 166). Such applications should not be surprising in view of a 1976 study that found a sample of bloodroot's aerial portions exerted *anti-inflammatory* effects; the roots were not tested (Benoit et al. 1976: 167).

Aside from the usage for tuberculosis, referred to above, various Native American tribes have cherished a spectrum of uses for bloodroot that we today would also classify under the heading of "antimicrobial." For example, the Malecite have steeped bloodroot, then boiled it down some more, then soaked a rag with it, and finally compressed this onto **infected cuts**, applying a fresh rag as soon as the previous one has dried (Mechling 1959: 246). Both Native Americans and southern whites have utilized bloodroot for **intermittent fevers**, such as malaria and dengue (Vogel 1970: 355). Not surprising, then, is that bloodroot's chief alkaloid, sanguinarine, has been demonstrated to possess significant and wide-ranging *antimicrobial* activity, including against both gram-positive and gram-negative bacterial strains, fungal pathogens such as *Candida*, and protozoa such as *Trichomonas* (sometimes a cause of vaginitis) (Godowski 1989; Mahady et al. 2003).

Another alkaloid in the root, chelidonine, which is also found in celandine (*Chelidonium majus*), has demonstrated *anti-HIV activity* in test-tube studies (Kakiuchi et al. 1987). Taking the clue from this and other research, certain scientists administered freeze-dried bloodroot and celandine to thirteen patients with **HIV infection**, with the result that marked improvements were noted in their CD8 values as well as in their persistent lymphadenopathy (D'Adamo 1992). A year later, a drug based on chelidonine was available to be injected into AIDS patients; it was found to markedly reduce their Kaposi's sarcoma lesions and to improve their CD4+ cells (Martinez et al. 1993: 401).

The Ojibwe of the Midwest have implemented a tea of bloodroot's rhizome for **abdominal cramps** (Densmore 1974: 344). John Scudder, quoted earlier, used it similarly, finding it "valuable in … atonic conditions of stomach and bowels with increased secretions of mucus" (Scudder 1870: 208). Bloodroot has also traditionally been used for both **amenorrhea** and **dysmenorrhea**. The Eclectic physician Finley Ellingwood wrote that "the tincture in full doses is an emmenagogue, restoring the menses when suppressed from cold," but that "it is not to be given if menstrual deficiency is due to anemia, although it is tonic and stimulant in its influence upon the reproductive organs" (Ellingwood 1983: 243). Further to what Ellingwood said about bloodroot's countering of the effects of "coldness," naturopathic physician Deborah Frances notes that a person who is generally chilly and who complains of cold hands and feet will respond best to bloodroot, regardless of the health condition being addressed (Frances 2009: 559).

Bloodroot also yields *emetic* and *cardiotonic* effects (Speck 1917: 318; Lewis and Elvin-Lewis 1977: 278; Newall et al. 1996: 42). The latter would seem to be due, at least partly, to the plant's content of protopine, which has an *antiarrhythmic* action (Lewis and Elvin-Lewis 1977: 191).

Renewed interest in the plant on the part of scientists occurred in the 1980s and 1990s, when numerous published studies demonstrated that sanguinarine helped to prevent and reduce **gingivitis** and **dental plaque**, evidently by killing the bacteria involved and by blocking enzymes that can degenerate gum tissue by the mechanism of destroying its collagen (Dzink and Socransky 1985; Mauriello and Bader 1988; Godowski 1989; Harper et al. 1990a; Harper et al. 1990b). As might have been expected, then, once these studies began to proliferate, several mouthwashes and at least one brand of toothpaste came to add sanguinarine to their lists of ingredients.

CAUTIONS

Bloodroot is contraindicated for use during pregnancy and lactation owing to the potentially toxic nature of its alkaloids and to their uterine stimulating potential. It is contraindicated as well with glaucoma. (Persons afflicted with such a condition should probably also avoid using toothpastes or mouthwashes containing sanguinarine.)

This is not a plant for the layperson to harvest and prepare, owing to its toxic potential! In addition, bloodroot is becoming somewhat scarce in the Midwest, making it further incumbent upon one to use only the commercial preparations grown from cultivated plants. Even when using commercial preparations, one needs to be very careful not to exceed the recommended dosages. Overdosing is very irritating to the system and can cause violent vomiting and possibly even death. (Not only that, but high doses simply *do not work* for the conditions delineated here; 1 to several drops of the tincture, or 1 teaspoon of the tea, repeated several times a day, is the effective dose.) Also, when taking bloodroot internally, one needs to take care to dilute it thoroughly, as it is most irritating otherwise. Bloodroot is also caustic when used externally, so it should likewise be diluted in these cases, and contact should be avoided with any area not being directly treated. All in all, I would advise that bloodroot only be used under professional direction. 🍃

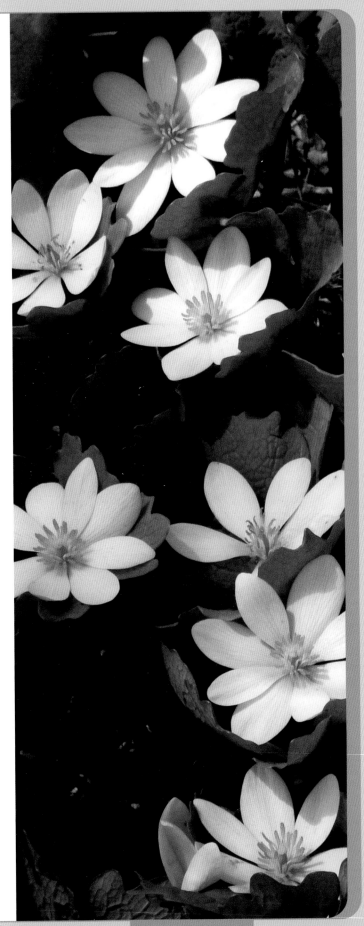

bloodroot

Bluebead Lily

CLINTONIA; CORN LILY

Clintonia borealis

DESCRIPTION

This gorgeous plant, whose genus was named after the famous governor of New York DeWitt Clinton (1768–1829), who was also a naturalist, adorns the northern woodlands.

Growing 6–18 inches tall, it has two to five (usually three) broad, shiny, succulent, parallel-veined basal leaves that reach 5–12 inches long.

Inflorescence consists of three to ten drooping, yellow-green, bell-like flowers on a leafless stalk 6–16 inches tall. The blossoms feature six stamens.

The fruit consists of oval-shaped, steel-blue berries, each about ⅓ inch in diameter.

RANGE AND HABITAT

Bluebead lily primarily flourishes east of the Mississippi River, from Newfoundland and Labrador south to Tennessee and Georgia. The preferred habitat is cool, rich, open woods with acidic soil.

MAJOR CONSTITUENTS

Little chemical work has been done on this plant. It is known, however, to contain chalcones; phytosterols (beta-sitosterol, stigmasterol, camposterol); and triterpenes (taraxasterol, alpha-amyrin, beta-amyrin). The fruits are known to contain sugars (levulose, dextrose) and acids (citric, acetic, tartaric). Diosgenin, a steroidal saponin, occurs in the roots.

FOOD

The young (still curled or newly unfurled) leaves are edible and delicious in a salad, tasting a lot like cucumber. As they age, however, they become tough, leathery, and bitter and leave an unpleasant aftertaste.

Bluebead lily can also be eaten as a potherb. Here the leaves are cooked for about ten minutes. The delightful foraging manual by Merritt Lyndon Fernald and Alfred Kinsey informs us that, prior to World War II, country residents of Maine relished this repast, calling it "cow's tongue" (Fernald and Kinsey 1958: 134).

HEALTH/MEDICINE

Although bluebead lily is largely neglected today as a medicinal plant, it has been widely utilized by Native Americans as such. First and foremost in this regard is its use as a *vulnerary*. For example, the Algonquin have implemented the leaves as a poultice for **bruises** and for **sores**, laying them on after either wetting or bruising them (Rafinesque 1828–30: 2:211). They have also poulticed them onto **infected open wounds** (Black 1980: 138). It is of interest here that an ethanolic extract of the leaves showed antimicrobial activity against *Staphylococcus aureus* (Jones et al. 2000). Indigenous tribes in the Quebec region found bluebead lily useful for the suppuration of **tumors** (Erichsen-Brown 1989: 346). The Ojibwe of the Midwest have used the plant topically for various kinds of skin injuries, including **burns** and **scrofulous sores** (Densmore 1974: 354–55). The Cowlitz from the region of Washington State have implemented the juice from a smashed plant of the western species, *Clintonia uniflora*, for topical application to **cuts** (Gunther 1973: 25).

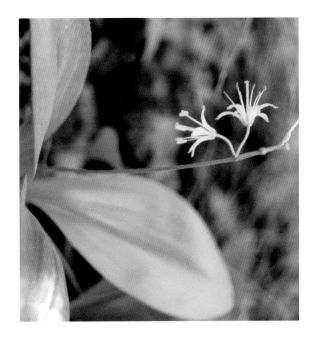

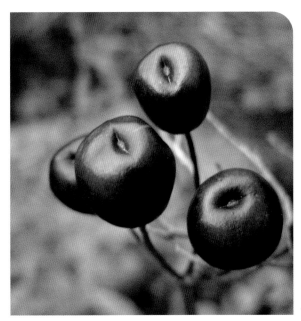

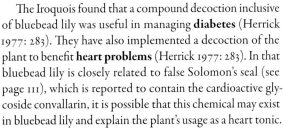

The Iroquois found that a compound decoction inclusive of bluebead lily was useful in managing **diabetes** (Herrick 1977: 283). They have also implemented a decoction of the plant to benefit **heart problems** (Herrick 1977: 283). In that bluebead lily is closely related to false Solomon's seal (see page 111), which is reported to contain the cardioactive glycoside convallarin, it is possible that this chemical may exist in bluebead lily and explain the plant's usage as a heart tonic.

The Micmac have appreciated bluebead lily when **urinary gravel** is present, for which they drink the expressed juice from the roots (Speck 1915: 317). Among the Flambeau Ojibwe, a root infusion has served an important role in **childbirth** (Smith 1932: 383). Might it be significant in this regard that the roots contain diosgenin (Marker et al. 1942), the precursor to the sex hormone progesterone? Or has the infusion instead simply been used because of its regenerative effects upon tissue, in the manner of its usual implementation (as a vulnerary)?

One use for bluebead lily still employed in the Midwest on occasion was gleaned from the Tête-de-Boule, who found that rubbing the crushed leaves on the face and hands largely protects those body parts from **mosquito molestation** (Raymond 1945: 126). Otherwise, sadly, this herb is mostly neglected nowadays. Yet, in view of its many uses as enumerated here as well as the inclusion of diosgenin in its chemical profile, I am inclined to agree with James Duke ("the Duke of Herbs") when he writes with a sense of

urgency regarding this plant: "Science should investigate!" (Foster and Duke 1990: 100)

PERSONAL AND PROFESSIONAL USE

Bluebead lily does not grow in my immediate area, but it flourishes in profusion in the woods of northeastern Minnesota, which I frequent in the summer and the autumn for food foraging, herb gathering, and wilderness solace. On these occasions, I feast heavily on bluebead lily's leaves, which I relish to no end! They are indeed reminiscent of cucumber in taste, but I find them even more palatable. In fact, I have eaten over twenty leaves on several occasions, and that with no ill effects.

I have also tried using the crushed leaves as a mosquito repellant. They seem to possess a mild ability toward that end, but my personal experience has been generally discouraging in this regard. Then again, nothing seems to deter skeeters from attacking me, as folks who have accompanied me out in the wilds can well attest, calling me a mosquito magnet. (I like to think that this is because I possess "rich blood"!)

CAUTIONS

Although some early American writers described the fruits, as Rafinesque did, as "sweetish" and "edible" (Rafinesque 1828–30: 1:211), they would actually seem to be inedible and perhaps even mildly toxic (Fernald and Kinsey 1958: 134–35). ⋘

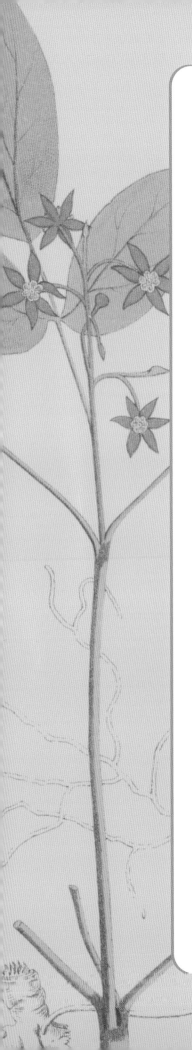

Blue Cohosh

Caulophyllum thalictroides

DESCRIPTION

Blue cohosh is a native perennial growing 1–3 feet tall. Its initially purple stem is covered with a whitish bloom until its leaves are fully opened, at which time the bloom vanishes, and the stem becomes green.

There are only two leaves, both of which are sessile and compound, possessed of wedge-shaped to egg-shaped leaflets. The upper leaf, which is the largest, is divided into seven to nine leaflets, while the lower leaf has twenty-seven leaflets, each growing 1–3 inches long.

The pretty green-yellow flowers are small—only about ½ inch in diameter. The corolla displays six small hood-shaped petals and six larger pointed sepals. Several blossoms can be found in loosely branched, terminal clusters.

What look like blueberries (being about their same size and color) appear in place of the flowers in the summer and are positioned on small, inflated stalks. These, however, are not the plant's fruits but rather its seeds.

RANGE AND HABITAT

This is a plant of moist, rich woods. It occurs in such environs throughout the Midwest but is not as plentiful as it used to be even a few decades ago.

MAJOR CONSTITUENTS

Blue cohosh rhizome contains quinolizidine alkaloids (N-methylcytisine [caulophylline], anagyrine, baptifoline, lupanine); isoquinoline alkaloids (including magnoflorine [thalictrine]); the glycoside leontin; triterpene saponins (including hederagenin and caulophyllosaponin); phytosterols; phosphoric acid; resin; citrullol; and tannin.

HEALTH/MEDICINE

Blue cohosh, possessed of *warming* and *drying* energies, is a powerful and important herb that has seen broad application in herbal medicine.

The Omaha have reverenced this plant as the best of all *febrifuges*, giving a decoction of the roots for **fever** (Gilmore 1991: 31). The Iroquois have likewise found it helpful for such—in fact for "*any* kind of fever" (Herrick 1995: 125). It has also been treasured by Native Americans as an *emetic:* the Midwest's Ojibwe have used it in such a manner (Smith 1932: 358), whereas the Iroquois have implemented an infusion of the smashed roots to help persons with gallstones to vomit (Herrick 1977: 333). Blue cohosh is a *vermifuge*, where the same principles may be at play (Wren 1988: 84; Fleming 1998).

Our herb is also *antispasmodic* (Smith 1999: 16–17) and has thus been used by the Ojibwe for both **stomach cramps** and **indigestion** (Densmore 1974: 342–44).

Blue cohosh has proven helpful for **arthritic pains**, especially when they occur in the fingers or in the toes (Winston 1999: 35). Another classic use has been for **rheumatism** (Wren 1988: 84), with tribes such as the Iroquois (Herrick 1977: 333) and the Cherokee (Hamel and Chiltoskey 1975: 30) using it for this malady. The Cherokee have also rubbed the leaves onto **poison oak rash** to achieve relief (Hamel and Chiltoskey 1975: 30). These uses are perhaps explainable by a study conducted in the mid-1970s, which found that blue cohosh significantly *inhibited inflammation* via the carrageenan-induced rat-paw edema model (Benoit et al. 1976: 163). The effect here may be due to the plant's content of leontin (Willard 1991: 41). *Diuretic* properties inherent in blue cohosh may also contribute to its success with rheumatism (Wren 1988: 84).

There appears to be some affinity for the respiratory system as well: the Ojibwe have found it helpful for **lung troubles**, making a decoction from two roots and 1 quart of water and dosing the tea at one swallow (Densmore 1974: 340–41). The Ojibwe have also taken a small quantity of the finely scraped root and squeezed it through a white cloth in warm water to treat **lung hemorrhages** (Densmore 1974: 346–47). The Eclectic physician Finley Ellingwood noted that blue cohosh had been used with repeated success in treating **bronchitis**, **pneumonitis**, and **whooping cough** (Ellingwood 1983: 481).

Blue cohosh seems to possess an affinity for the genitourinary system. The Meskwaki (Fox) have given it to men with problems in this system (Smith 1928: 205), while the Mohegan have used it for **kidney disorders** (Tantaquidgeon 1972: 71, 128–29). (As noted earlier, it appears to exert some diuretic effects.) The herb is best known, however, as a "female remedy": the Cherokee, for example, have esteemed it for a **uterine inflammation** (Hamel and Chiltoskey 1975: 30), while Ellingwood recommended it for "constant ovarian irritation" as well as for "chronic disease of the uterus or ovaries or of the cervix" (Ellingwood 1983: 481). Present-day herbalist Amanda McQuade-Crawford finds that it may sometimes shrink **uterine fibroids** (McQuade-Crawford 1996: 136). The Ojibwe have treasured it for **menstrual cramps**

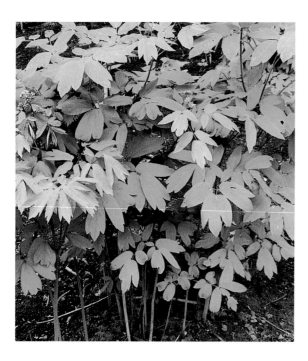

(Smith 1932: 358). Ellingwood agreed that "in painful menstruation it has an established reputation" (Ellingwood 1983: 481). The late, great Southwest American herbalist Michael Moore noted that it is most helpful for women with congestive dysmenorrhea who experience menstrual cycles of more than thirty days (Moore 1994b: 13.3; cf. Mills and Bone 2000: 242). The Menomini and Forest Potawatomi have boiled the roots to obtain a tea that is drunk to diminish **profuse menstruation** (Smith 1923: 28; Smith 1933: 43).

Blue cohosh's best-known use, however, is as a *parturient*. It was listed in the *United States Pharmacopeia* from 1882 until 1905 for just such a function. The root is, indeed, a labor aid par excellence, specifically for **stalled labor**, and studies conducted in the 1950s suggest that the active agent in its oxytocic is caulosaponin (Tyler 1993: 47). The Eclectics noticed that blue cohosh's action seemed to be especially helpful with "delicate women" (Felter and Lloyd 1898) and in cases where labor has been slowed by pain or fatigue, an observation shared by many modern herbalists (Willard 1991: 42; Moore 1994b: 14.2; McIntyre 1995: 26; Harrar and O'Donnell 1999: 37). The Eclectic physician John Scudder explained that it "exerts a very decided influence upon the parturient uterus, stimulating normal contraction, both before and after delivery. Its first use, in this case, is to relieve false labor pains; its second, to effect coordination of the muscular contractions; and third, to increase the power of these. The first and second are most marked, yet the third is quite certain. Still if any one expects the marked influence of Ergot, in violent and continued contractions, he will be disappointed" (Scudder 1870: 100). Scudder said that blue cohosh is best used as a tincture of the recently dried root (Scudder 1870: 99). Modern herbalist Susun Weed, in a discussion of the herb's parturient activity, recommends a dose of 10–20 drops of the tincture in a small glass of water, repeating hourly as needed to achieve delivery (Weed 1986: 65).

Blue cohosh's *oxytocic* properties have also been enlisted for starting, not merely assisting, labor. Even so, Weed's book stresses that its usage would only be effective once the cervix has ripened (Weed 1986: 60–61). In such a situation, she says, she has heard of good results with the application of a 200× homeopathic dose of blue cohosh, repeated every half hour for two hours. She herself particularly suggests, however, the use of 3–8 drops of the herbal tincture in a glass of warm water, repeated every half an hour until contractions are regular. She says that if labor is not underway after four hours, this dose can be increased to a dropperful under the tongue every hour up to four more hours until the contractions become powerful and reliable.

Very small amounts of the root—always in a formula with the renowned antiabortive herb black haw (*Viburnum prunifolium*) and several others—have traditionally been used to prevent miscarriage from the fourth to ninth months of gestation. One example of such a formula is the famed "Mother's Cordial" of the Eclectics. Ellingwood wrote that that formula's *Caulophyllum* component "prevents premature delivery by a superior tonicity, which it induces in all the reproductive organs. It has caused many cases to overrun their time a few days, and yet easy labors and excellent recoveries have followed" (Ellingwood 1983: 481).

However, a popular notion among some who possess but a casual familiarity with herbs is that blue cohosh should be used—either alone or merely in conjunction with black cohosh (*Actaea racemosa*)—for several weeks before the due date in order to tone the uterus and to keep the baby from running over term. Here it is true that *some* modern herbalists, including Susun Weed, have discussed the use of blue cohosh in this regard. Weed herself, however, sets a daily limit of 2 cups of tea or two divided doses of 20–30 drops of the tincture and advises use only when accompanied by black cohosh, quoting a midwife as saying that the use of blue cohosh alone can lead to "precipitous labor" (Weed 1986: 23). The Eclectics, with the possible exception of Ellingwood (Ellingwood 1983: 481), seem not to have used blue cohosh by itself as a partus preparator, but only in small amounts as one ingredient in a mixture of five herbs composing the Mother's Cordial, as noted above.

In view of the lack of any definable trend in historic use, then (see Bergner 2001), it is difficult to assess the reliability or safety of utilizing blue cohosh as a partus preparator, either alone or in conjunction with only black cohosh. There are, in fact, two modern cases that suggest it may not be appropriate: One woman who took three capsules of blue cohosh a day for three weeks before birth delivered a baby with heart problems (Jones and Larson 1998; Edmunds 1999). (The plant's saponins are definitely cardioactive; see

Cautions.) Another woman who used both blue cohosh and black cohosh prior to birth delivered a baby who experienced seizures (Gunn and Wright 1996; Baillie and Rasmussen 1997; Wright 1999). Until more is known about the margins of safety relative to the use of blue cohosh during pregnancy, its use as a partus preparator—especially by the layperson—is strongly discouraged.

CAUTIONS

Don't confuse this plant with any of the various meadow rues (*Thalictrum* spp.), which have similar leaves but quite different flowers and fruits.

Touching blue cohosh can cause dermatitis in sensitive persons.

The blue "berries" (actually the plant's seeds) are toxic and should not be consumed. Roasting them appears to eliminate or reduce the toxic elements (Spoerke 1990: 42), but there may be variables and intricacies of detail here that mandate preparation by a seasoned expert.

Blue cohosh should be avoided by persons with heart disease or high blood pressure owing to the effects of its chemicals N-methylcytisine (which increases blood pressure) and caulosaponin (which constricts coronary blood vessels) (Spoerke 1990: 42; Tyler 1993: 47).

Do not use blue cohosh root in the first trimester of pregnancy. If desirous of using it in the second trimester for any miscarriage-preventive effects, *do not use it alone*, and if at all, only in a commercial preparation (such as the Mother's Cordial referred to above) containing antiabortive herbs, including black haw (*Virburnum prunifolium*), and be sure not to exceed the maximum recommended dose.

For parturitive effects during stalled labor, this herb is best used under the guidance of a skilled herbalist or midwife. ❧

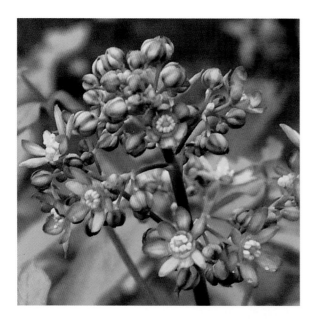

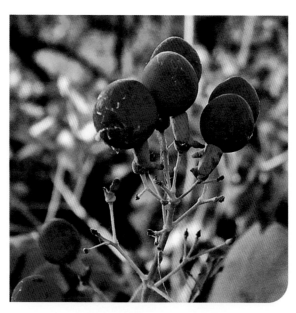

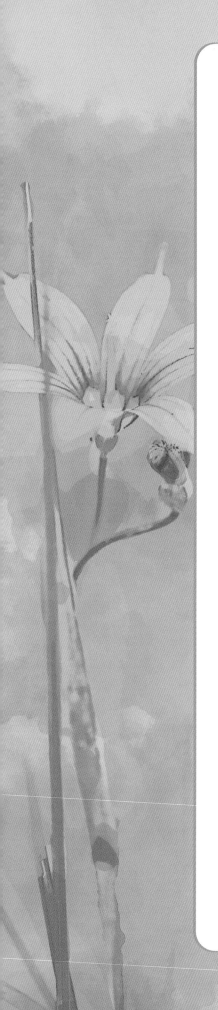

Blue-Eyed Grass

Sisyrinchium spp.

DESCRIPTION

This is a perennial plant with a stiff, grass-like appearance and fibrous roots. The stem is wiry and two-edged. The lovely flowers have yellow centers and six petal-like appendages (composed of three petals alternating with a like number of sepals), distinguished by their pointed tips.

Several species can be found in the Midwest, including the following:

Sisyrinchium campestre (prairie blue-eyed grass) has white or pale-blue flowers.

S. montanum (common blue-eyed grass) has flattened stems, deep-blue or violet flowers, short stalks, and leaves that are ¼–½ inch wide.

S. mucronatum (slender blue-eyed grass) has very slender stems and leaves (the latter only ¹⁄₁₂ inch wide!). In this species the leaves are shorter than the flowering stems.

RANGE AND HABITAT

This plant thrives in fields, meadows, and marshes throughout the Midwest.

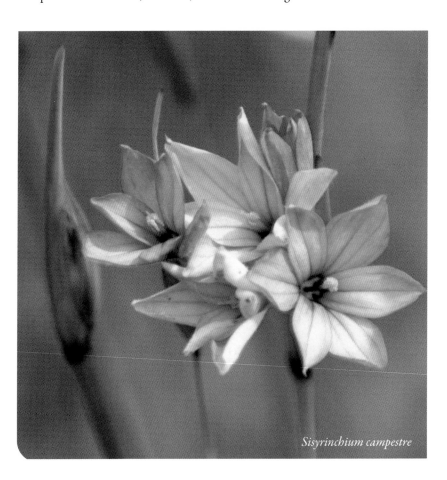

Sisyrinchium campestre

HEALTH/MEDICINE

The Meskwaki (Fox) have made a tea of *S. campestre* to treat **hay fever** (Smith 1928: 224). Blue-eyed grass has also been used in Appalachian folk medicine, in which it has been implemented for **fever** and **chills** (Crellin and Philpott 1990a: 105). Early American practitioners of botanical medicine used various species of the plant for *deobstruent*, *antiscorbutic*, *tonic*, and *laxative* purposes (Crellin and Philpott 1990a: 105).

As to the latter use, both the Cherokee and the Iroquois have used the plant to "keep regular." Here the Iroquois have imbibed a decoction of the root and of the stalks (½ cup roots and stalks in 1½ quarts of water) just prior to breakfast to ensure a morning bowel movement (Hamel and Chiltoskey 1975: 26; Herrick 1977: 288).

However, the steeped root of at least one species, *S. angustifolium*, has been used instead to quell **diarrhea**, especially that occurring in children (Hamel and Chiltoskey 1975: 26). The Iroquois have likewise used it for "summer complaint"—a nineteenth-century term describing the epidemic diarrhea that especially affected children during hot, humid weather (Herrick 1995: 247). Interestingly, in the early 1950s, this species was found to possess antimicrobial activity, inhibiting a virulent human strain of tuberculosis (Fitzpatrick 1954: 529). Might it also, then, inhibit the microbes that can cause diarrhea—so prevalent in children's daycare centers nowadays during hot, damp weather and analogous to the "summer complaint" of the nineteenth-century medical literature?

There would, indeed, seem to be some sort of positive effect upon the gastrointestinal tract, especially since both **stomachache** and **intestinal worms** are complaints that have been successfully addressed by the *Sisyrinchium* genus in the hands of the Mahuna (Romero 1954: 6). ᴀᴋᴋ

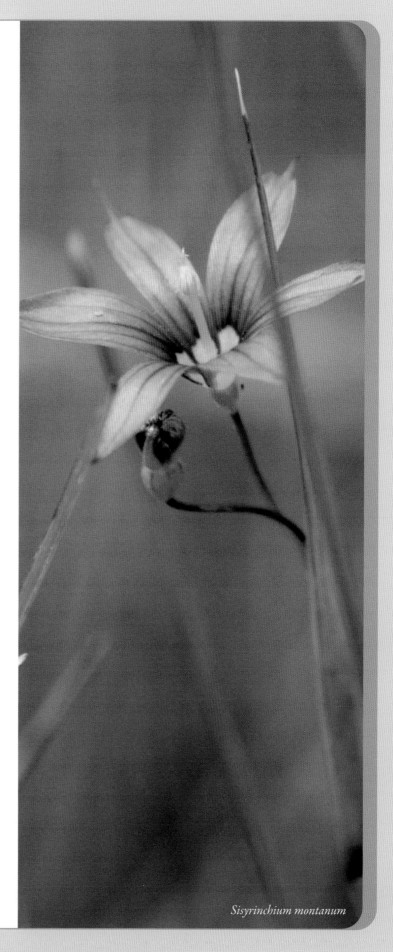

Sisyrinchium montanum

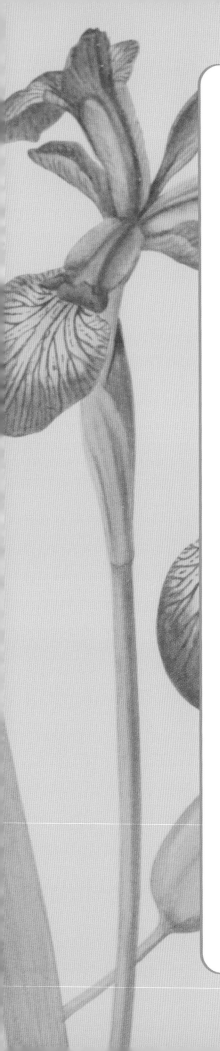

Blue Flag

Iris versicolor

DESCRIPTION

This is a divinely beautiful native perennial that reaches a height of about 3 feet. Its sturdy stem springs from a horizontal rhizome.

The plant's leaves are long (8–32 inches), flat, entire, toothless, and sword-like in shape. They arise from a common basal cluster.

The gorgeous blossoms, reaching some 3 inches in diameter, appear on branched stems. Each blossom displays what seem to be nine petals, in three whorls of three. However, only the middle whorl is composed of true petals—three small, ascending violet ones, blotched with yellow and white at their bases. The innermost whorl actually consists of three pale-violet, crest-like branches of the flower pistil, which are flared at their tips. Most showy, however, is the outermost whorl of three large sepals, which curve outward and then downward. The bases of these lovely structures are whitish with a blatant yellow blotch and bold purple veins running through this lighter coloration.

Long, erect green pods eventually replace the breathtaking blossoms.

RANGE AND HABITAT

Blue flag thrives throughout the Midwest in most woods, wet meadows, marshes, and ditches and on lakeshores and streambanks.

MAJOR CONSTITUENTS

Blue flag contains furfural, furfurol, ipuranol, heptacosane, the resin iridin (irisin), the triterpenoid iriversical, isophthalic acid, traces of other acids (salicylic, stearic, lauric, and palmitic), sterols, gum, and tannin.

HEALTH/MEDICINE

Formerly official in the *United States Pharmacopeia* (1820–95) and in the *National Formulary* (1916–42), the rhizome of blue flag is renowned as one of the very best of the *alterative* herbs (Smith 1999: 17; Mills and Bone 2000: 254) and thus often observed to be helpful in chronic skin conditions such as **eczema**, **psoriasis**, and dysfunction of the sebaceous glands (e.g., **acne**) (Smith 1999: 17).

North America's Eclectic physicians of the late 1800s and early 1900s noted here: "*Persistent ... psoriasis,* and *acne indurata* will usually present conditions calling for iris" (Felter and Lloyd 1898). An Eclectic physician writing a bit later, Finley Ellingwood, offered these observations: "In the treatment of certain cases of eczema of a persistent chronic character, as well as of other pustular and open ulcerating or oozing skin diseases, this agent, in from five to ten drop doses every two or three hours, will be found most useful. It may be diluted and applied externally also. Prurigo, crustalactea, and tinea yield readily to its influence at times" (Ellingwood 1983). In British herbalism, too, blue flag has been a much-treasured herb for chronic eczema (Hyde et al. 1976–79: 2:99). Southwest American herbalist Michael Moore found it most applicable to eczema accompanied by poor digestion of fats and dry skin (Moore 1994b: 11:7).

Blue flag has also been used by herbalists for **nonmalignant enlargement** of lymphatic structures or glands, especially the **thyroid gland**, the **spleen**, and the **lymph** nodes (Scudder 1870: 146; Clymer 1973: 67–68). It is universally agreed to be the herb of choice for these structures when they are soft and yielding to the touch (Smith 1999: 17) or where **lymphangitis** exists that is lingering and subacute (Moore 1994b: 21.6). (Moore noted, however, that for lymphatic conditions, our herb is better used in combination with other lymphatic herbs than by itself: Moore 1979: 40.)

Further as to its use for nonmalignant enlarged thyroid, the Eclectic scholars Harvey Wickes Felter and John Uri Lloyd observed: "It is one of the very few reliable drugs used for the cure of goiter, or enlarged thyroid. Indeed, for this condition it is our most direct and effectual remedy, whether the enlargement be constant, or whether it be simply a fullness due to menstrual irregularities. This use was early pointed out by Prof. King" (Felter and Lloyd 1898).

Because it exerts *diuretic* activity, blue flag can ably drain the lymph of impurities (Scudder 1870: 146; Ellingwood 1983: 313) so that it has often proven helpful in conditions such as **dropsy**, having been widely used for such by early American physicians (Rafinesque 1828–30: 2:232); **rheumatism**, as the Oklahoma Lenape (Delaware) discovered (Tantaquidgeon 1942: 30; Tantaquidgeon 1972: 118); **syphilis** (Scudder 1870: 146; Hutchens 1991: 57); **fluid-filled cysts** that are very boggy (Stansbury 1997); and **obesity**, especially where this problem is connected with poor glandular function (Tierra 1998: 100).

This plant is a *sialagogue*, increasing not only the secretions of salivary glands but also those of other glands and organs—including the pancreas, spleen, intestines, and especially the liver and gallbladder. It is most especially a *cholagogue*, and a very trustworthy one at that, indicated with poor hepatic management of bile as manifested by "biliousness" and specifically by the symptom set of a "sick" headache, dizziness, indigestion, nausea (especially after ingestion of fatty foods), and constipation with eventual clay-colored stools (Clymer 1973: 67–68; Moore 1994b: 8.1). Nineteenth-century medical botanist Laurence Johnson remarked: "In sick headache dependent upon indigestion, small doses, frequently repeated, often act most happily" (Johnson 1884: 271). When used moderately, it is a mild *laxative* for **constipation** attributable to poor biliary function (Millspaugh 1974: 694; Smith 1999: 17). In larger doses, however, it is *cathartic* as well as *emetic* (Wood et al. 1926: 597). Various Native American tribes discovered these physiological effects and have put them to good use when deemed appropriate (Smith 1932: 371; Bartram 1958: 288).

This plant has been widely implemented by Native American tribes, being used most prominently, in fact, as a *vulnerary* (Vogel 1970: 283). As such, a topical application of the rhizome has been used for **bruises**, **swellings**, **sores**, and **wounds**, including by the Ojibwe in the Midwest (Speck 1917: 315; Smith 1928: 224; Gilmore 1933: 126; Smith 1933: 60; Raymond 1945: 129; Densmore 1974:

366; Gilmore 1991: 20). In the early 1700s, an American colonel with the last name of Lydius was healed of horrible sores on his legs by Native Americans who poulticed the lightly boiled and crushed rhizome over his sores and washed his leg with the decoction (Kalm 1937: 2:606). These sores were probably **staph sores**, for which blue flag has traditionally been utilized (Moore 1979: 40). Indeed, the rhizome has been experimentally shown to manifest *antimicrobial* ability (Fitzpatrick 1954: 530). Further as to this effect, Charles Millspaugh, a practitioner and scholar of medicinal plants who lived and wrote in the late 1800s, pointed out that the pulped fresh root is justly considered to be one

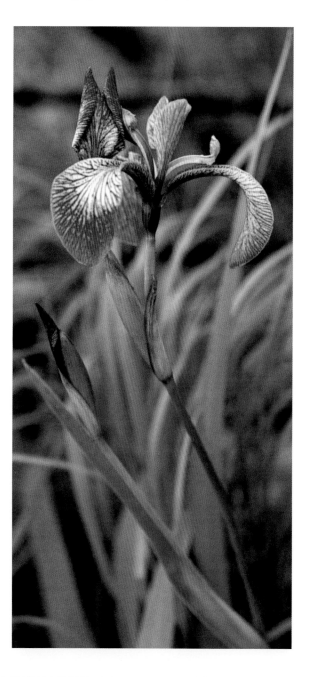

of the very best topical applications for a painful **felon** on the finger, typically the consequence of a bacterial infection (Millspaugh 1974: 694). Then, too, the Omaha-Ponca have mixed the pulverized rootstock with saliva and droppered this mixture into the ear to alleviate **earache**, which is also often a bacterial situation (Gilmore 1991: 20).

Energetically, blue flag is held to be *cooling* and *drying* and is thus appreciated as a plant for relieving stagnation (Holmes 1997–98: 2:689). As to form and dosage, a liquid extract (tincture) of the fresh rhizome is sometimes used (Millspaugh 1974: 694). The celebrated Eclectic physician John Scudder had utilized this sort of preparation, by way of a 76 percent alcoholic extract. Scudder strongly asserted that "the dried root ... possesses no more medicinal property than sawdust, and preparations from it ... are an imposition" (Scudder 1870: 146). In more modern times, Ed Smith, an herbalist from the western United States, is another who discusses using a tincture of the fresh rhizome, providing detailed guidelines for using his own commercial tincture of such in one of two ways: for regular, gentle use, mix 40–60 drops into ½ cup of water and imbibe 1 teaspoon of the mixture every one or two hours; for more intensive use, mix 10–20 drops into ½ cup of water, adding a bit of carminative and/or demulcent herbs, and drink immediately (Smith 1999: 17–18; see also Tierra 1998: 100).

Perhaps most herbalists, however, would choose not to use preparations of the fresh rhizome. Revered American herbalist John Raymond Christopher stressed that the fresh rhizome is "somewhat acrid and purgative, but the dried form retains its healing virtues, without the negative characteristics" (Christopher 1976: 76). Christopher therefore recommended using a liquid extract consisting of ½–2 fluid drachms of the dried rhizome (Christopher 1976: 76). With reference to the closely allied species *I. missouriensi*, Michael Moore encouraged the use of only the dried rhizome internally and even stressed that a tincture should never be made of the fresh rhizome (Moore 1979: 40). His recommended dose for a dried-rhizome tincture was 5–20 drops, to be used up to three times a day, but with caution (Moore 1994a: 14). Herbalist David Hoffmann describes the use of a decoction of the dried rhizome, which is accomplished by putting ½–1 teaspoon of the rhizome into 1 cup of water, bringing it to a boil, and then simmering it for ten to fifteen minutes, using up to 3 cups a day (Hoffmann 1986: 177). The official preparations in the *National Formulary* for 1942 and the twenty-first edition of the *United States Dispensatory* likewise preferred the dried rhizome.

PERSONAL AND PROFESSIONAL USE

There are certain areas in the wilderness where blue flag grows that I periodically visit just to sit and take in this plant's incredible beauty, which inspires such serenity in my soul!

In my clinical practice, I use blue flag most often for its thyroid-balancing effects, finding that a trial of use in a person with an enlarged thyroid often normalizes the size of this gland.

When there are thyroid nodules, I tend to combine it with cleavers (see page 86), an Ayurvedic herb called guggul (*Commiphora mukul*), and the lovely garden herb rosemary (*Rosmarinus officinalis* [syn. *Salvia rosmarinus*]), which formula I find quite helpful in shrinking—and sometimes even eliminating—the nodules. (I've found that ingestion of fish oil is often helpful here as well.)

So reliable is blue flag for an enlarged thyroid and in the above formula for thyroid nodules that its failure to affect either of these conditions suggests to me that malignancy might perhaps be present, which possibility can sometimes be either confirmed or excluded by a skilled endocrinologist.

I also use this herb a lot in formulas that I craft for persistent cases of skin conditions such as acne, psoriasis, and eczema.

CAUTIONS

Do not use blue flag when either pregnant or lactating.

The constituent iridin (irisin) allows for a toxic potential in the use of blue flag: even moderate overdoses may cause severe gastrointestinal blistering, facial neuralgia, nausea, vomiting, and diarrhea. Then, too, merely touching the plant can cause dermatitis in some people! Therefore, *extreme caution should be exercised in the use of blue flag.* This is not an herb that laypeople should wildcraft and prepare for themselves; only commercial extracts should be used, and even these should be diluted liberally and never implemented at a dosage greater than that recommended on the bottle. Naturopathic physician Francis Brinker points out that a mere 3 teaspoons of the tincture would be highly toxic, while herbalist Ed Smith cautions against using more than 60 drops in any twenty-four-hour period and even against utilizing the tincture for longer than a week (Smith 1999: 17; Brinker 2000: 122). 🌿🌿

Blue Vervain

WILD HYSSOP; AMERICAN VERVAIN

Verbena hastata

DESCRIPTION

Growing 1½–5 feet tall, this attractive wild plant has a stem that is square, erect, and grooved.

The leaves are opposite, narrow (lanceolate to oblong), and toothed (evenly to unevenly). Occasionally, the lower leaves possess three lobes. The length of the leaves varies greatly—all the way from 1½ inches to 7 inches!

The flowers are blue to reddish blue to bluish pink. They are clustered at the ends of the stalks in slender spikes that grow to 8 inches long. A helpful identifier is that they often blossom haphazardly, or in a loose band, advancing from the bottom of the spike toward the tip, leaving ripening grain behind.

RANGE AND HABITAT

Blue vervain grows in dry marshes, on the sides of streams, and in moist meadows, fields, pastures, and prairies. The plant can be found west, and slightly east, of the Mississippi River and in adjacent portions of Canada.

MAJOR CONSTITUENTS

Blue vervain contains iridoid glycosides (verbenalin, aucubin, hastatoside); phenylpropanoid glycosides (verbascoside, eukovoside); flavonoids (luteolin-7-diglucuronide); an unidentified alkaloid; essential oil (geraniol, verbenone, limonene); stachyose; tannin; and mucilage. Nutrients include vitamins (pro-vitamin A, C, and E), calcium, and magnesium.

FOOD

Several different Native American tribes have roasted the seeds of blue vervain and ground them into flour. The taste is somewhat bitter and the work involved quite tedious. Still, if the plant can be found growing in large patches, so that a quantity of the seeds can be gathered in a short time, the activity should not be readily dismissed. Here, as an emergency food source, the husked seeds can be eaten raw.

HEALTH/MEDICINE

Blue vervain is a mild to moderate *diaphoretic*, having been listed in the 1916 edition of the US *National Formulary* as such. It would also appear to possess a mild *galactagogue* effect, probably owing to its aucubin content (Oliver-Bever 1986: 239), and an *emmenagogue* effect. John Gunn, in his famed household medical guide published in the 1860s, noted of the latter: "The root ... is an excellent emmenagogue, one of the best and safest known, in all cases of suppressed menses; to be used freely in strong decoction ... half a teaspoonful or more, three or four times a day" (Gunn 1859–61: 875).

This plant's iridoid content allows it to serve as a gentle *laxative*, if used in higher than usual doses. Blue vervain also has *diuretic* and *lithotriptic* abilities, attributed to its saponins (Dobelis et al. 1986: 323; Grases et al. 1994: 507). Owing to this, the Menomini found that they could rely upon this plant to clear up urine when it was cloudy (Smith 1923: 58).

Styptic properties are in *Verbena*'s bullpen as well: the Ojibwe from the Midwest found that a snuff of the powdered blossoms serves as a remedy par excellence for halting a nosebleed (Densmore 1974: 294). This is understandable in that verbenalin, a glycoside found in significant quantity in this plant, hastens the coagulation of blood, according to scientific research (Duke 1985: 508). Internally, too, this glycoside is quickly transmitted to the brain, bringing feelings of peace and order, thus enabling blue vervain to prove useful both as a *nervine* and as a *sedative* (Mowrey 1986: 226; Wren 1988: 275). In harmony with this, a 2002 study found this herb to be a sleep extender (*hypnotic*) (Akanmu et al. 2002).

Not surprisingly, then, one of the herb's most dramatic uses is as an agent for easing **stomachaches** due to **stress** (Moore 1979: 160), an application that has been much appreciated by the Teton (Gilmore 1991: 59). **Headaches**, including some **migraines** (Holmes 1989–90: 1:133), often respond to blue vervain's magic as well, especially those triggered by stress or by exhaustion.

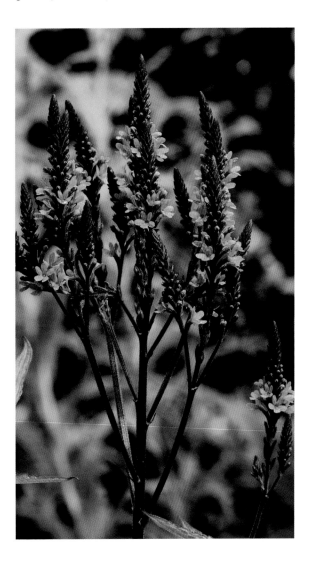

In accord with its nervine effect, herbalist Michael Moore suggests the tea for **fidgety children**, especially when first afflicted with a **cold** or the **flu** (Moore 1979: 160). The plant has a reputation for fighting colds and influenza per se, and even early-twentieth-century editions of the *National Formulary* held it to be an *expectorant*. *Antipyretic* activity has also been consistently attributed to it (Rafinesque 1828–30: 1:274); indeed, to such an end it has been used by the Cherokee, Lenape (Delaware), and Mahuna (Moerman 1986: 1:507). The herb's *antitussive* ability, confirmed for the related *Verbena officinalis* in a Chinese study (Gui 1985: 35), is also appreciated when colds are present. Then, too, the Eclectic writers Harvey Wickes Felter and John Uri Lloyd lauded its *tonic* effects in this regard: "Taken cold, the infusion forms a good tonic in some cases of debility, anorexia, and during convalescence from acute diseases" (Felter and Lloyd 1898).

A mid-1970s study found that blue vervain markedly inhibited inflammation in rats (Benoit et al. 1976: 169). Research conducted in Japan and elsewhere has confirmed that *V. officinalis* also possesses *anti-inflammatory*—even *analgesic*—properties (Sakai 1963; Deepak and Handa 2000). Both *V. hastata* and *V. officinalis* have been used for **gout** (Holmes 1989–90: 1:133) and have been found helpful for inflammation of the liver (**hepatitis**) and/or the gallbladder (**cholecystitis**) (Tierra 1988: 242; Wren 1988: 275), as the Houma discovered (Speck 1941: 65).

Any, or all, of blue vervain's nervine, emmenagogue, or anti-inflammatory properties may elucidate the plant's reputation in folk medicine as a treatment for **menopause** and for premenstrual syndrome where anxiety is the dominant complaint (i.e., **PMS-A**). Another possible factor is that a *luteinizing action* has been suspected for this plant by numerous clinicians. The likelihood of this may perhaps be gauged by the fact that *Verbena* is closely related to the popular marketed herb chaste-tree, or vitex (*Vitex agnus-castus*), which has a widely studied and heralded luteinizing action. In fact, so comparable are the two that vitex, like vervain, is also a galactagogue.

A widely observed and heralded *antispasmodic* effect on the part of blue vervain has long guided herbalists in using it for smooth-muscle tension, especially when experienced in the form of **menstrual cramps**, although herbalist David Winston points out that extracts made from the fresh plant are much more preferable in this regard than those made from dried material (Winston 1998). The antispasmodic effects presently lack detailed scientific confirmation, although in the mid-1980s it was reported that verbascoside assists the antitremor action of the Parkinson's drug levodopa (Oliver-Bever 1986). However, two studies of recent date have demonstrated anticonvulsant effects (as well as anxiolytic and sedative effects) for its close cousin *V. officinalis* (Khan et al. 2016; Rashidian et al. 2017). Long-standing clinical use leaves no doubt, going back (in the United States) to use by the Meskwaki (Fox), who are recorded as having implemented an extract of the root to successfully deal with **fits** (Smith 1928: 58). Independently—and apparently unaware—of Meskwaki use, the noted American herbalist Joseph Meyer studied this application thoroughly owing to a clinical report brought to him regarding its use in a long-standing case of epilepsy: "Its effects in that particular case were so remarkable, that I was led to study it more carefully. I found, after close investigation and most elaborate experiment that, prepared in a certain way and compounded with [three other herbs], and the best of whiskey, it has no equal for the cure of fits, epilepsy, or anything of a spastic nature" (cited in Shook 1978: 276). It is even listed as an antispasmodic in *Potter's Cyclopaedia of Botanical Drugs and Preparations* (Wren 1988: 275).

PERSONAL AND PROFESSIONAL USE

This is a plant on which I rely quite heavily as a nervine in my professional herbal practice and in which I have the utmost confidence. The red-letter indications to which I look for its use include (1) the predomination of a future-related anxiety; (2) tight or spastic muscles, especially in the upper back and shoulders; and (3) stools that tend toward constipation.

I have also found blue vervain to serve as an able spasmolytic or anticonvulsant, for which purposes I usually combine it with skullcap (see page 212) and sometimes also with other spasmolytics. Finally, I have observed it to function as a luteal tonic par excellence, especially when weakness in the system during this phase of the menstrual cycle allows for the manifestation of various afflictions otherwise only infrequently experienced or not experienced at all (e.g., herpes-sore eruptions, the onset of viral or other infections, epileptic attacks, headaches).

CAUTIONS

Because blue vervain has been shown, in animal studies, to stimulate the uterus (Farnsworth et al. 1975: 535–98), *any oral implementation of this plant should be strictly avoided during pregnancy.*

The glycoside verbenalin found in this plant is an emetic, so it should be borne in mind that drinking too much of the tea—or drinking it too quickly—could cause vomiting. ⟨⟨

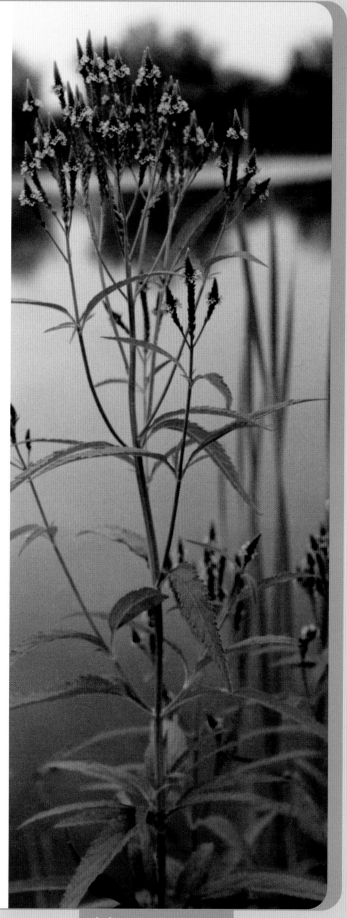

blue vervain

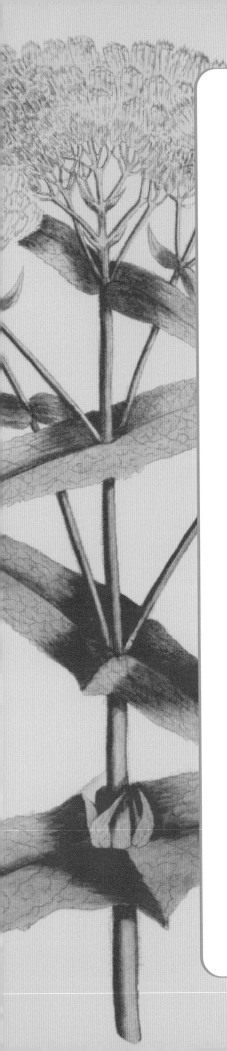

Boneset

DESCRIPTION

Boneset is a perennial plant indigenous to North America that can grow as high as 5 feet but usually tops off in the range of 2–4 feet. Its stem is erect, cylindrical, hairy, and branching at the top.

The wrinkled-looking, finely toothed leaves are 4 inches long or so toward the top of the plant but grow to around 8 inches toward the bottom of the plant. The undersides of the leaves are downy looking. Of curious interest is that the leaves are attached in an odd sort of fashion that makes identification of boneset fairly simple. The species name, *perfoliatum*, gives us the clue here, indicating that each set of leaves is united at their base—that is, they are joined across the stem, giving the appearance of but one long leaf *perforated* by the stem! This distinguishes it from its toxic cousin, white snakeroot (*Eupatorium rugosum*), whose leaves are stalked.

In midsummer, white florets grouped in flat-topped clusters appear at the top of the main stem and its branches. One can detect from these flowers only a weak odor. The eventual fruit is a tufted achene.

RANGE AND HABITAT

Boneset sometimes grows in very moist woods, but its preferred habitat is swampy regions and the borders of marshes and small ponds. It is found throughout the Midwest in such environs.

MAJOR CONSTITUENTS

Boneset contains sesquiterpene lactones of the germacranolide kind (euperfolin and euperfolitin) and of the guaianolide kind (eufoliatin and eufoliatorin); terpenes; diterpenes (hebeclinolide, dendroidinic acid, hebenolide); triterpenes (alpha-amyrin, dotriacontane); isohumulene; chromenes; polysaccharides (4-O-methyl-glucuronoxylans, inulin); flavonoids (eupatorin, kaempferol, kaempferol-3-rutinoside, quercetin, rutin, astragalin); sterols (sitosterol and stigmasterol); gum; resin; gallic acid; and tannic acid. It would seem also to contain two pyrrolizidine alkaloids, according to a 2018 analysis; but see below for further elucidation.

HEALTH/MEDICINE

With the possible exceptions of anise hyssop, plantain, and mullein, my cupboards are stocked with more boneset than any other medicinal plant. As I believe will become evident from the profile that follows, there are numerous good reasons for stocking up on this odd-looking marsh plant! Indeed, as Alabama herbalist Tommie Bass once so well put it: "It is as good a one as the Lord put out there" (Crellin and Philpott 1990a: 106).

Boneset was used with good success by early American settlers as a healing herb once the onset of a cold or flu was first suspected as developing. The brilliant Eclectic pharmacist John Uri Lloyd, who wrote a treatise on this herb in 1918, remarked that boneset was esteemed so valuable by early Americans for colds and the flu that it could be "found in every well-regulated household" of these times (Lloyd 1929: 137). The gifted author of *American Medicinal Plants*, Charles Millspaugh, further explained how, by the late nineteenth century, boneset could be encountered hanging from the rafters of nearly every woodshed and attic in the country, ready for use at the slightest symptom of a cold or of the flu (Millspaugh 1974: 312–14).

Such a therapeutic utilization of the plant seems to have been gleaned from Native Americans, in that available records evince numerous tribes—including the eastern Cherokee (Hamel and Chiltoskey 1975: 27), the Iroquois (Herrick 1995: 232), the Menomini (Smith 1923: 30), and the Mohegan (Tantaquidgeon 1928: 265)—also using the herb for treating **colds**, **influenza**, and **fevers**. The Lenape (Delaware) have used an infusion of the root, and sometimes of the leaves as well, for a fever with **chills** (Tantaquidgeon 1942: 28; Tantaquidgeon 1972: 33, 118–19). The Nanticoke have used it in combination with wild thyme for same (Tantaquidgeon 1972: 98, 126–27). The plant's implementation for colds and the flu in such a wide variety of cultures is abundant testimony as to its efficacy, although good clinical trials for boneset's abilities here have, surprisingly, not yet been undertaken. The lone clinical trial on record, published in 1981, showed that a homeopathic preparation of boneset (*Eupatorium perfoliatum* D2) was equally effective as aspirin in relieving the symptoms of a cold—both test groups showed equal improvement based on lab tests, body temperature, and subjective complaints (Gassinger et al. 1981).

Boneset tea was also a popular treatment in early America for various feverish, infectious diseases of a more serious nature than colds. It was, for example, the most popular treatment for **malaria** before the introduction of quinine (Bloyer 1901: 837; Felter 1924: 201; Hocking 1997: 296). Then, too, during the Civil War, when Peruvian bark, the source of quinine, became largely unavailable, boneset was recommended to Confederate troops for this illness by the prominent medical doctor Francis Porcher. As Porcher said, it was "thought by many physicians to be even superior to the dogwood, willow or poplar [the bark of which trees are febrifuges and are analgesic], as a substitute for quinine" (Porcher 1863: 9). One such physician was the noted John Sappington, who, in his classic work entitled *Theory and Treatment of Fevers*, published in 1844, identified boneset and dogwood as the best indigenous substitutes for quinine (Hall 1974: 527; cf. Jackson 1876: 234).

Then, too, early American physicians implemented boneset for **yellow fever** (Barton 1817–18: 2:135–37; Grieve 1971: 1:119; Millspaugh 1974: 314; Duke 1985: 188; Hocking 1997: 296). Benjamin Smith Barton, writing near the birth of the eighteenth century, reported that this herb was particularly instrumental in halting a yellow-fever epidemic that occurred in Philadelphia in 1793 (Barton 1900: 1:28; 2:22–26, 55). William C. Barton, writing just a decade and a half later, related of the work

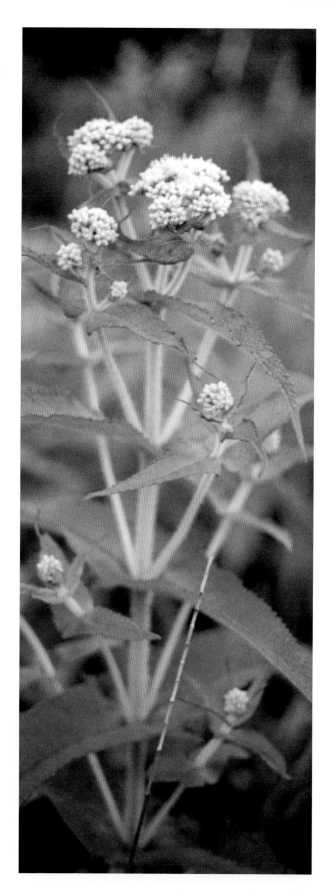

of Samuel C. Hopkins, of Woodbury, New Jersey, who had used *Eupatorium perfoliatum* most effectively as the sole treatment for typhus and for other serious fevers (Barton 1817–18: 2:136). Indeed, boneset was widely used for both **typhus** (Barton 1817–18: 2:135; Rafinesque 1828–30: 1:177; Millspaugh 1974: 314; Duke 1985: 188) and **typhoid fever** (Felter and Lloyd 1898; Bloyer 1901: 837; Grieve 1971: 1:119; Duke 1985: 188; Hocking 1997: 296).

Boneset's most famous historic role, however, unfolded during a dastardly plague that occurred during colonial times. With reference to this, Constantine Rafinesque, the noted compiler of a respected tome on medical botany published in the early 1800s, informs us that a medical authority he consulted, N. Chapman (the author of several works on therapeutics and material medica published from 1817 to 1822), "relates that it cured the kind of influenza called Breakbone fever" (Rafinesque 1828–30: 1:176). This so-called "breakbone fever" was a miserable viral contagion that produced joint and muscle pains so excruciating that its victims felt as if their bones were literally breaking—thus the virus's name! By checking this epidemic, *E. perfoliatum* earned the common name by which it is now most widely known, for in dealing with this virus, it was felt by the victims to have re-"set" their bones (thus, boneset). "Breakbone fever" is thought by historians of medicine to have been either a very powerful strain of **influenza** or a form of the mosquito-transmitted virus known as **dengue** (Millspaugh 1974: 314; Crellin and Philpott 1990a: 107).

As a result of its well-attested successes as enumerated here, boneset came to be widely implemented by nineteenth-century physicians. Rafinesque wrote of it in 1828: "It has been introduced extensively into practice all over the country ... and inserted in all our medical works" (Rafinesque 1828–30: 1:176). Asahel Clapp, in his 1852 report to the American Medical Association, emphasized that boneset "deservedly holds a high rank among our indigenous medical plants" (Clapp 1852: 791–92). By the 1870s, John R. Jackson, writing in the *Canadian Pharmaceutical Journal*, acknowledged that the herb was being "used by many physicians" (Jackson 1876: 234). The beloved boneset even received official pharmaceutical recognition, appearing in the *United States Pharmacopeia* (and that for over eighty years—from 1820 to 1916!) and in the *National Formulary* (for most of the first half of the twentieth century).

But how did boneset accomplish its task with breakbone fever—and indeed with the many other feverish viral contagions so prevalent in early America? In several ways, it seems. We note first that boneset has been used by the Mohegan for **general debility** (Tantaquidgeon 1972: 72) and that it was listed in the *US Pharmacopeia* (1820–1916) and *National Formulary* (1926–50) as a *stimulant* (cf. Bloyer 1901: 837; Culbreth 1927; Gathercoal and Wirth 1936: 721; Pedersen 1998: 55), so it no doubt proved to be of great benefit for the

severe lethargy that accompanied such feverish viral contagions. (I myself have witnessed it transform within one hour of use a person with a 102-degree fever who was flat on his back in bed and who thought he was dying into a person who proceeded to get up to do household chores and to go on to express a desire to go back to his job!)

Its strong *diaphoretic* properties were undoubtedly of great use as well, helping patients to "sweat out" the fever. Botanist and physician Laurence Johnson, writing in the 1880s, observed in this regard: "Taken warm in large doses, the infusion or decoction produces copious diaphoresis, and is employed in the acute stages of catarrhal affections and in fevers, especially of the intermittent or remittent type" (Johnson 1884: 173; cf. Wren 1988: 40; Fleming 1998). An interesting historical testimonial to its aid here survives from the pen of the British botanist Thomas Nuttall, who reported that when he was sick in 1819 with "intermittent fever," because none of the standard medicines were at hand, he "took in the evening about a pint of a strong and very bitter decoction, of the *Eupatorium cuneifolium*, the *E. perfoliatum* or Boneset, not being to be found in the neighborhood. This dose, though very nauseous, did not ... operate as an emetic, but acted as a diaphoretic and gentle laxative, and prevented the proximate return of the disease" (Nuttall 1905: 244).

Boneset is also a powerful *immunostimulant* (Fleming 1998), which was undoubtedly part of the reason for its success during the feverish contagions of colonial and pioneer times. Recent chemical analyses have revealed some fascinating information in this regard. For example, one of the plant's sesquiterpene lactones, eufoliatin, has experimentally been shown to exert strong immunostimulating activity of a general sort (Wagner et al. 1985c; Wren 1988: 40; Woerdenbag 1993: 180; Newall et al. 1996: 48). Then there are the polysaccharides in boneset, which have been demonstrated to possess potent immunostimulating effects as well. Here, several scientists employing three immunological test systems—carbon clearance, granulocyte, and chemiluminescence—found that the type of water-soluble polysaccharides occurring in boneset demonstrated a marked phagocytosis-enhancing effect, especially in the granulocyte test (Wagner et al. 1984; Wagner et al. 1985c; Vollmar et al. 1986). This means that they stimulated certain of the body's white blood cells to perform more effectively their job of phagocytosis, which involves an engulfing (through their cell membranes) of invading organisms so as to destroy them from the body. A similar study found this immune-enhancing effect to be equal to that possessed by the polysaccharides of the popular immune-enhancing herb echinacea (*Echinacea purpurea*) when both samples were in a concentration of 0.001 milligram per milliliter but *ten times stronger* when both were in a concentration of 0.01 milligrams per milliliter! (Wagner et al. 1985c; cf.

Wagner et al. 1984: 660) In another study, a combination of boneset, arnica (*Arnica montana*), wild indigo (*Baptisia tinctoria*), and *Echinacea angustifolia* showed over 50 percent greater immune stimulation than did *E. angustifolia* alone (Wagner and Jurcik 1991). My own careful observations over the last thirty-five years have convinced me that boneset is most efficacious as an immune enhancer over echinacea for type O blood, while echinacea proves to be as effective as boneset—or even more effective—for type A.

Aside from aiding immunity in a general sense, however, the plant seems to possess direct *antibacterial* and *antiviral* activity, judging by both clinical and experimental evidence. Activity against several kinds of bacteria has been reported for *E. perfoliatum* in lab experiments on several occasions (Mockle 1955: 89; Woerdenbag 1993: 180; Habtemariam and MacPherson 2000), as well as for other *Eupatorium* species (Croom 1983: 60 and references cited there). Moreover, two related species (*E. rotundifolium* and *E. squalidum*) have even been shown to exert a direct effect against the malaria organism (*Plasmodium*) in particular (Croom 1983: 62, ref. 131; Carvalho and Krettli 1991). In addition to this, a tincture of the related species *E. odoratum*, which has traditionally been used in Guatemala for **venereal diseases**, was shown in a test-tube study to be highly active against five strains of **gonorrhea** (Cáceres et al. 1995). Modern American herbalists have also effectively used boneset, alone or in formulas, against **herpes infections**, including genital herpes (Type 2) (Bergner 1995–96: 10). In this regard, it is of interest that early American physicians employed it against what was thought to be a "herpes" of sorts, the so-called James River ringworm (Barton 1817–18: 1:28, 2:22–26, 55). A study performed in Spain revealed some fascinating confirmatory evidence for these uses: scientists working at one of the universities there demonstrated that extracts of two species of *Eupatorium* (*E. articulatum* and *E. glutinosum*) are quite active against herpes simplex Type 1 (which was the only type tested) (Abad et al. 1999). We now have, however, published research verifying antiviral effects against influenza for our native boneset, *E. perfoliatum*. In 2016, the *Journal of Ethnopharmacology* published a paper by German scientists who used boneset to inhibit the growth of an influenza-A clinical isolate and to prevent that virus from attaching to host cells; the latter ability was attributed to the plant's polyphenolic constituents (Derksen et al. 2016). Thus, once again,

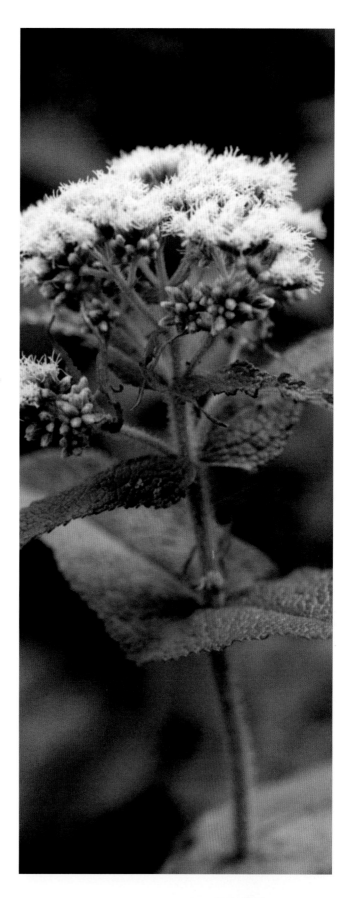

the traditional use of a plant has been verified by modern science.

Boneset possesses, as well, some *anti-inflammatory* potential (Benoit et al. 1976: 160; Fleming 1998; Habtemariam et al. 1998), possibly owing to its flavonoids (Newall et al. 1996: 48), so that it proves helpful where inflammation of the sinuses, ears, or bronchioles is involved. It is also *anti-catarrhal* (Bloyer 1901: 837; Grieve 1971: 1:119; Ellingwood 1983: 269; Santillo 1984: 92) and can work wonders with unyielding respiratory mucus, which it breaks up and expectorates most ably (Pedersen 1988: 55; Wren 1988: 40). In fact, the *expectorant* constituents in the related Asian species *E. fortunei*, used in Traditional Chinese Medicine (TCM), were identified as far back as the early 1980s (Cai 1983: 30). Thus, it is especially indicated where there is a *dry, irritable cough* corresponding to what TCM calls "lung wind-heat/dryness" (Holmes 1989–90: 1:131). Tommie Bass particularly appreciated boneset for the **cough** associated with **croup** (Crellin and Philpott 1990b: 187). America's Eclectic physicians of the late 1800s and early 1900s found that it "relieves chest pain and cough," especially in "bronchial pneumonia," serving as well to allay the "irritable after-coughing" often associated with this condition (Felter 1922: 201). They also found it to be invaluable in elderly or debilitated individuals when "there is an abundance of secretion but lack of power to expel it" (Felter 1924: 201). Here the Eclectics had a wealth of information and experience to draw upon, as numerous articles had appeared in the *Eclectic Medical Journal* outlining its history and efficacies, including one in 1924 that noted: "During the severe [Spanish influenza] pandemic of 1918–19 it was one of the safest and most successful remedies employed and contributed much to the successful management of the disease under Eclectic treatment" (Felter 1924: 201; Best 1928: 93).

But boneset has a plethora of uses aside from its legendary aid for those afflicted with infectious, febrile diseases. For one thing, the root has been used by both the Meskwaki (Fox) and the Ojibwe to treat **rattlesnake bite** (Smith 1928: 214). Then, too, it has long been employed as a *vermifuge*, even against the stubborn **tapeworm** (Mockle 1955: 89; Vogel 1970: 226; Grieve 1971: 1:119; Locock 1990: 229; Woerdenbag 1993: 179). One person who made this latter application somewhat famous in his own area of the country was a Meskwaki herbalist named John McIntosh, who used a tea of the leaves and of the flowers (Smith 1928: 214; Shemluck 1982: 330). Colonial physicians also often relied upon boneset as an *anthelmintic* (Christianson 1987: 73).

Owing to its very bitter sesquiterpene lactones, boneset also favorably *tones* and *stimulates* the digestive processes. Physician and botanist Laurence Johnson observed in this regard: "The infusion, taken cold in moderate doses, is tonic, and is employed in debility of the digestive organs and in convalescence" (Johnson 1884: 173). Early American

physician Jacob Bigelow had further pointed out: "Given in moderate quantities … in cold infusion or decoction, it promotes digestion, strengthens the viscera, and restores tone to the system" (Bigelow 1817–20: 1:36). It thus works well as an *appetite stimulant* and has been especially employed by herbalists to treat **lack of appetite in the aged** (Grieve 1971: 1:119; Spoerke 1990: 43; Hocking 1997: 296; Fleming 1998). Then, too, as Rafinesque observed, it is "particularly useful in the indigestion of old people" (Rafinesque 1828–30: 1:176).

In view of its bitter components, it is not surprising that boneset is *hepatic* (Grieve 1971: 1:119; Holmes 1989–90: 1:130). The Physiomedicalist physician William Cook explained that boneset is "relaxing to the hepatobiliary apparatus, promoting secretion of bile and also expulsion from the gallbladder into the digestive tract" (Cook 1985). Boneset's favorable effect upon the biliary system may further elucidate its classic and reliable implementation as a mild *aperient*, in that the free and proper flow of bile softens and moves stool through the colon (Felter 1922; Culbreth 1927; Wood et al. 1937: 446; Wren 1988: 40).

Despite this fine testimony as to boneset's liver-friendly effects, a chemical analysis published in 2018 claimed to have found low levels of two potentially hepatotoxic pyrrolizidine alkaloids (lycopsamine and intermedine) in boneset (Colegate et al. 2018). This study is problematic, however, in that all of the samples analyzed displayed hybridization with other *Eupatorium* species.

Indeed, many species in the *Eupatorium* genus do contain the potentially toxic pyrrolizidine alkaloids (PAs), including the widely used Eurasian species *E. cannabinum* and the two likewise often-used Asian species *E. fortunei* and *E. chilense*, as well as our resident joe-pye weed, formerly classified in the *Eupatorium* genus (see page 138). However, in none of these species has a toxic reaction with the liver been recorded. Moreover, a rat study employing three of the potentially toxic PA-containing species (*E. fortunei*, *E. japonicum*, and *E. chilense*) failed to show hepatotoxicity as against controls, *even after prolonged administration* (Zhao et al. 1987). And *E. cannabinum*, although possessed of several potentially toxic PAs (as we have seen), has actually been shown to be *hepatoprotective* against carbon-tetrachloride-induced hepatotoxicity (Lexa et al. 1989). Moreover, one of the authors of the 2018 study by Colegate et al. referred to above noted that commercial honey typically contains a greater concentration of PAs than did the boneset samples analyzed (Yearsley 2020).

Perhaps most important, however, is the widespread, two-centuries-old use of our *E. perfoliatum* in North America that has failed to yield a single case of hepato veno-occlusive disease (HVOD)—the liver disease chiefly associated with high amounts of these PAs—or any other liver damage, not to mention my own frequent use over the past three decades. Perhaps because of this widespread historical use and a lack of cases of liver damage connected with its use, the FDA has taken no action against the marketing of this herb as of this writing, approximately two years after the 2018 study by Colegate et al. All in all, it would seem, then, that the popular species known as boneset, *Eupatorium perfoliatum*, is safe to use as long as traditional dosages and cautions (see below, under Cautions) are observed.

As to yet other uses for boneset, our marsh-loving plant has demonstrated good success in treating **rheumatism** of a **neuralgic** or **muscular** sort (Barton 1817–18: 2:138; Rafinesque 1828–30: 1:177; Bloyer 1901: 837; Hocking 1997: 296). Boneset's anti-inflammatory potential, as noted previously, is undoubtedly of some aid here. However, the plant seems to be of assistance as a connective-tissue aid in other respects as well: for many years, for instance, the Iroquois used a cold, compound infusion of the herb's leaves as a poultice for broken bones (Herrick 1995: 232). Concordantly, in modern times, herbalist and naturalist Tom Brown Jr., who was mentored under the revered Apache herbalist Stalking Wolf, has offered his lifetime of personal experience with boneset as a connective-tissue aid, finding it most effective when a small amount of the herb is steeped for fifteen to thirty minutes in hot water (Brown 1985: 67).

Finally, a tincture of boneset leaves has been shown to manifest *cytotoxic* activity (useful against cancer cells) comparable to that of chlorambucil, a cytotoxic agent in regular use (Habtemariam and MacPherson 2000). In fact, boneset's flavonoid eupatorin has, by itself, been shown to be cytotoxic in laboratory tests (Kupchan et al. 1965; Midge and Rao 1975: 541; Herz et al. 1977; Heywood et al. 1977: 421; Vollmar et al. 1986: 377; Woerdenbag 1993: 179). The sesquiterpene lactones present in the herb have also been shown to produce similar effects against cancer cells (Cassady et al. 1969: 522; Herz et al. 1977), as have those of *E. cannabinum* (Woerdenbag et al. 1986) and *E. cuneifolium* (Kupchan et al. 1973).

As to manner of implementation, generally boneset is used today as a tincture, although some prefer to make the fully dried leaves into a tea—which, as we've seen, was the most common form of the herb taken in early America. The tea is drunk at various temperatures, depending on the situation: cold as a tonic, but hot or warm as a cold and flu combatant and/or as a diaphoretic.

It should also be noted that boneset tea taken in large doses during a short period of time serves as an *emetic*. This is probably largely due to the plant's concentration of the chemical eupatorin (Spoerke 1990: 43). Emetics can be useful at times, and it is of interest that the 1968 edition of the *Merck Index* (not to be confused with the *Merck Manual*) noted that eupatorin has been used in emergency medicine as an emetic in situations of poisoning in which gastric lavage is unavailable or inadvisable.

PERSONAL AND PROFESSIONAL USE

There are few plants that I have utilized more frequently in both my personal life and my clinical practice than this common resident of our swamps and marshes.

In my personal and family life, I have made use of boneset's benefits since at least the early 1980s, most often for fever, congestion, and lethargy occurring during bad colds or influenza, with predictably excellent results.

In my clinical practice, I've likewise used it often for the above complaints, as well as in formulas for persons manifesting a weakened immune response (especially with a low neutrophil count via laboratory analysis).

I've also found it to be helpful for food regurgitation. With reference to this latter application, I recall two different cases where it proved to be the only certain remedy.

CAUTIONS

If gathering boneset (*Eupatorium perfoliatum*) from the wild, be very careful not to confuse it with *its very deadly cousin*, white snakeroot (*E. rugosum*), to which it bears a close resemblance. Although white snakeroot flourishes in woodsy areas and boneset in marshy ones, the two plants *may be found growing together* where these areas intersect.

Both species have nearly identical flowers and a similar overall look to them—after all, they're closely related. However, white snakeroot's leaves, while opposite like those of boneset's, are not perfoliate like those of the latter but instead possess stalks.

White snakeroot was responsible for a horrible illness called "the trembles" that ravaged rural American areas in the early to mid-nineteenth century. This malady also came to be called "milk sickness" because it was eventually realized that a toxic component in white snakeroot (tremetol, a mixture of benzofuranoid compounds) became soluble in the milk of cows that consumed it and that when people drank the poisoned milk, the toxin was transmitted to them so that they became susceptible to "the trembles." Many died as a result, including Abraham Lincoln's mother.

In view of the discovery of potentially toxic PAs in boneset since the second edition of this book was published (2013), it would seem to be the course of wisdom that *it not be utilized during pregnancy or in infants or young children.* (That being said, however, I have known many pregnant women who have utilized the herb on a very short-term basis for a cold or flu without any harm having accrued to the embryo or fetus.) Even adults should, in view of the above-mentioned discovery, not use this herb on a long-term basis. Finally, persons with compromised liver function should most probably not use boneset at all. ⋘

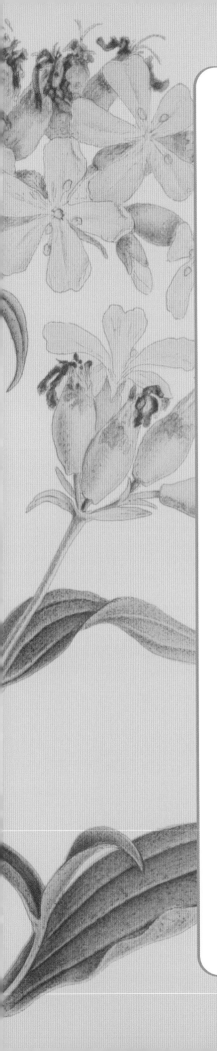

Bouncing Bet

SOAPWORT; LATHERWORT; FULLER'S HERB

Saponaria officinalis

DESCRIPTION

A European perennial that escaped from gardens during pioneer times, bouncing bet grows 1–1½ feet tall and tends to thrive in colonies (although I have come across many solitary specimens). Its stems are smooth but swollen at the nodes.

Bouncing bet's leaves are oval to lanceolate, 2–3 inches long, and prominently veined. They are entire and smooth edged, and they grow in pairs.

The plant's lovely flowers, which also often grow in pairs, are pink or white and possessed of five notched petals that are deflected downward. They are arranged in dense, terminal cymes.

RANGE AND HABITAT

This plant can be found in waste places and along the sides of roads and railroad tracks throughout the Midwest.

MAJOR CONSTITUENTS

Bouncing bet contains saponin (to 5 percent), saporins, flavonoids (including vitexin), resin, mucilage, gum.

HEALTH/MEDICINE

Bouncing bet is perhaps best known as an *expectorant* (Weiss 1988: 204) due to its large concentration of saponins. These irritate the stomach, causing reflex irritation to the respiratory mucosa so that any mucus therein is expelled. Research by Russian scientists shed much light on an *immunostimulating* aspect of these saponins (Bogoiavlenskii et al. 1999). Yet another line of research confirmed that the similar-sounding saporins in the plant are deadly to **lymphoma**, **leukemia**, **melanoma**, and **breast cancer** in vitro, although clinical studies are as yet lacking in confirmation (Siena et al. 1989; Gasperi-Campani et al. 1991; Tecce et al. 1991). There is some concern, however, that the saporins by themselves have been shown to be *hepatotoxic* to some extent (Stripe et al. 1987). Despite this, bouncing bet has classically been used to heal "liver affections," including **jaundice** (Chevallier 1996: 264), instead of cause them, so perhaps balancing agents in the plant serve to offset the toxic effect of the saporins to such an extent that the herb actually winds up being slightly supportive to the liver. In concert with this, America's Eclectic physicians of the late nineteenth and early twentieth centuries revered bouncing bet as "a remedy in the treatment of jaundice, liver affections" as well as an "alterative [for] syphilitic, scrofulous and cutaneous diseases." They also found it to be a fairly good *emmenagogue* (Felter and Lloyd 1898).

Bouncing bet has traditionally been taken by decoction (never by infusion—see below) of the dried and finely shaved root (Potterton 1983: 175), to the tune of 1 teaspoon per cup of water (Blumenthal 1998). Historically, the tea has been imbibed only by the teaspoon, with a total consumption of no more than 2–4 fluid ounces a day, owing to a toxic potential. *If allowed to macerate, the tea has the potential to cause paralysis and tremor.* Thus, boiling the root for only a few minutes and then straining right away has been considered the safest procedure for preparing the tea for internal use (Potterton 1983: 175).

External applications have also abounded, however. The Cherokee, for example, have poulticed **boils** with bouncing bet (Hamel and Chiltoskey 1975: 26). The herb has also classically been used—in both the European and the American herbal traditions—as a topical application for **erysipelas** (de Bairacli Levy 1974: 135). Since both boils and erysipelas are caused by bacteria (the latter usually by *Staphylococcus aureus*), the aforementioned applications are of interest in light of a scientific study finding bouncing bet to inhibit a virulent strain of *Mycobacterium tuberculosis* (Fitzpatrick 1954: 530). Such varied antimicrobial applications are understandable in light of the verified antimicrobial effects of the plant's saponins (Hiller 1987).

A topical wash made from a decoction of the plant's roots remains a time-honored treatment for **poison ivy**. It has been assumed that success here is due to a skin-cleansing ability on the part of the saponins (Dobelis et al. 1986: 118). Still, as the herb has been lauded as a treatment even after the rash has broken out, and not just prior to that time as a preventive, perhaps an *anti-inflammatory* aspect is involved, for indeed such an effect has been tapped in sundry ways by various cultures: Native Americans of California, for example, poulticed the ground, pulped leaves over an **inflamed spleen**, leaving them there for three to four hours (Romero 1954: 40). Then, too, the late, great European herbalist Juliette de

Bairacli Levy found bouncing bet to be useful as a rub for both **rheumatism** and **arthritis** (de Bairacli Levy 1974: 135).

PERSONAL AND PROFESSIONAL USE

I frequently borrow a few leaves here and there from colonies of bouncing bet when I'm out enjoying my wilderness activities, thereafter adding some spittle (or water from my canteen) and vigorously rubbing my hands with this combination in order to free them from dirt and grime. This natural soap works astonishingly well owing to the proliferation of the plant's saponins. (Please note that it is important to never wash one's hands in a body of water with bouncing bet, as saponins are extremely toxic to cold-blooded animals; just a small concentration can poison a wide area and kill many of our aquatic siblings very quickly.)

CAUTIONS

Due to the large concentration of saponins in this plant and the consequent possibility of toxicity from overuse or improper preparation and ingestion of it—manifested as gastrointestinal inflammation, diarrhea, and/or vomiting—any internal use should be left to skilled hands only. Furthermore, the herb's other major chemical constituent, saporin, appears to be hepatotoxic to some degree, as noted above (Stripe et al. 1987). ⋘

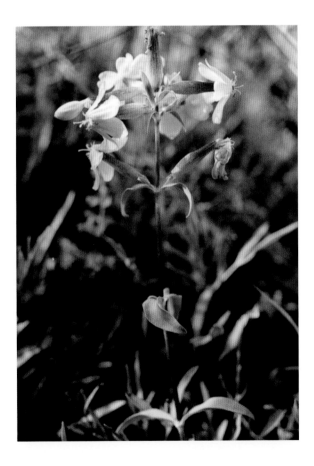

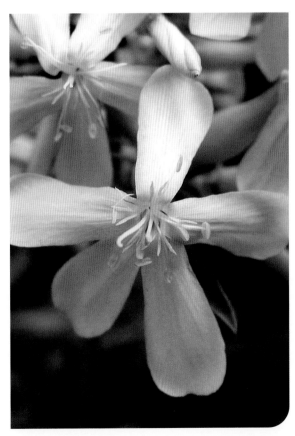

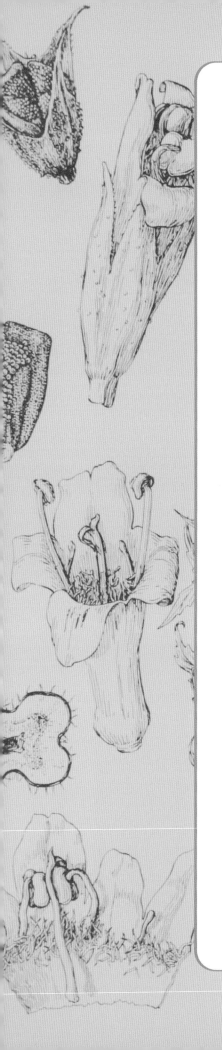

Bugleweed

DESCRIPTION

Bugleweed is a member of the mint family and, as such, is possessed of a square stem and paired leaves. Its flowers occur clustered along its stem at the leaf axils.

Species growing in the Midwest include the following:

Lycopus americanus (cut-leaved water horehound) grows 6–24 inches tall and has deeply lobed lower leaves and conspicuously toothed upper leaves.

L. asper (rough bugleweed, western water horehound) has sharply toothed leaves with ascending teeth. It is often hairy, thus yielding a rough feeling to the touch.

L. uniflorus (northern bugleweed, common water horehound) has hairless stems and fine-toothed leaves with short stalks (1–4 millimeters). Its small, whitish flowers are sessile and possessed of flared lobes. They appear in clusters of three to ten at the leaf axils.

L. virginicus (Virginia bugleweed) grows 6–24 inches tall and has dark-green—and sometimes purple-tinged—leaves that are narrow at both ends and sharply toothed. This species' calyx lobes are noticeably blunt.

RANGE AND HABITAT

One or more species of bugleweed flourish throughout the Midwest in rich, moist soil—especially along lakeshores, on riverbanks, and in or around swamps and marshes.

MAJOR CONSTITUENTS

Bugleweed is rich in tannin and in phenolic acids (including caffeic, chlorogenic, ellagic, gallic, lithospermic, and rosmarinic acids). It also contains flavone glucuronides of apigenin, acacetin, and luteolin. The plant's essential oil contains alpha-pinene, beta-pinene, camphene, caryophyllene, germacrene D, linalol, limonene, and pulegone. The triterpene ursolic acid also occurs. A glycoside, lycopin, is also present.

FOOD

Lycopus uniflorus has crisp tubers that are available from autumn until early spring. Native Americans have relished these tubers raw or cooked (boiled for ten to fifteen minutes), as do many modern foragers.

HEALTH/MEDICINE

Lycopus virginicus is one of several herbs—the others being motherwort, *Leonurus cardiaca* (see page 156), and lemon balm, *Melissa officinalis*—classically and presently used by herbal healers in the treatment of **hyperthyroidism**, including **Graves' disease** and especially when marked by tachycardia, a warm face and trunk, "morbid vigilance," wakefulness (including insomnia), and a sense of oppression in the chest that is accompanied by tight breathing.

Edgar J. George, a homeopathic physician practicing in Chicago, was one who came to an appreciation of bugleweed's power in Graves' disease. After failing to treat the disease successfully with homeopathic remedies, he found great success using a 5-drop dose of bugleweed tincture, given four times a day. He observed that cardiac and nervous symptoms were reduced after a short while and that after about one to two years of treatment, even the exophthalmus (the bulging eyes characterizing this disease) disappeared. He cautioned, however: "In giving the remedy for a continued period a change or rest should be allowed the patient from time to time, as the system becomes accustomed to the drug, which loses its effect" (George et al. 1911). The German phytotherapist-physician Rudolf Fritz Weiss, who practiced in the latter half of the twentieth century, also found this herb to be most helpful in Graves' disease but pointed out that its effects in reducing the subjective symptoms are not normally noticed until it has been employed for about one to two weeks (Weiss 1988: 279).

Bugleweed is the most scientifically studied of the known antithyrotropic herbs and has been shown to inhibit the binding of the pituitary-produced thyroid-stimulating hormone (TSH) to its receptor on the thyroid gland and also the ability of Graves' immunoglobulins to bind to the thyroid plasma membrane. Furthermore, it has been observed to reduce the levels of both thyroxine (T_4), the thyroid prohormone, and triiodothyronine (T_3), that gland's true hormone, but without resulting in a concomitant rise in thyroid-stimulating hormone (Deglmann 1955; Kemper et al. 1961; Samec 1961; Hiller and Kohrle et al. 1981; Auf'Mkolk et al. 1984; Auf'Mkolk et al. 1985; Winterhoff et al. 1988; Winterhoff et al. 1994; Vonhoff 2006). The active antithyrotropic components would appear to be rosmarinic acid,

ellagic acid, and luteolin-monoglucoside (Auf'Mkolk et al. 1984; Auf'Mkolk et al. 1985; Winterhoff et al. 1988).

As noted by George, above, bugleweed typically reduces the **rapid heartbeat** associated with Graves' disease, and it has been observed to do likewise with some other tachycardic etiologies as well, an effect that was greatly appreciated by America's Eclectic physicians of the nineteenth century (Scudder 1870: 156). Of especial value here is the fact that, as both George and the great medical botanist Constantine Rafinesque pointed out, bugleweed doesn't need to accumulate in the system to accomplish this effect, unlike some of the cardiac drugs used in orthodox medicine (Rafinesque 1828–30: 2:29; cf. Millspaugh 1974: 459).

We now also have two clinical trials in the scientific literature demonstrating efficacy of the European species, *Lycopus europaeus*, for mild hyperthyroidism. The first of these, published in 2008, showed a decrease in thyroxine (T_4) via an increase in urinary excretion as well as a reduction of symptoms in the trial participants (Beer et al. 2008). The second study, published in 2013, revealed a clinically relevant improvement of symptoms in a group of 403 patients, some of whom served as a control group (Eiling et al. 2013).

Because *L. virginicus*, at least, can lower prolactin levels (Brinker 1990), it is also often useful in **premenstrual syndrome**, in which elevated prolactin or a sensitivity to this

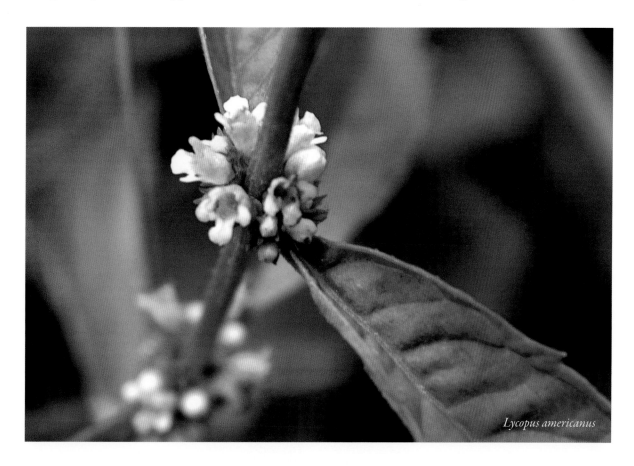

Lycopus americanus

hormone often exists and consequent **tension** and **anxiety** are the result (Fleming 1998).

Bugleweed is also a good *hemostat*, often looked to in **menorrhagia** and in **passive internal hemorrhage** (Millspaugh 1974: 459). The Natura physician R. Swinburne Clymer found it to be of particular value in **hemorrhage** of either the **lungs** or the **bladder** as well as in **urinary incontinence** (Clymer 1973: 150). In that herbal writers as diverse as Rafinesque and the twentieth-century folk herbalist Tommie Bass had also witnessed its successful use with **diarrhea** (Rafinesque 1828–30: 2:29; Crellin and Philpott 1990a: 120), we can assume that astringency is responsible for the above-noted effects on blood, urine, and stools.

Finally, research has discovered *antiallergic* effects from this herb, specifically in that it inhibits mast cell-derived, immediate-type allergic reactions and the involvement of proinflammatory cytokines (Shin et al. 2005).

PERSONAL AND PROFESSIONAL USE

I don't recall that I have ever used bugleweed for my own health. I have, however, recommended it on numerous occasions to clients with Graves' disease, often in combination with one or more of the following herbs, all of which besides lemon balm have their own entries in this field guide: lemon balm (*Melissa officinalis*), cinquefoil (*Potentilla* spp.) (see page 81), self-heal (*Prunella vulgaris*) (see page 201), and motherwort (*Leonurus cardiaca*) (see page 156).

My experience in the above regard has thus far been entirely positive. I have found Graves' disease to resolve after only six to eighteen months of treatment, confirmed by both lab results and the cessation of symptoms.

CAUTIONS

The use of this plant may not be without side effects. According to animal studies, bugleweed may, at the same time as inhibiting thyroid hormones, also inhibit some other hormones, including the pituitary hormones luteinizing hormone (LH) and follicle-stimulating hormone (FSH), which in turn stimulate production of the sex hormones (Winterhoff et al. 1988: 101; Brinker 1990). *Such effects may interfere with contraceptives and/or fertility medications and also clearly contraindicate the use of this herb during pregnancy, while its effects on prolactin contraindicate its use during lactation.*

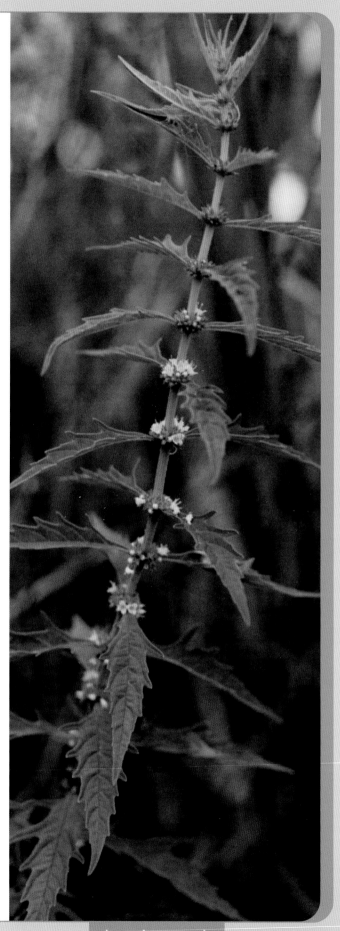

bugleweed

Bulrush

Scirpus acutus, S. validus, and related spp.

DESCRIPTION
Occasionally an annual but usually a perennial, the interesting bulrush plant grows 3–10 feet high and thrives in large colonies. The stem is erect and circular or triangular, and it fails to branch. Numerous small, drab flowers cluster on several pedicels just below the stem tip.

Several species thrive in the Midwest, but predominating are *Scirpus validus* (great bulrush, great American bulrush, or soft-stemmed bulrush) and *S. acutus* (tule, tule bulrush, or hard-stemmed bulrush).

The former has a soft stem, lacks leaves entirely, and possesses small, reddish-brown flowers on several stalked, drooping clusters. It is also characterized by a reddish and scaly rhizome. The latter possesses a stiff stem and has long, toothless, grass-like, pointed leaves arising from the base only. It is also bulkier than *S. validus*, and its flower clusters are cylinder shaped and grayish brown. The rhizome is also grayish brown.

The fruits are small, shiny black nutlets.

RANGE AND HABITAT
Bulrush is found throughout the United States and Canada (except within the Arctic Circle) in wet ground and in shallow, stagnant waters.

FOOD
The Thompson have collected the pollen from the flower spike of a species of bulrush to use as flour, mixing it with other flours to make biscuits or cakes (Steedman 1928: 484). Many non-Native wild-foods foragers follow suit.

The young stems are a valuable survival food; they can be peeled and eaten raw or cooked, as the Cheyenne discovered (Hart 1981: 8). The tender white heart at the base of the mature stem is very sweet and juicy and can be eaten raw or added to soups, just like the Gosiute have done (Chamberlin 1911: 381).

Younger (spring-collected) rhizomes can be peeled and eaten raw, as the Ojibwe have been known to do, after having pulled them in midsummer (Black 1973: 125). Alternatively, they can be sliced and added to salads. Crushed and boiled, they are full of natural sugar, yielding a sweet syrup when cooked over a good length of time. Another way to prepare them is to bake them for about two to three hours. Last but not least, the buds on the ends of the older rhizomes make a crispy, sweetish snack.

Bulrush seeds can be collected in the autumn and then parched, ground, and prepared with heated water to make a sort of mush—another useful survival food. They can also be combined with flour that can be secured from the rhizomes (by drying them, pounding them, and sifting out their fibers) and then pressed into cakes and baked. These are relatively sweet and sustaining.

I might add that Karl Knutsen, in his delightful foraging manual of the mid-1970s, provides a mouth-watering recipe for "Creamed Bulrush and Shrimp" that simply can't be beat! (Knutsen 1975: 46)

HEALTH/MEDICINE
The Ramah Navajo (Diné) and the Cherokee have coaxed *emetic* properties out of a decoction of this plant when needed (Vestal 1952: 19; Hamel and Chiltoskey 1975: 27). On the

other hand, *styptic* properties have been utilized by the Woods Cree, who have applied the pith of the stem of bulrush underneath a dressing to halt bleeding from **wounds** (Leighton 1985: 59). Likewise, burned and cooled ashes from the stalk have been applied by the Thompson to a newborn baby's navel to halt **bleeding** at this location (Turner et al. 1990: 115).

Bulrush's blood-stemming ability would seem to relate largely, if not entirely, to the plant's evident *astringency*, an effect noted by early American physicians (Porcher 1849: 851). Astringency also explains the use among Indigenous peoples of the Maritimes of bulrush as an agent for **sore throat** (Mechling 1959: 247) and likewise elucidates Bradford Angier's observation that the plant's chopped stems have long been applied to **sores** and **burns** and taken internally for **diarrhea** (Angier 1978: 73).

A 1976 study found three species of bulrush (*S. validus, S. americanus,* and *S. atrovirens*) to exert moderate *anti-inflammatory* activity (Benoit et al. 1976: 166). This may explain why the Malecite and the Micmac have been able to utilize the pounded root of a related species (*S. rubrotinctus*), after mixing it with water to make a paste, as a topical application to an **abscess** so as to ease it and reduce it (Mechling 1959: 247).

PERSONAL AND PROFESSIONAL USE

I have frequently enjoyed the tender white heart at the base of the mature stems as a sweet and juicy snack, although I have found that timing is everything in securing the best-tasting specimens.

In my professional herbal practice, I typically use astringents other than bulrush, due to the time involved in collecting and processing the plant and also to its limited market availability in the United States, where my practice is located. ⪡

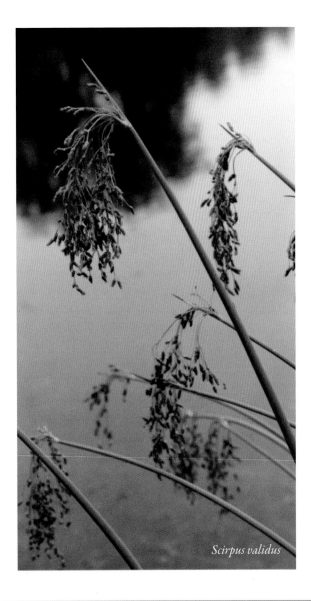

Scirpus validus

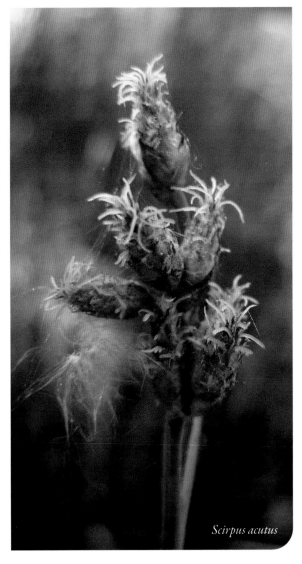

Scirpus acutus

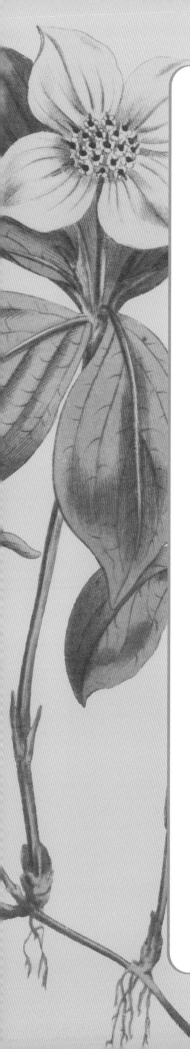

Bunchberry

DWARF DOGWOOD; DWARF CORNEL; PIGEON BERRY

Cornus canadensis

DESCRIPTION

Bunchberry is an attractive perennial that grows 2–9 inches tall. It tends to appear in dense colonies owing to the tendency of its rhizomes to spread. This tiny plant is of the same genus (*Cornus*) as dogwood trees and shrubs, hence its alternative common name of dwarf dogwood, although one would never guess it by the size differential!

The plant's leaves are pointed, egg shaped, prominently lined, and 1½–3 inches long. They appear about two-thirds of the way up the stem in a nearly sessile whorl of six (or occasionally four, if the plant is a nonflowering one). Upon careful inspection, one can find beneath this whorl—a little ways farther down the stem—another pair of smaller leaves.

In spring, the tiny plant bears what appears to be a solitary flower, ostensibly consisting of four white petals hugging a greenish-white center disk. However, the center section is actually a cluster of many minuscule, complete flowers, while the surrounding, white "petals" are really four large white involucral bracts (floral leaves).

Come late summer, the flowers are replaced with pea-sized, bright-reddish-orange "berries" (technically, drupes), which are usually tightly clustered in formation. Upon inspection, one can spot calyx remains at their tips. As with many fruits, they are soft when ripe.

RANGE AND HABITAT

As one of the plant's other alternative names, Canadian bunchberry, suggests, it is found pretty much throughout Canada (except for the very northernmost strip). But it also flourishes in the northern strip of the United States, dipping well into California in the West and into mountainous areas of West Virginia in the East. In the Midwest, it is found in the upper regions. The preferred habitat is cool, moist, coniferous woods—the type of environment where one might find bluebead lily (see page 31), wild strawberry (page 273), wild sarsaparilla (page 271), and the like.

SEASONAL AVAILABILITY

Fruits are available from August to September.

MAJOR CONSTITUENTS

The plant contains cornic acid, cornine, a variety of flavonoids, phenylethylamine, hydrolyzable tannins (including tellimagrandin I), and alpha- and beta-amyrin. The leaves alone contain astragalin, hexahydroxydiphenic acid, and juglanin, while the fruit alone contains cyanin. The fruit's seeds contain a goodly amount of all three of the major fatty acids: linoleic acid, linolenic acid, and oleic acid.

FOOD

Although the berries are edible, numerous foraging books and manuals describe the taste as "insipid." Naturalist Tom Brown Jr., after noting that this was a common assessment on the part of fellow foragers he had known, remarked in one of his books that the maligned little bunchberry really has a wonderful taste that comes through on a more subtle level if one gives it a chance (Brown 1985: 73–75). The problem, Brown intimates, is our MSG-laden society that demands strong seasonings on practically every food item, always clamoring for the ultratantalizing. Applying ourselves to savoring the taste of the bunchberry, he explains, forces us to slow down and to take a look at the finer things that life has to offer.

Native Americans have demonstrated the proper attitude in this respect by relishing these beautiful little rubies as good food—the Midwest's Potawatomi and Ojibwe, among other tribes, feasting upon them with great appreciation (Erichsen-Brown 1989: 304). The naturalist P. H. Gosse, while traveling through the Quebec wilds in the first half of the nineteenth century, also reminisced fondly of the bunchberries: "We ate many; they are farinaceous and agreeable" (Gosse 1971: 299).

Recipes abound for this fruit, but one of the best is bunchberry pudding—a good and healthful recipe for which can be found in the excellent foraging cookbook by Walter and Nancy Hall (Hall and Hall 1980: 323).

HEALTH/MEDICINE

Information on the medicinal properties of the various *Cornus* species is sorely lacking. This is regrettable in that some data exists to the effect that these species have been held in great respect by Native American healers. The Micmac, for example, have found bunchberry leaves, fruits, and roots useful in the treatment of **fits** (Mechling 1959: 256; Chandler et al. 1979: 56), while the Montagnais have implemented an infusion of the whole plant for **paralysis**

(Speck 1917: 315). Powdered, toasted leaves have been sprinkled onto **sores** by the Thompson (Steedman 1928: 458), while the Micmac have applied the leaves to **wounds**, primarily to stop bleeding and to hasten the healing process, for which application the plant material is first chewed and then further moistened (Lacey 1993: 80). **Kidney ailments** and **enuresis** in children have also been treated with an infusion of the plant by the Micmac (Lacey 1993: 80), which is interesting in that the related Asian species *C. officinalis* has long been used in Traditional Chinese Medicine to strengthen the urinary bladder's withholding power.

Boiled with wintergreen, the whole plant has been held by the Tête de Boule to be a valuable component in a bulwark against **colds** (Raymond 1945: 128). Similarly, the Iroquois have implemented a decoction of the whole plant for **cough** and for **fever** (Herrick 1977: 402; Herrick 1995: 177). The late Southwest American herbalist Michael Moore, who had good experience using bunchberry with clients, found the herb valuable for fevers; he emphasized that it works best with those that *tend to be chilling* in nature— that is, manifesting goosebumps and/or shivers (Moore 1993: 97). Moore also found the plant helpful for **headaches**, particularly those that were *clammy* in nature (i.e., accompanied by dampness of the neck and back and with slight nausea) (Moore 1993: 97). Interestingly, the Oklahoma Lenape (Delaware) have also implemented bunchberry as an *analgesic*, finding it useful for pain most anywhere in the body (Tantaquidgeon 1942: 26, 74).

Known constituents shed some light upon the uses summarized above. The cornic acid present in the plant, which has

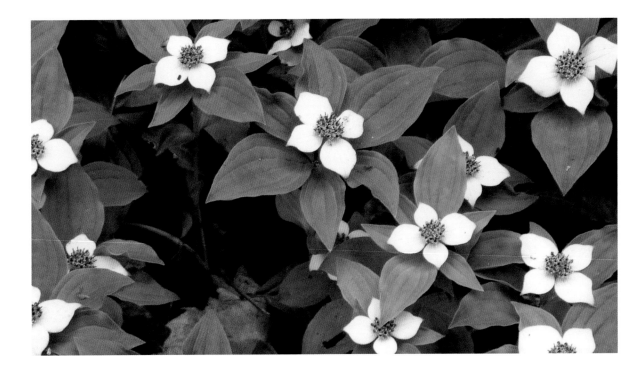

a known analgesic effect similar to aspirin (although milder), undoubtedly at least partly elucidates the usage of the fruits or dried plant as an infusion for **fever** or **headache**. Moore, in pointing out that both the cornine and the flavonoids are anti-inflammatory, suggested that such an effect, in conjunction with the herb's astringent tannins, would also lend bunchberry for use in treating **colitis**, **diarrhea**, **chronic gastritis**, and **flatulence** (Moore 1993: 97). Interestingly, a gastrointestinal symptom profile similar to this was recognized by several Native American tribes earlier in history as calling for bunchberry: the Flambeau Ojibwe, as one example, have infused bunchberry roots to treat **infant colic** (Smith 1932: 366–67), and the Micmac found the plant useful for certain **stomach problems** (Lacey 1993: 80). Not surprisingly, as well, in view of this species' *anti-inflammatory* and *astringent* properties as elaborated above, the Southern Carrier found an infusion of the plant (minus its fruit) to be an excellent eyewash for **sore eyes** (Smith 1929: 62).

Research from scientists at the University of Quebec has found extracts from the plant to be effective against **herpes simplex virus type 1** (**HSV-1**), which result these researchers found to be supportive of the traditional Native American use of this herb for viral infections (Lavoie et al. 2017).

Finally, a fascinating use for bunchberry is as an *appetite stimulant*. Here, the Scots have long called it the "herb of gluttony." Understandably, then, herbalists have long taken advantage of the plant's amazing appetite-stimulating properties to help those who have lost their desire for food, often by steeping the whole plant to produce a tea (Schofield Eaton 1989: 83).

UTILITARIAN USES

Wild-plant foraging author Joan Richardson says that the little bunchberry is widely rumored to serve as excellent bait for little fish (Richardson 1981: 53)—something that could be useful to know in a survival situation, since catching little fish provides a person with bait to catch bigger fish.

PERSONAL AND PROFESSIONAL USE

Bunchberry's renowned appetite-stimulating property is no myth: I recall how, on a trip to northern Minnesota, I once gorged myself on bunchberries and was immediately afterward so consumed with hunger that I proceeded to open a large can of tuna to make three sandwiches, which I then wolfed down in no uncertain fashion!

In my clinical practice, too, I have had occasion to put this amazing appetite-stimulating property to good use in individuals with cancer or other conditions that caused their appetite to be unhealthily reduced. I have also witnessed the fruit's bladder-strengthening effect on several occasions—both when used by itself and when used in formulas that I've crafted. I've also had occasion to add the herb to analgesic formulas that I've crafted to good effect.

The problem, however, is that neither the fruit nor the herbage is marketed in the United States. Hence, if my wildcrafted supply of the former runs low, I am constrained to use the fruit of the Chinese species (*Cornus officinalis*), which is commercially available in America from Chinese herb companies. However, I always prefer to use indigenous herbs whenever possible. ⋘

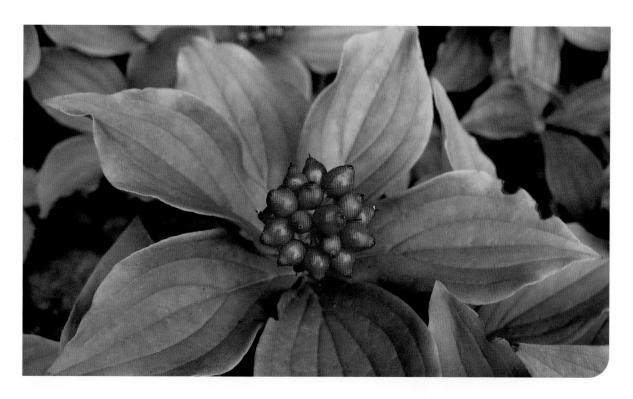

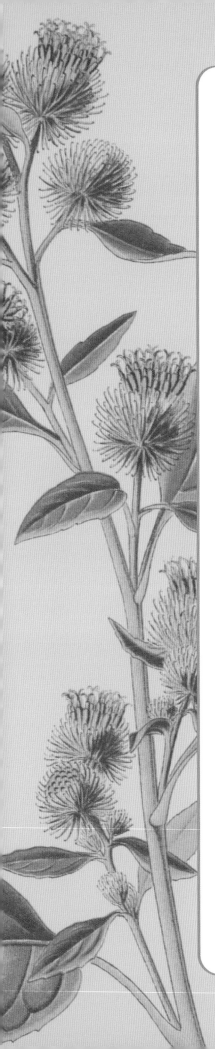

Burdock

Arctium minus, A. lappa

DESCRIPTION

Burdock is a biennial plant. During its first season, it appears only as a low-lying herb bearing long-stalked, heart-shaped leaves. These are quite large, at times growing to 18 inches. Other features are as follows: the leaves are dark green, wavy edged, possessed of a peculiar net-like surface pattern, and woolly underneath. A characteristic rank smell helps distinguish this plant from similar-looking species (such as rhubarb gone wild).

In the plant's second season, a branching stem (purple at its bottom) forms, eventually topping out at 3–5 feet. Stem leaves are alternate, ovate in shape, and smaller than the lower first-season leaves. Like those basal leaves, however, the stem leaves are also veiny and slightly velvet-like to the touch (especially on their undersides). Leafstalks are hollow in *Arctium minus* and filled with white pith in *A. lappa*.

Composite flowers—in the form of tubular florets—appear in the middle of the second season and are borne singly or in clusters at the upper part of the stem and branches. The flower head is ½ inch to 1 inch wide, very short stalked, reddish violet to amethyst in color, and bristly. It emerges from a spiny, ball-like bract (reminiscent of thistle, to which the plant is related). During autumn, these hook-tipped bracts transform into the infamous dry brown burs that so tenaciously stick to clothing and to fur.

RANGE AND HABITAT

Burdock is found throughout Canada and in the upper portions of the United States. The preferred habitat is disturbed areas, especially vacant lots, roadsides, old fields, and pastures.

SEASONAL AVAILABILITY

The root is available for harvest from the plant's first season to spring of its second season.

MAJOR CONSTITUENTS

Burdock root contains the polysaccharides inulin (to 45 percent!) and mucilage as well as lappin, tannin, polyacetylenes (fourteen of them!), nonhydroxy acids (lauric, stearic, palmitic), sterols, caffeic acid, chlorogenic acid, and essential oil. Nutrients in significant amounts include chromium, iron, magnesium, silicon, and thiamin. The leaves and stem contain arctiol, arctiin, arctigenin, taraxasterol, fukinone, alpha-amyrin, acetic and arctic acids, and arctiopicrin (a sesquiterpene lactone). The seeds contain 15–30 percent fixed oils, arctiin (a bitter glycoside), neoarctin, daucosterol, arctigenin, matairesinol, lappaol, and chlorogenic acid.

FOOD

The cooked roots of first-year plants are edible and nutritious, being sweetish to the taste. (Roots of second-year plants tend to be thin and woody, since they shrink in size as the plant begins to stalk. They are passable as fare if secured early in the spring, however.) Unfortunately, the roots are often entrenched several feet deep, where they tenaciously cling to the soil, so they must be dug out with a firm spade, at the least. (Euell Gibbons suggested that a posthole digger was ideal.) It requires some practice to get the hang of it. Then, too, one needs to be careful when the root pops out—the sheer force of the affair can fling loose soil toward the eyes!

Once successfully unearthed, burdock roots are best peeled, cut into chunks, and boiled in several changes of water (i.e., throwing off two waters and doing the final boiling in a third). They should be cooked in a glass or enamel pot if one wants to keep the chunks from turning dark (caused by anthocyanin pigments in the root darkening upon reacting with ions from a metal pot). The addition of a little baking soda helps break down the fibers.

Very early spring leaves—especially those of *A. lappa*—are enjoyed by some as a potherb (cooked for twenty minutes in two waters, with a pinch of baking soda added to the first).

HEALTH/MEDICINE

Burdock was adopted by Native Americans for medicinal purposes after it arrived in their lands as a weedy import. The Eclectics used it enthusiastically, and it found official status in the *United States Pharmacopeia* from 1831 to 1842 and 1851 to 1916 as well as in the *National Formulary* from 1916 to 1947. It is still official medicine in Germany, France, Belgium, and the United Kingdom and remains a favorite among herbalists of many heritages today. Moreover, it has attracted the attention of phytochemists (see below).

Both the plant's taproot and its seeds have long been looked to for *diuretic* effects (Bever and Zahnd 1979), which were a favorite application of this plant made both by the Eclectic physicians and the Iroquois (Herrick 1995: 229). Both plant parts—but especially the seeds—are somewhat *laxative* as well, lending themselves for use with **constipation**.

The Cowlitz have utilized a decoction of the root to treat **whooping cough** (Gunther 1973: 50). Other herbal traditions in America have similarly employed it for **cough**, **asthma**, and **pulmonary complaints**. The Ojibwe found the root invaluable for a hard, dry cough and have also drunk it after a coughing spell (Densmore 1974: 340–41).

Burdock is renowned as a *depurative* for helping the kidneys to eliminate harmful uric and other acids from the blood, and as such this plant is much appreciated by those afflicted with **rheumatic conditions.** Interestingly, the Iroquois use a burdock leaf poultice to treat rheumatic parts of the body, while the Lenape (Delaware) drink a

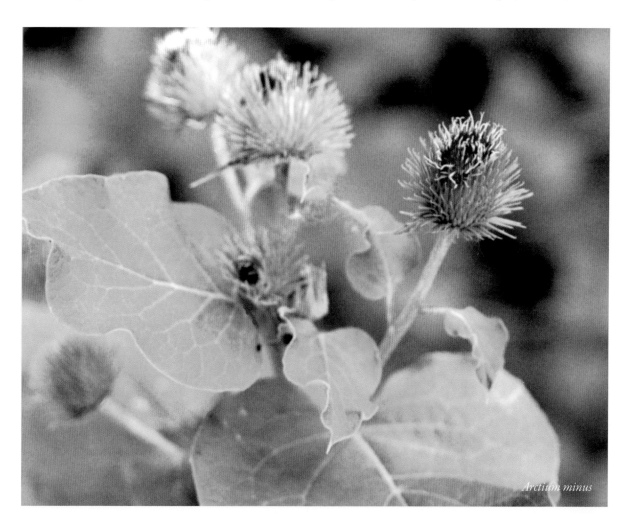

Arctium minus

decoction of the root for rheumatism (Tantaquidgeon 1942: 31; Herrick 1995: 229).

Anti-inflammatory principles in the plant, demonstrated via the rat-paw edema test (Lin et al. 1996), are no doubt partly responsible for these successes and have been elicited by various tribes in other respects. For example, the Iroquois found that a mashed-leaf poultice works wonders on a **bee sting**, a warmed leaf poultice eases pain from a **strained back**, and a root decoction eases the pain from **sore muscles** (Herrick 1995: 229).

The taproot is further known as a specific for both **dry eczema** and **psoriasis**, being listed in the *British Herbal Compendium* for internal and external use in these conditions. Perhaps its most famous use, however, is for **boils** (gleaned from Native tribes' usage: Smith 1933: 49; Tantaquidgeon 1942: 56; Shemluck 1982: 312) and a less common, more widespread, form of this condition, **furunculosis**. The herbal-minded physician Edward E. Shook once described in graphic detail how he witnessed the cure of a pronounced case of furunculosis by means of a decoction of burdock root used internally along with a poultice of the leaves that had been sprayed with eucalyptus oil (Shook 1978: 49). Whether Shook knew it or not, the Lenape (Delaware) tribe had also treated boils with a poultice of burdock, although they had used the leaf (Tantaquidgeon 1942: 56).

Burdock is also often used for **dermatosis** (not to be confused with dermatitis) and for many other **chronic skin problems** (Moore 1979: 45; Bruneton 1995: 151). The Iroquois have found it invaluable for big **pimples** on the face and on the neck (Herrick 1995: 229). The seeds, harvested in the fall after the burs have turned brown, are held by many herbalists to be the most efficacious part of the plant for this purpose—especially for **adolescent acne**, because it is thought that they interact well with testosterone. A decoction or a tincture of the seeds is taken internally and sometimes also mixed with a base paste and applied locally. Further as to the seeds, in the latter part of the nineteenth century a physician named W. H. Bentley found a tincture of them to be useful in the treatment of **epilepsy** (Bentley 1884).

Accumulated clinical and experimental evidence suggests that burdock *enhances hepatobiliary function* (Chabrol and Charonnat 1935). What is more, it has exhibited *hepatoprotective* properties against CC14-induced hepatotoxicity (Lin et al. 1996). Bitter principles in burdock also *stimulate gastric secretions*, improving a **sluggish appetite** and **poor digestion**.

Research on the part of German and other scientists has revealed that burdock's root—especially when fresh and not dried—has *antifungal* and *antimicrobial* properties, due at least in part to three of its fourteen polyacetylenes (Vincent and Segonzac 1948: 669; Schulte 1967). These chemicals have been shown to exert activity against gram-negative bacteria (Moskalenko 1986). A sesquiterpene lactone present in the leaves, arctiopicrin, also has demonstrated antibiotic activity but against gram-positive bacteria (Bever and Zahnd 1979). Together, the leaves and the flowers have shown activity against both gram-positive (*Bacillus subtilis*, *Mycobacterium smegmatis*, and *Staphylococcus aureus*) and gram-negative bacteria (*Escherichia coli*, *Shigella flexneri*, *S. sonnei*) (Moskalenko 1986). (The leaves' effects against *Staphylococcus aureus* may partly elucidate their previously

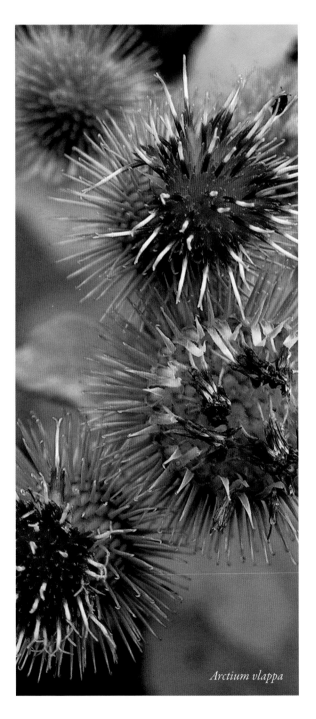

Arctium vlappa

mentioned healing of boils, which are usually caused by this gram-positive bacterium.) *Antiviral* properties are present as well: an *anti-HIV effect* has even been demonstrated in vitro (Duke 1997: 269).

Japanese studies suggest that burdock's root is *antimutagenic* (Morita et al. 1984; Morita et al. 1985; Ito et al. 1986). Additional research has isolated *antitumor* principles (Foldeak and Dombradi 1964; Dombradi and Foldeak 1966; Awale et al. 2006). A scientific study published in 2006 found that burdock's butyrolactone lignans inhibited the proliferation of leukemic cells and even caused these cells to self-destruct (Matsumoto et al. 2006).

The phytochemical arctiin, occurring in the seeds, has been shown to exert a protective effect against carcinogenesis of the pancreas, breast, and colon in rats (Hirose et al. 2000). Interestingly, the Potawatomi had used burdock to treat **cancer** many decades before these effects were verified by scientists (EthnobDB). Burdock is also one of four herbs in Canadian nurse Rene Caisse's Essiac formula, purportedly based upon information given to her by members of the Ojibwe tribe, which has a good track record in aiding some cancer victims and has shown antioxidant, DNA-protective, and antiproliferative effects in scientific studies (Richardson et al. 2000; Tai et al. 2004; Leonard et al. 2006). Burdock is likewise a component of the famed Hoxsey formula, which was also traditionally believed to exert activity against cancer and which has shown impressive results in a clinical follow-up study and in some other research (Austin 1994; Brinker 1995; Richardson 2001). Then, too, the scientist Jonathan Hartwell, in his mammoth study of the use of plants by Indigenous peoples for cancer, devoted a sizable section of his work to burdock's implementation against cancer by numerous cultures (Hartwell 1968: 71).

Hypoglycemic (blood-sugar-lowering) ability has also been demonstrated for this tenacious weed's root (Silver and Krantz 1931; Lapinina and Sisoeva 1964; Bever and Zahnd 1979; Leung 1980: 81).

PERSONAL AND PROFESSIONAL USE

I've enjoyed the taste of cooked burdock root on a number of occasions. Unfortunately, though, I am one of those who can get dermatitis if the leaf rubs against my skin.

In my clinical practice, I use burdock seed and/or root primarily for skin conditions (acne, eczema, psoriasis, and boils) and in alterative formulas for persons suffering from cancer.

CAUTIONS

As burdock has been shown to be a uterine stimulant (Farnsworth et al. 1975), *it should not be used during pregnancy.*

Burdock leaves should never be used if found growing near a road or factory, as they readily absorb pollutants.

Polyacetylenes in the plant can cause contact dermatitis in persons who have become sensitized to this chemical (Rodriguez 1995).

If one plans on sampling young burdock leaves as a salad ingredient or cooked repast, one needs to be careful not to confuse the plant with rhubarb (*Rheum rhaponticum*), which has similar-looking leaves (although burdock's are not as smooth and shiny looking and possess a net-like pattern on their surface) and which, having escaped from gardens of current or abandoned homesteads, sometimes encroaches upon wasteland, vacant lots, and fields. Rhubarb's leaves, which lack the rank smell associated with those of burdock, can be fatal if consumed. (Note that rhubarb's ripe stalk is red, unlike that of burdock—which, as will be recalled from the above information, is purple.) ✦

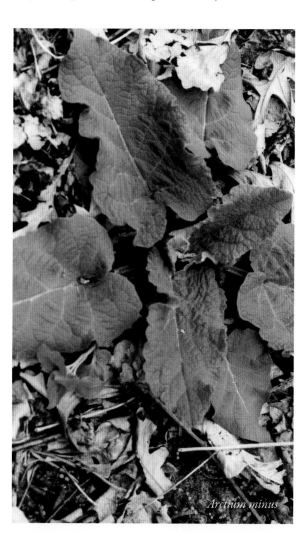

Arctium minus

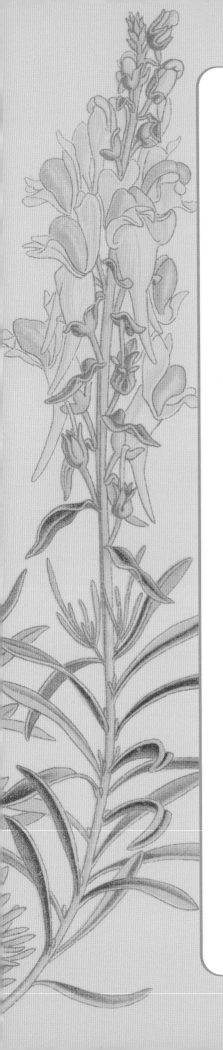

Butter-and-Eggs

Linaria vulgaris

DESCRIPTION

This odd-looking plant is a European perennial that reaches a height of 1–2 feet. Its leaves are numerous, entire, and narrow—even grass-like. Growing 1–2½ inches long, they tend to alternate on the upper part of the plant but to be arranged oppositely or in whorls on its lower portion.

The unusual yellow blossoms—clustered in dense, terminal, club-like racemes—are irregular and two-lipped, looking like those of a snapdragon: the upper lip is two-lobed and erect, while the lower one is three-lobed and spreading. The latter also displays a prominent orange inflation (thought to be a nectar guide for insects and to ensure that these visitors pick up pollen along the way). There is a long, curved descending spur at the flower base.

RANGE AND HABITAT

This is a ubiquitous weed, preferring dry and sunny places such as fields, roadsides, railroad embankments, and disturbed soils.

MAJOR CONSTITUENTS

Butter-and-eggs contains peganine (a quinazoline alkaloid), aurones (including aureusin and bracteatin-6-O-glucoside), phytosterol, iridoid monoterpenes (including antirrhinoside), flavonoids (linarin and pectolinarin), tannic acid, citric acid, choline, and goodly amounts of vitamin C.

HEALTH/MEDICINE

This pretty plant is possessed of *cooling* and *drying* energies. Physiologically, this takes the form of *anti-inflammatory* and *diuretic* properties. As to the former, the noted British herbalist Nicholas Culpeper pointed out: "The juice of the herb, or the distilled water dropped into the eyes, is a certain remedy for all heat, inflammation and redness in them." Well over a century earlier, horticulturist John Gerard observed that a decoction of toadflax "doth also provoke urine, in those that piss drop after drop, unstoppeth the kidneys and bladder" (Gerard 1975: 556). Scientific experiments have since verified the plant's traditional uses for **urinary-tract disorders** and **inflammatory conditions**, revealing that butter-and-eggs does indeed possesses *diuretic*, *anti-inflammatory*, *diaphoretic*, and mild *antimicrobial* properties (Fitzpatrick 1954: 530; Benoit et al. 1976: 168; Fleming 1998).

It is especially renowned, however, as a superb *hepatic*, with varied applications that seem to reveal its power only to those who truly suffer in extremis. Here its best-known use is for **jaundice.** Culpeper said here: "The decoction of the herb, both leaves and flowers, in wine, does somewhat move the belly downwards, open obstructions of the liver, and help the yellow jaundice" (Potterton 1983: 78). The renowned American herbalist Michael Moore found that a rounded teaspoon made into a tea and drunk three times a day rapidly brought rebound bilirubin levels back within parameters (Moore 1979: 153). He cautioned that it can be used for just a short while by itself because of its potential for irritation but allowed it for a longer period when combined with other hepatic herbs (Moore 1979: 153; Moore 1993: 301).

America's Eclectic physicians of the late nineteenth and early twentieth centuries likewise valued butter-and-eggs (referring to it under its alternative name of toadflax, as many did during that period) for hypertrophy of the liver as well as for the spleen. They preferred either a decoction of 1 ounce of the plant to 1 pint of water or a strong tincture dosed at 1–10 drops. They further emphasized that the plant should only be harvested while in flower, carefully dried, and then secured in airtight containers away from light (Felter and Lloyd 1898).

Because butter-and-eggs contains peganine, an alkaloid with *peristaltic* and *antispasmodic* effects, the herb has been found useful for **intestinal atony** (Kresanek and Krejca 1989: 118). The plant's bile-stimulating properties also help to ensure a smooth bowel movement in those persons troubled by **constipation** because of an insufficient flow of this fluid. On the other hand, the Iroquois found that an infusion of butter-and-eggs leaves helps to firm up **diarrhea** (Herrick 1977: 433). Why the difference? Moore explains that the herb only serves to stimulate bile *when it is insufficient* (Moore 1979: 153). Otherwise, the plant's astringent tannins are left unbalanced so as to firm up loose stools.

Being thus *astringent* (Wren 1988: 267), butter-and-eggs also has a good reputation as a **hemorrhoid** remedy (Fleming 1998), applied as an ointment. The Eclectic physicians often suggested that such be made from one part of the fresh, bruised plant to ten parts of an emollient base, such as hot lard or mutton tallow (Felter and Lloyd 1898). Another source suggests two parts fresh herb to five parts pork fat (Kresanek and Krejca 1989: 118).

PERSONAL AND PROFESSIONAL USE

I have had little occasion to use, or to recommend, this herb. On one occasion, however, a salve I made from butter-and-eggs, chickweed (see page 75), and cleavers (page 86) helped to heal a stubborn case of anal inflammation in a client.

CAUTIONS

Butter-and-eggs should be used with great caution, if at all, by the layperson, due to a toxic potential. It has also long been thought to be possessed of glycosides with the potential to cause cyanide poisoning, especially if the fresh or wilted plant—or an extract therefrom—is consumed internally and in too high an amount (Cooper and Johnson 1988: 107).

It is best used as a tea of the dried herb. The strongest preparation that I have come across is 2 teaspoons of the dried plant infused in ¾ cup water and sipped slowly throughout the day (Lust 1974: 417). Higher doses of 2–3 ounces at a time would seem to be safely imbibed of a much weaker infusion (a scant teaspoon infused in 1 cup of water), as long as the day's total intake of tea is kept to under 12 ounces (Moore 1994a: 15). Yet another source says to use only 1 teaspoon of the dried herb to two glasses of water, drinking only one-third to one-half glass (Kresanek and Krejca 1989: 118). A 1:5 tincture of the flowering herb, with 60 percent alcohol, is also sometimes used but should be kept to less than 20 drops at a dose, diluted well, and used no more than three times a day. John Lust cautions that as little as 20 drops of a strong tincture can give rise to unpleasant effects (Lust 1974: 417). ⬿

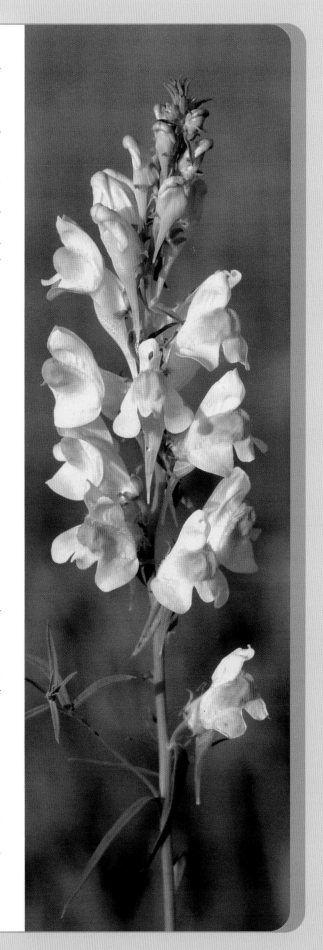

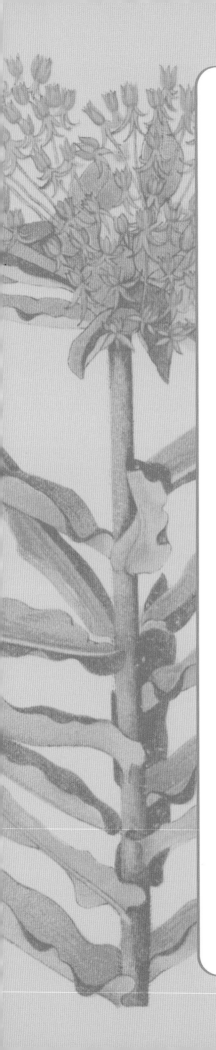

Butterfly-Weed

DESCRIPTION

Butterfly-weed is a native perennial that grows 1–3 feet tall. When in full bloom, it is one of the loveliest of plants in the Midwest.

Its single rough and hairy stem branches near the top. When damaged, it exudes a juice that is clear and not milky white as in other *Asclepias* species, such as common milkweed (see page 151).

The hairy leaves are ovate to oblong, sessile, toothless, and mostly alternate. They grow 2–6 inches long.

The brilliant orange flowers (sometimes more yellowish or more reddish) occur clustered into flat terminal heads that grow 2–3 inches long. Individual flowers have five downward-curved petals.

The ensuing seedpods are hairy, spindle-shaped structures, each growing to 5 inches long. These, like the preceding flowers, are grouped into clusters.

RANGE AND HABITAT

Butterfly-weed grows throughout the Midwest in sandy soil such as occurs in fields, meadows, and prairies. Owing to its beauty, it is often chosen for prairie restoration programs.

MAJOR CONSTITUENTS

Butterfly-weed contains a resin (inclusive of bitter principles such as asclepione); pregnane glycosides and cardioactive glycosides; essential oil; triterpenes (including alpha-amyrin and beta-amyrin); flavonoids (rutin, quercetin, kaempferol); beta-sitosterol; uzarin; caffeic, chlorogenic, gallic, and tannic acid; free-form amino acids; and choline.

HEALTH/MEDICINE

The dried rootstock of butterfly-weed has been valued as a medicine by both whites and Native Americans for centuries. Most often referred to by healers under its alternative common name of pleurisy root, it was listed in both the *United States Pharmacopeia* (1820–1900) and the *National Formulary* (fourth and fifth editions) and was noted in the *United States Dispensatory* to be an *emetic, cathartic, expectorant*, and *diaphoretic* (Wood et al. 1926: 1293). The *British Herbal Pharmacopoeia* says that it is *antispasmodic* as well (Hyde et al. 1976–79: 1:25). This makes sense when one considers that butterfly-weed has historically been used for **dyspepsia (indigestion)** (Millspaugh 1974: 540). Many herbalists have also implemented it for **spasmodic asthma** (Shook 1978: 301).

As to its expectorant properties (Lust 1974: 313; cf. Hyde et al. 1976–79: 1:25), it has been found helpful for **bronchitis** (Shook 1978: 301), especially when acute, hot, and dry (Moore 1994b: 4.3). Here, though, the Natura physician R. Swinburne Clymer said that it should be given by way of tincture in hot water for best effects and also combined with skullcap (see page 212), with the dosage being 15–40 drops of the former and 2–20 drops of the latter—or with boneset (see page 44) if skullcap is unavailable. He stressed that it should be provided every few hours until free perspiration is established, and then less frequently until the bronchioles are clear. He also urged that it be followed up with cayenne pepper and finally with goldenseal (*Hydrastis canadensis*) (Clymer 1973: 103).

Butterfly-weed is generally agreed to be most effective, however, for **acute lower respiratory tract infections** (Mills and Bone 2000: 216), serving to resolve **pulmonary catarrh** (Clymer 1973: 103; Shook 1978: 301). It is a specific when the catarrh is deep down and the chest feels oppressed but the upper respiratory tract feels dry. The sufferer's skin, noted Clymer, is also dry and hot (Clymer 1973: 104).

The plant is appreciated for a nonproductive **cough** that is acute and pulmonary or even when chronic, debilitating, and accompanied by indigestion (Christopher 1976: 222; Moore 1994b: 4.5). It has also been a favorite for **pneumonia** (Shook 1978: 301). Georgian folk medicine has used it thusly, adding it first to whiskey (Bolyard 1981: 46). It seems to be especially effective when the pneumonia is of the acute bronchial type, accompanied by vascular disturbance and fever, or when the person is recuperating but has difficult expectoration and the respiratory system is dry and tough (Moore 1994b 4.13).

Butterfly-weed has also long been used for **tuberculosis**, with observed benefits (Shook 1978: 301). Interestingly, in the 1950s, this classic application was elucidated when it was discovered that butterfly-weed was powerfully active in vitro against a virulent human strain of tuberculosis (Fitzpatrick 1954: 529). As the name pleurisy root would imply, however, our herb is perhaps most specific for **pleurisy** (Clymer 1973: 102; Hyde et al. 1976–79: 1:25) or for **intercostal pain** in general that occurs upon inhaling and is relieved by bending forward (Tilgner 1999: 96).

Unfortunately, butterfly-weed is little used these days. This is in contrast to the widespread use and recognition of benefits it achieved during the nineteenth century. For example, medical doctor Jacob Bigelow, writing in the early 1800s, remarked that it had been employed by practitioners in the "southern states in pulmonary complaints, particularly in catarrh, pneumonia, and pleurisy, and has acquired much confidence of the relief of these maladies." Elucidating the nature of its healing properties, he continued: "It produces effects of this kind with great gentleness and without ... heating ... relieving the breathing of pleuritic patients in the most advanced stages of the disease" (Bigelow 1817–20: 2:63). Medical botanist R. E. Griffith, although critical of many botanicals popularly used in his time, noted that it had "been employed with much benefit in [maladies] of the respiratory organs, and there is much ample testimony of its

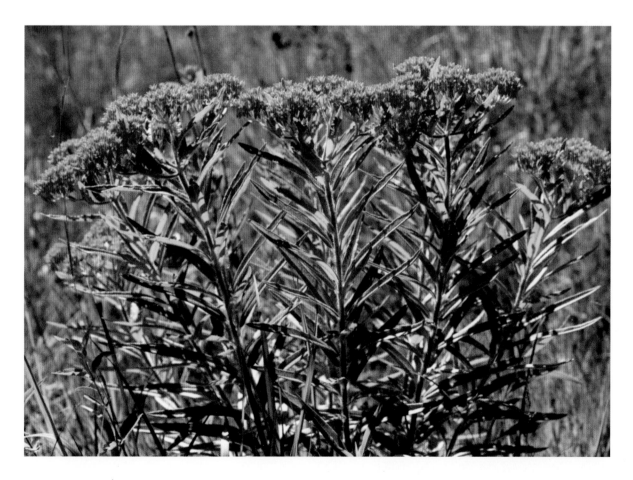

curative powers when judiciously administered for pulmonary ailments" (Griffith 1847: 455).

Butterfly-weed is a very strong and reliable diaphoretic and thus helpful for **fevers** (Elliott 1821–24: 1:77; Millspaugh 1974: 540; Shook 1978: 301). Also, as nineteenth-century physician and botanist Laurence Johnson explained, the "diaphoretic effects have been found useful in acute pulmonary and bronchial affections and in rheumatism" (Johnson 1884: 231). We have seen already the popularity of the botanical for pulmonary and bronchial complaints, but the application for **rheumatism** has also been widespread and well attested—both by whites and by Native American tribes (Tantaquidgeon 1972: 37, 116–17; Millspaugh 1974: 540; Shook 1978: 301; Bolyard 1981: 46).

This botanical was a favorite of the Eclectics for hypertension accompanied by a strong and vibratile pulse (Thomas 1907: 999). "It undoubtedly acts," said the Eclectic scholars Harvey Wickes Felter and John Uri Lloyd, "upon the general circulatory apparatus, lowering arterial tension" (Felter and Lloyd 1898).

As was true of so many plants, Native tribes have found this one useful as a *vulnerary*. Our own area's Menomini, for instance, have appreciated it for **wounds**, **cuts**, and **bruises** (Smith 1923: 25). The Omaha have poulticed the chewed roots onto both **sores** and **wounds** (Lewis and Elwin-Lewis 1977: 341; Gilmore 1991: 57). It has especially been revered as a **snakebite** remedy (Speck 1942: 13).

PERSONAL AND PROFESSIONAL USE

I tend to add butterfly-weed to a formula when a client has elevated blood pressure with a hard pulse and when their skin does not perspire normally.

I can also testify that it makes an excellent primary ingredient in formulas for pneumonia, pleurisy, and suchlike conditions of the lower respiratory tract, for which I sometimes even use it as a simple (i.e., by itself).

CAUTIONS

Butterfly-weed should not be used during pregnancy.

Do not use the fresh root, which is toxic and may cause vomiting. Overdosing of the dried root will also produce unpleasant side effects. Michael Moore notes that even as little as 1 tablespoon to 1 cup of water may cause nausea and vomiting (Moore 1979: 130). ᨑ

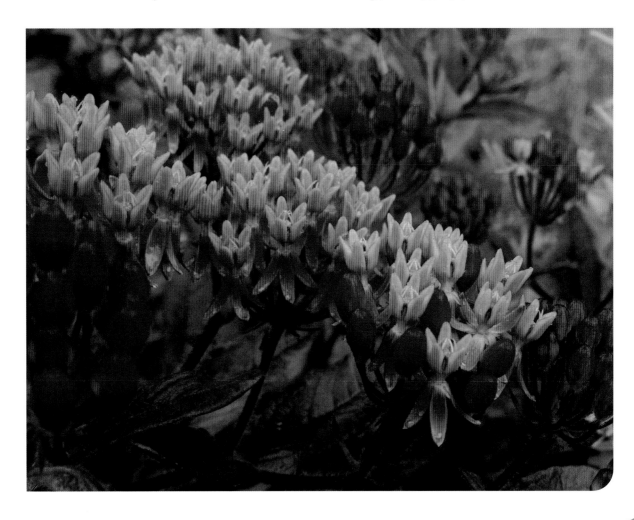

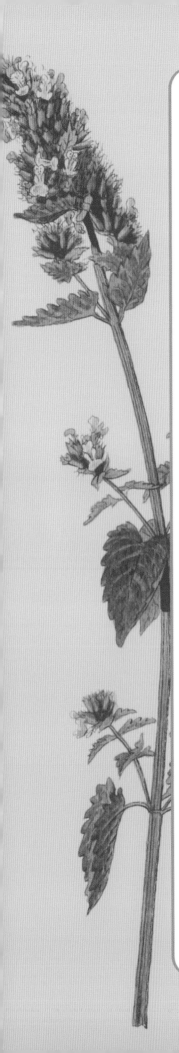

Catnip

CATMINT

Nepeta cataria

DESCRIPTION

This is a perennial herb that reaches a height of 1½–3½ feet. It possesses a distinctive musky mint sort of odor, especially when damaged. As a member of the mint family, its stem is square and branching; it is also ridged and hairy.

Catnip's leaves are opposite, heart shaped to arrowhead shaped, coarsely toothed, and covered on the lower side with what is best described as a mealy sort of down, giving them a gray-green sort of look and a very soft feel to the touch—like velvet. Leaf length is 1–2½ inches.

In midsummer, a number of ½-inch-long flowers appear, crowded into spike-like whorls 1½–2 inches long at the ends of the main stem and major branches. In color, the flowers are white to lavender to faint blue but almost always bear tiny purple spots. As is characteristic of mint flowers, they also possess two-lipped corollas.

RANGE AND HABITAT

Catnip was brought to North America from Europe as a plant of cultivation but escaped and is now widespread throughout the continent as a wild plant. In the Midwest, it is ubiquitous, except for a few counties in the upper-central to eastern parts of Minnesota and adjacent areas of northern Wisconsin. Its preferred habitat is disturbed ground—waste places, roadsides, trailsides, and old homesteads.

MAJOR CONSTITUENTS

Catnip essential oil contains nepetalactone (up to 90 percent, but some samples test at around 40 percent), nepetalic acid, nerol, carvacrol, citral, citronellol, limonene, piperitone, pulegone, camphor, thymol, humulene, myrcene, and beta-caryophyllene. The plant also contains tannins, iridoids (epideoxyloganic acid and 7-deoxyloganic acid), sterols, and notable amounts of the nutrients chromium, iron, manganese, potassium, and selenium.

FOOD

I enjoy the velvety-soft leaves fresh as a trail nibble, putting one in each cheek and slowly chewing the juice out of them as I go my way (an idea I gleaned from one of Euell Gibbons's books). Catnip tea is appreciated by many and can be made by pouring hot water over either fresh or dried leaves and steeping for 10–20 minutes. This makes an excellent bedtime beverage, being soothing and relaxing (see more on this below).

HEALTH/MEDICINE

At one time official medicine in America (the dried leaves were in the *United States Pharmacopeia* from 1842 to 1882 and in the *National Formulary* from 1916 to 1950), catnip is one of the more interesting wild plants owing to the contrasting effects that it has on felines and humans. Its stimulating effect on cats is well known, but its *calming effect* on humans is not so well known in North America (it is in Europe, however). As such, catnip is invaluable as a remedy for **tension headaches** and for **indigestion** induced by **nervousness** (Felter 1983: 281). Then, too, a tea made from the leaves makes an excellent sleep inducer (or sleep extender) for those who find it difficult to catch their forty winks. This has been confirmed in nonfeline animal studies (Harney et al. 1978: 369, 373; Sherry and Koontz 1979). The soothing effect also combines with the herb's cooling energies to provide a marvelous treatment for hot, inflamed conditions. For such, herbalist and naturalist Tom Brown Jr. recommends a tea of half catnip and half boneset, *Eupatorium perfoliatum* (see page 44), for **sore**, **strained muscles** (Brown 1985: 66).

The warm infusion is also a remarkable *diaphoretic* (Felter 1922: 281; Fleming 1998) and has thus been utilized by the Ojibwe and Menomini tribes here in the Midwest for **fever**

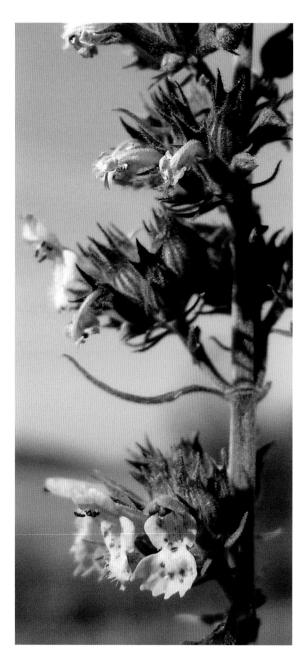

(Densmore 1932: 132; Densmore 1974: 354–55), especially for treating conditions that are eruptive (e.g., measles, chicken pox) or intermittent (e.g., malaria) in nature (Holmes 1997–98: 1:167). The Menomini have even been known to apply a poultice of the leaves to the chest of a person afflicted with **pneumonia** (Smith 1923: 39). The Iroquois found that drinking a cup of catnip tea serves as a *decongestant* when the upper respiratory system is congested with mucus (Herrick 1977: 423).

Catnip has classically been used by herbalists to *promote menstrual flow* and to ease **painful cramps.** With reference to the former, the Eclectic physician Harvey Wickes Felter noted: "When marked nervous agitation precedes menstruation in feeble and excitable women and the function is tardy or imperfect, this simple medicine gives great relief" (Felter 1922: 281). With reference to the latter, the plant's nepetalactone content has been shown to exert an *antispasmodic* effect (Leung 1980: 137), so that this chemical may be largely responsible for providing the relief from menstrual cramps that has long been witnessed by herbal practitioners. Concordantly, this herb has classically been used in formulas for **tremors** and **convulsions** (especially in infants, with whom it has a special affinity) (Holmes 1997–98: 1:168). It is thus most appropriately called a spasmolytic in the most recent edition of the authoritative *Potter's Cyclopaedia* of herbs (Wren 1988: 66). Indeed, such an effect is undoubtedly largely responsible for its reputation as a *carminative*—especially noted with respect to its effect upon **infant colic**, as the Mohegan came to appreciate (Tantaquidgeon 1928: 266). Felter, too, called catnip "a splendid quieting agent for fretful babies" and listed its specific indications as follows: "Abdominal colic, with constant flexing of the thighs; writhing and persistent crying; nervous agitation" (Felter 1983: 281).

The tea is likewise the herb of choice for **infant diarrhea**, an application that the Iroquois have greatly appreciated (Herrick 1977: 422). Scientific evidence supports this application, since an aqueous extract of catnip leaves has been shown to inhibit *Escherichia coli*, which has led to the suggestion that the tea be used as oral replacement therapy for infant diarrhea (Crellin and Philpott 1990a: 140).

The herb's renowned, although curious, affinity for youngsters reveals itself yet again in its observed ability to relieve **bull hives** in babies (symptomatized by "red spots on the face" and "a cross disposition")—a use long appreciated in Appalachian communities (Bolyard 1981: 89; Crellin and Philpott 1990a: 140). Catnip's efficacy as a nervine for **restless**, **agitated children** is likewise often most marked (Holmes 1997–98: 1:168), as the Iroquois discovered (Herrick 1995: 209). In this latter regard, too, the Alabama-based herbalist Tommie Bass cherished catnip for toddler frustrations during **teething** (Crellin and Philpott 1990a: 140). Herbalists have also long recommended a cup of catnip tea before bedtime for youngsters who are plagued by **nightmares** (Grieve 1971: 1:74). Finally, the Iroquois have used small amounts of the tea to help assist a **fever** to do its work and thus more quickly resolve in infants (Herrick 1995: 209).

UTILITARIAN USES

Catnip is a demonstrated **insect repellent**, owing mostly to its nepetalactone content. James Duke reports on a test of it involving twenty-seven insects in which an impressive twenty were rebuffed (Duke 1985: 325). Thomas Eisner detailed a fascinating array of insect experiments in which catnip oil repelled thirteen out of eighteen kinds of insects, acting like an impenetrable barrier around impregnated food, while controls were eagerly seized (Eisner 1965: 1318). Ants seemed especially dissuaded by the herb, a conclusion confirmed by another study conducted two years later (Regnier et al. 1967: 1281). In a 2001 study performed by the Department of Entomology at Iowa State University, catnip essential oil exhibited "excellent spatial repellency" against the mosquitoes that transmit yellow fever and did so at a lower concentration than did DEET! (Peterson and Coats 2011) Interestingly, a 2009 study found catnip essential oil to repel not only mosquitoes but also the nymphs of black-legged (deer) ticks (*Ixodes scapularis*), prime carriers of Lyme disease (Feaster et al. 2009).

PERSONAL AND PROFESSIONAL USE

In the late 1970s, my infant son was miserably beset with painful colic while my wife and I were visiting a friend in Duluth. Our host suggested the use of a few tablespoons of catnip tea, which calmed my little one instantly and eased him into restful sleep. This was a key incident in sparking my own interest in the use of herbs for health.

Since then, in my professional herbal practice, I've recommended the use of catnip to hundreds of youngsters—not only for the type of colic as described above but also for infant and toddler diarrhea, fever, insomnia, nightmares, and teething pains.

Sadly, this herb is vastly underutilized by the public, who remain largely unaware of its multitudinous applications.

CAUTIONS

As is true of most mints, *catnip should not be used during pregnancy*. It is, as we've seen, an emmenagogue, and it contains pulegone, which is the same chemical in pennyroyal that contraindicates the use of that relative of catnip during pregnancy.

When making a tea from wildcrafted catnip for infant use, such must be carefully strained so as to remove any solid particles. Paper coffee filters are especially useful here.

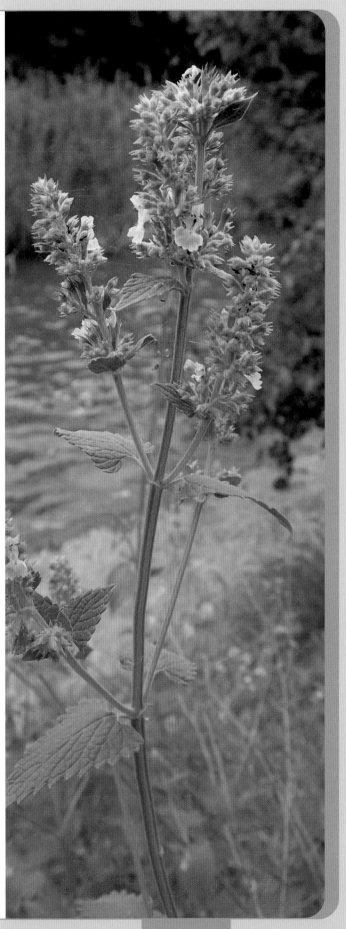

catnip

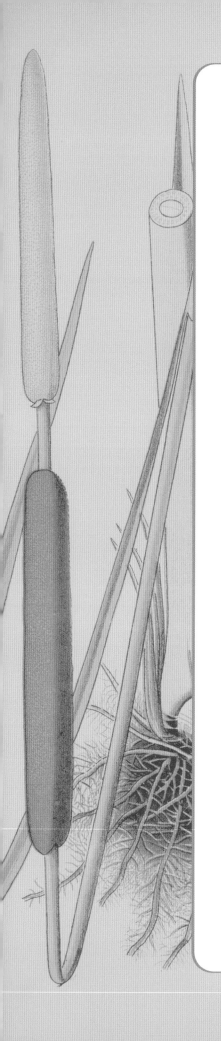

Cattail

Typha latifolia, T. angustifolia

DESCRIPTION

The familiar cattail is a tall (4–10 feet) perennial plant that grows in thick colonies in marshes and swamps and on the perimeters of ponds and lakes. Its very long stem is tough, round, and smooth.

The plant's leaves are basal, enwrapping the lower portion of the stem. They are also long, flat (strap-like), and pointed. Because they spiral several times, an onlooker gazing at this plant on a sunny day can sometimes see what appear to be alternating light and dark bands on the green leaves.

A pair of 6-inch heads—sausage-like in shape and wrapped in a papery husk—finds form at the top of the stem. The lower one is composed entirely of a cluster of female flowers, while the upper one is a male appendage that enriches with vibrant yellow pollen during the month of June. This latter head eventually releases its load and shrivels away thereafter, leaving behind simply a bare stem situated above the female head (which by this time has turned dark brown in color). Buried in the muck below is the horizontal white rhizome.

Two main species predominate in the Midwest: narrow-leaved cattail (*T. angustifolia*) and common (or broad-leaved) cattail (*T. latifolia*). The former's parts are thinner than the latter's, and, most distinctly, there is a space between *T. angustifolia*'s heads that does not exist between those of *T. latifolia*.

RANGE AND HABITAT

This is a plant that is nearly ubiquitous throughout our area (although, surprisingly, unrecorded in a few counties). The habitat is, of course, swamps, marshes, roadside ditches, and the perimeters of both ponds and lakes.

SEASONAL AVAILABILITY

Various edible or medicinal portions are available from late April through mid-October.

MAJOR CONSTITUENTS

Cattail pollen contains isorhamnetin-3-*O*-neohesperidin, typhaneoside, sitosterol, and nutrients such as protein and pro-vitamin A. The rhizome contains saponins, flavonoids, coumarin derivatives, more protein than can be found in either corn or rice, more starch than is contained in a potato, and a good supply of fatty acids. Other nutrients include a high amount of potassium and a moderate amount of phosphorus. Both the stem and the seeds contain leucanthocyanidin. There is a higher amount of omega-3 fatty acids in the seeds than in any comparably sized source.

FOOD

One of the most utilizable of wild plants, the cattail offers a variety of culinary delights for the adventuresome forager.

Initially available are the plant's shoots, which can be collected by firmly grasping the stem inside the enwrapping leaves as far down as possible and then pulling the stalk from the ground (some recommend twisting it first). The roots and the rhizome will usually stay behind. Once the prize has been unearthed, simply cut the bottom 12 inches or so free; this portion can be peeled to reveal a white core that can be eaten raw or cooked (simmered not more than ten or fifteen minutes). This delightful repast has been called "Cossack's asparagus," although the taste is not really like asparagus but more like raw cucumber, watercress, or parsnips. As the shoots mature, they become less tasteful. Even at this stage, however, they can still be cut into segments and added to stews.

The next segment available for food is what has been called "cattail corn on the cob," with reference to the sausage-like head situated at the very top of the plant (the male appendage). As it begins to appear, it is green and wrapped in a papery husk. At this stage, it can be cut free and prepared as a potherb—immersed for five to ten minutes in rapidly boiling water, salted or not. Alternatively, it can be cooked for five minutes in boiling water and then allowed to sit for ten more minutes after the pot has been removed from the heat. Both the shape of this head and the method of eating it—and, to some extent, even its taste—reminds one of corn on the cob.

In a survival situation, the lower female head can, at the same (green) stage in its own development, be prepared in similar fashion. It is only deemed a survival food, however, because (1) it has very little substance to it, (2) it is not nearly as tasty as the male spike, and (3) it is a lot messier to consume! Either head, too, can be boiled for just a few minutes and then packaged and frozen for later use. Bear in mind that both heads become inedible after they lose their green coloring (with the exception of some of their constituents—see below).

The next segment to become available is the golden pollen that saturates the male appendage in June, appearing on that head as if it has been dusted with yellow chalk. This pollen can be collected into a bucket, bowl, or paper bag by bending the cattail stem so that the pollen head rests against the side of the collecting implement, after which it is gently beaten or rubbed off into the container. Thereafter, it can be separated from the large amount of chaff (also unavoidably collected) by means of a flour sifter. One can then dry it and store it for future use or simply use it like flour right away in a variety of recipes, including in bread, corn bread, cookies, or pancakes. (It is most often used for the latter.) As the pollen tends to resist wetting, however, it is best used half and half with domestic flour, such as wheat or corn. Used alone and simmered in water for half an hour, however, it can thicken into a pretty good oatmeal substitute.

Available in late summer are tiny seeds enwrapped in the female head, which can be acquired by removing the fluff from the brown head. This can be accomplished by laying this downy material on a flat and inflammable surface (such as a rock) and then igniting it, which serves to burn away the fluff, leaving the parched seeds ready to eat. (One will usually need to winnow the remaining chaff first—either by blowing on the mass or by letting the wind do the job.)

In autumn, the starch from the rhizomes can be acquired by first digging out the latter with a firm stick or long stone.

Then, simply chew it out after roasting the rhizome in the slow embers of a campfire, which produces a very pleasant and sweetish taste. (Never consume raw rhizomes; having been submerged in swampy water for some time, they may harbor parasites or other harmful microorganisms.) The starch can also be separated from the fibrous part of the rhizome and then used like flour for muffins, bread, and so on. Two main methods for doing so have evolved among wild-foods connoisseurs: The first calls for one to dry the rhizomes in the sun for several days or in an oven set at about 200 degrees Fahrenheit for a few hours. Using two large stones or a grinder, one then simply pulverizes the dried rhizomes. Next, the fibers are picked out by hand or sifted, and the resultant flour is used immediately or stored for later use. The second method of preparation involves washing and peeling the rhizomes, cutting them into small segments, and putting them into a large bowl of cold water. Next, the material needs to be vigorously worked over with one's hands in an endeavor to separate the starch from the fiber with the aid of (clean!) fingernails and a sloshing of the rhizome segments in the water. When the starch seems to have largely separated from the core segments, the latter is discarded. Next, one strains the resultant fluid through a coarse sieve to remove any fiber segments, after which the remaining liquid is allowed to sit for one-half hour, during which time the starch settles to the bottom of the container. Then, the water and any remaining chaff on the surface are carefully poured off so that only the starch is left at the bottom of the bowl. The container is then refilled with clean water and the process repeated to further purify the starch. Finally, it is repeated one more time. Then the cattail "dough" is wrapped around a stick and cooked over a campfire or fireplace for a tasty treat. Alternatively, the material can be used in a recipe or dried in the sun (or in an oven) and stored for later use.

HEALTH/MEDICINE

While most people are acquainted with some of the uses of cattail as an edible plant as described here, very few are aware of its medicinal applications. However, such uses are legion.

The Alabama herbalist Tommie Bass once remarked that since grasses and aquatic plants are generally *diuretic*, cattail, as a grass-like plant, should likewise be possessed of this physiological effect, although he was not personally aware of any such use for the plant. Interestingly, however, history has recorded a few applications for the genitourinary system—for example, the Oklahoma Lenape (Delaware) have used it to treat **urinary gravel** (Tantaquidgeon 1942: 80–81; Tantaquidgeon 1972: 122–23).

The prolific early American medical botanist Constantine Rafinesque highlighted some of cattail's other physiological functions in noting that the roots are "sub-astringent" and "febrifuge" (Rafinesque 1828–30: 2:270). America's Eclectic physicians agreed, stressing the *astringent* quality and adding that the rhizome was *emollient* (King 1882: 840). As to cattail's astringency, the French have traditionally used it for **chronic dysentery** (Porcher 1863: 544–45). The Cheyenne found that a decoction of the pulverized, dried roots and of the white base of the leaves is useful for alleviating **stomach cramps** (Hart 1981: 13).

The plant's astringent and other properties have rendered it useful as a *vulnerary*. Ojibwe from the Midwest pound the rhizome for use as a poultice on **sores** (Hoffman 1891: 200), while the Malecite and Micmac grease a leaf and lay it onto these as well (Mechling 1959: 246). The Algonquin of southwestern Quebec poultice the crushed rhizome onto both **infections** and **wounds** (Black 1980: 132). The Potawatomi have implemented cattail for **swellings**, **wounds**, and **burns** (Smith 1933: 85). As to the latter, pharmacist Heber W. Youngken, an aficionado of Native American medicine, wrote of cattail's use by the Omaha: "The root was powdered, wetted and spread as a paste over the scald. The ripe blossoms were then applied as a covering and the injured part bound, so as to hold the dressing in place" (Youngken 1924: 499; Gilmore 1991: 12).

The rhizome seems to provide medicinal benefits when ingested as well. In a 2013 scientific study employing a rat model of colitis, the inclusion of cattail rhizome flour as 10 percent of the rodents' diet not only prevented intestinal inflammatory processes but did so on a scale comparable to the steroid drug prednisolone. The authors concluded that cattail rhizome holds promise for the prevention and treatment of ulcerative colitis in humans (Fruet et al. 2012).

Naturalist and herbalist Tom Brown Jr. points out that the sticky juice found between the leaves yields a powerful *anesthetic* that, in a wilderness situation, can be used to dull the pain of a toothache or even a tooth extraction (Brown 1985: 91).

Cattail pollen is an important medicine in Traditional Chinese Medicine, in which it is used to relieve blood stagnation manifested by stabbing **dysmenorrhea** or **stomach pain**. In harmony with this usage, scientific research has demonstrated an *anticoagulant* effect (Gibbs et al. 1983). Interestingly, though, when cooked, its properties reverse, and it becomes a *hemostat*.

PERSONAL AND PROFESSIONAL USE

I have partaken of cattail as a food (raw or cooked) every year since 1973 and have relished each and every one of these repasts. In my herbal practice, I've sometimes used the raw pollen as a blood mover. Occasionally, I've carried the charred pollen with me in the wilderness as a potential hemostat.

CAUTIONS

Cattail is easily recognized once it has flowered but should be used cautiously by the amateur prior to flowering due to a possibility of confusing it with the poisonous wild iris (blue flag, page **38**), which also grows in marsh-like environments and bears similar-looking leaves. Should the two be found growing together, one will note that wild iris's leaves are wider and more sword-like than cattail's; also, iris shoots are flattened where they meet the base, whereas cattail's shoots remain rounded.

Do not harvest any cattail growing near roads, as the plant collects pollutants from auto exhaust like a magnet (Erickson and Lindzey 1983). Do not eat cattail rhizomes without cooking them first, due to possible parasitical contamination from having been submerged in swampy environs.

Use of cattail pollen as a medicine, or heavy consumption of it as a food, should be *avoided during pregnancy* due to an emmenagogue effect. Also, those with pollen allergies should probably not use it in any fashion. ⤶

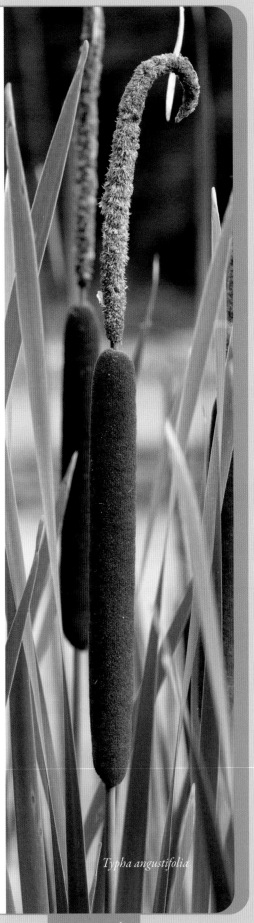

Typha angustifolia

cattail

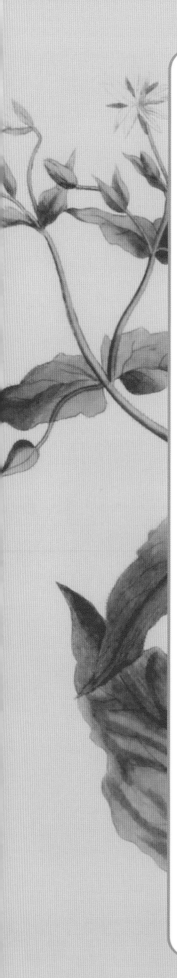

Chickweed

Stellaria spp.

DESCRIPTION

This is a small to medium-sized annual or perennial plant (depending on the species) possessed of white, star-like flowers—hence the Latin genus name, *Stellaria*. It is often found growing in clumps or mats. Several species occur in the Midwest, as follows:

Stellaria media (common chickweed) is a common sprawling, scrawny plant with weak, delicate stems. It typically grows only 4–8 inches tall. Small pairs of toothless, pointed, egg-shaped leaves up to 1 inch long grow along the thread-like stem. Lower leaves are often stalked, but upper leaves are frequently sessile. Its stem has one line of hairs running down its length, switching sides at each node.

Stellaria aquatica or *Myosoton aquaticum* (water chickweed) is a perennial plant that is more upright than the former species, growing 8–16 inches high. Its stem, unlike that of *S. media*, is entirely hairy. Its opposite leaves are ovate, growing at times to 4 inches long and to 1¼ inches wide. They are mostly or entirely sessile, although some may be stalked toward the bottom of the plant. White flowers appear on the forked, upright branches.

Stellaria longifolia (long-leaved chickweed) has hairy sepals and very long, thin leaves that are oppositely situated. It flourishes in moist woods. Although widespread in the Midwest, it is not well known or appreciated by foragers.

All chickweed species have white flowers (*S. aquatica*'s are the biggest) with five sepals and five petals that are notched so deeply that it looks as if the plant actually possesses ten petals (especially so with *S. aquatica*). However, *S. media*'s petals are shorter than its sepals, whereas *S. aquatica*'s are longer than its sepals. The blossoms of all *Stellaria* species open only on sunny days.

Chickweed's fruits find form as oval-shaped, bump-covered capsules.

RANGE AND HABITAT

S. media is found in most parts of Canada and practically ubiquitously in the United States, including throughout the Midwest. Its preferred habitat is lawns, gardens, and waste places. *S. aquatica* is found throughout much of the Midwest in moist woods, streams, ponds, and ditches—almost always in partial shade. *S. longifolia* is found in moist woods in parts of our region (especially Minnesota).

SEASONAL AVAILABILITY

Chickweed is available year-round, even in early winter! This is because of its renowned ability to survive under mild winter snows, which is facilitated by the mechanism of its leaves closing over both its delicate flower buds and its developing leaflets.

MAJOR CONSTITUENTS

Chickweed contains triterpenoid saponins; phytosterols (beta-sitosterol and daucosterol); coumarins; anthraquinones (emodin, physcion); mucilage; flavonoids (including apigenin and rutin); anthocynidine; esters (hentriacontanol, cerylcerotate); and carboxylic and octadecatetraenic acids. Nutrients include protein; unsaturated fatty acids (linoleic, gamma-linolenic, oleic); saturated fatty acids (palmitic and stearic); pro-vitamin A (as beta-carotene), several B vitamins (thiamin, niacin, and riboflavin), vitamin C (very high—0.10–0.15%!), and vitamin K_1 (phylloquinone); and minerals, among them

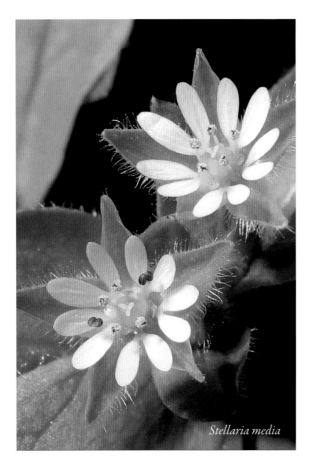

Stellaria media

rake back the leaves to reveal fresh chickweed greens for the pickin'. This generally works as long as the ground hasn't frozen too thoroughly in the area.

HEALTH/MEDICINE

Chickweed provides a much-appreciated *anti-inflammatory* effect. Internally, **ulcers**, **arthritis**, **rheumatism**, and **gout** are improved thereby. **Urinary tract inflammation** is also eased, especially by fresh chickweed juice. Externally, a tea for washing **inflamed, sore eyes** has been frequently utilized. Also, a crushed-plant poultice (especially when warmed) has long been used for exterior inflammation of almost any kind, including **arthritic joints**, **hemorrhoids**, **sores**, and especially **itchy rashes**. Such anti-inflammatory action may also help explain chickweed's long-appreciated use as a *vulnerary* for many kinds of **wounds**. (The fragile plant can easily be mashed with a fingernail, lending it to ready use for **cuts** and for **scrapes**.)

The anti-inflammatory effect here may be due to the saponins, which perhaps help solubilize the toxins in abscesses and rashes (Pedersen 1998: 73). A possible explanation for the increase in efficacy when the plant is warmed is proffered by John Heinerman: "A volatile oil present in the herb permits a chemical change in the basic compound structure of the ... glycosides under conditions of warmth and heat. In other words, chickweed's best virtues are brought out when subjected to an influence of heat, either internally or externally" (Heinerman 1979: 186).

Chickweed is also revered as a first-rate *demulcent* and *expectorant.* Here it appears that the mucilage is primarily responsible for the former and the saponins for the latter. In addition, mild *antibiotic* activity against certain respiratory pathogens has been found (Fitzpatrick 1954: 531). No wonder that the herb has been praised by many for its aid in dealing with **coughs**, **bronchitis**, and **hoarseness**, as numerous Native American tribes discovered (Scully 1970: 212–13). Tom Brown Jr. adds that the congestion-relieving properties are especially appreciated because they perform this function *without drying up the passages*, unlike many stronger herbs (Brown 1985: 98–99). Indeed, this plant is preeminently a *moistening* herb (Holmes 1997–98: 1:458).

Another of chickweed's assists lies in its *depurative* ability. This herb is thought to help rid the liver and kidney of wastes and is eagerly looked to by many each spring as a "tonic" along such lines.

Our herb is also a blood builder, being high in iron and thus historically used to help offset **anemia**. The plant's exceptionally high vitamin C content helps to assure absorption of the iron.

A treasured cooling (*refrigerant*) herb, chickweed is known for its mild *antipyretic* action. Such a cooling action may also elucidate its value in treating the "heat" conditions highlighted above. In addition, herbalist Peter Holmes

calcium and potassium salts, magnesium, manganese, silicon, sulfur, zinc, phosphorus, and an extraordinary supply of iron—one of the highest known in the herb kingdom.

FOOD

Most forms of chickweed are delicious picked straight from the wilds and eaten raw. It is also extremely nutritious, being high in vitamins and minerals. Thus, it makes a fine ingredient to include in a healthful "green drink" or wild salad or simply as a trail nibble. Chickweed can also be prepared as a potherb. (In fact, the hairy mouse-eared chickweed should always be cooked.) It should be boiled in salted water for two to eight minutes. One needs to pick double the amount one plans to eat, as chickweed cooks down in size quite a bit. Many equate the taste with that of spinach. One naturalist claims that it adds a "special touch" to a rabbit stew.

The plant's fascinating ability to survive under winter snows allows one to gather it in the winter if snowfall is not too deep and one knows where to find this herb. I enjoy winter foraging and always strive to make chickweed a menu item during this time. Those not so inclined, however, can try this: Cover known chickweed patches with oak leaves (about 6 inches deep) after the first frost but before the ground freezes. Lay a flat covering, such as a board, over the leaves to compact them. When hungry, lift up the board and

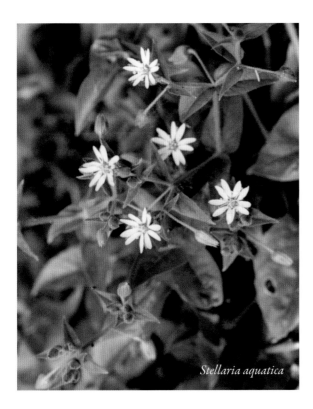

Stellaria aquatica

recommends it for **heat exhaustion** and for **dehydration** (Holmes 1997–98: 1:458).

This plant is further an important, although underrated, *laxative*—especially the roots. Brown tells a story of its *anticonstipational* power, relating how he accidentally over-treated a case of constipation with it and thereby precipitated three days straight of diarrhea! (Brown 1985: 97–99)

This versatile weed has frequently been cited as an aid to help offset **obesity**. Clinical experience suggests that it gently *stimulates the thyroid* (Holmes 1997–98: 1:459), which may be one mechanism in how it achieves this result. Scientific studies published in 2011 and 2012 reveal that chickweed definitely exerts an *antiobesity* effect in mice, seemingly in part by inhibiting pancreatic amylase and lipase, and reduces low-density lipoprotein (LDL) cholesterol and triglycerides. Its activity in these regards would seem to be due to any or all of its content of saponins, beta-sitosterol, and flavonoids (Chidrawar et al. 2011; Rani et al. 2012).

PERSONAL AND PROFESSIONAL USE

I've probably dined on more chickweed than on any other wild plant, as I so relish its rich, spinach-like taste!

In my herbal practice, I typically suggest its use with thyroidal sluggishness marked especially by constipation, anemia, elevated cholesterol, and weight gain.

I've found a salve of chickweed useful as an antipruritic (anti-itch agent), but I find the results to be even more pronounced if I incorporate cleavers (see page 86) and butter-and-eggs (page 64) into the mix. ⤺

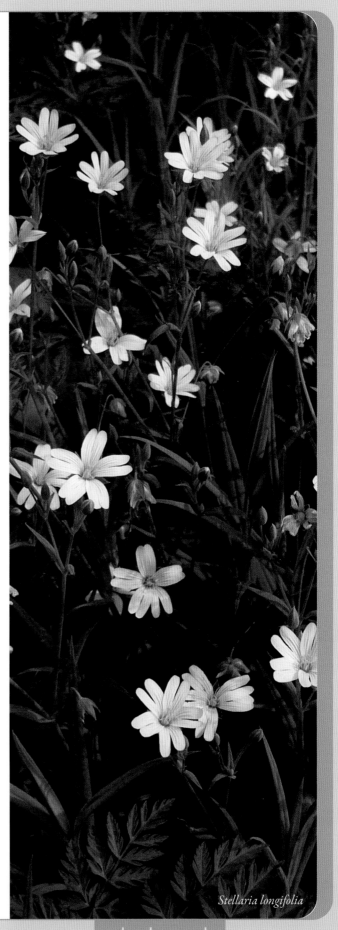

Stellaria longifolia

chickweed

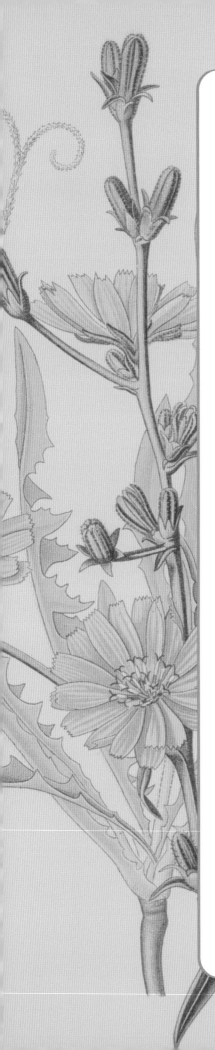

Chicory

Cichorium intybus

DESCRIPTION

This perennial European import, a close relative of the cultivated endive, is erect, 1–3 feet tall, and possessed of a milky sap that exudes from the stem when damaged. The plant emerges from a very large and fleshy rootstock.

Chicory's initial appearance is as a basal rosette of spatula-shaped leaves that grow 3–6 inches long. These have edges that are cut, lobed, or toothed, and they are often curled as well. Once the stem sprouts, smaller leaves—oblong to lanceolate—appear on it, clasping it tightly with their bases.

The flower heads, occurring along the upper stem from May to October, are sessile, generally situated two at a spot, 1–1½ inches across, and usually of a beautiful blue color (thus the plant's alternative common name of blue sailors), although sometimes they are white or pink. The petal tips are square and marked by notches that make them appear ragged (thus the other common name of ragged sailors). The flowers open only in the first part of the day and close around noon. The great botanist Carolus Linnaeus found that the process was so reliable in his area—opening at 5:00 a.m. and closing at 12:00 p.m.—that he could even use the plant as a clock!

RANGE AND HABITAT

This is a weedy plant that is most frequently found on roadsides, railroad rights-of-way, waste areas, and fields. It is most common in the southern half of the Midwest.

MAJOR CONSTITUENTS

Chicory root contains sesquiterpene lactones (including lactucin, lactupicrine, and intybin); taraxasterol; coumarins (esculetin, umbelliferone, cichoriin); essential oil; fatty oil; tannin; inulin (15–58%); and pectin. The flowers also contain cichoriin and esculetin. The leaves contain flavonoids (including hyperoside), unsaturated sterols or triterpenoids, catechol tannins, tartaric acid, and glycosides. Nutrients include vitamins such as pro-vitamin A (4000 imperial units per 100 grams), C, K, thiamine, choline, and folic acid (50 milligrams per 100 grams) and minerals such as potassium (a whopping 430 milligrams per 100 grams), iron, calcium, magnesium, and phosphorus.

FOOD

Chicory's early-spring shoots have long been valued as a salad bitter, especially the whitened, developing leaves situated just below the visible leaves. After the plant flowers, its leaves become too bitter to the palate, but at this time it can still be prepared as a potherb. Here, boiling it for ten minutes in two waters is usually preferable and seems to effectively reduce the intense bitterness to an acceptable level. Blanching the plant before harvesting by covering it for a week or more with a box or a pail can even further reduce the bitterness.

Blanched chicory leaves can be acquired throughout the winter, as well, by "forcing" them. This can be accomplished as follows: Gather some plants in autumn just before the ground freezes hard. Cut the leaves back to within an inch of the root, then place the plants in a container filled with sand (or sandy soil) and put that away in a very dark place—a closet or basement is ideal. Finally, water your secreted chicory every few days. If you've performed your task with skill, you'll discover very pale leaves emerging in just a few weeks.

Chicory crowns are edible as well. They can be boiled for five minutes and then served with butter for a tasty treat. These crowns, along with the lovely flowers, also make decent salad ingredients. The flowers can even be made into jelly.

The small white center portion of the root, dug early in the spring, is edible. However, the most revered use of the roots is as the world's most famous coffee substitute. One accomplishes this by digging the roots anytime from midsummer until the following spring, thoroughly scrubbing them, and then cutting them into long, thin strips and finally into quarters. Next, one either allows these segments to dry in a warm place for a few days or roasts them on a baking sheet in an oven at 250–300 degrees Fahrenheit for two to four hours until they snap easily and are dark brown inside. Finally, the roots are ground and brewed the same way as regular coffee, using 1½ teaspoons chicory root to each cup of water. Alternatively, the powdered root may be mixed with ground coffee.

HEALTH/MEDICINE

This plant has many of the same benefits as its close lookalike and tastealike dandelion (see page **99**). First, chicory is similar to dandelion in being a *diuretic*. In this regard, plant scientist Jean Bruneton remarks that chicory enhances the ability of the kidneys to eliminate water—so effectively that it has often been used in weight-loss regimens (Bruneton 1995: 78). Likewise similar to dandelion is chicory's reputation of being, as the second-century Greek physician Galen once put it, "a friend of the liver." Indeed, chicory has been found to be both a superb *hepatoprotective* (Sultana et al. 1995; Zafar and Ali 1998: 227) and a *cholagogue* (Fleming 1998: 745), being most especially used to treat **liver enlargement** and **jaundice.** Its sesquiterpene lactones are undoubtedly most responsible for these celebrated hepatic assists (Vuilleumier 1973), including the bile-stimulating effects, which enable chicory to serve as a valuable *tonic*, as the *United States Dispensatory* once noted (Wood et al. 1926: 1256). Hence, it has long been valued as a treatment for **dyspepsia.** Interestingly, too, chicory has been thought to possess the ability to rid the gastrointestinal tract of phlegm-like material that can plug the intestinal villi so that efficient nutrient absorption is hampered. **Sclerosis of the spleen** has also been treated with chicory, especially by the Germans (EthnobDB).

Chicory has traditionally been used in European herbalism as a *refrigerant*. The noted herbalist Nicholas Culpeper found that it "helps the heat of the reins and of the urine," that it is "good for hot stomachs ... heat and headache in children," and that it "allays swellings, inflammation" (Culpeper 1983: 186). An aqueous distillation of the flowers

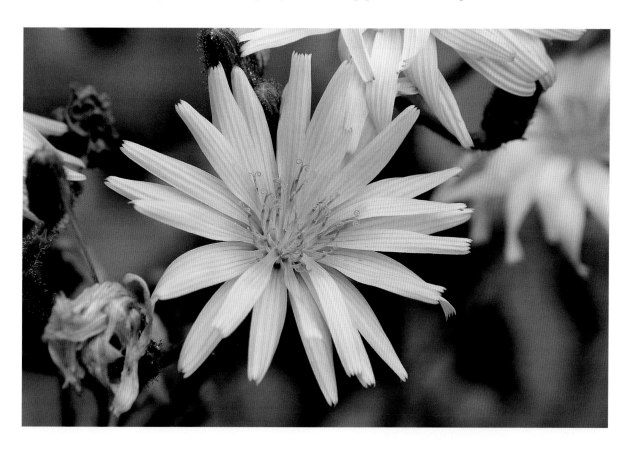

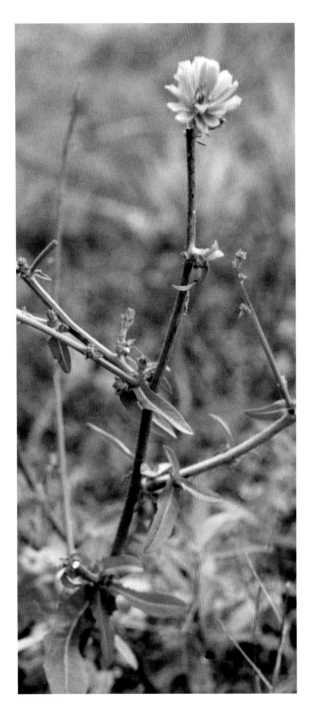

rat-paw edema model found chicory to be *anti-inflammatory* (Benoit et al. 1976: 164).

Scientific studies have also shown that chicory favorably affects lipid metabolism and even prevents oxidation of low-density lipoprotein (LDL) (Kim and Shin 1998; Kim and Yang 2001). Then, too, several animal studies have shown that our herb depresses the heart rate in a fashion similar to the alkaloid quinidine from cinchona bark (Balbaa et al. 1973: 133), so that it has been used to treat both **tachycardia** and **arrhythmia** (Fetrow and Avila 1999: 163). The Cherokee, in fact, have used it directly as a *nervine* (Hamel and Chiltoskey 1975: 29). In fact, chicory has long been thought to be mildly *sedative* and, as such, useful in offsetting the stimulating properties of coffee—with which, as noted earlier, it is often mixed. This sedative effect would appear to derive from principles in chicory's white latex—similar, in this respect, to the more widely familiar sedative principles in the latex from the related wild lettuce (*Lactuca* spp.).

British herbalists say that a syrup made from chicory (produced by simmering equal parts root juice and honey until a syrupy consistency is reached) serves as a useful *laxative* in children, appreciated because it does not cause irritation (Grieve 1971: 1:198). This preparation has been dosed at 1 teaspoon and repeated twice during the day. The laxative effects have also been appreciated by the French, German, and Iraqi peoples (EthnobDB).

Chicory has traditionally been used by way of decoction, to the tune of 1 ounce of the root to 1 pint of water, boiled five minutes and then infused for ten to fifteen more minutes. Herbalist Michael Moore noted that the decoction has been typically, and best, used in a dose of 3–6 ounces, repeated up to four times a day (Moore 1994a: 8).

PERSONAL AND PROFESSIONAL USE

I very much enjoy the rich taste of hot chicory tea, which I drink from time to time, purely for pleasure. Therapeutically, I often recommend chicory when I want the services of a good hepatoprotective, such as in hepatitis, cirrhosis, or conditions in which pro-oxidants or toxins are threatening the liver.

I also treasure chicory for its neurocardiac effects, finding that it often serves to relax a nervous heart producing a rapid heartbeat. I recall here one case where it worked better than anything else that was tried—even classic neurocardiac herbs such as motherwort (see page **156**), hawthorn (*Crataegus* spp.), and bugleweed (page **52**).

CAUTIONS

For some people, simply touching chicory can cause dermatitis, owing to its content of sesquiterpene lactones (Malten 1983: 232). ⋘

has long been used as a wash for **inflammation of the eyes** (Grieve 1971: 1:199). For countless generations, too, herbalists have recommended that the boiled leaves and flowers, lightly wrapped in a cloth, be applied to painful inflammations on the body (Lust 1974: 156). In this regard, naturalist and herbalist Tom Brown Jr. vividly relates how his Apache herbal mentor, Stalking Wolf, used just such a poultice to heal his family dog, Butch, from a painful abscess accruing from a fight with another dog (Brown 1985: 93). It certainly comes as no surprise, then, that a 1976 lab study using the

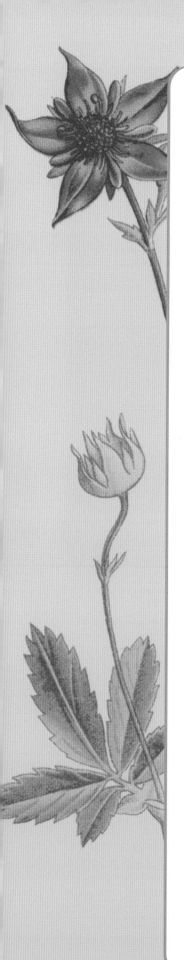

Cinquefoil

DESCRIPTION

Members of the *Potentilla* genus usually possess flowers with five petals and leaves with five finger-like leaflets (hence the common name of cinquefoil, which means "five-leaved"). A number of species flourish in the Midwest, including the following:

P. anserina (silverweed) is a hairy, prostrate perennial with feather-like basal leaves (4–8 inches long) divided into seven to thirty-one toothed leaflets (1 inch long) that are green above and silvery white beneath. It bears solitary flowers on separate stalks. The fruits that eventually replace them resemble dry strawberries.

P. argentea (silvery cinquefoil) is an erect perennial, growing 5–12 inches high. Its five leaflets are wedge shaped and have edges that are rolled back. The undersides are downy, and the stem and its branches are woolly.

P. arguta (tall cinquefoil) can reach a height of 1–3 feet and has a stem that is covered with clammy brown hairs. Its seven to eleven toothed leaflets are hairy on their undersides. The flowers are not fully yellow, as they are in most other cinquefoil species, but creamy white with yellow centers. They are grouped into loose clusters at the tips of the branching stems.

P. norvegica (rough cinquefoil) reaches a height of 5–36 inches and has a stout, hairy stem. This species bears leaves possessed of only three leaflets, not five as is typical of the *Potentilla* genus. Its flowers have five pointed sepals (calyx lobes), which are longer than its petals.

P. palustris (marsh cinquefoil, purple cinquefoil) grows 6–24 inches tall, but its stem manifests a sprawling tendency. Its star-shaped flowers are large and crimson (or purple) and grow on slender stalks. The leaves of this species have five to seven toothed leaflets.

P. pensylvanica (prairie cinquefoil) tops off at about 1–2 feet tall and sports pinnate leaves that have lobes resembling those appearing on the leaves of white oaks. Like some of the other species in this genus, it is downy all over.

P. simplex (five fingers, old field cinquefoil, common cinquefoil), one of the most common species in the Midwest, reaches a height of 6–20 inches and is possessed of alternate, toothed, palmate leaves with five finger-like leaflets that grow to 2½ inches long. Its flowers—borne singly like those of *P. anserina*—manifest rounded petals.

Other species growing in the Midwest include *P. paradoxa*, *P. tridentata*, and *P. fruticosa*. The latter, a species quite common in our region, has toothless leaves that are rolled over at the edges and reddish-brown woody stems that bear thin, loose bark that tends to peel in shreds.

RANGE AND HABITAT

Most of the above species are found throughout the Midwest and thrive in dry, open soil in fields and on trailsides. *P. anserina* can be spotted on lakeshores and riverbanks, whereas *P. palustris* makes its home in marshes.

MAJOR CONSTITUENTS

P. anserina (and probably most other species) contains tannins, flavonoids, and hydroxycoumarins (umbelliferone, scopoletin).

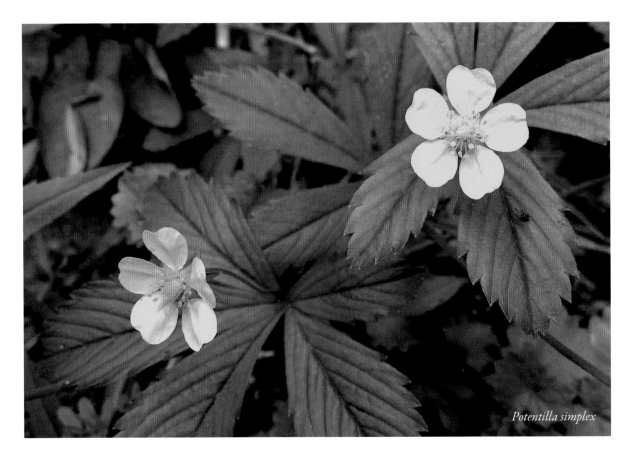

Potentilla simplex

FOOD

The very young leaves of most, if not all, *Potentilla* species are edible. As cinquefoil plants mature, however, they accumulate a large amount of chemicals that render their aerial portions unpalatable.

The thick rhizomes of *P. anserina* (silverweed) are edible and possessed of a parsnip-like (some would say a sweet potato-like) taste. They can be eaten raw and are quite pleasant as such. Alternatively, they can be scraped, sliced, and cooked in water for about forty-five minutes. Steaming is the method that best preserves the flavor. Quite sustaining, these rhizomes once supported inhabitants of the Hebrides and Scotch islands for months during a food scarcity. Rhizomes of some other species are reputed to be edible as well.

HEALTH/MEDICINE

Astringency is the *Potentilla* genus's most famous and pronounced effect, elucidating the implementation of this plant by the Kayenta Navajo (Diné) for **burns** (Wyman and Harris 1951: 26). The astringent property also sheds light on the Ojibwe custom of using a decoction of *P. norvegica*'s root and stalks to soothe a **sore throat** (Densmore 1974: 342). Famed and much-loved European herbalist Juliette de Bairacli Levy noted that such a preparation is also helpful for relieving **chronic respiratory catarrh** and as a syringed injection up the nostrils for **sinus problems** (de Bairacli Levy 1974: 135).

Astringency probably largely explains why the cinquefoils are *styptic*, for which property the Ojibwe have implemented the dry or moistened root of the tall cinquefoil as a topical application to **bleeding wounds** (Densmore 1974: 32).

Writing in the early 1800s, the American naturalist Constantine Rafinesque further explicated the genus's astringent applicability in noting that species such as *P. reptans*, *P. canadensis*, and *P. fruticosa* were "mostly used in weak bowels, hemorrhage, agues, menorrhea, & c." (Rafinesque 1828–30: 2:253).

As to "weak bowels," the Cherokee have employed a tea of the roots of *P. simplex* for **dysentery**, while the Ojibwe have done the same with *P. arguta* (Densmore 1974: 350). The Iroquois have utilized cinquefoil for **diarrhea** in general (Herrick 1995: 164), as have the Okanogan (Turner et al. 1980: 127). Such an application is still popular in many lands and has even received the approval of the German Office of Health, which recommends cinquefoil for "acute, nonspecific diarrhea" (Pahlow 1993: 162). Both the astringent and the antimicrobial activity of the tannins are undoubtedly at play here and no doubt explain why the Cherokee have had success in using a cinquefoil-root mouthwash for sore or **spongy gums** as well as for **oral thrush** (Hamel and Chiltoskey 1975: 26). Extracts of two different European species, *P. alba* and *P. erecta*, have been scientifically tested to determine their antimicrobial effects: the alcoholic extracts of both species manifested activity against *Escherichia coli*, while their aqueous extracts inhibited *Staphylococcus aureus* (Grujic-Vasic et al. 2006). Shrubby cinquefoil (*P. fruticosa*) has demonstrated antimicrobial activity against *Candida albicans* and *Bacillus cereus* (Jurkstiene et al. 2011).

Juliette de Bairacli Levy, earlier mentioned, pointed out that the name for cinquefoil's Latin genus derives from the Latin term *potens*, meaning "powerful," and such she found it, deeming it a reliable *nerve sedative*, even with applicability to **epilepsy.** Nicholas Culpeper also used *Potentilla* for epilepsy, advising use of the plant's juice and stressing that it needed to be taken to the tune of 4 ounces at a time, with such a regimen continuing for at least a month before results could be expected (Potterton 1983: 46). Certain species of Potentilla, most especially *P. anserina* (silverweed), appear to possess a marked *antispasmodic* property, and perhaps it is this quality that is primarily at play in the alleged aid for those with epilepsy.

In Ukrainian herbalism, this botanical has traditionally been used to heal persons afflicted with **Graves' disease**, an autoimmune disorder in which the immune system attacks the thyroid gland, resulting in a dangerous increase of metabolism in the body. In a clinical trial, a dosage of 1–3 tablespoons of the tincture of *P. alba* per day reduced **goiter**, **tachycardia**, **blood pressure**, and **tremor** in nineteen test subjects afflicted with this condition. The authors of this study further observed: "In [contra]-distinction of many modern drugs used for the treatment of thyroid diseases, *Potentilla alba* L. does not produce any unfavourable side effects" (Smyk and Krivenko 1975). Cinquefoil is rich in the glycoside aucubin, which has a verified effect against the hormone prolactin (Phytochem DB), elevated levels of which are associated with autoimmunity.

PERSONAL AND PROFESSIONAL USE

Cinquefoil tea is a first-rate astringent that I have found to be quite serviceable for soreness in the oral cavity.

I also find cinquefoil to be most effective for rotavirus infections in children. Here I use the tincture—a few drops diluted in a bit of fluid that will not exacerbate diarrhea, such as flat mineral water or, better yet, a tea of fragrant giant hyssop, which is also excellent for gastrointestinal infections (see page 120). I will also use drops of the tincture in a tea of fragrant giant hyssop for use as a wash or as a compress for oral thrush.

I frequently include cinquefoil in formulas to reduce hyperhidrosis (excessive sweating), usually with good results. Finally, I've had many clients with Graves' disease for whom this herb—in combination with others that may include bugleweed (page 52), lemon balm, motherwort (page 156), or self-heal (page 201)—has enabled total and permanent resolution of this serious autoimmune disorder after only nine to eighteen months of use.

CAUTIONS

Due to cinquefoil's high tannin content, neither the plant nor its extracts should be used (especially as a simple) for an extended period of time in high amounts. ⤺

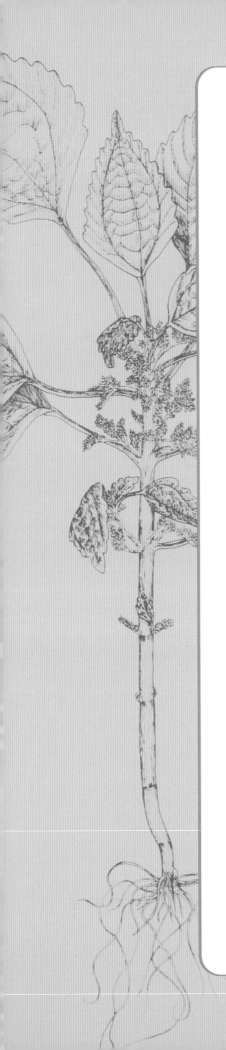

Clearweed

RICHWEED

Pilea pumila

DESCRIPTION

Clearweed is an annual herb that grows 3–24 inches high. Tending to grow in colonies, it is related to the well-known stinging nettle (see page **226**) and therefore looks a lot like that herb. It lacks the stinging hairs, however.

The stem is translucent and juicy. The opposite, smooth, lustrous, egg-shaped, coarsely toothed leaves grow 1–5 inches long. They each have three conspicuous veins.

As with stinging nettle, clearweed's tiny green flowers are clustered in the plant's axils. They are of a darker green color than are nettles', however, and are short, curved, and drooping.

RANGE AND HABITAT

Clearweed thrives throughout much of the Midwest, often growing in large colonies. For habitat, it prefers three things: rich soil, moisture, and shade. If you come across this combination of particulars, you may well find clearweed.

SEASONAL AVAILABILITY

Clearweed is available from July through mid-October.

MAJOR CONSTITUENTS

No data available.

FOOD

Foraging author Steve Brill recounts meeting a family that had been digging and eating clearweed plants all summer long under the mistaken impression that it was stinging nettle! (Brill and Dean 1994: 243) Prior to this encounter, Brill had always assumed that clearweed was inedible, in harmony with the impression given by most foraging authors. However, writing in the 1940s, Merritt Lyndon Fernald and Alfred Kinsey had opined that clearweed might prove to be a genuine wild edible since a related species had long been heartily consumed in Asia (Fernald and Kinsey 1958: 166). Euell Gibbons, in personal experiments with our American species during the 1960s and 1970s, found this to be the case but said that palatability depended upon our native *Pilea* being cooked only briefly, as is necessary with its close relative, stinging nettle. He discovered the taste to be rather bland but suggested that that characteristic could prove to be valuable in a vegetable medley to offset the taste of stronger greens (Gibbons and Tucker 1979: 73).

HEALTH/MEDICINE

Little is known about this succulent plant. However, several Native American tribes have a history of using it.

The Cherokee have found that an infusion of clearweed makes a fine pacifier for children with **excessive hunger** (Hamel and Chiltoskey 1975: 53). (This may suggest that this plant possesses an unusually high content of protein, like stinging nettle—see page **226**.) They have also rubbed the herb's stems between **itching toes**. If such itching is owing to **athlete's foot**, as seems likely, one wonders whether clearweed might possess some sort of *antifungal* potential.

The Iroquois have inhaled juice squeezed from the stem to alleviate **sinus problems** (Herrick 1977: 308; Herrick 1995: 133). The plant's *anti-inflammatory* potential, demonstrated in a 1976 lab study (Benoit et al. 1976: 164), could be a major factor in its ability to soothe troubled sinuses. However, as recurrent sinus infections have been demonstrated by scientists to be connected with a fungus in the sinuses, could this be yet another clue that clearweed may exert antifungal activity?

PERSONAL AND PROFESSIONAL USE

I frequently consume up to two handfuls of raw clearweed plants on my forays into open, wet woods from July through October. The taste is strong—but, to my palate, enjoyable.

In my clinical practice, I've used clearweed as an ingredient in sinus support formulas, with favorable testimony. I have one client who adds a few drops of the tincture to the salt-and-water mixture she uses in her neti pot, concluding that it works better to keep her sinuses clear than just the salt-and-water mixture alone.

On one occasion, I used a few drops of juice squeezed from a clearweed stem as a topical treatment to a long-standing fungal infection in the outer portion of an ear canal, to good effect: the rash faded, and the itching subsided.

These results suggest to me that clearweed may indeed exert antifungal effects. It would be interesting to see scientific studies designed to test that hypothesis.

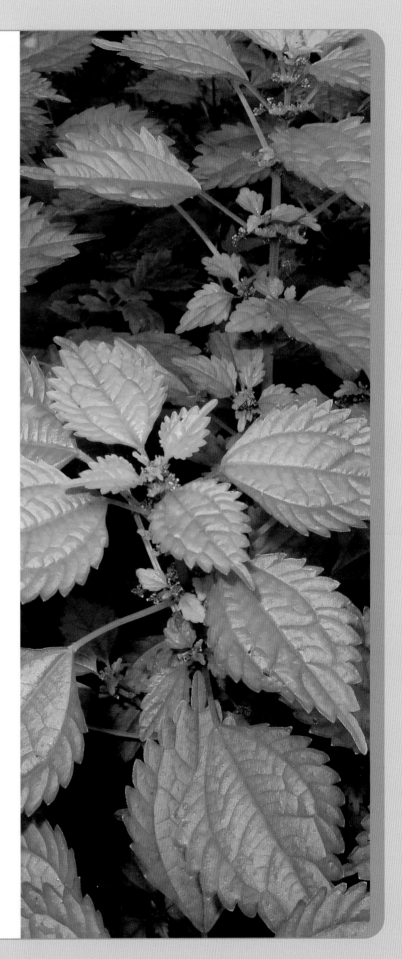

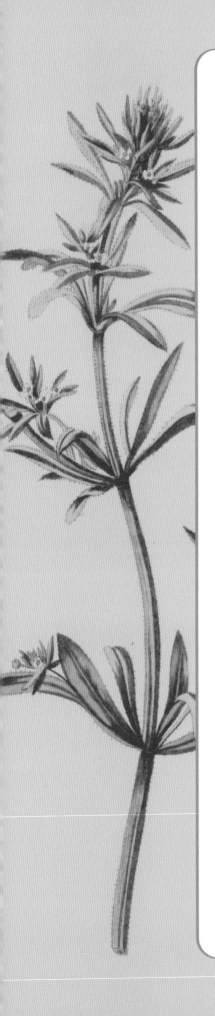

Cleavers

Galium aparine

DESCRIPTION

This is an annual weed growing 1–6 feet tall. It possesses weak, square stems that frequently latch on to other plants (especially bushes) for support, so that this herb is often appropriately referred to as a "climber." Cleavers often grows in colonies, forming clumps.

Whorls of six to eight leaves appear every so often along the stem. These leaves are narrow and lance shaped, grow ½–3 inches long, and are nearly sessile. They are rough all over because they are covered with many tiny, backward-hooked bristles (likewise with the stem, which has four rows of these tiny hooks).

Clusters of two or three very small white flowers appear on stalks arising from the leaf axils. Star-like and four-petaled, they lack sepals.

The blossoms are replaced by twinned fruits in summer. These are covered by hooked bristles, which cling easily to clothes and to fur. The burs are globular in shape.

RANGE AND HABITAT

Cleavers is a cosmopolitan weed, found throughout the United States and in Canada from Newfoundland to British Columbia. Its preferred habitat is rocky woods and rich thickets, meadows, fence rows, trailsides, roadsides, and waste places (usually in partly shaded areas).

SEASONAL AVAILABILITY

Cleavers is available from spring through autumn, but the seeds are obtainable only from late summer onward.

MAJOR CONSTITUENTS

Cleavers contains the iridoid glycosides asperuloside (rubichloric acid) and monotropein; benzylisoquinoline alkaloids (including protopine); quinazoline alkaloids; coumarins; starch; citric, caffeic, gallic, salicylic, tannic, *p*-hydroxybenzoic, and *p*-coumaric acids; *n*-alkanes; and flavonoids (including luteolin). Nutrients include high amounts of vitamin C.

Anthraquinones occur in the roots.

FOOD

Cleavers can be eaten as a potherb but must be boiled or steamed longer than other plants (more than fifteen minutes) so as to reduce the toughness of the barbed stems.

The bristly autumn fruits of this plant make an excellent dry-roasted coffee substitute. This is not surprising, in that cleavers belongs to the coffee family! One proceeds by first baking the fruits at 275–375 degrees Fahrenheit till brown, then grinding them with a grinder, blender, or mortar and pestle. Next, about ¾ cup of the ground fruits is simmered in 1 quart of water until the water turns dark brown. When finally ready, the caffeine-free coffee substitute is strained and served. In a camping or survival situation, one can improvise by simply grinding the seeds between rocks, placing the meal in a drink container, pouring boiling water over it, and steeping for about fifteen minutes.

HEALTH/MEDICINE

Cleavers is a powerful *antiscorbutic*, due to its high vitamin C content, and is a renowned *diuretic blood purifier*, working in conjunction with the lymphatic system. This herb is considered to be one of the finest *tonics for the lymphatic system* and one of the few that is safe for children. Cleavers stimulates this system, helping it to eliminate toxins and wastes via excretion through the urine. It is one of the best herbs for so-called "swollen glands" (i.e., **swollen lymph nodes**) and even helpful for more heavyweight afflictions such as **tonsillitis**, **lymphedema**, **lymphadenitis**, and **scrofula**. Interesting, in the latter regard, is that a 1954 study found cleavers to exhibit significant activity against the **tuberculosis** bacterium (Fitzpatrick 1954: 530). In China, it is even used to treat **leukemia** (EthnobDB).

Strong *anti-inflammatory* activity with relation to the urinary tract has been demonstrated for cleavers, and the plant has a long history of use by Native American tribes in this regard, including the Micmac, Ojibwe, and Penobscot (Moerman 1986: 1:192). This ability, coupled with its diuretic potential, has allowed the plant to be frequently employed for the alleviation of **cystitis** and **scalding** or **bloody urine**;

in these cases, it is recommended to be taken about one hour before meals (Moore 1979: 57). It is even used in cases of **urine stoppage** (Ellingwood 1983: 432), in which capacity it has been particularly appreciated by the Flambeau Ojibwe (Smith 1932: 386). A nineteenth-century Eclectic physician had elucidated here: "The first use of *Galium* is to relieve irritation of the urinary apparatus, and increase the amount of urine. ... One of our best remedies. In dysuria and painful micturition, it will frequently give prompt relief" (Scudder 1870: 126). Not surprisingly, then, the plant is also famed as an aid to the reduction of **gravel**. Teaspoonful doses of the juice have also been implemented in the East Indies to help treat **gonorrhea** (Tierra 1988: 221), as was done in bygone days by the Micmac, the Penobscot, and other Native American tribes (Moerman 1986: 1:192).

A tea made from cleavers is held to be one of the best skin washes for **psoriasis**, **dandruff**, and other **dry-skin conditions**. (The *British Herbal Compendium* lists it as official medicine in this regard.) The Iroquois even use it as part of a topically applied compound infusion to soothe **poison ivy rash** (Herrick 1977: 439; Herrick 1995: 219). The Eclectics found it indicated for "nodulous growths or deposits in skin

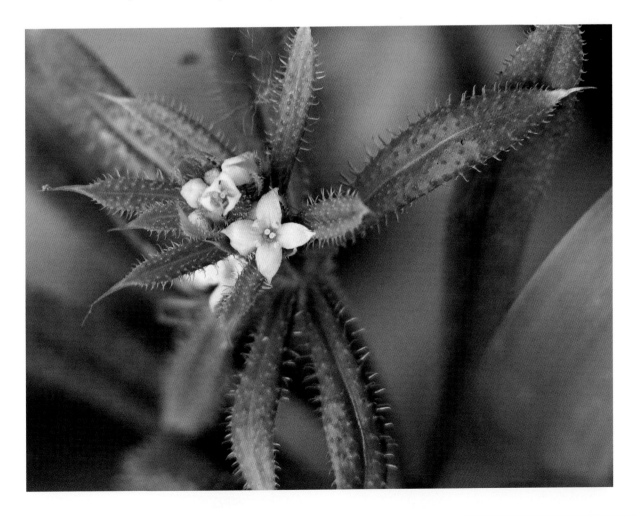

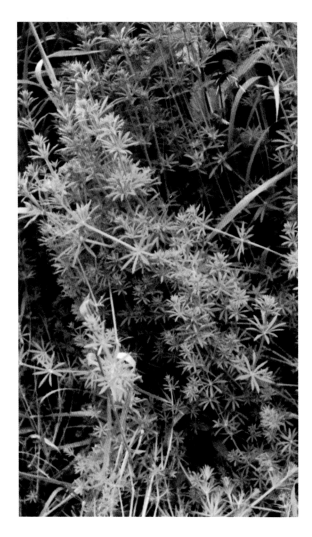

Astringent factors are likewise responsible for its traditional use in halting **diarrhea**. Nicholas Culpeper noted that a cleavers poultice worked well as a *styptic* (Potterton 1983: 48), undoubtedly due to the astringent principles in the plant but also probably to its asperuloside content. Various Native American tribes (including the Micmac and the Penobscot) also implemented the herb to stop the "spitting up of blood" that sometimes occurred after a messenger's long run (Moerman 1986: 1:192).

Modern herbalists hold cleavers to be helpful with **liver problems** and thus sometimes include it in herbal regimens for **hepatitis**. Moore noted that it is not irritating to the liver in such a case, unlike most other hepatics (Moore 1979: 57).

Herbalists of earlier times found cleavers to be helpful in the reduction of **obesity**. For example, John Gerard, writing in the late 1500s, commented: "Women do usually make pottage of clevers with a little mutton and otemeale, to cause lankness and keepe them from fatnesse" (Gerard 1975: 963–64). Culpeper concurred (Potterton 1983: 48). A few modern herbalists, such as the famed Alabama herbalist Tommie Bass (Crellin and Philpott 1990a: 155, 235), revived this tradition, often combining (or interchanging) cleavers with chickweed, which was also implemented in bygone days for weight reduction (see page **75**). The principle or principles involved here have not been isolated, but possibly with *Galium* it is as Eleanor Viereck suggests—that the acids in cleavers may serve to speed up the metabolism of the body's stored fats (Viereck 1987: 19).

Truly, the herb's applications are legion. Culpeper maintained that cleavers juice, droppered into the ears, relieved the pain of **earache** (Potterton 1983: 48). Numerous herbalists say that drinking a cup of cleavers tea before bed promotes sound, restful sleep; thus, it is recommended for **insomnia** (Grieve 1971: 1:207). A cleavers infusion applied to the armpits has been held to be an effective *deodorant*. A study done in the 1940s found that our herb had a *hypotensive* effect when administered intravenously to dogs (Delas et al. 1947: 57).

As is apparent from the above, cleavers is an interesting and widely applicable herb. Notably, the effects are clearly strongest if the plant is used by way of an infusion as opposed to a tincture (Scudder 1870: 126). Here, too, the use of the fresh herb is preferable. If the dried herb is used, it must be infused for at least two hours (Gunn 1859–61: 776).

PERSONAL AND PROFESSIONAL USE

I've had numerous occasions to use cleavers relative to its classic lymphatic, urinary, and dermatological indications as elaborated above. I find it to be helpful—especially if used with other, synergistic herbs in a formula. (However, it works fine by itself for scalding urine and for many nodulous growths.) ⪦

or mucous membranes" (Felter and Lloyd 1898). Scudder, as one of such, even pointed out that "a case of hard nodulated tumor of the tongue, apparently cancerous, is reported in the *British Medical Journal* as having been cured with it" (Scudder 1870: 126).

A renowned *refrigerant* herb, cleavers is appreciated in most conditions that require cooling. For example, the plant makes a soothing wash for **sunburn**. It is also revered as a *febrifuge*, a use frequently employed by the Mazatec of Mexico. The Eclectic physician Finley Ellingwood noted here that it "impresses the temperature greatly, stimulates the excretion of all urinary constituents and the fever is shortened by its use" (Ellingwood 1983: 432). The combination of its refrigerant nature and its *astringent* factors (owed to a high tannin content) renders this herb useful as a poultice for **burns** and for **scalds**. Michael Moore offered the thought that slow-healing burns might heal better if soaked in a tub of cleavers tea; he also added that such a bath is often helpful for **inflamed stretch marks** (Moore 1979: 57).

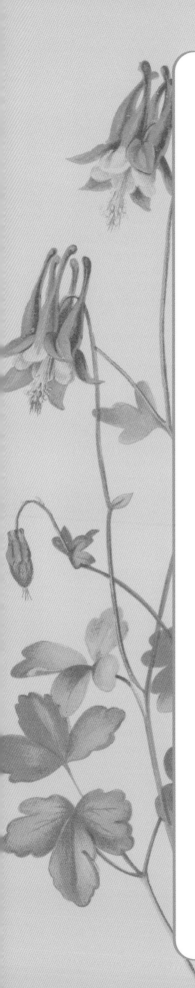

Columbine

DESCRIPTION

This is a lovely native perennial plant, growing 1–3 feet tall.

Columbine's long-stalked leaves reach a length of 4–6 inches. They are compound, each being divided into three leaflets and then subdivided into three more. They occur both basally and as scattered along the stem.

The gorgeous blossoms, situated singly on slender stalks arising from the leaf axils, give the appearance of drooping bells. Growing 1–2 inches long, they are composed of five yellow-and-red funnel-shaped petals and five long, red tubular sepals. The latter are spurred and terminate in a knob. Five yellow pistils, along with numerous stamens, extend beyond the length of the petals.

RANGE AND HABITAT

Columbine thrives in partial shade throughout the Midwest in environs such as open woodlands, forest edges, rocky cliffs, and clearings.

MAJOR CONSTITUENTS

The flowers are rich in flavonoids. The leaves contain isocytisoside and other flavonoids and most likely cyanogenic glycosides, which occur in *A. vulgaris,* the Old World cousin of our species. (The flavonoid content in the flowers of the two species has been found to be identical, suggestive of a very close chemical profile overall between them, as indeed typically occurs between species of the same genus.) The root of *A. vulgaris* contains alkaloids, including aquileginine, berberine, magnoflorine, and others. These most likely occur in *A. canadensis* as well, and for the same reason as explained above, but also given the historical applications of the root, as described below, and with the clarification provided there.

HEALTH/MEDICINE

The Pawnee have crushed and dried columbine seeds and then steeped the powder as a treatment for **fever** (Gilmore 1991: 30). Likewise, America's Eclectic physicians of the late 1800s and early 1900s found the root to be *diaphoretic* (Smith 1932: 383). Scientific research since these times has confirmed that at least the seeds possess this property and has also evinced that the leaves and the stems are *diuretic* and *antiscorbutic* (Mockle 1955: 41). As to the latter, the Iroquois steeped a handful of the roots in 1 quart of water and imbibed 6 ounces of this tea three times a day to treat **kidney problems** (Herrick 1995: 119). Then, too, the Meskwaki (Fox) in the Midwest have included columbine in a compound herbal formula for "when the contents of the bladder are thick" (Smith 1928: 238–39).

The Cherokee have valued columbine for **flux** (Hamel and Chiltoskey 1975: 30). The Meskwaki have likewise chewed the root for **stomach and bowel troubles** and boiled the leaves and root into a tea to treat **diarrhea** (Smith 1928: 238). The Pillager Ojibwe have similarly considered columbine root to be invaluable for **stomach troubles** (Smith 1932: 383). Members of the Gosiute tribe yearned for a decoction of the roots when they were "sick all over" or when presenting with **abdominal pains** (Chamberlin 1911: 563). Of

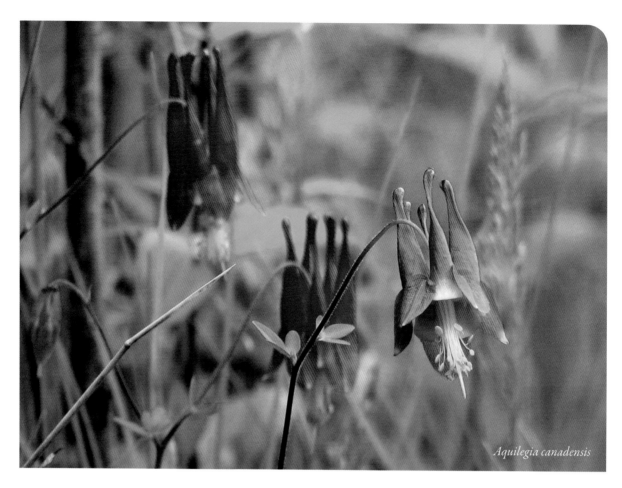

Aquilegia canadensis

possible interest in the above regard is that the scientific panel known as German Commission E affirmed that the European species, *A. vuglaris*, is a *cholagogue* (Blumenthal 1998).

Some of the above-described ethnobotanical uses, too, are perhaps of significance in the light of a 1954 study that demonstrated columbine possesses *antimicrobial* activity (Fitzpatrick 1954: 530). If the roots of our North American species contain berberine, as does *A. vulgaris* (and this is most likely, given their similar chemical profile in other respects, as noted earlier), this chemical, which has been shown to be a powerful antimicrobial, may have been the factor that stymied troublesome microorganisms in the guts of those Native Americans who were afflicted with diarrhea and abdominal pains.

Finally, to control **hair-lice infestation**, some Native American tribes have rubbed the crushed seeds of this plant into the hair of one so afflicted (Foster and Duke 1990).

CAUTIONS

Our North American species of columbine is most likely possessed of cyanogenic glycosides, like its European cousin (*A. vulgaris*), and is thus potentially poisonous. The *PDR for Herbal Medicines* notes that toxicity from ingestion of the leaf preparations of *A. vulgaris* has not been observed, presumably because the level of hydrocyanic acid that is releasable from the leaves is negligible (Fleming 1998). However, it is important to bear in mind that there can be variation among species and that most authorities regard our American species as more potent than the European species. In fact, seeds of the latter are reported to have caused deaths in children (Lewis and Elvin-Lewis 1977: 30).

The above having been said, how do we explain the many and varied internal applications implemented by Native Americans, as detailed throughout this profile? First of all, it should be noted that although we know Native tribes have, in fact, used columbine internally, we don't know the circumstances; their applications may have involved preparation techniques that somehow obviate any cyanogenic effects, such as the use of dried seeds or roots only (in that cyanogenic glycosides are typically inactivated upon drying).

All things considered, it seems prudent to urge that internal applications of columbine not be implemented by the layperson. If and when such applications might become necessary, such would be most wisely undertaken *only under the direction of a seasoned herbalist who is skilled in the use of this plant.* ⋘

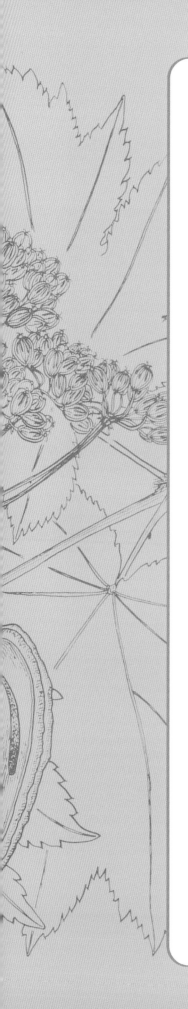

Cow-Parsnip

MASTERWORT; GIANT HOGWEED

Heracleum lanatum [alternatively, *H. maximum, H. sphondylium* ssp. *montanum*]

DESCRIPTION

This is a huge plant, topping off at 5–10 feet, with a stem that is grooved, hairy, hollow, and up to 2 inches thick at its base.

The alternate, palmate leaves are also huge, often reaching beyond 1 foot in length, and possessed of three oval leaflets. The base of the leafstalks has a large, inflated sheath, which is an important identifier distinguishing cow-parsnip from toxic plants that otherwise bear some similar features.

The tiny white flowers are arranged in flat-topped clusters that reach a diameter of 6–8 inches. The notched petals are often tinged with purple.

Cow-parsnip emits a rank odor when bruised.

RANGE AND HABITAT

This plant thrives throughout the Midwest in wet or moist soil, such as on riverbanks, lakeshores, and the borders of swamps and marshes.

MAJOR CONSTITUENTS

The aerial portions contain pimpinellin, sphondin, imperatorin, psoralen, bergapten (5-methoxypsoralen), angelicin, phellopterin, and xanthotoxin. The root contains vaginidiol, scopoletin, umbelliferone, apterin, ferulic acid, and paracoumaric acid.

FOOD

If you can get past this plant's rank odor and take a few safety precautions, you may be rewarded with some decent wild fixings. The first-year root, as one instance, is quite edible; it can be boiled or roasted, then peeled and consumed. The taste is somewhat reminiscent of a rutabaga.

Blackfoot Native Americans have also peeled and roasted the young stems (Hellson and Gadd 1974). If instead boiled, as some prefer, the spring shoots need to be cooked in two changes of water to lessen their otherwise rank taste and smell. Even thus properly prepared, a hint of rankness may remain. (But this is the wilderness, bucko—not a candy shop!)

Woods Cree tribes have peeled the leafstalks of older plants and eaten the naked petioles. They have also peeled the main stem, split it, roasted it, and then scraped out the pith, which they have then consumed (Leighton 1985: 40). The older stems do, indeed, need to be peeled before being eaten, as the peel contains furanocoumarins, chemicals that can cause blisters on the lips and the skin (Szczawinski and Turner 1980: 81; Leighton 1985: 40).

HEALTH/MEDICINE

This majestic and conspicuous plant has served a wide array of Indigenous tribes as a valuable *vulnerary*. The Inuit heat leaves and apply them to **sore muscles** and to **minor cuts** (Smith 1973: 327). So do the Quinault tribe of the Pacific Northwest (Gunther 1973: 42). The Meskwaki (Fox) of the Midwest have poulticed the stem (peeled, presumably) onto

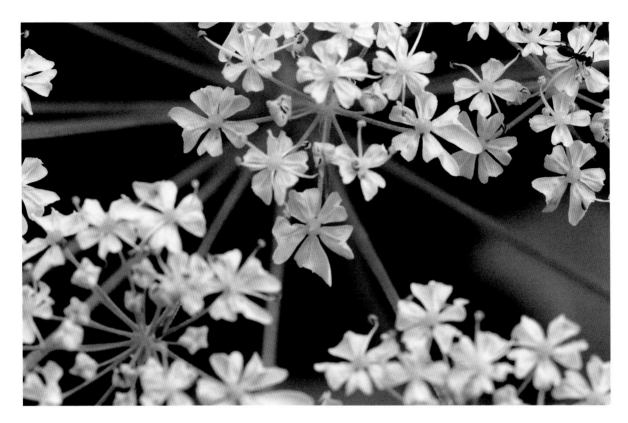

wounds (Smith 1928: 249). The Ojibwe of the Midwest have poulticed the pounded fresh roots onto **sores** (Smith 1928: 390; Smith 1932: 390). They have also used a decoction of the root as a gargle for a **sore throat** (Densmore 1974: 342–43) and applied the boiled and pulped root to **boils** to force them to a head (Densmore 1974: 350–51). The latter application has been appreciated by a wide range of tribes: The Cree and Gitksan have utilized the root for boils as well as for various swellings (Smith 1929: 61; Beardsley 1941: 484). The Pawnee have scraped the root, pounded it thoroughly, boiled it, and then applied a compress of the decoction to the painful eruption (Gilmore 1991: 55). The Bella Coola have crushed and baked the roots and then applied them to boils (Smith 1929: 61).

To relieve **gum discomfort** caused by loose teeth, the Coast Salish tribes of the British Columbia area have sprinkled powdered cow-parsnip root onto the gums (Turner and Bell 1971: 63–99). However, the Cree have appreciated its use in the case of a **toothache** per se: they have applied a 1-inch-square portion of the root to the aching tooth, making sure not to swallow any of the juice (which they have instead spit, as it is toxic) (Beardsley 1941: 491). It has also been widely used as a poultice for rheumatism. Here, a mild anti-inflammatory effect may have derived from the scopoletin content of the roots.

The plant tops have been used by the Winnebago (Ho-Chunk) as a smoke treatment for **seizures** (Gilmore 1991: 55) as well as internally (or in some cases, simply the roots were used) by the Eclectics and other physicians before them for **epilepsy** (Rafinesque 1828–30: 2:227; Scudder 1870: 138; Smith 1928: 390; Lewis and Elvin-Lewis 1977: 167). Cow-parsnip's internal application was pioneered by early American physician Joseph Orne, who found that a daily decoction of the dried and pulverized roots followed by a bedtime infusion of the dried leaves and tops prevented epileptic attacks. (Interestingly, too, Orne [1791] found that it worked best in patients who were flatulent!) Research in the 1980s verified that angelicin, a furanocoumarin found in cow-parsnip, possesses powerful antispasmodic properties (Patnaik et al. 1987). A later study found that the seed of a related species exhibited anticonvulsant activity in mice (Sayyah et al. 2005).

Undoubtedly at least partly owing to the above-delineated antispasmodic property, the root decoction has also been used internally for **colic**, **flatulence**, and **indigestion** by various Native American tribes and by the Eclectic physicians (Rafinesque 1828–30: 2:227; Smith 1928: 390; Krochmal and Krochmal 1973: 12; Hellson and Gadd 1974: 67, 76). It was even listed in the *United States Pharmacopeia* (from 1820 to 1863) in reflection of these uses. As late as 1926, in fact, the *United States Dispensatory* made note of its *carminative* property (Wood et al. 1926: 1330). The seeds are especially carminative, as well as *stomachic* and *antiemetic*.

Cow-parsnip also has been experimentally shown to possess *antifungal* properties (McCutcheon et al. 1994), so herbalists find it to be especially indicated when flatulence, colic,

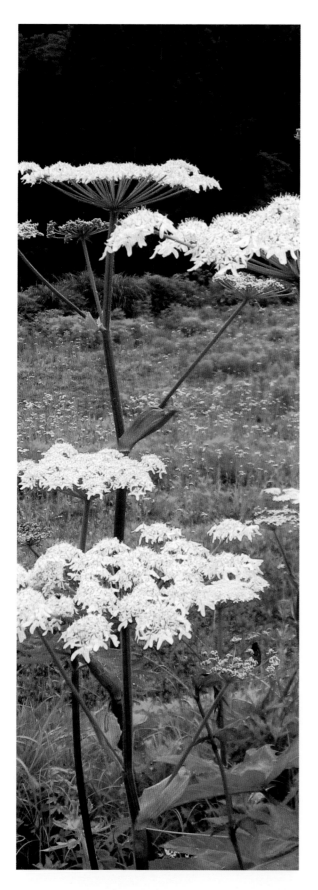

or nausea is accompanied by overgrowth of yeast or other fungi in the gastrointestinal tract.

This dovetails with what Eclectic physician Finley Ellingwood observed in 1919 about the need for cow-parsnip (or "masterwort," as the Eclectics called this herb) when the system was overloaded with filth so that "the tongue is heavily coated with a pasty coat or furred. ... The breath has a bad odor. ... The patient is, drowsy, and there is general capillary stasis." As to its effects on the system, he wrote that it "stimulates the pulse, and strengthens the capillary circulation. ... Its antispasmodic influence seems to be exercised independent of the alterative influence the agent would exercise." He further lamented that "the remedy has not received general attention" (Ellingwood 1983).

Cow-parsnip also possesses *stimulant* (Wood et al. 1926: 1330; Lust 1974: 268), *emmenagogue* (Lewis and Elvin-Lewis 1977: 330; Stuart 1982: 73), and *purgative* properties, the latter of which the Thompson peoples have especially appreciated, drinking a decoction of the root when needed (Turner et al. 1990: 45).

Finally, it has been reported that the seeds are an *aphrodisiac* (Stuart 1982: 73). Interestingly, the roots of a related species growing in far-off Nepal are similarly used (Lewis and Elvin-Lewis 1977: 328).

PERSONAL AND PROFESSIONAL USE

I always receive the most wonderful testimonials from clients when I recommend cow-parsnip seed as a carminative for troublesome intestinal gas.

I've used the plant for epilepsy accompanied by flatulence—the plant's red-letter indications—which seems to reduce the frequency and severity of the attacks. However, cow-parsnip is getting harder and harder to find on the market, necessitating that I wildcraft it nowadays, which is cumbersome and time consuming in that one must wear protective gloves to prevent the plant's juice from contacting the skin (see Cautions). As a result, I don't get the chance to use this unique and interesting plant as much as I have done on previous occasions—something that is most disappointing!

CAUTIONS

Handling the fresh plant can produce dermatitis in susceptible individuals. Exposure to the sun after handling may even result in sunburn, blistering, and possible permanent purple pigmentation due to the concentration of the plant's phototoxic chemicals (pimpinellin, bergapten, sphondin, angelicin). This plant should only be collected and processed with disposable gloves. Better yet would be to locate a tincture of the seeds from commercial sources, thereby bypassing any safety concerns.

This plant is *contraindicated during pregnancy* because of its emmenagogue potential. Its toxic potential would contraindicate its use during lactation as well. ⮜⮜

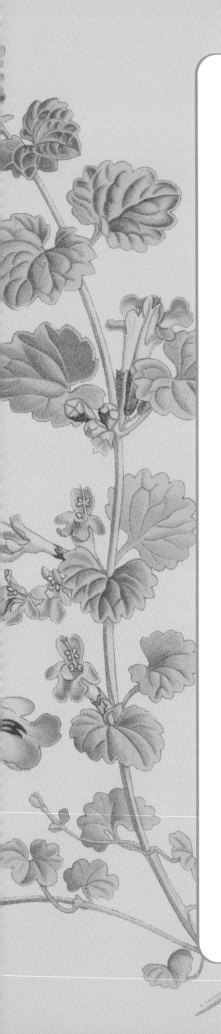

Creeping Charlie

GROUND IVY; GILL-OVER-THE GROUND; ALE HOOF

Glechoma hederacea

DESCRIPTION

Creeping Charlie—or ground ivy, as it tends to be called outside the Midwest—is an ivy-like creeper that can grow to a height of 8 inches. It bears the characteristic square stem of the mint family, to which it belongs, and it creeps owing to the fact that each of its stem nodes roots to the ground.

Like all mints, creeping Charlie's leaves are paired. In this particular case, they are also long stalked, kidney shaped, and possessed of highly scalloped margins. Growing ½–1½ inches long, they often display a purplish tinge.

Three to seven blue-violet flowers bear two-lipped corollas, also characteristic of the mint family. In creeping Charlie's particular case, however, the lower lip possesses three lobes. There are four stamens.

Like many mints, creeping Charlie emits a powerful musky mint odor when bruised—sometimes even when just brushed!

RANGE AND HABITAT

Creeping Charlie thrives in moist and shady areas throughout our region, especially in lawns, waste places, fields, moist woods, and roadsides.

MAJOR CONSTITUENTS

Creeping Charlie contains glechomine; essential oil (including borneol, limonene, pulegone, linalool, myrcene, alpha-cadinol, p-cymene, alpha-terpineol); resin; bitter principles (sesquiterpenes, including glechomafuran); flavonoids (including apigenin, rutin, luteolin); diterpene lactone (marrubiin); beta-sitosterol; caffeic, ursolic, and rosmarinic acid; and tannins. Stachyose is in the roots. Nutrients include choline, silicon, iodine, iron, sulfur, phosphorus, copper, zinc, potassium, molybdenum, and a very high amount of vitamin C.

HEALTH/MEDICINE

Who would have suspected that this aggressive, much-cursed weed that can rapidly take over Upper Midwest lawns is actually a valuable medicine? But such it is, and such are most common weeds. In fact, creeping Charlie's uses are legion, and it has been vastly appreciated and utilized by herbalists in a great many areas of the Western world.

Firstly, the *British Herbal Pharmacopoeia* notes that creeping Charlie is a specific for *tinnitus aurium*, that mysterious ringing in the ears that is increasingly affecting a wider and wider range of people, to their extreme discomfort (Hyde et al. 1976–79: 1:149). Although we tend to think of **tinnitus** as a modern condition, it really isn't; it's been with humankind for millennia! Fortunately, the use of creeping Charlie to combat it has also been traditional for quite some time. Thus, way back in the late 1500s, John Gerard observed that "ground ivy is commended against the humming noyse and ringing sound of the ears, being put into them, and for them that are hard of hearing" (Gerard 1975: 201). Herbalist David Hoffmann says that it can be used *orally* for tinnitus as well, but that it proves to be especially helpful when such is caused by catarrh (Hoffmann: 1986: 199).

Creeping Charlie, in fact, has been long revered in European herbalism for **chronic catarrh** and especially for **bronchitis** (Hyde et al. 1976–79 1:149), and it was used here in the United States by the Cherokee for **colds** (Hamel and Chiltoskey 1975). Our herb has also been popularly used in both British herbalism and Appalachian folk medicine for **moist coughs** (Bolyard 1981: 83; Bradley et al. 1992: 121) and was implemented by the Physiomedicalists for "sub-acute coughs" (Cook 1985). The plant's *expectorant* activity in these regards has variously been attributed to its content of marrubiin, flavonoids, triterpenoids, and/or essential oil (Bradley et al. 1992: 121). Creeping Charlie also *decongests* respiratory mucus with its essential oil and dries it up owing to its *astringent* powers (Ody 1993: 138, 156–57). The latter effect, attributable not only to its tannins but also to its rosmarinic acid (Newall et al. 1996: 154), lends its use as well for combating **sore throat** (Lust 1974: 212), **hemorrhoids** (Hyde et al. 1976–79: 1:149), and **diarrhea** (Lust 1974: 212; Hyde et al. 1976–79: 1:149; Kresanek and Krejca 1989: 100). Even **flatulence** is vanquished by ground ivy (Potterton 1983: 13), undoubtedly owing to the herb's essential oil.

Modern scientific research has elucidated many of these classic applications. A 1987 study utilizing the rat-paw edema test revealed *anti-inflammatory* activity for this botanical (Mascolo et al. 1987), which may accrue from any combination of its plant acids, tannins, flavonoids, and exceptional amount of vitamin C (PhytochemDB), the latter elucidating why creeping Charlie has also been a revered *antiscorbutic* (Wren 1972: 141). A 1987 study isolated a fatty acid, 9-hydroxyoctadecadienoic, which was found to regulate the adenylate cyclase activity of human platelet membranes (Henry et al. 1987). A 2002 study evinced *free-radical-scavenging* and *antibacterial* activities for our herb (Kumarasamy et al. 2002). A 2006 study found the herb to be effective against macrophage-induced inflammation in mice (An 2006). These findings may also account for some of creeping Charlie's traditional respiratory uses (Sévenet 1991). The antibacterial finding is interesting in that this herb has further been used as an aid in **tuberculosis** (de Bairacli Levy 1974: 73), and here a 1954 lab study found it to be mildly active against a virulent human strain of such (Fitzpatrick 1954: 530).

As to applications other than to the respiratory system, creeping Charlie's anti-inflammatory effects have been put to good use by means of a poultice for **contusions** (Stuart 1982: 70). *Glechoma* is a *digestive tonic* as well, largely owing to its bitter principles (Lewis and Elvin-Lewis 1977: 390). It is helpful for overall **digestive troubles** in that it stimulates digestive juices (Lust 1974: 213; Kresanek and Krejca 1989: 199). It may also serve to ease both **gastritis** and **catarrhal enteritis** (Lust 1974: 213; Hyde et al. 1976–79 1:149).

Diuretic properties can be found here as well, making it useful for **gout**, as we have noted. Creeping Charlie has also

proven its merit for **cystitis** and for certain kinds of **venereal diseases**. It is *antilithic* to **gallstones** and has long been used by country folk for **jaundice**.

Our herb's uses do not stop here, however. Kentucky folk medicine has long mixed a small amount of creeping Charlie with catnip (see page **69**) for relieving "bull hives" on children, characterized by red spots on the face and a cross disposition (Bolyard 1981: 82–83). Alabama herbalist Tommie Bass used a tea of the fresh or dried leaves for **nervous headaches** (Crellin and Philpott 1990a: 238). European herbalism has long appreciated that the plant helps to expel a **retained placenta** (de Bairacli Levy 1974: 73). Herbalist Susun Weed writes of her own and others' experiences in using the plant to expel the afterbirth in both humans and animals, where a dose of 1 cup of the infusion or ⅓ to 1 teaspoon of the tincture has typically been given to (human) mothers immediately after giving birth (Weed 1986: 70). Scientific research has also confirmed *antitumor* effects, attributable to the plant's content of ursolic and oleanolic acids (Ohigashi et al. 1986; Tokuda et al. 1986).

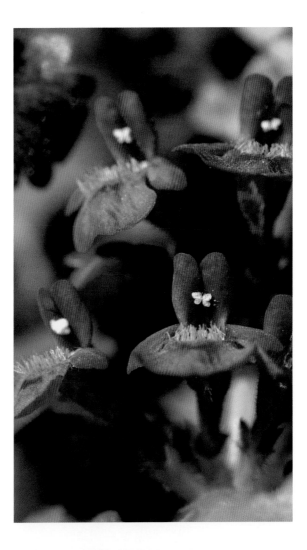

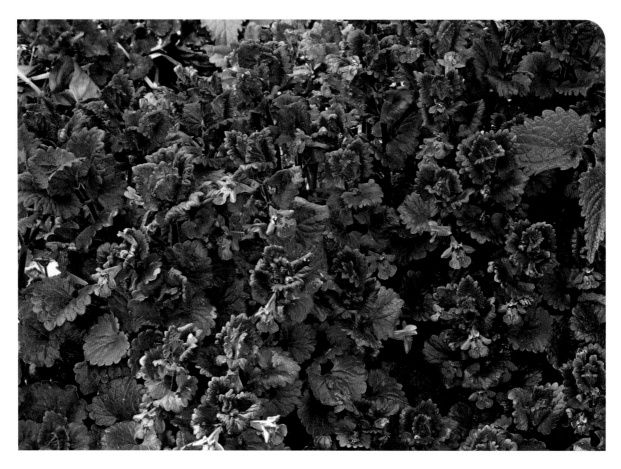

Probably creeping Charlie's most unusual application has been for offsetting **lead poisoning**, for which an infusion of the fresh plant has been used, drunk a wineglassful at a time and taken fairly frequently (Grieve 1971: 2:443; Bolyard 1981: 83; Carse 1989: 104). Amazingly, herbalists have used it for many years to great success (as confirmed by laboratory results) with painters and others who have manifested this insidious poisoning. Many have assumed that the plant's high vitamin C content explains its results in this regard (e.g., Dobelis et al. 1986: 204), and a monograph in the *Journal of the American Medical Association* powerfully underscored the value of ascorbic acid in reducing levels of lead in the blood (Simon and Hudes 1999). Other plants with an even higher content, however, do not appear to exert the same effect. I would guess, then, that at least one other chemical in the plant must either enhance or augment the vitamin C effect.

PERSONAL AND PROFESSIONAL USE

I've always marveled at the anticatarrhal effect achieved by this herb, especially with reference to fluid accumulation in the ears. Here I usually recommend oral use of 10–40 drops of a tincture mixed half and half with plantain (see page 180), sometimes advising that 1 or 2 drops of the mixture be put into the ears as well—but only if the problem persists, which it seldom does!

I've had occasion to use creeping Charlie to chelate lead out of the system as well, with three different people. On the first two occasions, it worked marvelously, confirmed by hair analysis done before and after treatment. On the third occasion, it seemed to be working up to a certain point, but when the hair analysis was eventually repeated, it revealed an even *greater* content of lead than previously—a mystery, until careful questioning revealed that the client was unwittingly reexposing himself to large amounts of lead dust periodically through his line of work!

CAUTIONS

Don't use creeping Charlie (ground ivy) if pregnant or lactating. It has also traditionally been contraindicated for persons afflicted with epilepsy.

The plant contains an irritant oil that is toxic to horses (Fuller and McClintock 1986: 181–82). Some authorities say that potentially harmful effects are increased after the first frost. Persons who use creeping Charlie would best not collect it after the first frost and should always stay within standard dosing: for the infusion, that would be ½ cup three to four times a day and for the tincture, 30–40 drops three times a day. ⤛

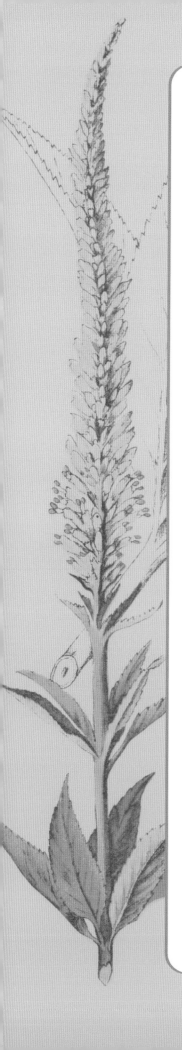

Culver's Root

Veronicastrum virginicum [formerly *Leptandra virginica*]

DESCRIPTION

This attractive plant is a tall (2–7 feet), striking, native perennial that tends to branch at the top.

The leaves are lanceolate and sharply toothed and typically grow 2–6 inches long. They are short stalked and arranged in whorls at intervals along the stem in groups of three to eight. (The plant's very bottom leaves are often in pairs, however.)

The tiny (¼-inch-diameter) flowers are creamy white, tube-like, and possessed of four to five fused petals with an equal number of pointed green sepals. Two conspicuous stamens extend beyond the length of the petals, possessing yellowish to reddish-brown tips.

Many of the flowers are arranged in one to five vivid, terminal, spiked clusters that tend to taper at their tips. Owing to the beauty and unusual design of these racemes, Culver's root is often a plant of choice in prairie restoration programs.

RANGE AND HABITAT

Culver's root tends to grow in colonies in moist meadows, mesic prairies, open savannas, rich woods, thickets, and railroad rights-of-way. It can be found scattered throughout the Midwest but seems to be more heavily concentrated in the southern portion.

MAJOR CONSTITUENTS

Culver's root contains bitter principle (leptandrin), resin, essential oil, phytosterols, saponins, citric acid, cinnamic acid, paramethoxycinnamic acid, tannin, and D-mannitol.

HEALTH/MEDICINE

Culver's root is a classic and most effective *hepatic*. It is most specific for **torpidity of the liver**, especially when associated with **headache** (Clymer 1973: 147; Ellingwood 1983: 312). The Eclectic physician Finley Ellingwood noted here: "It certainly increases the discharge of bile and stimulates and gently improves the function of the liver" (Ellingwood 1983: 312). For such purposes, it was at one time official in the *United States Pharmacopeia* (from 1820 to 1840 and from 1860 to 1916) and in the *National Formulary* (from 1916 to 1955). However, Culver's root can resolve not only a situation involving too little bile but also one involving too much of it, serving to rid the body of its excess, as the Iroquois discovered (Herrick 1995: 217). This is because when one is "all biled up," as the British say, stimulating the flow of bile will also stimulate its elimination via the intestines. Interestingly, the cinnamic acid found in Culver's root has indeed been shown in lab experiments to act as a *choleretic*, thus shedding a spotlight on the herb's traditionally understood effects on the flow of bile (Galecka 1969; Das et al. 1976; Fleming 1998).

Culver's root has likewise proven its mettle for **cholecystitis** and for **nonobstructive jaundice** (the latter especially when accompanied by pale and dry skin, a thick-coated tongue, and moderate liver pain: Moore 1994b: 9.9). It can also be of aid in **hepatitis** (Tilgner 1999: 56), and it is specific for this condition when it is accompanied by hot skin, cold feet, abdominal congestion, a white-coated tongue, bad breath or a bad taste in the mouth, and pain in the right hypochondrium that is referred to either shoulder

(Moore 1994b: 8.7). Malaise is also present, while the conjunctivae of the eyes are yellowish.

This herb has a cherished reputation as a *laxative* as well (Fleming 1998). It is a specific for constipation with symptoms of liver congestion (Hyde et al. 1976–79: 2:225). Although the fresh root is violently purgative, the dried root is a gentle laxative that removes excessive mucus from the gastrointestinal tract and stimulates liver function to soften stool and to increase peristalsis (Smith 1999: 28). Herbalist David Lytle says that in his experience, the most effective dose of the tincture is 2 drams (¼ ounce) mixed with an equal part of neutralizing cordial. With this dosage, he says, the stools are softened without watery discharge, cramps, or other discomforts (Lytle 1992: 103). Even the dried root, however, can be cathartic in high doses (1 gram or more) (Fetrow and Avila 1999: 80). This latter effect has sometimes been sought by Native American tribes, including the Seneca (Lewis and Elvin-Lewis 1977: 284) and our own area's Menomini and Ojibwe (Smith 1923: 54–55; Densmore 1974: 346–47). The latter group accomplishes such a task by steeping five roots of Culver's root in 1 quart of water to make a tea.

As to the herb's physiological effects, the Eclectic physician John Scudder explained: "The Leptandra exerts a gentle stimulant influence upon the entire intestinal tract, and its associate viscera, and in medicinal doses strengthens functional activity. Its action in this direction is so persistent that it might be called a gastrointestinal tonic" (Scudder 1870: 151). Herbalist Ed Smith notes that it can be beneficial with atony of the gastrointestinal tract, even serving to restore lost function (Smith 1999: 28). The late, great herbalist Michael Moore found it to be of value in **dyspepsia**, especially when such was connected with indigestion of fats and/or of proteins (Moore 1994b: 10.9). Charles Fetrow and Juan Avila note that the herb has been shown to exert an inhibitory effect upon the gastric enzyme system, thus resulting in *antisecretory* and consequent *antiulcer* effects (Fetrow and Avila 1999: 80).

The Meskwaki (Fox) found Culver's root to be helpful for **urinary gravel** and even to stymie **fits** (Smith 1928: 247). The Dakota and Winnebago (Ho-Chunk) discovered that it was helpful in treating snakebite (Andros 1883: 118).

CAUTIONS
Not to be used in pregnancy or where there is bile-duct obstruction, such as gallstones.

The fresh root is toxic. Only dried roots (aged one year) are to be used. ⤺

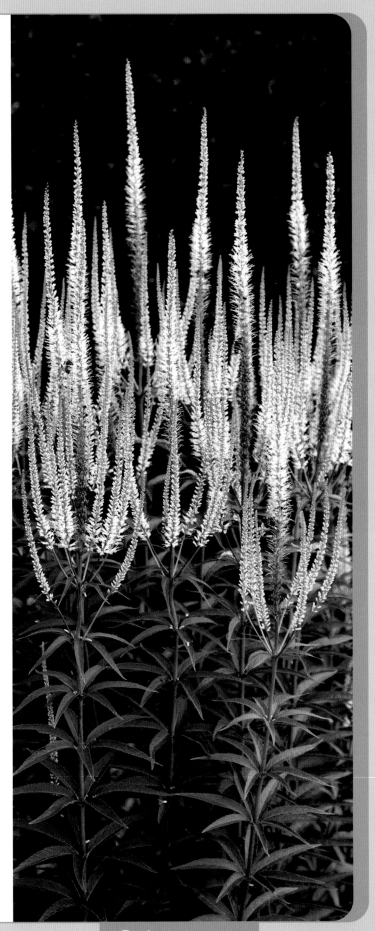

Culver's root

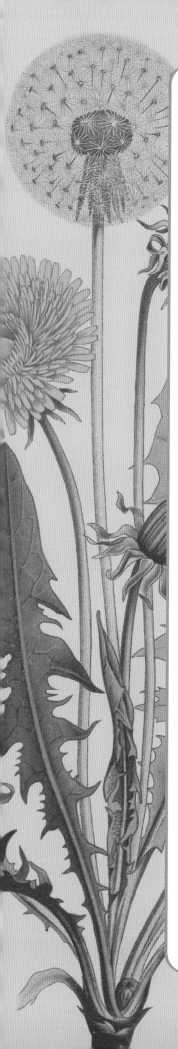

Dandelion

LION'S TEETH; PISS-A-BED

Taraxacum officinale

DESCRIPTION

It is highly doubtful that a description of this plant is needed, but for the sake of consistency, here goes: a biennial or perennial herb growing 2–18 inches tall, the dandelion has a thick taproot and an unbranched, hollow stem that exudes a milky, latex-like juice when broken or cut.

Leaves are entirely basal, forming a rosette. They are oblong, 3–16 inches long, ½–5½ inches wide, and pinnately lobed so that the teeth are coarse (although when young, the leaves are almost entire). Like the stem, the leaves exude a milky juice when damaged.

The blossom is a composite flower, opening only on sunny days. It is solitary and sits at the tip of the stalk. Its strap-shaped ray flowers are a golden yellow, and each is possessed of a five-notched tip (the flower's petals). There are one hundred to three hundred of these ray flowers per flower head.

Conspicuous bracts rest underneath the flower head. These are brown to green, thin, pointed, and reflexed downward.

The eventual fruits are dry, one-seeded structures, each attached to a feathery tuft. Together, they form a conspicuous, globular head that gives the impression of a delicate silky ball. Eventually, they release themselves to the slightest wind, whereby they are blown hither and thither.

The dandelion can be differentiated from a number of lookalikes by four characteristics taken together: (1) a milky sap, (2) reflexed bracts, (3) an unbranched flower stem, and (4) leaves that are only slightly pubescent as opposed to being blatantly hairy.

RANGE AND HABITAT

As is well known, the dandelion is a cosmopolitan weed, growing throughout the United States except in its extreme southeastern portions. The preferred habitat consists of fields, pastures, roadsides, wasteland, disturbed sites, and lawns (in which latter habitat they should be treasured, not cursed; cultivated, not exterminated; and utilized, not discarded).

SEASONAL AVAILABILITY

For medicinal uses, the root is collected in the fall, when the inulin content is highest. For food use, the leaves, crown, and roots are collected in the spring or in the fall, depending on personal preferences as to bitterness.

MAJOR CONSTITUENTS

Dandelion flower contains lecithin, beta-amyrin, and carotenoids (flavoxanthin, cryptoxanthin, violaxanthin). The leaves contain phytosterols (including beta-sitosterol); triterpenes (beta-amyrin, taraxol, taraxerol); sesquiterpene lactones (eudesmanolides); hydroxycinnamic (phenolic) acids (cichoric, chlorogenic, caffeic); organic acid (tartaric acid); coumarins (esculin, cichoriin); and flavonoids (luteolin, apigenin). The roots contain sesquiterpene lactones (both eudesmanolides and germacranolides, including taraxacin); an essential oil (largely consisting of triterpenes such as taraxol and taraxerol); taraxacerine; phenolic acids; fatty acids (palmitic, linoleic, linoleic, stearic, oleic, myristic, lauric); phytosterols (stigmasterol, beta-sitosterol); asparagine; inulin (up to 40 percent in autumn-harvested samples!); flavonoids (luteolin, apigenin); fructose (up to 18 percent in spring samples); coumarins (esculin, cichoriin); mucilage; levulin; tannin; pectin; and the enzyme tyrosinase. Nutrients include pro-vitamin A (up to 7,100 imperial units per cup of fresh greens!) and vitamins B_1, B_2, B_3, choline (only in the root), C, and D and minerals such as calcium, magnesium, zinc, boron (only in the leaf), selenium, and silicon in moderate amounts; there is an especially high amount of iron, manganese, phosphorus, sodium, and potassium.

FOOD

People are often amazed when I tell them that the commonest of weeds, as opposed to exotic wildflowers, provide the very best in food and medicine. There could be no greater example than the common dandelion! Indeed, all parts of the plant except for the flower stalk are edible, nutritious, and very tasty. In fact, the Apache valued dandelion so highly that they would scour the surrounding countryside for days in order to satisfy their prodigious appetite for this herb.

Dandelion leaves are wonderfully tasty as a salad herb, especially if they are taken from well-shaded plants growing in rich soil. The leaves of the sunned plants, however, are sometimes too bitter. That bitterness aids digestion, but if you just can't tolerate it, look for the leaves that are not deeply toothed, since this is a visual clue that these are the ones that consistently get the most shade during the day. Also, give prime attention to those plants lacking flower heads (i.e., existing merely as rosettes), which indicates that they get a lot of shade, since sun-drenched plants will almost invariably grow a flower stalk.

Rather than merely harvesting leaves, it is often preferable to take the whole plant, not only because you may want to utilize other parts of it but also because dandelions are often gritty, and the whole plant is much easier to clean than just the leaves. Such a cleaning can be accomplished by rinsing the plants under the faucet or, often even more effectively, by dunking them up and down in a container of water.

Dandelion greens can be enjoyed as a cooked vegetable, too. Here they can be steamed in a nonaluminum pot in just enough water to cover them for about three to five minutes. Some foraging manuals urge that the usual cooking procedure for greens of immersing them in already boiling water should be reversed for dandelions, and that they should be started in cold water that is then heated to a boil. Some feel that this method most effectively removes any excess bitterness, especially if a water change—again starting with cold water—is implemented halfway through the boiling period. Bear in mind, however, that dandelion's bitterness has health benefits, as mentioned above (and discussed in more detail below), so removing all aspects of bitterness may not always be desirable.

The greens can be frozen for winter use but should first be given a two-minute blanching. Dandelions—like nettles (see page 226), chicory (page 78), and some other plants—can also be "forced" through the winter in one's house, so that one has access to a fresh crop throughout the cold season. How so? Gather some whole plants in autumn, right before the ground freezes hard, and cut the leaves back to within an inch of the root. Then, place the plants in a container filled with sand (or sandy soil) and put the whole thing away in a very dark place—a closet or basement is often ideal. Water your secreted dandelion remnants every few days. If you've performed your task with skill, you'll discover some very pale leaves emerging in just a few weeks! "Blanched" like this, they are less bitter than outdoor dandelions.

And you're not through yet: cut them back as initially and keep watering them every few days, and you may find yourself harvesting another two to three crops before winter's end! It's a lot of fun, even though it doesn't work with every plant. If you like the taste and texture of these blanched dandelions, you can also blanch the ones growing outside during the warmer seasons, too. Simply cover them with a plastic pail (or some other structure) that will block the sunshine yet allow them space to grow and thrive. In about a week, they will be paled to readiness.

The roots of dandelions are likewise edible, nutritious, and delicious. Moreover, they are a renowned survival food, having at one time kept alive the sizable population of a Mediterranean island after locusts had destroyed the cultivated food crops. Those from older plants should be peeled before being consumed, however, and such are especially tasty after being cooked. Here they can be baked (at 375 degrees Fahrenheit for about thirty minutes) or boiled (in two waters, for about twenty minutes total, with a pinch of baking soda added to the first water). After being cooked, they usually taste even better if they are chilled, in which condition one is tempted to employ them as a salad ingredient.

The roots can also be oven-roasted until dry (about four hours) and then ground and brewed into a caffeine-free coffee substitute. Many persons, however, simply prefer them raw, chopping them up and mixing them into salads. Some digestive tracts react with flatulence to the raw roots, as they contain inulin, a soluble fiber that is not digested but only metabolized in the colon (where it promotes the growth of beneficial bifidobacteria that are resident there).

The flower heads are also edible and sweetish to the taste. To remove them from their stalks, simply twist them off (as opposed to pulling or cutting them). They are most often dropped into pancake batter to add a hint of sweetness to the resultant flapjacks. They may also be eaten raw, as a trail nibble or in salads, although some find them too sweet when consumed in this fashion. (Those with known reactions to pollen should exercise caution when contemplating any consumption of flowers.) Or they can be steamed for five minutes, stirred, and then let stand for a few minutes prior to serving.

In the opinion of many, the prize dandelion part is the crown, located just under the surface of the ground where the stem and leaves meet the taproot. Cut this structure from the plant and cook it until tender (three to five minutes), then top it with your favorite dressing. (You can make your own "wild" dressing from vinegar and the seedpods of peppergrass—see page **173**.) Unlike the leaves, the crown doesn't become excessively bitter with age. Developing buds, hidden inside the crowns of new dandelions, are also cherished; these need to be boiled for just a few minutes and then can be buttered and served.

HEALTH/MEDICINE

Possessed of *cooling* and *drying* energies, this "weed" so castigated by North American civilization has so many healing benefits for humankind that the dogged attempts to eradicate it from suburban lawns are nothing short of criminal!

First, in view of its bitter sesquiterpene lactones, dandelion is a revered *tonic* for **poor digestion**, especially when attributable to **hypochlorhydria.** The sesquiterpene taraxacin has especially been demonstrated to stimulate saliva, gastric juice, and appetite (Kuusi et al. 1985). The Potawatomi, among other Native American tribes, have greatly treasured its benefits in this regard (Smith 1933: 54). The Pillager Ojibwe found a root tea helpful for **heartburn** (Smith 1932: 366). The Eclectic physician John Scudder noted that this botanical "exerts a stimulating influence upon the entire gastrointestinal tract, promoting functional activity" (Scudder 1870). An Eclectic colleague writing almost one-half century later, Finley Ellingwood, highlighted its applicability in **chronic**, **nonerosive gastritis** (Ellingwood 1983). The root has long been a staple in British herbalism for **atonic dyspepsia** coupled with **chronic constipation** (Hyde et al. 1976–79: 1:197).

A botanical that has long been relied upon by various cultures to enhance liver function, dandelion's high choline content, in conjunction with its sesquiterpene lactones, appears to be highly contributory to its revered role as a *hepatic*. Indeed, countless thousands of people throughout history have benefited from dandelion's gentle but effective nature in this regard. In the mid-nineteenth century, for instance, the American physician Asahel Clapp reported that dandelion was widely used during his time for **chronic liver disease** (Clapp 1852: 806), and it also has a long pedigree of use in this regard in Europe. Various clinical trials during the last fifty years have confirmed that dandelion can be most helpful for liver-related conditions such as **hepatitis**, **cirrhosis**, **congestive jaundice**, **chronic liver congestion**, **nonalcoholic fatty-liver disease**, and **cholecystitis** (Kroeber 1950; Faber 1958; Hyde et al. 1976–79: 1:197; Sankaran 1977; Susnik 1982; Davaatseren 2013).

Dandelion's assistance with these problems has been shown, through a variety of animal studies, to be attributable to *cholagogue* and *choleretic* abilities possessed by the plant, as herbalists have long surmised (Chabrol et al. 1931:

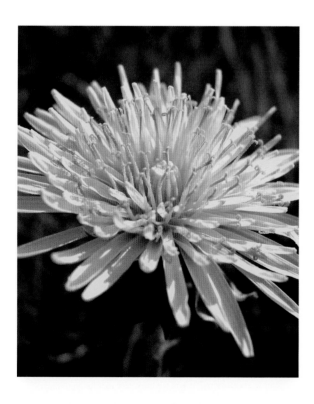

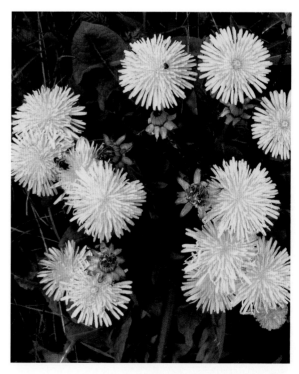

1100; Chabrol and Charonnat 1935; Bussemaker 1936: 512; Bohm 1959; Benigni et al. 1964; Popowska et al. 1975: 491).

In view of the preceding information, too, dandelion has understandably proven to be invaluable for chronic constipation, especially when associated with poor bile flow. Such a *laxative* effect, appreciated as well by the Lenape (Delaware) (Tantaquidgeon 1972: 39), seems at least partly due to the plant's essential oil (Pedersen 1998: 78).

This greatly despised lawn weed is also a treasured *depurative* for both **eczema** and **acne**, including the juvenile forms of such (Scott 1990: 56). Eclectic physicians esteemed the root as "a laxative-alterative in autointoxications giving rise to skin disorders and aphthous ulcers [canker sores]," but with the caveat that "the best preparation is an extract of the fresh root" (Niederkorn 1905; Felter 1922; Ellingwood 1983: 326). In the Physiomedicalist herbal tradition, the root has been esteemed as a helpful therapy for **eczema** and other **chronic skin diseases** (Clymer 1973: 125, 213). Likewise, in Russian herbalism, dandelion root is one of the most popular ingredients in formulas for eczema (Zevin 1997: 67). As for acne, some modern Western herbalists find the root to be more applicable to whiteheads than with red, "angry" acne.

Dandelion's effect for autointoxication seems largely to be due to its bitter flavonoids, but detoxification may also ensue owing to its content of both mucilage and inulin—which, respectively, absorb toxins and regulate the beneficial intestinal microflora that generate chemicals that kill or inhibit harmful bacteria (Pedersen 1998: 79; Winston 1999: 39). Such a regulatory function with respect to the microflora may at least partially explain the herb's help in vanquishing canker sores, since research has connected these aphthous ulcers with depressed quantities of the specific B vitamins manufactured by the colon's bifidobacteria (Wray et al. 1978; Porter et al. 1988; Palopoli and Waxman 1990; Mills and Bone 2000: 173).

Dandelion's regulatory effect upon the intestinal microflora may also explain why a clinical study revealed that the herb (in combination with lemon balm, calendula, fennel, and St. John's wort) helped sufferers of chronic, nonspecific **colitis** (Chakurski et al. 1981), in that reduced quantities of beneficial intestinal microflora have been found in colitis sufferers (Murray and Pizzorno 1998: 593). Dandelion's aid toward improving human microflora activity, coupled with a study that showed direct activity against the yeast *Candida albicans* (Duke 1985: 476), suggests that it can be an important weapon in any ongoing battle against **chronic yeast infections**.

Additionally, dandelion may directly fight colitis's inflammation, since *anti-inflammatory* effects have been verified for the plant (Mascolo et al. 1987). This makes it invaluable, as well, for other inflammatory conditions, such as **mastitis**, for which practitioners of Traditional Chinese Medicine often successfully use a compress of a dandelion-root decoction

(Yanchi 1995: 64). Still others (Hoffmann 1986: 190) use dandelion to treat **muscular rheumatism**, an application that had a long tradition in Europe and has even been recommended in the *British Herbal Pharmocopoeia* (Hyde et al. 1976–79: 1:197).

Both dandelion's leaves and its root are *diuretic* (not for nothing have the French long called dandelion *piss-en-lit*—piss-a-bed!), although studies have shown that the former are much more pronounced in this effect (Rácz-Kotilla et al. 1974). The reason (or reasons) for dandelion's diuretic effect is not known for certain. Good arguments can be presented for such an action owing to: (1) its bitter flavonoids (Pedersen 1998: 78), (2) an ability to inhibit sodium reabsorption by the kidneys (Tilgner 1999: 57), (3) its high potassium content, and/or (4) the action of its sesquiterpene lactones (Duke 1997: 83; Blumenthal et al. 2000: 80). Unlike pharmaceutical diuretics, however, dandelion leaves replace potassium lost through diuresis by means of their own rich contribution of that mineral to the system (Rácz-Kotilla et al. 1974; Hook et al. 1993). The diuretic effect, perhaps together with other actions of the plant, helps to eliminate metabolic toxins—such as uric acid, responsible for **gout** (Ellingwood 1983: 326; McQuade-Crawford 1996: 142). Dandelion leaf is also commonly used by herbalists to alleviate **edema** resulting from cardiac disorders or **hypertension** (Winston 1999: 38) and is, in fact, one of the few herbal diuretics entrusted to such a task owing to its ability to replace potassium lost through diuresis.

The diuretic effect, combined with the hepatic properties outlined above, makes dandelion the herb of choice for PMS-H, a subtype of **premenstrual syndrome** in which a woman gains five or more pounds of water weight just prior to her menstrual period. Here the plant's diuretic effect leaches out the excess fluid, while the hepatic effect helps the liver to process the estrogens causing the water retention in the first place. Further with reference to reproductive issues, herbalist Amanda McQuade-Crawford finds the root helpful for **uterine fibroids** (McQuade-Crawford 1996: 142).

Because dandelion contains generous amounts of the coumarin esculin, it can improve the quality of the veins by supporting their structure (Williams et al. 1996), so it often proves useful for **varicose veins**—including the anal form, **hemorrhoids** (Brooke 1992: 103; McQuade-Crawford 1996: 142). It has also shown *anti–platelet aggregating* action (Neef et al. 1996). Dandelion has traditionally been used to offset **dizziness** (Brooke 1992: 103; McQuade-Crawford 1996: 142) and **sleepiness** (de Bairacli Levy 1974: 57), but whether this has anything to do with stimulation of circulatory function remains unclear.

Dandelion has been used by various cultures for **pulmonary complaints.** The Meskwaki (Fox), for example, have used the herb for "pain in the chest" after the usual remedies had failed (Smith 1928: 218). A test-tube study conducted in the 1950s even demonstrated some effects against a virulent human strain of the tuberculosis organism (Fitzpatrick 1954: 531).

Extracts of dandelion have inhibited growth of **cancer** cells and have produced antibodies to tumor polypeptides (Kotobuki 1979; Kotobuki Seiyaku 1981; Salvucci et al. 1987). One study found a hot-water extract to display *antitumor* activity (Baba et al. 1981). One Asian species, *Taraxacum japonicum*, has likewise shown anticarcinogenic activity (Takasaki et al. 1999), giving credence to the widespread use of that herb for breast cancer in Traditional Chinese Medicine. (Probably dandelion's sesquiterpene lactones are a prime factor in such activity, as they have been shown to be crucial in the tumor-fighting capacities of other plants possessing them.) From 2008 to the present, PubMed displays over a dozen more studies in which either our *T. officinale* or the Chinese species *T. mongolicum* was used to beneficial effect against **prostate cancer**, **breast cancer** (including the triple-negative form), **leukemia**, **gastric cancer**, **colorectal cancer**, **pediatric cancer**, and **melanoma** (Sigstedt et al. 2008; Chatterjee et al. 2011; Ovadje et al. 2012; Oh et al. 2015; Ovadje et al. 2016; Li et al. 2017; Rehman et al. 2017; Zhu et al. 2017; Menke et al. 2018; Rahmat and Damon 2018; Saratale et al. 2018; Nguyen et al. 2019).

Dandelion has further been experimentally shown to restore damaged nitric oxide production by the body, an important factor in both bloodflow and immune function (Kim et al. 1998). It has also demonstrated *hypoglycemic* effects in lab animals (Farnsworth and Segelman 1971; Yamashita et al. 1984). This latter effect might suggest that it could have potential for treating diabetes, but another animal study showed that it only decreased blood-sugar levels in nondiabetic animals and *not* in diabetic ones (Akhtar et al. 1985).

The German physician-phytotherapist Rudolf Fritz Weiss used to give 2 cups of dandelion root, in addition to some fresh leaves as a salad, once a day to his patients suffering from chronic degenerative joint disease, substituting juniper fruits in the autumn. His clinical impression was that this program improved their joint mobility, reduced their joint stiffness, and improved their overall sense of well-being (Weiss 1988: 260–61). As noted above, dandelion manifests alterative effects, increasing the flow of both bile and urine to rid the system of toxins. (Weiss attributed its usefulness to these effects as well as to an ability to favorably influence both interstitial tissue and cell function.)

The latex in dandelion's stem and leaves has been a revered topical folk remedy for **warts**, traditionally applied three times a day for ten days, after which the wart has been observed to blacken and fall away. My own experimentation with this treatment has shown it to be useful, but not

as effective as the latex from milkweed, *Asclepias syriaca* (see page 151), another folk remedy for warts. Dandelion root, as noted above, however, contains tyrosinase, an enzyme that also occurs on the inside of overripe banana peels and is another folk remedy for warts. Here I've found that the topical application of the inner part of dandelion root is even more helpful in ridding warts than is the latex. (Milkweed's success is likewise attributed to an enzyme that it possesses.)

Dandelion root was official in the *United States Pharmacopeia* from 1831 to 1926 and in the *National Formulary* from the first edition until 1965. It was listed as *tonic*, *diuretic*, and *aperient*. The root is still official in the British, German, Austrian, and Czech pharmacopeias.

PERSONAL AND PROFESSIONAL USE
From April through November, I munch on some dandelion leaves almost daily in my forays into the wilds. I *really* love the taste!

Among its many medicinal uses, I probably use dandelion the most to offset premenstrual bloating, which typically works admirably. I also frequently use a tincture of both the root and the leaf in formulas to support optimal blood pressure in persons prone to hypertension, to stimulate hydrochloric acid and bile in persons with suboptimal digestion, and to detoxify persons afflicted with autointoxication as manifested by frequent canker sores and a geographic (or mapped) tongue.

All in all, dandelion is probably in my top twenty most commonly utilized herbs.

CAUTIONS
Never collect dandelions from lawns or other cultivated areas where herbicides or chemical fertilizers are suspected of being used.

Persons sensitive to sesquiterpene lactones who handle this plant may develop contact dermatitis. (Only a very small segment of the population is sensitive to these chemicals, which predominate in the daisy, or aster, family.)

Persons with active ulcers or acute gastritis should be aware that bitter foods such as dandelion leaves will stimulate an abundance of hydrochloric acid, which may irritate the condition.

Persons with known or suspected gallstones larger than 1.5 millimeters should avoid using dandelion root, which has the potential to move the stones into the biliary ductwork, where they could become stuck and create tremendous pain—a medical emergency known as "biliary colic."

Emaciated persons should avoid ingesting dandelion leaf or its extracts, owing to its diuretic effects. ⤺

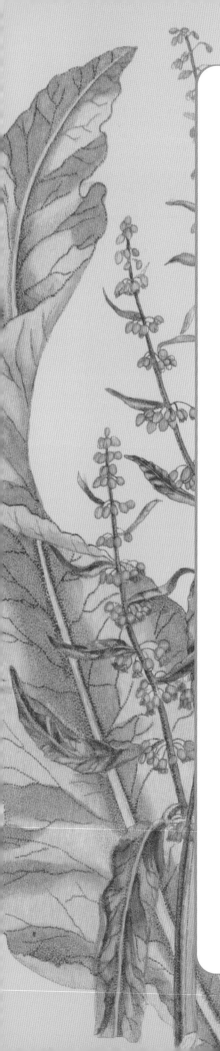

Dock

DESCRIPTION

Dock is a familiar perennial that begins life in the spring as a rosette of wavy, curly-edged leaves 4–13 inches long. The summer plant shoots up to a height of 1–5 feet, developing an upright, smooth, ribbed stem that becomes rigid and hollow as the plant fully matures. Branch stems may or may not appear. If they do, it is only toward the top of the plant.

The stem leaves are dark green, oblong to lanceolate, and pointed at the tip, growing alternately along the stem. They are about half as long as the basal leaves and display strongly curled and wavy margins, responsible for one of the plant's common names, curly dock. They show a strong vein down the central axis, with a number of veins branching off from it that angle toward the edge and then curve back to join other branch veins. Finally, a papery, straw-colored sheathing membrane can be found around the stem where the leaves attach. It is sometimes slimy to the touch.

In early summer, an abundance of tiny green flowers (with a slight reddish or purplish tinge) are densely clustered along the upper part of the stem in wand-like fashion. In late summer, these flowers transform into winged, three-angled brown achenes, reminiscent of tobacco, and present a more striking appearance than the previous green flowers.

Dock's taproot is long and carrot-like. It is noticeably yellowish red when cut open, giving rise to the plant's alternative common name of yellow dock.

RANGE AND HABITAT

This plant, castigated as a weed, is almost as ubiquitous as the dandelion. It is common to roadsides, wasteland, vacant lots, ditches, and fields throughout North America.

MAJOR CONSTITUENTS

The root contains resins; an essential oil; anthraquinone glycoside derivatives (including nepodin, chrysophanic acid, emodin, physcion); rumicin; fatty acids (stearic, palmic, erucic); sugars (fructose, dextrose); tannin; and yellow pigment. Aboveground portions contain flavonoids (avicularin, quercetin, quercitrin, hyperoside); calcium oxalate; oxalic acid; chrysophanic acid; and tannin. They also contain the following nutrients: pro-vitamin A (very high—a 100-gram portion contains 12,900 imperial units!); vitamin C (119 milligrams per 100 grams); B vitamins (niacin, riboflavin, and especially thiamine); phosphorus (41 milligrams per 100 grams); potassium (338 milligrams per 100 grams); and iron (1.6 milligrams per 100 grams); and some manganese, zinc, selenium, and sodium.

FOOD

This abundant herb is widespread and easily recognized, which is fortunate, considering that it allows for a variety of repasts.

The curled leaves can be consumed raw, sparingly—see the Cautions section—but some are too bitter, especially during certain times of the year, and any plants growing in soil known to be high in nitrates should not be eaten. Well-chosen plants, however, yield delightfully sour leaves, similar in taste to the closely related sheep sorrel, *Rumex acetosella* (see page 204).

Dock also makes a delicious cooked vegetable. To prepare it, boil the leaves in two changes of water—about five minutes in the first and about ten in the second. (The extra pot of water is necessary only if the leaves are bitter.) Recipes appear in several weed cookbooks. One recipe I especially enjoy is "Clam Soup with Dock," provided in Karl Knutsen's informative foraging manual (Knutsen 1975: 37).

Unfortunately, dock is one of those very tender wild veggies that is difficult to keep by freezing. Successful efforts relate to careful preparation. One foraging guide (Young 1993: 26) suggests cutting the dock leaves into smaller pieces, putting them into a pot with 1 cup of water for each quart of dock, bringing the water to a boil, and then cooking the contents for three minutes, stirring occasionally. Thereafter, it is suggested that the segments should be ladled into 8-ounce plastic or glass containers with 1-inch headspace and then cooled in a pan of ice water (ensuring that the ice water does not get into the containers). Finally, it is urged that the containers be capped and frozen.

The fully husked and winnowed seeds can be ground into flour for bread, but the vision of work involved is too prohibitive for most persons.

HEALTH/MEDICINE

Possessed of *cooling* and *drying* energies, yellow dock has long been regarded as a superb *alterative* and *hepatic*. Not surprisingly, then, the Southwest American herbalist Michael Moore noted that a tea made from dock root can often be of service for **bilious problems** (it has been used as such by the Oklahoma Lenape [Delaware]) and particularly for the **poor digestion of fats**. His recommended dose is a teaspoon of the chopped root, boiled (not steeped) in water, taken twice a day—but see Cautions (Moore 1977: 166). The Lenape (Delaware) have even used dock for **jaundice** (Tantaquidgeon 1972: 33).

The Cherokee found that dock, rather curiously, possesses both *astringent* and *laxative* properties (Hamel and Chiltoskey 1975: 32). The tannin-rich leaves, stems, and fruits are all astringent. Kuskokwagmiut cured persons afflicted with severe cases of diarrhea by feeding them dock leaves and stems as a potherb in the morning before any other food and also before bedtime (Oswalt 1957: 24). The root is usually thought of as laxative owing to the anthraquinone glycosides and because of the plant's favorable effect upon the liver's activation of bile. Yet because the latter also contains tannins, there is a balancing effect therefrom, which results in dock being much less powerful and irritating a laxative than other anthraquinone-containing plants, such as rhubarb (even though dock has higher anthraquinone content than that plant does), cascara sagrada, or senna. Some cultures, such as the Tarahumara (Kay 1996: 240), have even coaxed an astringent effect from the root so as to allow it to serve as an antidiarrheal as well (Kay 1996: 240). James

Duke, a former economic botanist with the US Department of Agriculture, asked whether the body, in its wisdom, might be able to choose which effects it desires, depending upon its need at the time (Duke 1985: 413).

Dock also serves as a wonderful *depurative*, and it has been made use of in this fashion by numerous Native American tribes, including the Cherokee, Lenape (Delaware; Oklahoma), Mohegan, Paiute, Rappahannock, and Shoshone (Moerman 1986: 1:421–22). The Eclectic physician Finley Ellingwood held it to be "a renal depurative and general alterative of much value when ulceration of mucus surface or disease of the skin results from impure blood" (Ellingwood 1983: 378). Even the nineteenth-century physician and botanist Laurence Johnson, who was generally critical of plant remedies in vogue among the Eclectics, acknowledged that dock's "properties render it useful in a variety of chronic affections, such as scrofula, obstinate cutaneous diseases, ... syphilis, etc., in which an alterative and depurative effect may be desired for a long time" (Johnson 1884: 238). Charles Millspaugh made note of the popular use of a dock-root ointment as a *discutient* for "indolent glandular tumors" (Millspaugh 1974: 576).

One of dock's most renowned uses, however, is as a salve for **skin rashes**, for which it has been employed by the Cherokee (Hamel and Chiltoskey 1975: 32) as well as by European American herbalists. The specific indication for its use here is a skin rash accompanied by signs of liver stagnation and constipation (Hyde et al. 1976–79: 1:171). The chrysophanic acid is thought to be the most important constituent toward the dermatological assists, and James Duke notes that as late as 1977 chrysarobin was used in orthodox medicine as a topical agent for skin disorders, proving particularly effective against **psoriasis** (Duke 1985: 415). (Chrysarobin is also widely regarded as a fungicide.) Undoubtedly, the tannins and perhaps other constituents are important in this regard as well.

In fact, yellow dock is a classic herb for **pruritus** of most any kind (McQuade-Crawford 1996: 182; Harrar and O'Donnell 1999: 81). Our own area's Ojibwe apply the powdered root via a wetted cloth to itchy areas on the skin (Densmore 1974: 350–51). Interestingly here, a mid-1980s lab study found that leaves of the related species, *Rumex nepalensis*, significantly reduced itching, which was attributed to *anticholinergic*, *antibradykinin*, and *antihistamine* properties (Aggarwal et al. 1986).

Topical application of dock has also been heralded for parasitic skin infections such as **scabies**, **ringworm**, and **urticaria (hives)**, and here it is thought that the constituent rumicin, possessive of an *antiparasitic* effect, is largely responsible (Krochmal and Krochmal 1973: 193; Stuart 1982: 128; Duke 1985: 415). An *antibacterial* effect from the anthraquinones may further explain its aid in these and other skin conditions (Anton et al. 1980). One study has shown effects against *Escherichia coli, Mycobacterium smegmatis, Shigella*

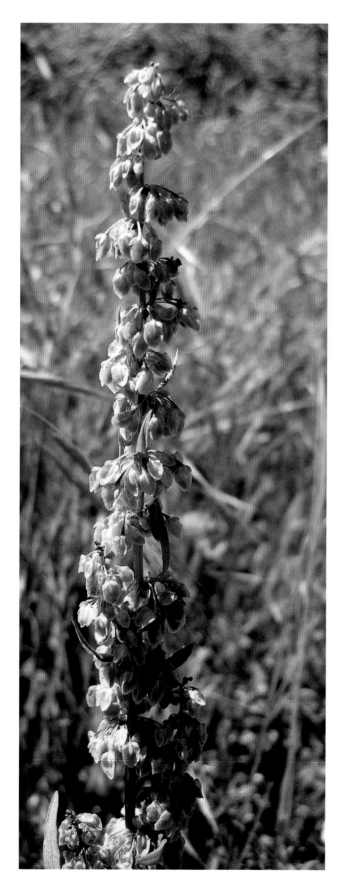

sonnei and *S. flexneri*, and *Staphylococcus aureus*, although this was from an extract of the aerial portions, not the root, and attributed to the plant's essential oil (Miyazawa and Kameoka 1983). Another study on the leaves has shown a moderate effect against a virulent human strain of the tuberculosis organism (Fitzpatrick 1954: 530).

Crushed leaves of this weed—also those of jewelweed (see page **136**), mullein (page **161**), and plantain (page **180**)—have long been held to be efficacious for relieving the **sting** produced from **nettles** and even, to some extent, the **rash** accrued from **poison ivy**. I cannot vouch for poison ivy, but my own experience has convinced me that rubbing with the leaves of this plant does relieve the sting from nettles.

A large variety of Native American tribes have employed dried, powdered dock root or leaves as a sprinkle for **cuts** and **wounds**, including the Flambeau Ojibwe (Smith 1932: 381) and tribes of the Nevada region (Train et al. 1957: 87). The Teton Dakota have crushed the plant's leaves and poulticed them onto **boils** so as to suppurate them (Gilmore 1991: 25). Undoubtedly the tannins largely account for dock's long-standing reputation as a **burn** remedy, a function likewise seized upon by various tribes, including the Paiute and Shoshone.

Astringent properties undoubtedly account as well for dock's aid in helping to heal **spongy gums** (Millspaugh 1974: 576). Thus, too, a cold infusion of the leaves swished in the mouth sometimes helps to relieve the discomfort caused by **canker sores**, which has been appreciated by the Navajo (Diné) and Ramah Navajo (Diné) (Mayes and Lacy 1989: 33). Mexican Americans sometimes gargle a root infusion to soothe a **sore throat** (Kay 1996: 240).

Exciting new research out of Korea suggests that dock increases osteoblast production and decreases osteoclast production in bones, suggesting to the study authors that it possesses potential for counteracting **osteoporosis** (Shim et al. 2017).

Dock has potential against some heavyweight afflictions, too: an Egyptian study found that it may be useful in the war against **AIDS**, since an extract of its fruits inhibited HIV reverse transcriptase (el-Mekkawy et al. 1995). Emodin, a quinone found in the roots of our own *Rumex crispus*, has also shown pronounced *antitumor* activity (Harborne and Baxter 1993: 499).

In view of the material we have thus far considered, it should come as no surprise that yellow dock was listed in the *United States Pharmacopeia* from 1863 to 1905 and in the *National Formulary* from 1916 to 1936, initially as an *alterative* and later as a *laxative* and *tonic*. It is also official in some European nations.

PERSONAL AND PROFESSIONAL USE

From spring to autumn, I relish the taste of dock leaves as a trail nibble. In the winter, I occasionally make mush out of the husked and winnowed seeds.

In my professional herbal practice, I turn to dock root when the dyad of constipation and chronic skin affliction exists, using it either as a simple or as the chief ingredient in a formula.

CAUTIONS

Because dock leaves contain a significant amount of oxalic acid and its salts, which can hinder calcium absorption in the body by chelating with this mineral, they should *not be consumed as a regular staple* but only every once in a while at most. Further underscoring this caution is that the calcium oxalate crystals that can be formed from the combination as mentioned above are excreted through the kidneys and, if bunched up in quantity, can cause mechanical damage there. The potential problem is negligible for occasional consumption as long as it is in moderation. Then, too, cooking breaks down the oxalate, so this may well be the best way to go for most dock repasts.

Animals have died from eating dock, possibly because they ate too much of it so that their systems could not process the oxalates and/or perhaps because amounts of nitrates toxic to these creatures were present (Duke 1985: 415; Panicera et al. 1990). In the late 1980s, a man with insulin-dependent diabetes died from consuming a large amount of dock soup, equaling approximately 500–1,000 grams of the plant (Reig et al. 1990). It was estimated that his total consumption of oxalic acid was 6–8 grams, which is in accord with the mean lethal dose (set at 5–30 grams). Any human consumption should therefore be undertaken with care, as outlined above, and in moderation.

Medicinally, the plant is *not to be taken internally during pregnancy*, owing to dock's laxative effects, which could precipitate a miscarriage. As the purgative anthraquinones can make their way into breast milk, dock is also *contraindicated during lactation*. Owing to its content of oxalic acid and oxalates, it should also not be used by those with kidney failure, diabetes, or electrolyte abnormalities nor concurrently with drugs known to lead to hypocalcemia. ↞

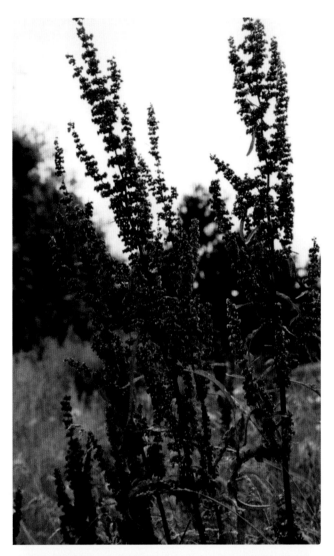

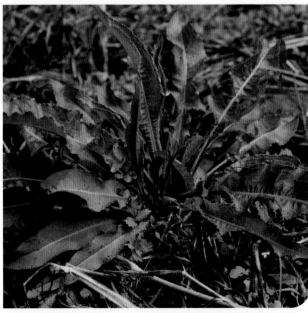

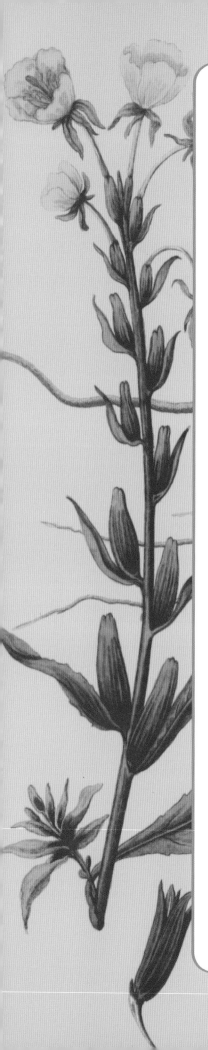

Evening Primrose

SUNDROPS; GERMAN RAMPION

Oenothera biennis

DESCRIPTION

This pretty plant is a hairy biennial that can grow to 6 feet tall in its second year. It starts off as a basal rosette of thick, wavy-edged leaves—sometimes with a dab of red here and there. Growing to 8 inches long, these leaves each display a prominent midrib that is either white or red.

In the summer of the second year, the flowering stem appears, crowded with many alternate lanceolate leaves. Next to appear are the showy yellow flowers, which are four-petaled and possessed of a characteristic cross-shaped stigma. They occur clustered at the end of the stem. These flowers open only in the afternoon and close before dawn of the next day, giving rise to the plant's common name of evening primrose. (I like to call it the night owl of the plant world because it prefers to get up late and stay up late.)

The fruits consist of thick, horn-like capsules that jut upward—the skeletons of which remain throughout the winter, allowing for easy recognition even during this season.

RANGE AND HABITAT

Evening primrose flourishes in waste places, fields, meadows, railroad embankments, and riversides. It grows throughout the Midwest except for the very northern strip of Minnesota.

MAJOR CONSTITUENTS

The plant contains oenotherin, oenothein B, gallic acid, mucilage, resin, bitter principle, phytosterols, caffeic acid, digallic acid, ellagic acid, neochlorogenic acid, *o*-coumaric and *p*-coumaric acids, and flavonoids (quercetin, kaempferol, delphinidin). Nutrients include vitamin C, calcium, magnesium, and potassium in significant amounts. The seed contains gramisterol, obtusifoliol, tryptophan, phenylalanine, beta-sitosterol, and a fixed oil of which about 70 percent is cis-linolenic acid, 9 percent is gamma-linolenic acid (GLA), and the rest a mixture of oleic, palmitic, and stearic acids. Nutrients in the seed include boron, copper, iron, zinc, sodium, and a variety of free amino acids, such as arginine.

FOOD

The plant's taproots, known as German rampions, are edible and can be collected from first-year plants in the fall or in the spring. Eaten raw, they have a powerful, turnip-like afterbite. Fortunately, proper cooking renders them more palatable. This should be done in three different waters, for a total cooking time of about one-half hour. (Europeans often prefer to boil them for two hours, however.) The roots should be peeled—either before being cooked or afterward.

Some say the taste is like parsnips, while to others it is more like turnips or salsify. Be forewarned that the roots will have an unpleasant, peppery, biting quality if under-cooked or if harvested too early in the fall or too late in the spring. However, the peppery quality can still be useful as a spicy ingredient in soups or stews, and so the chopped roots are sometimes added to such. The pungent leaves can also be added—in moderation—to these repasts.

Euell Gibbons felt that the rosette's central crown also makes a decent cooked vegetable (Gibbons 1973: 97).

HEALTH/MEDICINE

In 1903, Professor of medical botany B. B. Smythe listed evening primrose's root as possessing the physiological properties of an *alterative*, an *astringent*, and a *demulcent* (Smythe 1903: 202). The demulcent properties at least partly explain why it has traditionally been a soothing **cough** remedy (Lust 1974: 187). Because our herb is also *antispasmodic*, it has traditionally been employed most especially for **whooping cough**, as well as **hiccups** and **spasmodic asthma** (Wood and Ruddock 1925; Smith 1932: 376; Mockle 1955: 65). To make a cough medicine, Southwest American herbalist Michael Moore said to chop up the fresh or dried root and then to boil it slowly in twice the amount of honey, thereafter giving 1 tablespoon every three to four hours as needed (Moore 1979: 74). (Never give honey to a child younger than one year old, however.) Naturopathic doctor John Lust, in his detailed book on herbal remedies, wrote of making a syrup from the flowers instead, which he suggested to help ease whooping cough and asthma (Lust 1974: 187).

Herbal authorities G. P. Wood and E. H. Ruddock spoke of evening primrose as being "an efficient remedy as a nervine and sedative to quiet nervous sensibility, well adapted to neuralgia" (Wood and Ruddock 1925). As to the sedative effect mentioned, which Michael Moore notes as being stronger in some people than in others (Moore 1979: 74), perhaps this is at least partly due to the high tryptophan content.

Evening primrose is also a much-appreciated *vulnerary* (Millspaugh 1974: 60). The Flambeau Ojibwe utilized the "whole plant soaked in warm water to make a poultice to heal bruises" (Smith 1932: 376). Constantine Rafinesque, an early American authority on medicinal plants, described an application popular in his day wherein the leaves were "bruised and applied to wounds" (Rafinesque 1828–30: 2:247).

This plant has a history of use as an external application in "infantile eruptions" (Millspaugh 1974: 60). In the mid-1800s, R. E. Griffith wrote: "Some years since, hearing of the efficacy of a decoction of the plant in infantile eruptions, I made a trial of it in several cases of an obstinate character, which had resisted other modes of treatment and became satisfied that it was highly beneficial; and this opinion has been confirmed by subsequent experience" (Griffith 1847: 304).

The Cherokee have used a tea of the plant for "**overfatness**" (Hamel and Chiltoskey 1975: 33). They have also utilized a hot root poultice as an application to **piles**, while the Iroquois have employed an infusion for the same affliction— boiling one evening primrose root with one root each of wild mint (see page **264**) and self-heal (page **201**) in 1 quart of water, then drinking 2 cups of the brew and using the rest as a wash (Herrick 1995: 175).

Evening primrose has also had a place in treating gastrointestinal problems. Charles Millspaugh, in his classic work on American medicinal plants, wrote of a certain Dr. Winterburn as one who found the plant helpful for "gastric irritation and chronic exhaustive diarrheas" (Millspaugh 1974: 60). A Canadian researcher likewise detailed the plant's use in his country's folk medicine to "soothe gastrointestinal disturbances" (Mockle 1955: 65). Griffith wrote of it as having been "a favorite emollient in ulcers" (Griffith 1847: 304). The Montagnais have implemented evening primrose for **bowel pain** (Tantaquidgeon 1928: 267). Wood and Ruddock list it as being helpful for "pains of the lungs, stomach, heart, liver, bowels and womb" (Wood and Ruddock 1925). British herbalists have traditionally used it to offset **dyspepsia**, theorizing that it finds success in this regard by improving liver function.

Traditional forms and dosage for most of the above conditions have been to infuse 1 teaspoon of evening primrose in 1 cup of water and then to imbibe 1 cup a day, a little at a time. A tincture of the plant has been used to the tune of 5–40 drops a day, as needed (Lust 1974: 187).

The seed oil, available commercially and rich in the essential fatty acid known as gamma-linolenic acid (GLA), has been the subject of over three hundred studies. GLA supports the production of a series of prostaglandins (PGE-1), which modify inflammatory processes, lower blood pressure, and inhibit platelet aggregation (thereby reducing blood clotting, which in turn can help prevent **heart attacks** and **stroke**). This being so, the seed oil has been put to good use in the treatment of a wide variety of inflammatory conditions. Numerous clinical trials in a variety of research centers have shown positive results for **atopic eczema**, sometimes better than with the use of steroids (Morse et al. 1989; Stewart et al. 1991; Hederos and Berg 1996). James Duke, a former economic botanist with the US Department of Agriculture, suggests that the phenylalanine content may be significant in the treatment of **migraines** (Duke 1997: 235). A Scottish trial showed improvement in **rheumatoid arthritis** in 60 percent of patients, many of whom were even able to quit their antiarthritic drugs (Jäntti et al. 1989; Leventhal et al. 1993). Numerous studies have shown efficacy for **premenstrual syndrome** and **dysmenorrhea**, including at least three double-blind ones (Brush et al. 1982: 155–61; Horrobin 1983; Puolakka et al. 1985; Ockerman et al. 1986; Budeiri et al. 1996). Because essential fatty acids are crucial to the health of the myelin sheathes that protect the nerves, the oil may be beneficial to those with **multiple sclerosis**, a condition in which those structures degenerate (Field 1978). One study showed improvement in characteristic tremors of **Parkinson's disease** in 55 percent of people taking the equivalent of 2 teaspoons a day for several months (Duke 1997: 353).

Other conditions that may be treated with evening primrose oil include **mastalgia** (Pashby et al. 1981; Pye et al. 1985;

Gateley et al. 1992; Mellanby et al. 1996); **Sjogren's syndrome** (Campbell and MacEwen 1982: passim; Horrobin 1990; Giuffrida et al. 2000); **scleroderma** (Horrobin 1984); **asthma** (Hederos and Berg 1996); **ADHD** (as rated by parents) (Aman et al. 1987; Puri and Martins 2014); **schizophrenia** (see the studies cited in Mills and Bone 2000: 369); the pain and nerve damage of **diabetic neuropathy** (although James Duke recommends using the crushed seeds instead of the extracted seed oil since little tryptophan is available in the latter: Duke 1997: 348; Mills and Bone 2000: 367); and **blood-sugar problems** and **alcoholism**, two conditions that, since the pioneering research of endocrinologist John Tintera, have been known to be directly related (Tintera 1966). (See the research summary in Mills and Bone 2000: 364–65, 368–69, 370–71.) A Scottish study even showed that evening primrose oil aided the regeneration of livers damaged by alcohol (Mabey et al. 1988: 89). Later research found benefits to the nervous system and to body systems and structures damaged by alcohol (Glen et al. 1987; Corbett et al. 1992; Duffy et al. 1992).

Finally, the oil is widely used to bring back a healthful sheen to dry hair and skin and sometimes rubbed into the vaginal area by individuals experiencing menopause-induced dryness in this region. (However, its effect, while often quite helpful, doesn't hold a candle to regular, pulse-pounding sex, which can dramatically improve blood flow to this region and thereby enhance its tone and lubrication.) At a minimum dosage of 3,900 milligrams per day, the oil was shown, in one scientific study, to be effective for **nocturnal hot flashes** in menopausal women (Chenoy et al. 1994).

PERSONAL AND PROFESSIONAL USE

I recommend the commercial softgels of evening primrose oil quite a bit to clients afflicted with any of the conditions mentioned in the preceding section. My experience has been that it is a most effective measure in the majority of these complaints—especially menstrual cramps (dysmenorrhea), breast tenderness (mastalgia), menopausal hot flashes (especially nocturnal ones), vaginal dryness, alcohol-damaged livers, and infantile eczema.

It is usually the treatment of choice in the latter situation, especially if the baby has not been breastfed or if the complaint develops after weaning from breastfeeding. Why? Because in these situations, the baby is not able to derive the significant quantity of GLA that can be available from breast milk, and its ability to enzymatically convert cis-linoleic acid into GLA from any other food source is inefficient. Sometimes, too, even if the baby is breastfed, the breast milk is deficient in GLA owing to nutritional deficiencies on the part of the mother.

I have also witnessed the oil to enhance the quality of life in many clients afflicted with autoimmune diseases such as

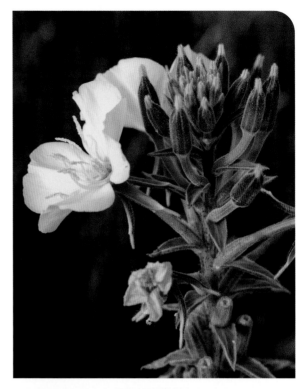

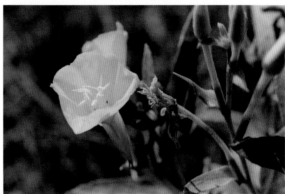

MS, rheumatoid arthritis, and Sjogren's syndrome, although the results are less predictable than with the earlier mentioned conditions.

My clinical observation, which accords with most of the scientific studies, is that the effective dose of evening primrose oil is 2½–6 grams a day. Note that this is five to ten softgels of the typical 500-milligram size; at least two companies offer it in a 1,300-milligram size, however. Using just one or two of the 500-milligram softgels a day, as many laypeople do, should not be expected to produce any positive results.

CAUTIONS

As animal research suggests that evening primrose oil may be somewhat of a uterine stimulant, it would be *best not to use it during pregnancy.*

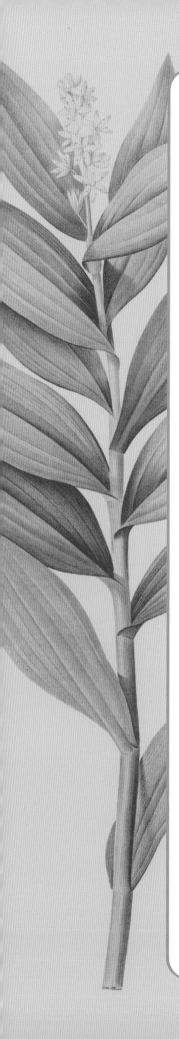

False Solomon's Seal

Smilacina racemosa, S. stellata

DESCRIPTION

The number of Solomon's seal lookalikes (see page **218** for the true plant) can be quite bewildering to the neophyte, though one eventually learns to distinguish among the more common varieties. The two species listed in the heading above, both perennials, are each commonly referred to as false Solomon's seal by various sources, so one should learn their respective scientific names and distinguishing features.

The first plant, *Smilacina racemosa*—variously called false spikenard, wild spikenard, or Solomon's plume—is the larger of the two species (1–3 feet tall) and the one that most resembles true Solomon's seal, being generally of the same height and bearing similar-sized oval, alternating leaves that are 3–6 inches long and have prominent veins. The leaves, however, are not as waxy looking as those of true Solomon's seal. Most noticeably, the berries do not dangle under the plant's stem from the leaf axils as they do on the true Solomon's seal but are borne in a branched, pyramidal cluster at the tip of the stalk, replacing tiny creamy-white flowers. (True Solomon's seal flowers are greenish-yellow bells and are much larger than *S. racemosa*'s flowers.) The berries are at first white and gold, later a blotchy pink-red, and finally pure red (never blue like those of true Solomon's seal). Finally, the arching stem of *S. racemosa* is constructed of a curious zigzag design—giving rise to yet another common name for this plant, Solomon's zigzag—in contrast to the nonzigzag stem of true Solomon's seal.

The other species, *Smilacina stellata*, is smaller (1–2 feet high) and more graceful in appearance. The leaves, thinner and more upswept than in *S. racemosa*, usually have a slight bluish hue to them, and their bases seem almost to wrap themselves around the plant's stem in that they are sessile (that is, stalkless). The six-petaled flowers—giving rise to the alternative common name star-flowered false Solomon's seal—are, unlike those of *S. racemosa*, arranged in unbranched clusters. They are thus fewer (three to fifteen) but individually larger in size than those of their cousin. Otherwise, this species shares the feature of the placement of the berries (and, earlier in the season, the flowers) with the larger *Smilacina* species. As to those berries, they change color as they grow: first, a blotchy sort of red; second, green with red-brown stripes; and finally, in August and September, an attractive dark ruby red. Eight or more seeds can be discovered in each berry.

RANGE AND HABITAT

False Solomon's seal can be found throughout the Midwest in deciduous woods, coniferous woods (especially *S. stellata*), thickets, clearings at the edges of woods, sandy banks, and the areas along streams and rivers.

MAJOR CONSTITUENTS

Very little research has been done on either species, although berries of both are presumed to contain large amounts of vitamin C due to the fact that they have been known historically as scurvy berries. A purgative principle is also to be inferred, owing to their laxative effects. In addition, *S. racemosa* is known to contain several saponins, the flavonoid

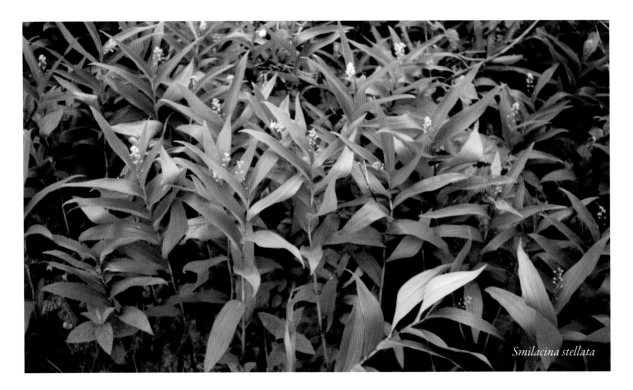

Smilacina stellata

asparagin, mucilage, sitosterol, and the cell-proliferant allantoin. Older literature listed the presence of the cardioactive glycoside convallarin.

FOOD

The ripe berries of both *S. racemosa* and *S. stellata* are edible. In that they sometimes persist late into autumn on both plants, they should be committed to memory as being possible rations for survival predicaments. The berries of *S. stellata* are the best tasting, their flavor being strongly reminiscent of molasses. Those of *S. racemosa* are slightly bitter, possessing a milder molasses taste. (Interestingly, in early New England, the berries of the *Smilacina* species growing there were called treacle berries because their taste was adjudged to resemble an English molasses by that name.) In small amounts, the berries are gently laxative, so obviously they should not be consumed in large amounts in their raw state. Many say that they taste best simmered, which also reduces the purgative principle.

The early-spring shoots and leaves of *S. racemosa* may also be eaten raw or as a potherb (boiled in water, preferably salted, for ten minutes). The rootstocks are toxic as is but can be prepared in such a way as to make them edible. The process is involved and depends upon the availability of lye, so it will not be detailed here.

HEALTH/MEDICINE

Although neither species is used much by modern herbalists, available records reveal that the Native Americans have made use of both in numerous ways. This has led some herbalists to begin looking at the genus more closely (see more on this under Personal and Professional Use).

Available records inform us that the Paiute and other western Native tribes have dried, sliced, and powdered the roots of *S. stellata* for use as an emergency *styptic*. From experience, they found that such a powder, when thrown onto a **wound**, would clot it instantly! (Train et al. 1988: 93; Kindscher 1992: 282) The Washoe have done the same, believing the root to be *antiseptic* for **blood poisoning** (Train et al. 1988: 93). On the other hand, the Southern Ojibwe prefer *S. racemosa* as a *stypic*, employing a poultice composed of its fresh, smashed leaves (Hoffman 1891: 199).

Because this genus possesses *anti-inflammatory* properties, an important use of *Smilacina* rootstock (either fresh or powdered and dried) has been as a poultice for wounds and sores as well as for **burns**, **sprains**, **boils**, **swellings**, **insect bites** and **stings**, **poison ivy rash**, and other **inflammatory states** (Zigmond 1981: 64; Train et al. 1988: 92). This has even included **inflamed eyes** and **ears.** As to the former, the Shoshone would soak the rootstocks in water, mash them, and apply the resultant liquid (presumably strained) to inflamed peepers (Train et al. 1988: 93). As to the latter, the Paiute of Lake Tahoe would sometimes treat this situation by forcing pulped material of *S. stellata* through a cloth, thereby straining it, and into the afflicted ear (Train et al. 1988: 93). **Rheumatism** was another sort of inflammation for which the plant has been found helpful. For this condition, the Thompson would drink a decoction of the leaves two or three times a day (Turner et al. 1990: 129). The Gitksan have preferred a decoction of the "roots," presumably dried

(Smith 1929: 53), while the Gosiute have pounded such for topical application (Chamberlin 1911: 382).

Michael Moore, an American herbalist who manifested interest in the *Smilacina* genus for healing, found that the dried root of *S. racemosa*, when prepared as a decoction—1 teaspoon of dried, finely chopped rhizome in 1 cup of water, boiled fifteen minutes or more—proved useful for **frontal headaches** caused or accompanied by **indigestion**. He also used it to soften and to expectorate **respiratory mucus**. Moore even further used the rootstock decoction for the inflammatory stages of **infections of the lungs** and of the **throat** (Moore 1979: 77). The Menomini have used the plant for catarrh but instead have ground up the rootstock, mixed it with water, and then heated it to release steam that was inhaled by the sick person (Smith 1923: 41).

The Lenape (Delaware; Oklahoma) and Shoshone have decocted the root of *S. stellata* for treating **venereal diseases** (Tantaquidgeon 1942: 80; Moerman 1986: 1:458). A quite different application affecting the reproductive system has been implemented by the Nevada, among whom women would drink ½ cup of the leaf tea daily for one week as a most effective *contraceptive* (de Laszlo and Henshaw 1954; Trease and Evans 1957: 92). The Costanoan have employed the root of *S. racemosa* for the same purpose (Bocek 1984: 28). The Thompson have used a decoction of the latter species as a postpartum aid and to offset **painful menstruation** (Turner et al. 1990: 129).

Interestingly, the Potawatomi have implemented a smudge of the rhizome of *S. racemosa* on hot coals to revive a person in a **coma** (Smith 1933: 63). One cannot help but wonder whether such a procedure might find some success today with persons trapped in a comatose state.

PERSONAL AND PROFESSIONAL USE

I've relished the molasses-like taste of the ripe (reddened) fruits of false Solomon's seal since the mid-1970s. I also enjoy sharing this taste with students who accompany me on wild-plant identification walks. As the fruits can exert laxative effects, however, one must keep the quantity eaten to just a few at any one time to avoid any stool urgency. On the other hand, this lends use of the fruits to treat stubborn constipation, which I did on one occasion in the mid-1990s—to the great relief of the sufferer! Otherwise, I have made little use of this lovely woodland plant.

CAUTIONS

The fresh belowground portions of *Smilacina* are toxic when ingested unless treated per the procedure mentioned in the text above.

Eating too many berries will result in diarrhea. ⮜⮜⮜

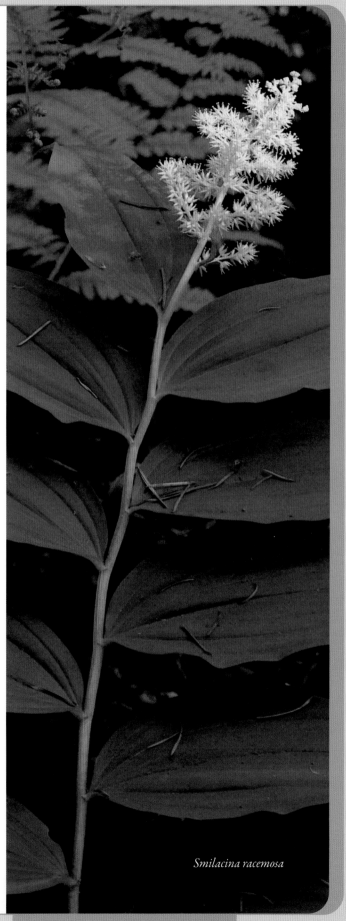

Smilacina racemosa

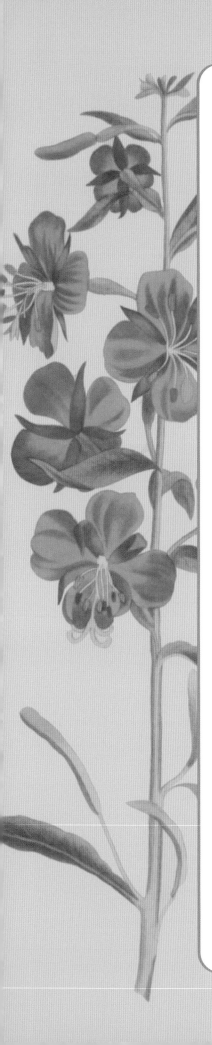

Fireweed

DESCRIPTION

Fireweed is a perennial, 2–6 feet high with a single smooth, erect stem. Its leaves are narrow and lance shaped, even willowy, giving rise to the alternative name of great willow herb. They grow alternately along the stem and tend to be 2–8 inches long and 1–1½ inches wide. They are shiny green on their topsides but dull green on their undersides, either toothless or minutely toothed, and nearly sessile.

Beautiful four-petaled pink-purple flowers are stalked on a showy, spike-like raceme. (Note for the novice: The number of petals is a quick means of distinguishing fireweed from purple loosestrife—see page 191.) Like mullein and blue vervain (page 161 and 41, respectively), fireweed's flower spike is never entirely in bloom. This is because the blossoms begin opening at the bottom of the stem, with the process climbing upward, so that one often encounters a triple treat: seedpods at the bottom of the spike, blossoms in the middle, and buds at the top!

This being as it is, it is not difficult to conceive why many—myself included—find this plant to be one of the most attractive of our native flora. Here, too, fireweed seems to induce a sense of deep serenity, thus being a wonderful plant simply to behold to ensure one's dose of sublimity for the day.

By late summer, the slender, bean-shaped red seedpods—ever angling upward—split into four segments, folding back in spirals to reveal fluffy white seeds with long, silky hairs (reminiscent of down). Once windborne, these seeds whiten the surrounding landscape. Prior to being released, they give the plant a very shaggy look, allowing it to be easily identified during this stage of life.

RANGE AND HABITAT

Fireweed is an inhabitant of roadsides, open woods, clearings, dry soils and fields, and rich, wetter soils along streams. It invariably seems to spring up in areas that have been burned over, since the seeds need a high temperature in order to germinate. In fact, fireweed grows so quickly after a fire that some persons claim to have witnessed it emerging from the soil even before the smoke has cleared!

This beautiful plant flourishes in the southern four-fifths of Canada and throughout much of the northern third of the United States—dipping deep into the southern states in the west and into mountainous areas of Georgia in the east. In the Midwest, it thrives in the upper portions, except for the extreme western strip.

MAJOR CONSTITUENTS

Fireweed contains chlorogenic acid; ursolic acid; oenothein B (an ellagitannin); gallic acid; flavonoids (including kaempferol, quercetrin, quercetin, and myricetin-3-O-beta-D-glucuronide); palmitic acid; beta-sitosterol; and pro-vitamin A and vitamin C.

FOOD

Very young leaves and flower buds can be eaten raw in small amounts. They, as well as slightly older ones, can also be boiled and eaten, although one or more waters may need to be thrown off. The Kuskokwagmiut tribe even add the leaves to stews (Oswalt 1957: 22). Otherwise, the leaves—either fresh or fully dried—can be made into a tea, which is very distinctive in taste and so delectable that I often curse myself because I never seem to gather enough of them to carry me through the winter!

The pith inside the stalks can be eaten raw. In the opinion of many, however, boiling the young stems provides the tastiest of fireweed treats. Older stems can be boiled and eaten, too, but they should first be stripped and cut into chunks. As with the leaves, however, one may need to throw off one or two waters.

HEALTH/MEDICINE

A tea made from the leaves is reported to be *tonic* to the human system. Fireweed is also a powerful and revered *astringent* and *anti-inflammatory*. The former is due to its tannin content; the latter is possibly due to several factors, including the plant's acids and its flavonoids, especially 3-O-beta-D-glucuronide, which is well evidenced as an anti-inflammatory (Hiermann et al. 1991). Both physiological functions render it immensely practical as a wash for **mouth sores** and as a gargle for **sore throat**—uses heartily implemented by the Snohomish and other Native American tribes (Gunther 1973: 41; Moerman 1986: 1:163).

The abovementioned physiological functions also enable fireweed to serve ably as an aid in **gastritis**, an application appreciated by the Kayenta Navajo (Diné) (Wyman and Harris 1951: 32); certain **stomachaches**; **piles**, for which it is used internally and topically after steeping the flowers and leaves in olive oil; **bowel hemorrhage**, a use implemented by the Cheyenne (Grinnell 1972: 181); **ulcerative colitis** (Moore 1993: 138); **gastroenteritis**, especially in children (Fearn 1923); and **chronic diarrhea**, especially when pasty and green or yellow in color (Moore 1993: 138). The antidiarrheal use was an especial favorite of the Eclectic physicians, who recommended it when there was "a dry, red tongue, with ... the abdomen ... contracted and the evacuations ... very painful. ... There is enfeeblement and many disturbing colicky pains; discharges [that] are frequent and feculent, not watery" (Felter and Lloyd 1898; Bloyer 1899: 276). In addition, Michael Moore recommended the tea as a wash for infants possessed of **inflammation** in the region of the **anal opening** (Moore 1993: 138). A pediatric application has also been utilized by the Blackfoot, who have administered an enema of an infusion of the inner cortex and root to babies who had **difficulty eliminating** (Hellson and Gadd 1974: 66).

Scientific studies have demonstrated anti-inflammatory effects for fireweed (Hiermann et al. 1986; Juan et al. 1988), which may explain many or all of the above-delineated applications.

The plant is also widely appreciated as a *vulnerary*, and a poultice made from the grated root has been found to be useful in treating **ulcerated sores**, as widely used by Native tribes including the Cree and Thompson (Leighton 1985: 38; Turner et al. 1990: 235). It has also been used for **burns**, owing at least partly to the tannin content. The latter use is especially of interest because, as Canadian herbalist Terry Willard notes, this plant also heals the burns of the earth—i.e., it grows in burned-over ground (Willard 1992a: 146). The Ojibwe have poulticed the leaves onto **bruises**, as well as onto **slivers** to draw them out (Densmore 1974: 352–53), while their relatives of the Flambeau band have poulticed the pounded root onto boils or carbuncles to draw out the inflammation (Smith 1932: 376). The Bella Coola also have used the smashed root as a poultice for **boils** (Smith 1929: 60). The Iroquois have used a fireweed poultice on **swollen knees** (Herrick 1977: 389–90).

The plant is thought to have an affinity for the *genitourinary system*, having long demonstrated its value for **uterine hemorrhage**, **menorrhagia**, **leukorrhea**, and **urethritis**. (It has been much used by the Iroquois for the latter condition: Herrick 1977: 389–90; Herrick 1995: 174.) It especially has a cherished reputation for **prostatic swelling**; scientific research has confirmed here that oenothein B, a chemical occurring in significant amounts in our plant, inhibits the enzymes 5-alpha-reductase and aromatase, which are understood to be responsible for prostatic swelling (Lesuisse et al. 1996; Ducrey et al. 1997). Moreover, an in vitro study published in 2001 found that a fireweed extract inhibited the growth of human prostatic epithelial cells in all tested conditions (Vitalone et al. 2001). A 2019 Chinese study verified the effects against benign prostatic hypertrophy (Deng et al. 2019).

Further scientific research has confirmed *antiproliferative* effects against several different cell lines of **prostate cancer** and has shed light on several mechanisms by which fireweed inveighs against this merciless killer (Vitalone et al. 2003; Kiss et al. 2006b; Schepetkin et al. 2009; Stolarczyk et al. 2013a; Stolarczyk et al. 2013b).

It has also been shown that oenothein B is a powerful *antiviral*, significantly reducing replication of **HIV** (Okuda et al. 1989) and strongly inhibiting **herpes simplex (HSV-1)** (Fukuchi et al. 1989). The Snohomish even used fireweed to combat **tuberculosis** (Gunther 1973: 41), while a Finnish study published in 2000 found it to possess powerful *antibacterial* properties, attributed to its polyphenols (Rauha et al. 2000). Additional research has found that both a tincture and an aqueous extract of the plant display activity against a number of common infectious microorganisms in vitro, including *Staphylococcus aureus* (including MRSA), *S. albus*, *Bacillus subtilis*, *Pseudomonas aeruginosa*, *Micrococcus luteus*, *Escherichia coli*, *Saccharomyces cerivisae*, and *Candida* (*C. albicans*, *C. tropicalis*, and *C. dubliniensis*) (Fleming 1998; Battinelli et al. 2001; Webster et al. 2008; Bartfay et al. 2012; Kosalec et al. 2013). Hungarian scientists found that topical preparations are especially effective (Silló et al. 2014).

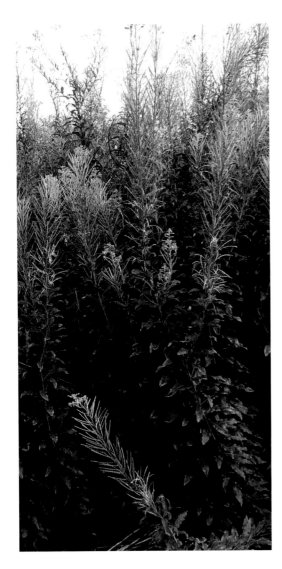

Fireweed is usually used as a tea because of its very pleasant taste. The Eclectic physicians specified that 1 ounce of the leaves be infused in 1 pint of water and dosed at 2–4 fluid ounces, repeated four or five times during the day (Felter and Lloyd 1898).

PERSONAL AND PROFESSIONAL USE

I so relish the unique and pleasant taste of fireweed tea! Then, too, when I am on wilderness outings in northern Minnesota, I often enjoy cutting the pith from the stems and eating it.

In my clinical practice, I employ fireweed most frequently for prostate issues—not only for swelling but also when there is a risk of cancer. I've also relied upon it for soreness or inflammation anywhere in the alimentary canal or in the genitourinary system. I've observed excellent results in all of these conditions, no doubt at least partly because the pleasant taste of the tea tends to result in such good compliance. ⤎

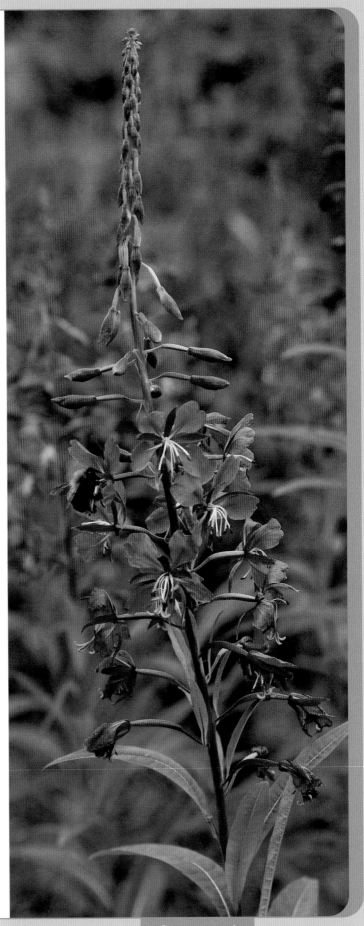

fireweed

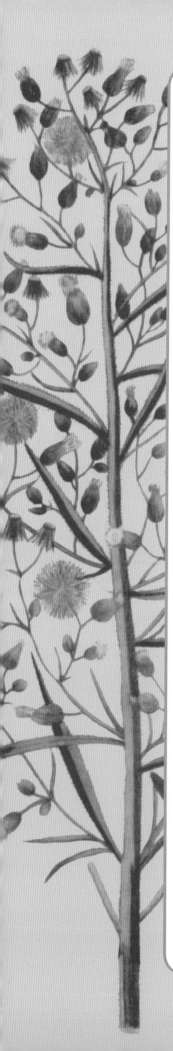

Fleabane

Erigeron spp.

DESCRIPTION

Fleabane is a weedy member of the Asteraceae (Compositae) family of plants that is often confused with aster (see page 24). However, the former blooms in early summer to midsummer while the latter spreads forth its petals first in late summer. The *Erigeron* genus is represented in the Upper Midwest by about half a dozen species, the chief of which are as follows:

E. annuus (annual fleabane, daisy fleabane) is a native annual growing to 4 feet tall and possessed of a stem with spreading hairs. Its alternate leaves are wide, ovate to lance-olate, and coarsely toothed; they grow to about 5 inches long, with their bases clasping the stalk. The plant's composite flowers have a yellow center with many (70–120) thin, tightly clustered ray flowers that are white or lavender in color.

Another native annual is *E. canadensis* (horseweed), also known as *Conyza canadensis*, which can reach a height of 5 feet, though 2–3 feet is average. Its stem is bristly and does not branch from its lower half but tends to do so from its upper half. The alternate leaves are dark green, hairy, and minutely toothed: they grow 1–4 inches long and are short stalked or even sessile. Horseweed's flowers—composed of yellow disks surrounded by inconspicuous greenish-white ray flowers—are situated on narrow, pointed bracts and occur in panicled clusters on stalks arising from the leaf axils.

E. philadelphicus (common fleabane, Philadelphia fleabane, daisy fleabane) is a hairy perennial or biennial growing 6 inches to 2½ feet tall. Its alternate, spatula-shaped leaves are serrated and grow to 4 inches long. They are sessile and conspicuously clasp the stem. The flower heads have a yellow center disk surrounded by up to 150 thread-like rays that may be lavender, pink, or white.

E. strigosus (rough fleabane, daisy fleabane) is an annual or biennial plant that reaches a height of 3 feet and is possessed of a stem covered with hairs that lie flat. Its leaves are alternate, narrow, and toothless (or barely toothed). Its flower heads are the smallest of those of the *Erigeron* species listed here (only ½ inch across) and marked by forty or so white ray flowers surrounding a yellow center.

RANGE AND HABITAT

The fleabanes are widespread in fields, meadows, roadsides, and disturbed ground. They can be found throughout the Midwest in such places.

MAJOR CONSTITUENTS

Most fleabane species contain an essential oil (generally inclusive of terpenes such as lim-onene, germacrene, camphene, myrcene, beta-pinene, linalool, dipentene, terpineol); a variety of flavonoids (including apigenin, luteolin, and quercetin); sterols; sphingolip-ids; and vanillic, caffeic, succinic, gallic, and tannic acid. In addition, 3-beta-erythrodiol (a triterpene) has been found in at least one species.

FOOD

The Miwok eat the pulverized raw leaves and tops for food. The flavor is onion-like.

HEALTH/MEDICINE

The various species of fleabane are all *astringent* and *styptic* to a large extent (Millspaugh 1974: 319). In fact, they are among the Midwest's most notable plants in these regards! Both Native American healers and white herbalists have used these species for a variety of health problems, especially where the tissues need tightening. For example, the Thompson toast the leaves, mix them with grease, and use them as a salve on **sores**, **swellings**, and **wounds**; they also use the fresh plant for same (Turner et al. 1990: 46). Kayenta Navajo (Diné) apply a lotion containing crushed horseweed leaves to **pimples** (Wyman and Harris 1951: 47, 50). Miwok place the chewed root in tooth cavities to alleviate **toothache** (Strike and Roeder 1994: 58). A decoction of the upper part of *E. canadensis* has traditionally been used for **sore throat** (Krochmal and Krochmal 1973: 93); **internal hemorrhage**, especially **uterine hemorrhage** (de Bairacli Levy 1974: 68–69); **hemorrhoids**, especially those that are congested as opposed to those that are inflamed (Moore 1989: 23); **childbirth hemorrhage** (Johnston 1987: 56); **bleeding ulcers** (Moore 1994b: 10.15); **bloody stool** (Moore 1994b: 10.9); and **ulcerative colitis** (Moore 1989: 23). The Cree have valued a decoction for plain old **diarrhea** (Holmes 1884: 303; Youngken 1925: 172). The Houma have employed a species of fleabane for **leukorrhea**, drinking a decoction of the root as hot as could be tolerated (Speck 1941: 64). The Southwest American herbalist Michael Moore found it useful for **irritable bowel syndrome** when it possesses a well-established cholinergic phase and when the episodes of diarrhea are painful and aching (Moore 1989: 23).

The extracted oil from *E. canadensis* was official in the *United States Pharmacopeia* during the last half of the nineteenth century for hemorrhages. Its terpenes would seem to be the chief hemostatic agents (Stuart 1982: 58). The *United States Dispensatory* even noted the oil's ability to stymie **hemoptysis** (Wood et al. 1926: 1293). The Eclectic physician Finley Ellingwood recommended erigeron oil for "menorrhagia with profuse flow of bright-red blood" and for "dysmenorrhea with blood clots, bloody lochia increased by movement, epistaxis, haemoptysis, hematuria, haematemesis … in all passive hemorrhages where there is no fever or constitutional irritation" (Ellingwood 1983: 352). Herbalist Ed Smith markets a tincture compound of the oils of erigeron and cinnamon based upon an original formula constructed by Ellingwood; it not only works well as a hemostat but also smells very nice! (However, see the Cautions section regarding sensitization to the oil by some persons.)

The various fleabanes are *diuretic*, too, even having been recognized in the *US Pharmacopeia* as such (from 1820 to 1882 for *E. canadensis*, from 1831 to 1882 for *E. philadelphicus*, and from 1831 to 1882 for *E. heterophyllum*). *E. philadelphicus* possesses the most pronounced ability in this regard, however; early American botanist Constantine Rafinesque informs us that it was once demonstrated to "have increased the daily evacuation of urine from 34 to 67 ounces" (Rafinesque 1828–30: 1:166).

The Lakota have utilized the plant's ability in this regard to assist adults who have **difficulty urinating** (Munson 1981: 234). Then, too, Laurence Johnson, a nineteenth-century physician and botanist who was often critical of botanicals then in use, acknowledged: "It has been used beneficially in diseases of the urinary organs and in dropsies" (Johnson 1884: 175), an observation echoed by both Charles Millspaugh and John R. Jackson, who each specifically highlighted Philadelphia fleabane's benefits in **dysuria**, **strangury**, **urethritis**, and **dropsy** (Jackson 1876: 235; Millspaugh 1974: 319).

The herb's combination of astringent and diuretic actions has lent its use as well for **urinary stones** (Barton 1810: 2:46; Jackson 1876: 235) and for certain kinds of **kidney disease** (Potterton 1983: 78). European herbalist Juliette de Bairacli Levy stated that she found it helpful for both **scalding urine** and **enuresis** (de Bairacli Levy 1974: 69).

The plant is also "a powerful emmenagogue," noted Charles Millspaugh (Millspaugh 1974: 308). At least *E. canadensis* has been used by our own area's Ojibwe for "female weakness" (Densmore 1974: 356–57). The Maidu and Houma have also utilized fleabane for **menstrual problems** (Speck 1941: 62; Strike and Roeder 1994: 58). Rather than serving simply to stymie menorrhagia, however, as the oil was used, the whole plant achieves a more comprehensive effect upon the body system by balancing astringency with other properties. Thus, the Thompson discovered that the decoction quickly eliminated **cramps** and **backache** associated with **menstruation** (Turner et al. 1990: 180). The Cherokee found the plant to be helpful for **amenorrhea** (Hamel and Chiltoskey 1975: 35). Fleabane has historically been used against **venereal disease**, too (Lewis and Elvin-Lewis 1977: 333).

Early American physician Benjamin Barton said that the combination of the herb's diuretic effect with a seeming *sudorific* effect explained the reports made to him by patients that fleabane was useful for both **urinary gravel** and **gout** (Barton 1810: 2:46). The Cherokee have also used it for the latter, exceedingly painful, condition (Hamel and Chiltoskey 1975: 35). Horseweed (*E. canadensis*), rough fleabane (*E. strigosus*), and annual fleabane (*E. annuus*) have all demonstrated *anti-inflammatory* activity, perhaps shedding light on the plant's reported effects on inflammatory conditions like gout (Benoit et al. 1976: 165; Lenfeld et al. 1986; Jo et al. 2013). This may also explain how the Kayenta Navajo (Diné) could report successfully using a hot poultice of *E. canadensis* on an **earache** (Wyman and Harris 1951: 47) and perhaps why the Kawaiisu could effectively implement a decoction of the root as a wash for **headaches** (Strike and Roeder 1994: 58) and the Cherokee a poultice of the fresh plant for same (Hamel and Chiltoskey 1975: 35). The Okanogan-Colville found that they could get headache relief, however, simply by drinking an infusion of the leaves and the blossoms (Turner et al. 1980: 83). As for the sudorific property mentioned by Barton above, this allowed the plant to be used to treat **fevers**, as the Pillager Ojibwe were fond of doing (Smith 1932). The Miwok have utilized Philadelphia fleabane and the related species *E. foliosus* to treat **fevers** with **chills** (Strike and Roeder 1994: 58).

Tommie Bass, an Appalachian herbalist of note, recommended a washing of **lice**-infested hair with fleabane tea (Crellin and Philpott 1990b: 153). It has classically been used to deter fleas as well, as its common name suggests, by way of burning the plant in order to drive them away (Vogel 1970: 305).

Writing about *E. canadensis* (horseweed) in the *Canadian Pharmaceutical Journal*, John R. Jackson observed: "An infusion of the powdered flowers is considered antispasmodic, and is used in cases of hysteria and affections of the nerves" (Jackson 1876: 235). The Cherokee have even used *E. philadelphicus* for **epilepsy** (Hamel and Chiltoskey 1975: 35).

This latter species has also shown experimental *hypoglycemic* activity (Lewis and Elvin-Lewis 1977: 218). This is interesting in that, in the 1870s, Eclectic physicians had found it useful for **diabetes** (Scudder 1870: 119). Then, too, obesity, which is often associated with Type 2 diabetes, was found to be attenuated by annual fleabane (*E. annuus*) in an animal study (Zheng et al. 2019). This species, as well, yielded isolates that were active in vitro against the production of advanced glycation end-products and aldose reductase, factors involved in the formation of **diabetic cataracts**. Moreover, opacity of lenses in rats was significantly prevented when they were pretreated with one of the compounds from this plant (Jang et al. 2010).

Yet another scientific study revealed that a European species, *E. linifolius*, demonstrated *antifungal* activity (Nene and Kumar 1966). Then, too, a 2012 Hungarian study revealed that the essential oil of *E. canadensis* showed moderate to strong activity against a variety of fungal strains (Veres et al. 2012). This latter species has long been used for **ringworm** in Africa (EthnobDB).

Several fleabane species manifest *antineoplastic* activity. When Hungarian scientists tested a variety of plant extracts against three different cancer cell lines (cervix, breast, and skin epidermoid carcinoma), they found eleven plants to be active against all three, including *E. canadensis* and *E. annuus* (Réthy et al. 2007). Chinese scientists also found a triterpene from *E. canadensis* to markedly inhibit gastric cancer cell proliferation, and that by several different mechanisms (Liu et al. 2016).

PERSONAL AND PROFESSIONAL USE

I once had a client whose nighttime sleep was severely hampered by a terrible dysuria and strangury that led to frequent nighttime trips to urinate, which was tentatively diagnosed by his physician as what was then known as

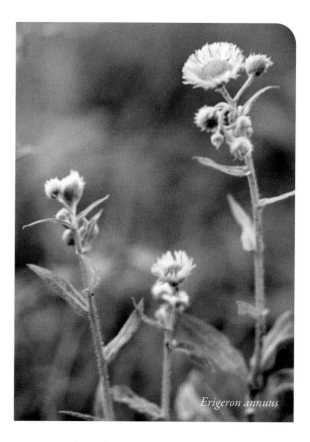

Erigeron annuus

Reiter's syndrome (laterly called "reactive arthritis"). After seeing several health-care providers, he found the only thing that took the edge off of this situation was the regular use of a tea made from Philadelphia fleabane, which I wildcrafted for him.

I've observed that painful, aching, watery diarrhea is often eased by horseweed, as the Eclectics found to be true. Still, in holistic medicine, we always look for the cause and then reverse that: with a symptom set such as the above, such a cause may be lactose intolerance, gluten intolerance, inflammatory bowel disease, or an infection—all of which must be investigated via laboratory testing and sometimes also by a scoped inspection. In the interim, however, I've found that horseweed tea often provides some welcome relief.

I've seen horseweed combined with cinnamon make a profound difference for acute menorrhagia—although if that problem is chronic, I usually try to nip it in the bud by implementing shepherd's purse (see page 208) and/or yarrow (page 282), starting about five days before the anticipated menstrual flow and continuing into menses.

CAUTIONS

Certain sensitive persons may develop dermatitis from handling this plant, especially the leaves, which are saturated with an essential oil rich in sesquiterpene lactones.

Fleabane is *contraindicated during pregnancy* due to emmenagogue and other effects produced by this plant. ⫷

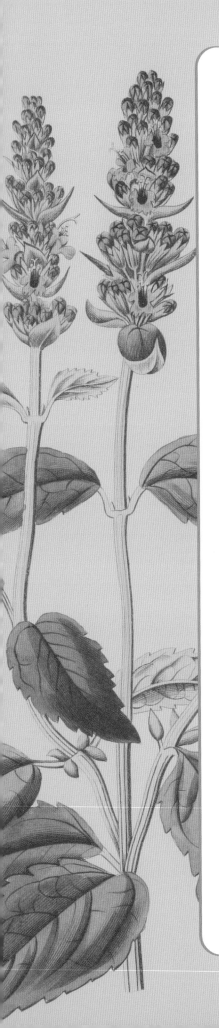

Fragrant Giant Hyssop

Agastache spp.

DESCRIPTION

Fragrant giant hyssop is an attractive, native perennial that grows 2–5 feet tall. It is possessed of a square, smooth, and branching stem. The entire plant possesses a faint anise scent that comes through much more strongly when its leaves are crushed.

Speaking of its leaves, they are opposite, shiny, ovate, coarsely toothed, and tapered at their apex. They are downy on their undersides, with the topsides being hairless but rough. The leaves of *Agastache foeniculum* are small (1–3 inches long and 2 inches wide) and short stalked, whereas those of *A. scrophulariaefolia* (purple giant hyssop) are larger (2–6 inches long) and have longer petioles. The latter species also has purple stems with whitish hairs.

The small purplish-blue flowers appear in whorls on dense, terminal, spiked clusters that are 1–4 inches long. Each flower bears four stamens, occurring in two protruding pairs, with these pairs crossing each other and one of them curving upward. Many tiny black seeds evolve from the flowers.

RANGE AND HABITAT

Fragrant giant hyssop can be found in prairies, fields, meadows, and open upland woods, growing in sandy and well-drained soil. It prefers sun but will tolerate some shade.

MAJOR CONSTITUENTS

Fragrant giant hyssop contains an essential oil (0.1–0.3 percent of the plant) consisting chiefly of methylchavicol, alpha-limonene, beta-caryophyllene, and germacrene B and D but also trace amounts of alpha-pinene, eugenol, camphene, beta-myrcene, linalool, and pulegone.

FOOD

The leaves of this anise-scented plant make both a nice trail nibble (the Lakota call it *wahpe yatapi*, meaning "leaf that is chewed") and a pleasant-tasting tea. The plant can be dried, powdered, and stored for use as a licorice-like flavoring and sweetener in baking, in the tradition of certain Native American tribes (Gilmore 1991: 113). The seeds of some *Agastache* species, such as *A. urticifolia*, have also been reported to be edible (Kirk 1975: 80).

HEALTH/MEDICINE

The Ojibwe have utilized a poultice of the leaves or stalk of this plant to treat **burns**. Thus implemented, it is thought to "prevent blister and take out the fire" (Densmore 1974: 352–53). They also utilized fragrant giant hyssop for chest pain and for the cough of an "internal cold with tendency to pneumonia" (Densmore 1974: 340–41). The Cheyenne have likewise appreciated that a cooled infusion of this plant is useful for **chest pains**, including those from **excessive coughing** (Grinnell 1905: 42). Likewise, the Woods Cree found this herb to be invaluable in treating the **coughing up of blood** (Leighton 1985: 26).

Interestingly, Traditional Chinese Medicine (TCM) uses the related Asian species *Agastache rugosa* (called *huo xiang* in Chinese) for "oppression in the chest" (Reid 1992: 106). TCM practitioners understand this species to be one of the very best remedies to fight off what they call "damp summer heat," finding it to be powerfully drying. They therefore use it to offset **heat stroke** and **summer colds** (Reid 1992: 106). Likewise, halfway around the world, the Cheyenne have used the American species similarly, rubbing the powdered leaves on the body of a person engripped by a **high fever** (Hart 1981: 27).

The Cheyenne, it is of interest, have also appreciated fragrant giant hyssop to help offset a **dispirited heart** (Hart 1981: 27). I find this fascinating in that a related mint, lemon balm (*Melissa officinalis*), possessing an essential oil with a terpene profile similar to that of fragrant giant hyssop's (they both contain linalool, limonene, etc.), is used by contemporary herbalists to offset **melancholy**. I use the latter extensively and have found it to be marvelously effective in most cases, especially for teenage girls.

Other uses for *Agastache* species include the topical application of the tea to **yeast infections** and oral use of it for both **nausea** and **vomiting** (Yanchi 1995: 78; Belanger 1997: 582–83). Scientific research has shed light on the former usage in verifying antifungal activity in *A. rugosa*'s essential oil (Shin and Kang 2003: 111; Shin 2004: 295). Published studies have also confirmed **anti-HIV activity** in the roots of *A. rugosa*: rosmarinic acid was identified to be an active agent in one study (Kim et al. 1999), while two diterpenoid compounds were found to be responsible in another investigation (Min et al. 1999).

PERSONAL AND PROFESSIONAL USE

Although this herb is not readily obtainable from the herb market, I have wildcrafted lots of it over the years and have both used it myself and recommended it to relatives, students, and many, *many* clients—all of whom have been most appreciative!

When I get a summer cold—which is rare—I always rely on this herb, chewing the fresh leaves straight from the fields where they grow. Their delicious, licorice-like taste makes this a not unpleasant experience, although the leaves are so dry that I always bring a bottle of water with me to keep them from getting caught in my throat on the way down! Amazingly, this treatment has never failed to vanquish the cold for me most speedily, sometimes on the very day on which I have consumed the leaves! Many of my students and clients have reported similar results.

I have also used a wipe and a gentle squeeze of gauze soaked with the tea for oral thrush in infants, with marked success.

Most often, however, I have sought fragrant giant hyssop's antinauseant effects. Here, it has seldom failed me, my clinic assistants, my students, or my clients when nausea, vomiting, and/or diarrhea have ensued from food poisoning, "stomach flu," or other infectious agents.

I couldn't even imagine what life would be like without this wonderful plant—one of my all-time favorites! ⋘

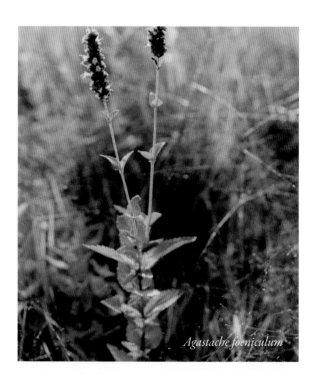

Agastache foeniculum

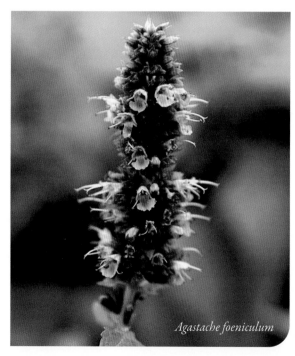

Agastache foeniculum

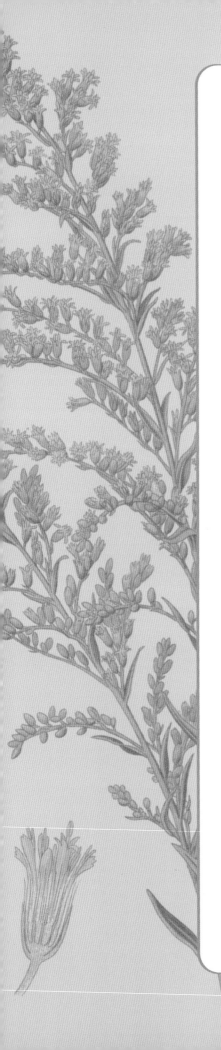

Goldenrod

Solidago spp.

DESCRIPTION

Goldenrod is a genus of native perennials that is represented in the Midwest by almost twenty different species!

Solidago is marked by alternate leaves and golden flowers, as the common name implies—these often being situated in a "rod" as well. The Midwest's more important species are as follows:

Solidago canadensis (Canada goldenrod) grows 2–4 feet tall and possesses a stem that is hairy on the upper, leafy part and often afflicted with insect galls. Its sharply toothed leaves grow to 6 inches long and display three main veins. The small yellow flowers are clustered terminally in long plumes, with the tip of the chief cluster nodding to one side.

S. flexicaulis (zigzag goldenrod) tops off at 1–3 feet and is characterized by a zigzag stem. Its alternate, ovate leaves are pointed and coarsely toothed. They grow 1–3 inches long and are attached to the stem by short leafstalks. This species is unusual in the sense that its yellow flowers are arranged in small rounded clusters (1–2 inches) in the axils of the upper leaves.

S. gigantea (late goldenrod) is 5–6 feet tall with a smooth, shiny stem that is green or purplish red. Like *S. canadensis*, this species has an arching flower stalk and tends to accumulate insect galls on its stem.

S. hispida (hairy goldenrod) has, as its common name implies, hairy stems. Its elliptical leaves are blunt and taper toward the base. The flower heads are narrow, ascending, and orange-yellow in color.

S. missouriensis (Missouri goldenrod) grows 1–2 feet tall and has a smooth stem. Its stem leaves are narrow, toothed, and somewhat erect. All of its leaves are markedly three-veined.

S. nemoralis (gray goldenrod) likewise grows to 1–2 feet. Its slender stem is densely hairy, as is the rest of the plant. This species has large basal leaves and small, narrow stem leaves. There is also a pair of tiny leaflets in the axils of its upper leaves. The golden flowers are arranged in an arching plume that nods to one side.

S. rigida (stiff goldenrod) grows ½–4 feet tall and has short hairs that cover the entire plant. This species sports rough basal leaves that reach a length of 10 inches as well as round, clasping, stem leaves. There are numerous flower heads appearing as wide clusters, several inches across.

S. speciosa (showy goldenrod) reaches a height of 1–3 feet. Its stout stem is smooth on the lower end but rough above. The leaves are elliptical and barely toothed. Both the basal leaves (growing up to 10 inches long) and the lower stem leaves are stalked, while the upper stem leaves lack stalks. The terminal flower cluster looks like a fat plume, although it is sometimes more pyramidal in shape.

Other species common to the Midwest include *S. ptarmicoides* and *S. uliginosa*.

RANGE AND HABITAT

Most of the species in this genus prefer dry, sunny ground such as is found in fields, prairies, and meadows. It is very common throughout the Midwest in such locales.

MAJOR CONSTITUENTS

Goldenrod contains phenolic glycosides (including leiocarposide); flavonoids (rutin, quercetin, astragalin, quercetrin); carotenoids; an essential oil (which includes borneol); polyacetylenes; hydroxylbenzoates; tannic acid; pseudotannins; organic acids; saponins; and polysaccharides.

HEALTH/MEDICINE

Goldenrod is a medicinal plant with a long tradition of use by a wide range of healing communities. It has, as one example, been treasured by Native Americans as a *vulnerary*: the Costanoan have used a decoction of the leaves of *Solidago californica* as a wash for **sores** and for **burns**, and they have also sprinkled toasted and crumpled leaves onto **wounds** (Bocek 1984: 255). The Midwest region's Ojibwe have implemented the pulverized and moistened root as a poultice for **boils**, the flower as a poultice for **burns**, and the stalk or root as a poultice for **sprains** marked by severe swelling (Densmore 1974: 348–49, 362–63). Russian healers have traditionally applied powdered flowers to slow-healing wounds (Hutchens 1991: 143). Herbalist and naturalist Tom Brown Jr., who was mentored by Apache medicine man Stalking Wolf, related how when he was a youngster, his mentor once eased a bevy of **yellowjacket stings** with a salve made from goldenrod tea and tallow, on top of which the medicine man had poulticed some chewed leaves. Brown says that this treatment took away his pain almost instantly (Brown 1985: 123).

The soothing effects achieved with these conditions have no doubt been due at least in part to the plant's tannins, which explain, as well, why the Cree could effectively utilize a decoction of the root for **diarrhea** (Turner et al. 1990: 50). Such *astringent* properties would also elucidate goldenrod's many applications to the oral cavity. Thus, a decoction of *S. virgaurea* has been used in England to help fasten **loose teeth**, while the flowers have been chewed to combat **pyorrhea** (Lewis and Elvin-Lewis 1977: 261). In the Ozarks, various species of *Solidago* have been placed on **teeth** with **caries** (Lewis and Elvin-Lewis 1977: 258). The Miwok found that a decoction of the plant, held in the mouth, relieved **toothache** (Strike and Roeder 1944: 148). The Cherokee have swished goldenrod tea in a **sore mouth** (Hamel and Chiltoskey 1975: 36). The Zuni have chewed the crushed blossoms and swallowed the juice to soothe a **sore throat** (Stevenson 1915: 60). The Blackfoot have relished goldenrod tea for **sore throat**, **throat constriction**, and **nasal congestion** (Hellson and Gadd 1974: 74).

Astringency would also explain goldenrod's demonstrated assistance for **minor internal hemorrhages**—but only partly, since the plant has also been shown to decrease the fragility of capillaries, no doubt owing to its flavonoids (Kresanek and Krejca 1989: 180). At any rate, the Cherokee have been grateful for its aid when afflicted with **bowel hemorrhage** (Hamel and Chiltoskey 1975: 36). The Ojibwe

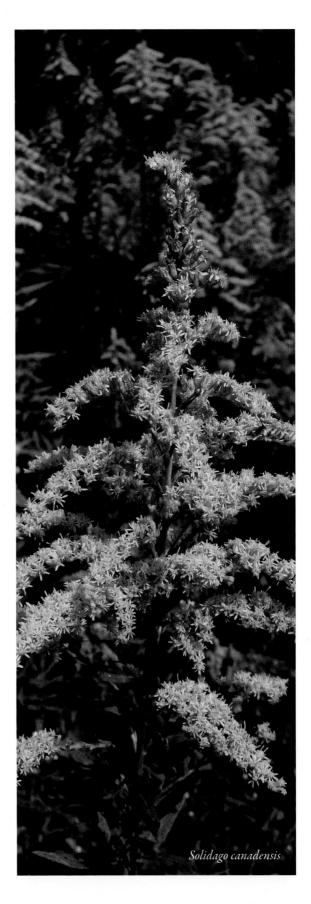

Solidago canadensis

also employed a cooled decoction made from one root of *S. rigiduscula* and 1 quart of water to check **hemorrhage** coming from the mouth when a tribal member had been wounded (Densmore 1974: 352–53; cf. 340–41). In fact, one or another species of *Solidago* has been famed as a wound herb in numerous cultures throughout history. The beloved European herbalist Juliette de Bairacli Levy noted that the ancient Saracens would refuse to go into battle without this herb at their side! (de Bairacli Levy 1974: 72) The famous horticulturist John Gerard perhaps summed it up best when he wrote that goldenrod "is extolled above all other herbs for the stopping of blood in wounds" (Gerard 1975: 109).

Our herb's many vulnerary applications might be partly elucidated by at least three different scientific studies that have demonstrated powerful *anti-inflammatory* properties for a variety of goldenrod species, including *S. canadensis, S. rugosa, S. flexicaulis, S. virgaurea,* and *S. gigantea* (Benoit et al. 1976: 165; Okpanyi et al. 1989; el-Ghazaly et al. 1992; Leuschner 1995). Such an ability has since been acknowledged by the scientific panel known as German Commission E (Blumenthal 1998). This effect, which seems largely due to the plant's content of leiocarposide (Metzner 1984: 869) and perhaps, as well, to its flavonoids, undoubtedly sheds light on why the Zuni could imbibe an infusion for practically

any sort of **body pain** (Stevenson 1915: 60) and why many herbalists have esteemed goldenrod for **chronic eczema** and have used it as an *antiallergic* (Stuart 1982: 138). While some may balk at this last use and claim that goldenrod pollen produces, rather than stymies, allergic reactions, many researchers have noted that the plant's pollen is not wind-borne, so it is most unlikely to prove a nasal allergen as commonly believed. These researchers point out that ragweed blooms at the same time as goldenrod and that the former is most likely the real culprit when goldenrod is implicated (Wunderlin and Locky 1988).

A rat study has found this herb to be *antispasmodic* (Leuschner 1995), an effect that perhaps explains why the Ojibwe could soothe **stomach cramps** by poulticing the heated root onto the stomach (Densmore 1974: 344–45) and why the Cherokee could obtain relief from **facial neuralgia** by holding the root tea in their mouths (Hamel and Chiltoskey 1975: 36).

A tincture of goldenrod is also *diuretic*, which has been confirmed by several lab studies (Chodera et al. 1985; Kresanek and Krejca 1989: 180; Chodera et al. 1991; Leuschner 1995) and attributed again to the herb's content of leiocarposide (Duke 1997: 208) as well as to its array of flavonoids and saponins (Fetrow and Avila 1999: 299). The plant's

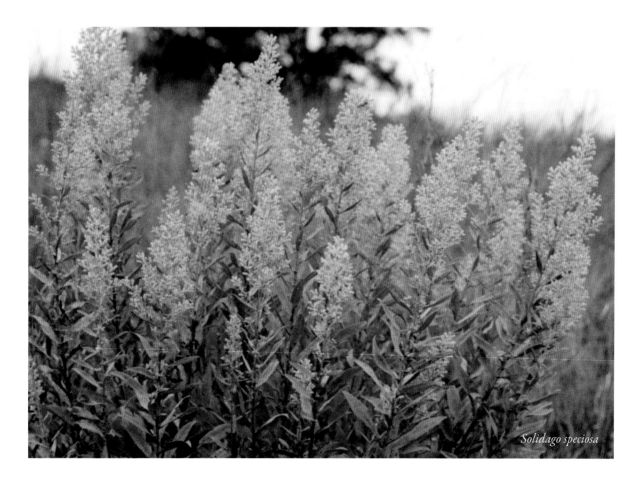

Solidago speciosa

historic uses for **rheumatism** and **gout** are thus explained through a combination of these anti-inflammatory and diuretic activities (Kresanek and Krejca 1989: 180; Pahlow 1993: 171).

Goldenrod has also been used for both **urinary tract inflammation** and **urinary stones** (Kresanek and Krejca 1989: 180; Pahlow 1993: 171; Blumenthal 1998; Melzig 2004). M. Grieve's herbal reports that in 1788, a ten-year-old boy who had been drinking the infusion for months wound up passing large amounts of gravel, including fifteen large stones and fifty others that were a bit larger than a pea! (Grieve 1971: 1:361) The Eclectic physician Finley Ellingwood listed the herb's specific indication for the urinary system as follows: "Difficult and scanty urination, where the urine is of dark color, and contains a heavy sediment. Where there is nephritis, either acute or chronic. It is useful where there is suppression of urine in infants, or retained urine, which causes general depression, with headache; urinary obstructions from any character" (Ellingwood 1983: 452). Modern herbalists, such as Oregon's Ed Smith, often find it helpful for **kidney pain**, associated **backache**, and even **ulceration of the bladder** (Smith 1999: 35). Herbalist Peter Holmes regards it as a genuine trophorestorative to the kidneys (Holmes 1997–98: 1:190). However, goldenrod should probably not be used for edema associated with either kidney failure or heart failure in that its unique diuretic effects induce chiefly water, and not salts, to be excreted (Tilgner 1999: 70).

The genitourinary system as a whole seems to benefit from goldenrod's power. A decoction of *S. spathulata* has been drunk by the Thompson for **syphilis** (Turner et al. 1990: 48). The plant's saponins are active against *Candida* organisms—those tiny but common bodily inhabitants that can aggressively get out of control and induce **vaginal yeast infections** (Bader et al. 1987: 140; Blumenthal 1998). It is also a classic *emmenagogue*, used in Belarus for **amenorrhea** (Hutchens 1991: 143). The Cherokee have likewise treasured goldenrod for "female obstructions" (Hamel and Chiltoskey 1975: 36). The Ojibwe have implemented it to alleviate a **difficult labor** (Densmore 1974: 358).

Goldenrod is also a cherished digestive *tonic* (de Bairacli Levy 1974: 72), having often demonstrated its benefits for conditions such as **gastric catarrh** and excessive **fermentation** (Kresanek and Krejca 1989: 100). Then, too, the Thompson have used a decoction of *S. spathulata* to *stimulate the appetite* (Turner et al. 1990: 44). Physician and botanist Laurence Johnson noted that "goldenrod is gently stimulant, diaphoretic, and carminative. It has been used in domestic practice to produce diaphoresis, to relieve colic, and to promote menstruation" (Johnson 1884: 176). The Houma have drunk a decoction of *S. nemoralis* for **jaundice** (Speck 1941: 66), while the Iroquois have treated this same condition with an infusion of *S. juncea* (Herrick 1995: 237).

The diaphoretic effects that Johnson mentioned, and to which the pharmaceutical literature also attests (Wood et al. 1926: 1484), probably derives from the plant's essential oil. This constituent, along with goldenrod's supply of saponins, which are possessed of an expectorant effect, probably explains why goldenrod is widely regarded as one of the first herbs to consider for **upper respiratory catarrh**, whether acute or chronic (Hoffmann 1986: 197). Diaphoresis no doubt also largely explains the plant's traditional use for **fever**, such as implemented by Native American tribes as diverse as the Cherokee (Hamel and Chiltoskey 1975: 36), Forest Potawatomi (Smith 1933: 53), Lenape (Delaware) (Tantaquidgeon 1972: 122–23), Iroquois (Herrick 1995: 237), and Ojibwe (Densmore 1974: 354–55). From the standpoint of energetics, goldenrod's cooling and drying energies would be most appropriate for the above-delineated conditions (Holmes 1997–98: 1:188–90).

Last but not least, scientific research of late has carved out a possible role for goldenrod with reference to **cancer**. Scientists from Southern Illinois University School of Medicine found that an extract of *S. virgaurea* leaf exhibited powerful cytotoxic activities on various tumor cell lines, including breast (MDA435), melanoma (C8161), human prostate (PC3), and small-cell lung carcinoma (H520). Their conclusion was that it was "promising as an antineoplastic medicine with minimal toxicities" (Gross et al. 2002).

PERSONAL AND PROFESSIONAL USE

I've recommended goldenrod's astringent, anti-inflammatory, urinary, hemostatic/styptic, and anticancer effects on various occasions and have seldom been disappointed. I'm thinking now, as I write this, however, that I really should be implementing it much more often, given its broad spectrum of applications and its commonality in my own area.

CAUTIONS

Do not use goldenrod during pregnancy owing to its emmenagogue effects.

As this plant can easily absorb high levels of harmful nitrates from the soil, never harvest from areas where fertilizers have been used. ⥽

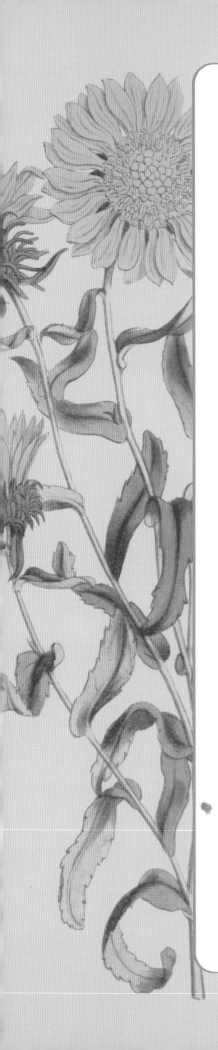

Gumweed

GUMPLANT; GRINDELIA; ROSINWEED

Grindelia squarrosa

DESCRIPTION

The *Grindelia* genus is composed of some thirty species, but only one predominates in the Midwest: *G. squarrosa*. It is a low, branching perennial or biennial plant with many flower heads that grows 1–2 feet tall.

Gumweed has alternate, toothed, linear-oblong, stiff, and leathery leaves that are somewhat aromatic and grow 1–2 inches long. They are each covered with translucent glands that look like tiny dots. The upper leaves clasp the stem. The lower leaves disappear when the plant begins to flower.

Gumweed is appropriately named: its many yellow, dandelion-like flower heads—each growing 1–1½ inches wide—arise from rough, sticky burs composed of five to six rows of extremely gummy, cup-like bracts, the tips of which curl downward and then recurve outward. Even the flower heads are sticky to the touch and, prior to their opening (i.e., in bud form), are also smothered with a white "stickum."

RANGE AND HABITAT

Gumweed grows from British Columbia to Minnesota and dips southward in the west to California and Texas. Originally native to the United States west of the Mississippi, it is now rapidly spreading eastward. In Minnesota, as an example of a state from our region, it has been recorded in all quarters of the state but currently can be confirmed in only about one-half of the counties. Its preferred habitat is open, dry areas, such as prairies, waste places, railroad rights-of-way, roadsides, and dry fields.

MAJOR CONSTITUENTS

The resin in gumweed (20 percent of the plant!) contains diterpenoid acids and grindelic acid; an essential oil (consisting of borneol, alpha-pinene, beta-pinene, limonene, and other components); grindeline (a bitter alkaloid); matricarianol acetate; flavonoids (acacetin, kumatakenin, quercetin, luteolin, and others); triterpenoid saponins; and phenolic acids (including *p*-coumaric, vanillic, caffeic, chlorogenic, *p*-hydroxybenzoic, ferulic, gallic, and ellagic).

HEALTH/MEDICINE

The dried leaf and flowering tops of this herb were official medicine in the *United States Pharmacopeia* from 1882 to 1926 and appeared in the *National Formulary* from 1926 all the way up to 1960. It is still official in some European pharmacopeias. Because of its tough, resinous nature, a decoction has been preferred over an infusion; tinctures and fluid extracts have also been employed.

This plant yields *antispasmodic* and *expectorant* effects and thus has primarily been employed as a respiratory aid, especially for highly spasmodic conditions such as **asthma**, **whooping cough**, **pneumonia**, and **bronchitis**. It relaxes and opens bronchial tubes and helps expel phlegm, at least partly owing to its saponin content. In that its resinous nature also helps moisten the respiratory tract, it is held by herbalists to be especially useful for **dry**, **hacking**, **unproductive**, and **spasmodic coughs** (Moore 1994b: 4.5; Smith 1999: 37) and has been used as such by various Native American tribes (Shemluck 1982:

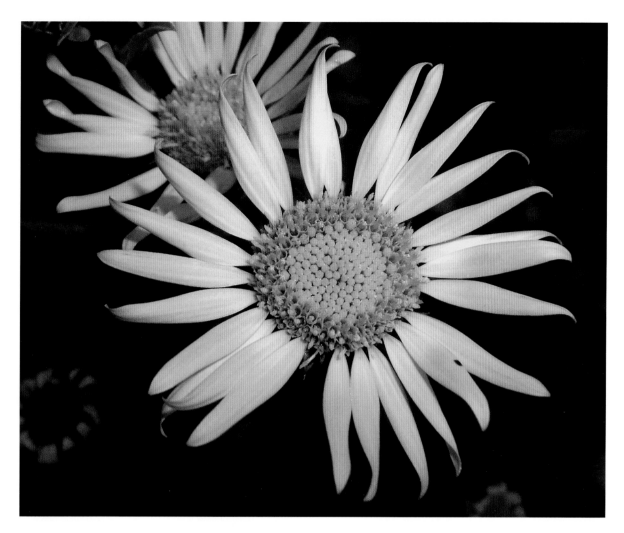

333; Smith 1999: 37). Gumweed's uses for the respiratory tract were pioneered by the Shoshone, Paiute, Crow, and Flathead (Salish) tribes (Vogel 1970: 313; Kindscher 1992: 120). The Ponca even implemented it to treat **tuberculosis** (Gilmore 1991: 81). Interestingly, skilled herbalists, both white and Native, have always insisted that only the top one-third of the plant should be used when treating respiratory problems. Further, the Southwest American herbalist Michael Moore felt that a tea was preferable to a tincture when treating these afflictions (Moore 1979: 80).

Gumweed's antispasmodic properties also have led to the plant's use with **postpartum pain**, for which the Crow have used an infusion of the flowers (Shemluck 1982: 333); **toddler colic**, utilized by the Teton (Gilmore 1991: 81); **indigestion**; and **headache**. The latter application was especially valued by America's Eclectic physicians of the late nineteenth and early twentieth centuries. Finley Ellingwood, as a representative of such, noted that gumweed was the herb of choice when there was "headache accompanied with dizziness, and some nausea" and also when the headache was "persistent, day after day, and there is dullness, drowsiness,

and dizziness ... lassitude, and the patient tires easily. A dull headache is present when he awakes in the morning, and with some exacerbations continues all day" (Ellingwood 1983: 320).

Verified *anti-inflammatory* activity (Benoit et al. 1976: 164; Krenn et al. 2009; La 2010; Gierlikowska et al. 2019) may largely explain two other popular uses of this plant, as a *vulnerary* and as a *dermatology aid*. In Native American medicine, it has been poulticed on all sorts of afflictions, including **wounds**, **cuts**, **sores**, **broken bones**, and **burns** (Shemluck 1982: 333; Moerman 1986: 1:208–9; Strike and Roeder 1994: 67). Yet its most famous implementation has been as a remedy for **poison ivy rash**, a use established by various Native American tribes (Vogel 1970: 313; Shemluck 1982: 334; Strike and Roeder 1994: 67). This remedy was brought to the attention of the medical profession in 1863 by C. A. Canfield of California, who personally witnessed the successes of the Native treatment (Vogel 1970: 313). Later, it was incorporated into the official and semiofficial American pharmacology manuals; thus, the *United States Dispensatory* of 1926 (twenty-first edition) noted: "It has considerable use

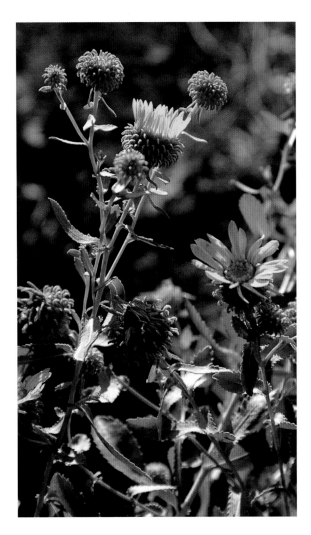

especially if applied three times a day (Jones 1911: 204). Herbalist Peter Holmes sees it as valuable also in **running sores**, **skin ulcers**, **dermatitis**, and **insect bites** and **stings** (Holmes 1997–98: 1:511–12).

Gumweed's anti-inflammatory effects may also partially elucidate its traditional aid for **genitourinary afflictions**, which has been widely appreciated by several Native American tribes (Moerman 1986: 1:208–9; Train et al. 1988: 55). Holmes finds it called for in the Traditional Chinese Medicine syndrome known as "kidney *qi* stagnation," manifested by cystitis, malaise, fatigue, and skin rashes (Holmes 1997–98: 1:511–12). Moore noted that the tincture is preferable for the urinary afflictions, suggesting that, for an adult, ¼ teaspoon be given in a little water every four hours (Moore 1979: 80). Various Native tribes—including the Navajo (Diné), Shoshone, and Montana—have even implemented gumweed to treat **venereal diseases** (Shemluck 1982: 333; Moerman 1986: 1:208–9; Mayes and Lacy 1989: 48).

The plant has long been a cherished folk remedy for two types of **cancer**—that of the **spleen** (the plant, in fact, is a spleen tonic par excellence: Ellingwood 1984: 320) and that of the **stomach**.

The Karok have used a decoction of the western species, *Grindelia robusta*, to kill **hair lice** (Strike and Roeder 1994: 67). Investigations have verified that highly resinous substances (such as mayonnaise, an old folk treatment) smother the lice, so it is understandable why this treatment might work from that respect. There may be other factors involved, however, such as the plant's essential oil.

Finally, the herb is understood to be a *heart relaxant*—capable of slowing a rapid heartbeat and moderating blood pressure. Holmes points out that it is most effective with what Traditional Chinese Medicine calls "heart *qi* constraint," manifested by a nervous, rapid heartbeat (Holmes 1989–90: 1:202). Moore noted that it is not always dependable in this regard, however (Moore 1979: 80). Holmes and other herbalists point out that gumweed can also act as a *circulatory stimulant* to help relieve a situation such as acute pulmonary **edema** (Holmes 1997–98: 1:511–12).

PERSONAL AND PROFESSIONAL USE

In my clinical practice, I haven't used gunweed much for respiratory conditions but have used it topically for itchy skin conditions—most often for poison ivy rash but also for lichen and some others. I've always found it to be most effective in the above regards.

CAUTIONS

The twenty-eighth edition of *Martindale: The Extra Pharmacopoeia* (1982) warns that large doses may irritate the kidneys. This is because of the large amount of resin in the plant. ⃬

... as a local application in the treatment of *rhus* poisoning" (Wood et al. 1926: 537–38). Although this application was later abandoned by the medical profession (which, however, has yet to come up with anything comparable), it is still utilized by some of today's herbalists, by way of various applications. The flowers may be crushed or pounded and then poulticed onto the rash; a wash may be made from a tincture mixed with a little water or from a fifteen-minute decoction, the latter of which is said to be as effective as fluid extracts of the plant (Moore 1979: 80; Weiner 1980: 109); or a commercial spray may be utilized. Finally, it should be noted that a 2005 clinical trial verified Canfield's observations on its efficacy for poison ivy rash (Canavan and Yarnell 2005: 709).

Other beneficial uses for the skin have been coaxed out of this plant as well, so that it has been found useful as a topical application for itchy skin conditions such as **impetigo**, **vaginitis**, and **eczema** (Wood et al. 1926: 537; Hutchens 1991: 147). Here, too, the Eclectic physician Eli Jones found that a mixture of one part fluid extract of grindelia with three parts water was the most effective topical application for **lichen**,

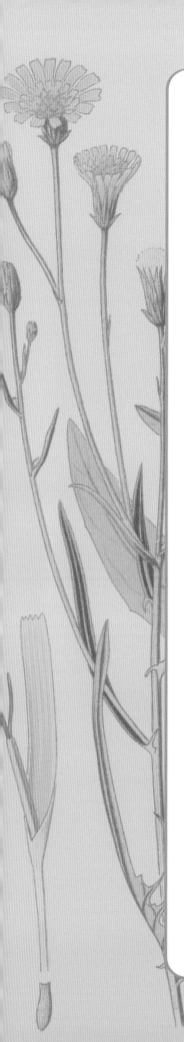

Hawk's Beard

Crepis tectorum, C. runcinata

DESCRIPTION

This is a weedy annual or perennial growing 1–3 feet tall and possessed of a slender stem filled with a milky juice. It displays both basal leaves and very narrow stem leaves.

The dandelion-like flower heads are yellow, about ½ inch in diameter, and arranged in spreading clusters. These eventually give rise to tufted achenes (similar to those produced by dandelions when they go to seed). Two species occur in the Midwest: *Crepis tectorum* and *C. runcinata*.

RANGE AND HABITAT

Hawk's beard is found throughout the Midwest in open, disturbed soils.

MAJOR CONSTITUENTS

Hawk's beard contains sesquiterpene lactones, flavonoids, and chlorogenic acid.

FOOD

I could find no record of either of our two native species ever having been used as food. However, the leaves of what is now considered a subspecies of *C. runcinata, C. glauca*, which edges into our area from the western United States, were consumed by the Gosiute (Chamberlain 1911: 367), and the peeled stems of *C. acuminata* have been eaten as greens by the Karok (Schenck and Gifford 1952).

HEALTH/MEDICINE

The Meskwaki (Fox) have viewed *C. runcinata* as a powerful topical medicine, strong enough to open a **carbuncle** and even a **cancerous growth** so that either could easily be excised (Smith 1928: 213). The particular application utilized is simply a poultice of the entire plant.

Homesickness and lonesomeness have been viewed as amenable to an infusion of the young plant of this same species by the Keres of the western United States (Swank 1932: 40). Western tribes have also used an indigenous species, *C. scopulorum* (*C. modocensis*), as an eyewash, implementing a decoction of the root (Train et al. 1988: 41). **Caked breast** has also been treated by a poultice of the mashed plant of this species as well as that of *C. modocensis* (Train et al. 1988: 41). Even the latex of *C. scopulorum* has been utilized by these tribes, who have applied it to **bee stings** and to **insect bites**, for which afflictions it appears to have greatly reduced the discomfort (Train et al. 1988: 41). ⋘

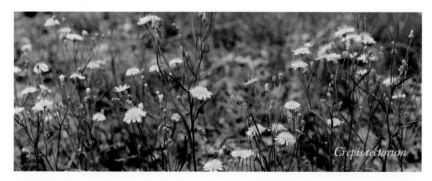

Crepis tectorum

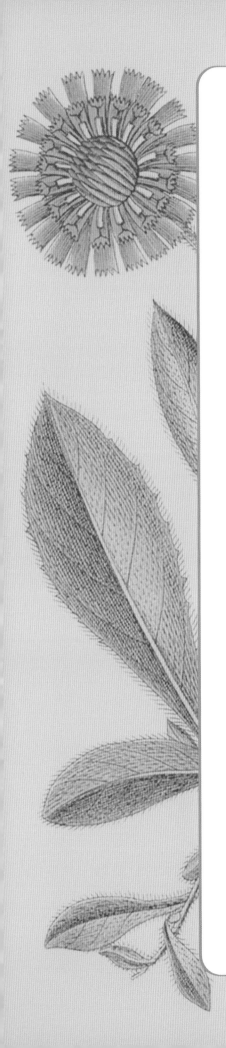

Hawkweed

Hieracium spp.

DESCRIPTION

This is a weedy, perennial member of the Asteraceae (Compositae) family, possessing ray flowers with squared-off tips and hairy herbage. The several important species in the Midwest include the following:

Hieracium aurantiacum (orange hawkweed, devil's paintbrush) grows ½–1½ feet tall and possesses a slender, very hairy stem that is conspicuous in that it is entirely leafless. There is, however, a cluster of long basal leaves, which—like the stem—are very hairy, aside from being entire and spatula-shaped. Inflorescence is in the form of a terminal, spreading cluster of two to ten reddish-orange flower heads, each about ¾ inch across. There are ten to twenty ray flowers but no ostensible disk flower. The ends of the rays are abruptly squared. The green bracts cupping the flower heads are covered with black, gland-tipped hairs.

H. kalmii (Kalm's hawkweed) (some prefer *H. canadense*—[Canada hawkweed] or *H. umbellatum* [Northern hawkweed]—the Latin names are currently in contention) reaches a height of 1–3 feet and possesses a stem that sprouts many sessile, clasping leaves that can range from elongate-elliptical to oval in shape. They are usually coarsely toothed and grow to about an inch long. The basal leaves, 2–5 inches long, disappear by flowering time, which sees the opening of four to ten yellow, dandelion-like flower heads sporting twenty to thirty ray flowers.

Other species in the Midwest include *H. pilosella* (mouse-eared hawkweed), which has a white bloom on the underside of its leaves, *H. longipilum, H. scabrum,* and *H. scabriusculum.*

RANGE AND HABITAT

Hawkweed thrives in dry, sunny places: open woods and fields, roadsides, clearings, pastures, and disturbed soils. In the Midwest, its range is from central to northeastern Minnesota into adjacent areas in Wisconsin.

MAJOR CONSTITUENTS

Hawkweed contains umbelliferone (a hydroxylated coumarin derivative), essential oil, and tannins.

HEALTH/MEDICINE

This plant has *diuretic* and *astringent* properties, as noted in the 1926 edition of the *United States Dispensatory* (Wood et al. 1926: 1332). As such, the Rappahannock have chewed *Hieracium scabrum*, or prepared a tea from it, to treat **diarrhea** (Speck 1942: 27). A species outside of the Midwest, *H. fendleri*, has been used by the Navajo (Diné) for **cystic stones**, **pelvic pain**, **anuria**, **hematuria**, and **venereal disease** (Wyman and Harris 1951: 60). The Cherokee have utilized a species of hawkweed in their area, *H. venosum*, for **trouble in the bowels** (Hamel and Chiltoskey 1975: 37).

These Native uses parallel the European usage for that continent's species, *H. murorum*, such as that by the seventeenth-century herbalist Nicholas Culpeper. He wrote of that species: "The juice in wine helps digestion, dispels wind, hinders crudities abiding in the stomach, and helps the difficulty in making water. ... The decoction of the herb and Wild Succory with wine cools heat, purges the stomach, increases blood, and

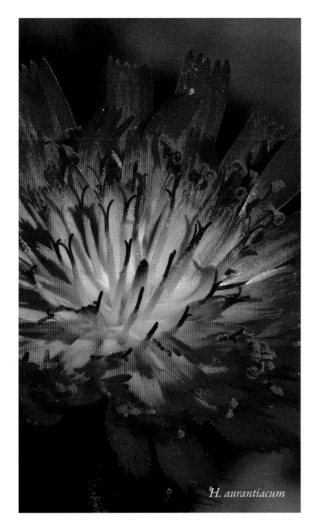

H. aurantiacum

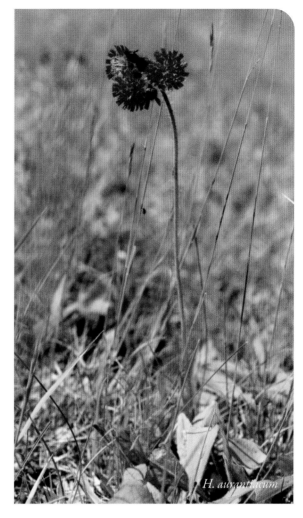

H. aurantiacum

helps diseases of the reins and bladder" (Culpeper 1983: 91). Culpeper also found hawkweed invaluable for **respiratory complaints**: "The decoction of the herb in honey digests phlegm, and with Hyssop helps the cough" (Culpeper 1983: 91). His predecessor in British herbalism, John Gerard, claimed that the hawkweeds were "good for the eyesight, if the juice of them be dropped into the eyes" (Gerard 1975: 300). This idea has been perpetuated in herbal practice ever since.

The veiny hawkweed, *H. venosum*, has been renowned as a remedy for **rattlesnake bites**. (In fact, an alternative common name for this species is rattlesnake weed.) So convincing was the evidence accumulated by the end of the first quarter of the nineteenth century that a Pennsylvania physician, Richard Harlan, felt compelled to weigh the evidence in experimental fashion: he subjected animals to serpentine attacks and then endeavored to see whether the remedy would take effect. Such a crude (and cruel!) methodology did not prove out the treatment, however, which is understandable given the plentitude of variables involved (Harlan 1830; Vogel 1970: 223).

Hawkweed has also been implemented by the Cherokee as one of several plants in a formula to treat what has been called "deer disease" (Mooney 1890). This term is not explicated in ethnobotanical texts, but I can't help but wonder whether this might have been what we now know as the deer tick–transmitted Lyme disease. It is of interest here that hawkweed has pronounced *antimicrobial* activity, although it has not been tested specifically for spirochetes. A 1954 screening of plants for antibacterial activity found the fresh flowers of *H. praeaeltum* to most strongly inhibit *Mycobacterium tuberculosis*, while its leaves and those of *H. venosum* mildly inhibited it (Fitzpatrick 1954: 530). Then, too, relative to the "floating arthritis" that Lyme disease can produce, a 1976 study found *H. unctate* and *H. florentinum* to produce an *anti-inflammatory* inhibition of 24 percent and 19 percent, respectively, in the rat-paw, carrageenan-produced edema test (Benoit et al. 1976: 164). ⤺

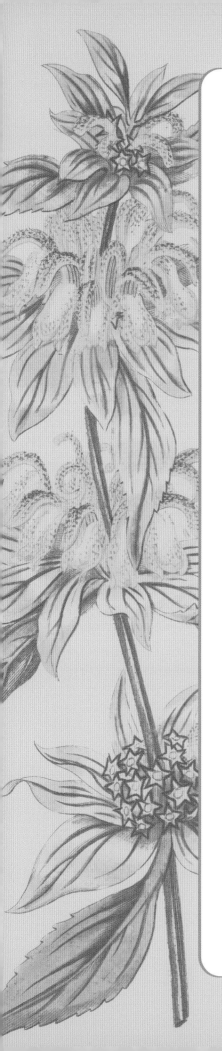

Horsemint

DESCRIPTION

This highly scented plant (it smells like perfume to me) is a perennial growing to 2 feet tall and possessed of a strong, erect, square stem.

The paired leaves are lanceolate, 2–4 inches long, and covered with dotted glands on their undersides. The upper leaves are somewhat white or even lavender in color.

The flowers emerge in the axils of the upper leaves in dense whorls and are yellow with purple flecks. They are surrounded by white to pale-purple leaf-like bracts.

RANGE AND HABITAT

This plant flourishes in the eastern two-thirds of the United States—in the alkaline, sandy soil of dry fields where it can get a lot of sun. In Minnesota, it is found in Anoka County on down through the southeastern counties.

MAJOR CONSTITUENTS

Horsemint contains glucuronide (a flavonoid) and an essential oil, known as monarda oil, composed of thymol (60 percent), cymene, carvacrol, thymohydroquinone, D-limonene, camphene, heptanal, pulegone, and a trace of formaldehyde. This plant has the highest known amount of both thymol (much higher than in thyme) and carvacrol (Duke 1994: 12).

HEALTH/MEDICINE

Like all mints, horsemint proves useful for expelling gas from the colon (i.e., it is a *carminative*), and it was recognized in the 1926 and 1937 editions of the *United States Dispensatory* for just such activity. This source also made mention of *stimulant* qualities possessed by the herb, which may explain why Carolina moms have tended to use it as an aid in **postpartum recovery** (Morton 1974: 97). Indeed, too, the Fox are even documented to have used horsemint as a *nasal stimulant* to rally a person who was slipping into death! (Smith 1928: 225, 226) Some modern herbalists also use a stimulating cup of horsemint tea to dispel **nasal congestion**, as have the Fox and Nanticoke tribes (Moerman 1986: 1:298).

While stimulating in certain respects, the herb has traditionally been used to unwind the mind after a day filled with too many thoughts and/or activities. Horsemint's most pronounced effect, however, is an *antiemetic* one, which was appreciated by the Eclectics (Felter and Lloyd 1898; Ellingwood 1983: 281). Jacob Bigelow, a prominent physician of the early 1800s, was most enamored of this property, along with the herb's carminative effects (Vogel 1970: 338).

As noted, horsemint is the highest known source of thymol, a powerful *fungistatic* and *bacteriostatic* chemical (Didry et al. 1993) that is the major component of the plant's essential oil, called monarda oil. Toxicologist David Spoerke notes that because 50 percent of this oil is excreted in the urine, it might serve as a urinary *antiseptic*, although he feels that the proteins present would limit the bacteriostatic potential (Spoerke 1990: 91). The clinical experience of herbalists, however, suggests otherwise; likewise, the Eclectics found it to be highly useful in "urinary disorders" (Felter and Lloyd 1898). Thymol also serves as an antiseptic for the throat and has thus long been an ingredient in Listerine. A 2014 scientific study found the plant's essential oil to damage or kill (depending on the concentration used) a variety of respiratory pathogens, especially *Streptococcus pyogenes* (Li et al. 2014).

Owing to the thymol content, too, the essential oil was formerly used as an *anthelmintic*, especially for **hookworm**, but the dosage required was so high as to be dangerous (Weiner 1980: 23). However, such use of the oil may have been unnecessary, as simple infusions of the plant were popularly used as anthelmintics by physicians in colonial America (Christianson 1987: 73). Monarda oil was also used, in times past, as a *rubefacient* for **rheumatic** joints (Vogel 1970: 338; Bolyard 1981: 88); for **neuralgia** (Felter and Lloyd 1898); and, what is especially of interest, for **deafness** (Vogel 1970: 338; Bolyard 1981: 88). Yet as it tended to blister the skin if left on too long (Felter and Lloyd 1898), it is no longer being utilized.

The British herbalist M. Grieve observed that horsemint has been widely utilized as both an *emmenagogue* and a *diaphoretic* (Grieve 1971: 2:546). As to the former application, the Eclectic writers Harvey Wickes Felter and John Uri Lloyd noted similarly: "The warm infusion … has acquired some reputation as an emmenagogue" (Felter and Lloyd 1898). In modern times, even the *PDR for Herbal Medicines* lists dysmenorrhea as an indication for the use of this odoriferous plant (Fleming 1998). Horsemint's sweat-inducing ability has been noted by numerous sources as well and strongly contributes to its renowned *antipyretic* property, which has been implemented by Native tribes as diverse as the Lenape (Delaware) (Tantaquidgeon 1972: 73, 130), the Mohegan (Tantaquidgeon 1942: 54), the Creek (Taylor 1940: 54), and the Navaho-Ramah (Vestal 1952: 42) whenever fever broke out. The antipyretic effects are what originally impressed an E. A. Atlee, in the early nineteenth century, who brought the herb to the attention of the medical profession in 1819, demonstrating it to be useful for various low forms of **fever** as well as topically in a liniment for both neuralgia and rheumatism (Atlee 1819; Crellin and Philpott 1990a: 252).

In a fascinating article published in 1994, James Duke pointed out that horsemint contains four ingredients—thymol, carvacrol, pulegone, and limonene—demonstrated by Austrian scientists to prevent the breakdown of acetylcholine in the brain, a process understood to be overactive in **Alzheimer's disease**. Since at least some of these compounds reportedly pass through the blood-brain barrier, Duke asks whether a shampoo made with horsemint might prove useful for Alzheimer's sufferers (Duke 1994).

PERSONAL AND PROFESSIONAL USE

I occasionally drink horsemint tea in the evening to unwind my mind after a frazzled day—which it does nicely, ensuring a good night's sleep. I've also used it, for both myself and clients, as an antinauseant, always with excellent results.

CAUTIONS

Because of the high content of both thymol and carvacrol and the classic use as an emmenagogue, *this herb should be excluded from use during pregnancy.* ⤶

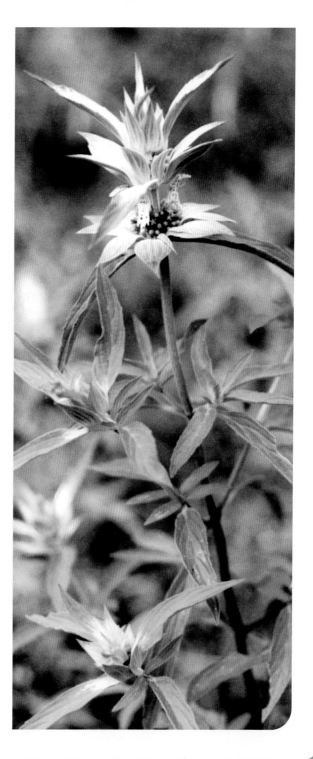

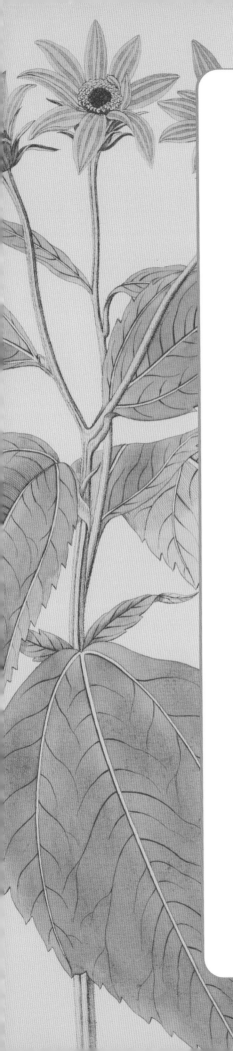

Jerusalem Artichoke

DESCRIPTION

This is a lovely perennial plant growing up to 12 feet (7–9 feet is average, however). The stem is hairy and branches considerably toward the top.

The long-stalked leaves are oblong to oval in shape, sharply pointed, and coarsely toothed. They grow 6–10 inches long and 2–4 inches wide. They are usually trident veined (i.e., with two branching veins from the midrib forming what looks like a trident), starting at the base of the leaf. As with the stem, stiff hairs envelop the leaves so that a rough, bristly feeling is experienced when running one's hand along them. Interestingly, too, while the upper leaves are alternate, the lower leaves are often opposite.

The plant's gorgeous yellow-orange blossoms appear at the tip of the main stem and its branches (up to eighteen blossoms per plant!). These bloom in September and are 2–3 inches across. Botanically, they are composite, which means that they consist of a central disk flower (which in this case is yellow) and ten to twenty ray flowers (which are also yellow).

The rhizome has numerous large tubers, each possessing opposite buds.

This plant, being a member of the *Helianthus* genus, is a sunflower and thus resembles other sunflowers to a large degree. This being as it is, it is often frustrating for the amateur to try to distinguish it from other sunflowers. Here, however, the following pointers can be borne in mind: Jerusalem artichoke has blossoms that open later in the year than do those of most other sunflowers; it has more branches, and consequently more flower heads, than do most other species; it has longer leaves than do most other species; and its leafstalks are winged.

RANGE AND HABITAT

A lover of wet soil and disturbed ground, Jerusalem artichoke grows pretty much throughout the Midwest.

SEASONAL AVAILABILITY

Tubers are available in October (after the blossoms have fallen) as well as in the winter (in still-unfrozen ground) and in the spring (before the shoots start popping up again).

MAJOR CONSTITUENTS

The tubers contain carbohydrate in the form of inulin. Nutrients include high amounts of iron.

FOOD

Sometimes called sunchokes, the tubers of Jerusalem artichoke are widely known to be edible. Locate them by scouting patches in September when the plants are flowering and then returning to harvest them in late fall (after the first frost, when the flowers have disappeared) or early spring before the shoots start up again. Those dug in the spring are sweetest because the sugar content is highest at this time.

Many feel that the tubers, when peeled of their unpleasant-tasting rind, taste like Chinese chestnuts. There's only one problem: because of the inulin content, they are

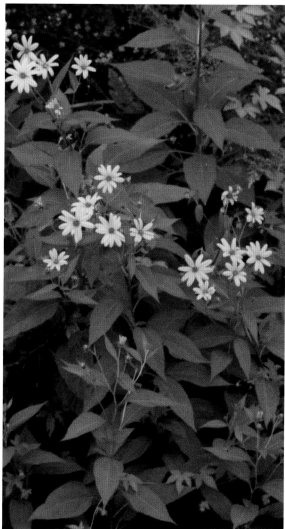

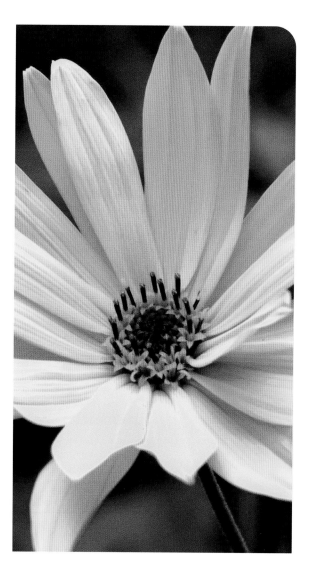

somewhat indigestible, so those with weaker digestive systems tend to experience flatulence after eating them. Cooking, however, greatly reduces the gassiness that the tubers can induce and renders the taste potato-like.

Sunchokes can be stored in the fridge for up to two weeks but then spoil rapidly, becoming mushy.

HEALTH/MEDICINE

Jerusalem artichoke has *tonic*, *diuretic*, and *hypoglycemic* activities (Porcher 1849: 798–99; Lewis and Elvin-Lewis 1977: 218). Not surprisingly, then, its fleshy tubers have proven useful for those with **diabetes**. This is because, as previously noted, they contain inulin, a carbohydrate that is not a starch and so does not raise blood-sugar levels.

A tincture of Jerusalem artichoke blossoms has been used for **bronchitis**, especially when there is **chronic bronchial dilation** (Angier 1978: 150).

PERSONAL AND PROFESSIONAL USE

I've partaken of Jerusalem artichoke tubers that I've dug from the ground on a number of occasions. The taste is a bit too strong for my palate. Notwithstanding, however, they've proven a welcome addition to my diet when on survival excursions during the late fall or early winter.

CAUTIONS

Be absolutely sure of identification, since these tubers resemble those of several highly poisonous plants.

Be aware that eating raw Jerusalem artichokes may cause flatulence. ⤜⤜

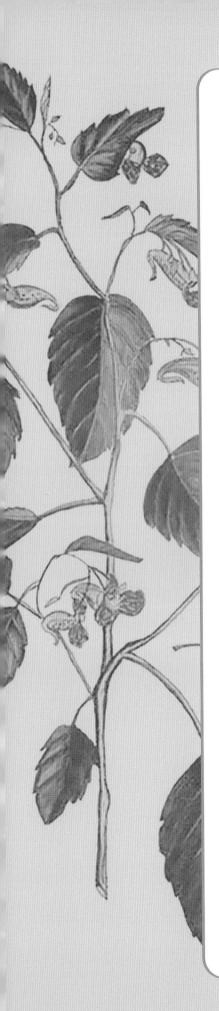

Jewelweed

TOUCH-ME-NOT; SILVERWEED

Impatiens capensis [alternatively, *I. biflora*], *I. pallida*

DESCRIPTION

Jewelweed is a succulent annual herb that reaches a height of 2–5 feet. The branched stem is smooth, characteristically translucent, and very juicy.

The ovate leaves have rounded teeth and grow 1½–3½ inches long. They are densely covered with small hairs. In fact, if submerged in water, they glisten, from which fact the plant's alternative name of silverweed derives. The uppermost leaves are alternate, while the lower leaves are sometimes opposite.

Snapdragon-like flowers appear on slender stalks arising from the leaf axils. These flowers are bilaterally symmetrical, sporting three petals emanating from a bell-shaped corolla that terminates in a spur. The flowers of *Impatiens capensis* are orange with reddish-brown spots, while those of *I. pallida* are pale yellow. As a further point of distinction, the spur of *I. capensis* extends backward, while that of *I. pallida* extends downward.

RANGE AND HABITAT

Jewelweed flourishes in moist ground (streamsides, perimeters of marshes and swamps, wet woods) throughout the Midwest.

MAJOR CONSTITUENTS

Jewelweed contains lawsone; tannin; minerals (selenium, calcium oxalate); saponins; and probably 2-methoxy-1, 4-naphthoquinone (which occurs in *I. balsamina*).

FOOD

This is an edible and tasty plant if used when less than 6 inches tall and properly prepared. To do this, separate the stems from the rest of the plant and cut them into string-bean-size pieces. Then, boil these for ten to fifteen minutes in two changes of water. When done, shake off all of the water before consuming. (However, the water, while having extracted mildly toxic principles from the plant, can still be saved and frozen for skin applications—see below.) Many wild-foods authors stress that jewelweed is too powerful for the system if consumed alone and should therefore have its potency moderated by being mixed with other vegetables before being eaten. One can do this after cooking as outlined above or alternatively, after only five minutes of simmering, the stem segments can be mixed into stir-fry dishes.

When jewelweed seeds are ripe, they are edible and can be eaten as a trail nibble, tasting a bit like walnuts. However, because they are rapidly discharged from their fruits when the plant is brushed, their efficient collection requires some manual dexterity and a large collection device (a shopping bag is ideal). Additionally, before the seeds can be eaten, their jettison coils must be removed.

HEALTH/MEDICINE

The crushed, juicy plant is an age-old topical treatment for a wide variety of skin ailments. The Lenape (Delaware) have applied it to **burns** (Speck 1915: 320), and **ringworm, impetigo, contact dermatitis,** and **athlete's foot** have all been successfully combated via topical

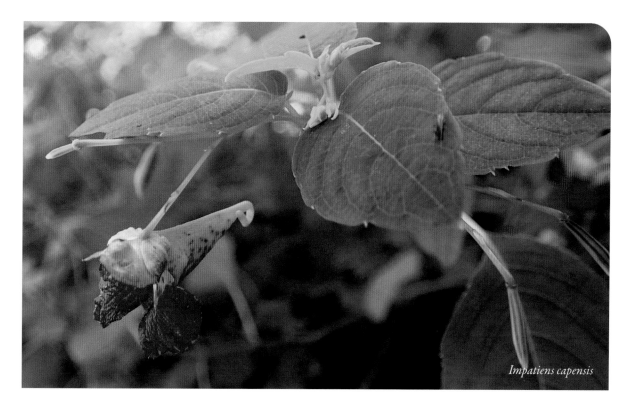

Impatiens capensis

use of this plant. A powerful *antifungal* chemical, known as 2-methoxy-1,4-naphthoquinone, has been confirmed in the related species *I. balsamina* and may in fact be present here, shedding light on the above delineated applications.

The Meskwaki (Fox) and the Potawatomi have rubbed the juice onto **nettle stings** to bring relief (Smith 1928: 205; Smith 1933: 42). James Duke reported that a chemical called lawsone extracted from the plant is the active agent in this nullification process, which he confirmed via personal experimentation with the extracted chemical on both himself and volunteers who subjected themselves to nettle stings (Duke 1997: 262).

The Omaha have treated **rash** and **eczema** with jewelweed (Gilmore 1991: 49). Here the most celebrated topical use of this plant, however, has been for **poison ivy rash**: the Potawatomi have reverenced the use of jewelweed for this miserable affliction (Smith 1933: 42), as have the Cherokee, who prefer rubbing the juice from seven flowers on just such a rash (Hamel and Chiltoskey 1975: 41). Although two published studies (Guin and Reynolds 1980; Long et al. 1997) declared such treatment ineffective, others have suggested efficacy. One late-1950s clinical study following a physician's treatment of 115 patients with jewelweed noted its success with an impressive 108 of these—a 94 percent success rate! (Foster and Duke 1990: 136)

Yet while there is conflicting evidence for jewelweed's effect on a full-blown poison ivy dermatitis, evidence for positive *prophylactic* efficacy is not generally contested and has been demonstrated in a published clinical trial (Abrams Motz et al. 2012). Rutgers University chemist Robert Rosen offered the thought that the active ingredient in jewelweed's prevention of poison ivy–induced rash is lawsone, which binds to the same receptor sites on the skin as the troublesome vine's active agent, urushiol, and beats the latter to those sites if applied quickly after initial contact with the resin; the net effect is that the urushiol is "locked out." James Duke adds that the greatest concentration of lawsone is in the reddish protuberances at the base of jewelweed's stem (Duke 1997: 359). However, more recent research has failed to correlate lawsone content with rash prevention and has demonstrated that the plant's saponins are the effective agents (Abrams Motz et al. 2012; Motz et al. 2015).

As for other topical uses, the ethnobotanist Huron Smith observed that the Potawatomi would boil down an infusion of this plant into a thick mass to apply to **sprains**, **bruises**, and **sores** (Smith 1933: 116). Naturalist and herbalist Tom Brown Jr. finds jewelweed to be soothing to **insect stings**, **blisters**, and **sunburn** (Brown 1985: 132).

PERSONAL AND PROFESSIONAL USE

I enjoy the beauty of this plant, especially the yellow-flowered species. Although that species is not commonly found in my area, I am familiar with two different areas where it does grow and where I will go to view it. I also treasure the rich taste of jewelweed seeds in the fall.

CAUTIONS

Jewelweed's high content of minerals with toxic potential suggests that consumption of this plant should be limited. ⤷

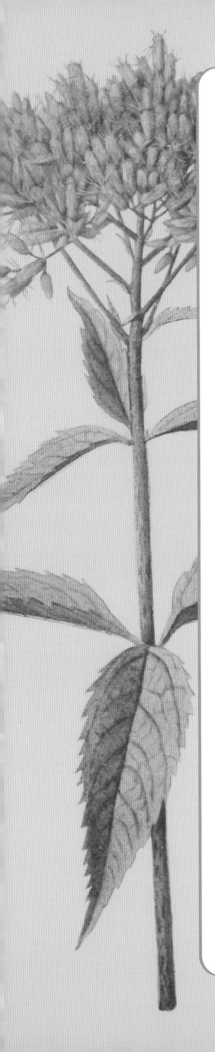

Joe-Pye Weed

GRAVEL ROOT; QUEEN OF THE MEADOW; PURPLE BONESET

Eutrochium [formerly *Eupatorium*] *purpureum, E. maculatum*

DESCRIPTION

Joe-pye weed is a tall plant (2–7 feet) with an erect, rigid, unbranched stem.

It is possessed of lanceolate leaves that are rough above and downy below. These are positioned in whorls of three to six at intervals along the stem.

The flower head is in the form of clustered blossoms resting at the tip of the stem. The blossoms are solely disk flowers and are pink-purple in color—thus the alternative common name purple boneset, in distinction from its white-flowered relative, boneset (see page 44).

In early autumn, a fluffy seedhead replaces the flowers.

Several species flourish in North America, but those growing in the Midwest are *Eutrochium maculatum* (spotted joe-pye weed) and *E. purpureum* (sweet joe-pye weed, gravel root, queen of the meadow). The former has a purple or purple-spotted stem and somewhat flat-topped flower heads. The latter has a hollow green stem with a purple band or spots at the leaf nodes only, a more dome-shaped florescence, and flowers and leaves that exude a very pleasant vanilla-like odor (especially when crushed).

RANGE AND HABITAT

Joe-pye weed thrives in marshes, ditches, shores, damp meadows, and open and wet woods. *E. maculatum* flourishes throughout the Midwest, while *E. purpureum* grows principally in areas east of the Mississippi.

MAJOR CONSTITUENTS

Joe-pye weed contains benzofurans (including euparin, euparone, and others); cistifolin; eupurpurin (an oleoresin); sesquiterpene lactones; unsaturated pyrrolizidine alkaloids; and an essential oil.

HEALTH/MEDICINE

Joe-pye weed has served most prominently as a reliable *diuretic* (Mockle 1955: 90) and was listed as such in the 1820–1830 editions of the *United States Pharmacopeia*. John C. Gunn, in his famous household medical guide of the latter half of the nineteenth century, said here: "The root is the part used, and is regarded by botanic physicians as a valuable diuretic ... highly esteemed in dropsical affections ... and affections of the kidneys and urinary organs. ... [Implemented are the] bruised roots in water ... given in doses of from half to a teacupful three or four times a day" (Gunn 1859–61: 846).

Joe-pye weed is more than just a diuretic, however—it is more broadly a *urinary* and hence is renowned as being a specific for **hematuria** (Tierra 1988: 220; Willard 1993: 171) as well as serving as a very powerful *lithotriptic* (hence its alternative common name of "gravel root"). As to the latter use, however, Canadian herbalist Terry Willard notes that, in his experience, it sometimes has eliminated kidney stones too quickly, causing a lot of pain. He therefore recommends its use for this purpose only when accompanied by a demulcent herb, such as marshmallow root (*Althea* spp.), and further stresses that joe-pye weed should not be taken in large quantities (Willard 1994: 6:9).

Further explicating its diuretic/urinary applications, early-twentieth-century botanical writer Charles Millspaugh wrote—in reflecting upon comments in the materia medica of the Eclectic physician John King—that the root of joe-pye weed seems "to exert a special influence upon chronic renal and cystic trouble, especially when there is an excess of uric acid present" (Millspaugh 1974: 309). Therefore, a decoction has often been used by herbalists for **joint stiffness** and for **lumbago** when either is known or suspected to be caused by uric acid deposits (Hutchens 1991: 255). Such a tea has, in like accord, been used by the Cherokee for **gout** and for **rheumatism** (Hamel and Chiltoskey 1975: 42), while our own area's Ojibwe have preferred a lukewarm decoction as a wash for those painful joints (Densmore 1974: 348–49). A late-1990s study identified the chemical cistifolin as being one active agent in preventing rheumatic inflammation. It was found that this chemical inhibited integrin-mediated cell adhesion (Habtemariam et al. 1998).

Joe-pye weed is also a *nervine* (Wren 1972: 140; Tierra 1988: 220) and, as such, is especially thought to be helpful for genitourinary conditions of an "irritable" nature. The Natura physician R. Swinburne Clymer noted here: "It is of much value in irritable conditions of the bladder and in kidney conditions accompanied by aching in the small of the back. In irritated conditions of the female organs, it is most helpful" (Clymer 1973: 158). Western American herbalist Ed Smith points out that one should especially think here of the **uterus**, including the **atony** or **displacement** of such, as well as **chronic endometriosis** (Smith 1999: 37). Not surprising in view of the latter is that joe-pye weed is a fair *emmenagogue*, especially being applicable to **painful amenorrhea** (Ody 1993: 57). It is also often helpful for **pelvic inflammatory disease** (Mabey et al. 1988: 48).

British herbalist Mary Carse also finds the decoction valuable for **spermatorrhea**, dosed at 1 teaspoon every three waking hours (Carse 1989: 119). Others would list it for **prostate problems** as well, especially for a boggy prostate (Christopher 1976: 254; Willard 1993: 171; Smith 1999: 37). One champion of the latter application was the legendary Alabama herbalist Tommie Bass, who cited several examples of his successful use in this regard, including one case of a client who had prostate trouble so bad that his doctor had urged an operation. Bass noted that this man proceeded to drink 2–3 cups of the tea a day for a while and then submitted to his physician's exam, upon which he was thrilled to get a clean bill of health as well as his doctor's strong urging: "I don't know what you have been doing, but keep doing it" (Crellin and Philpott 1990a: 274–75).

Joe-pye weed has also historically been used to help deal with **diabetes**. Lab experiments have verified *hypoglycemic* activity for *Eutrochium* (at the time called *Eupatorium*) *purpureum* (Lewis and Elvin-Lewis 1977: 217–18). Tommie Bass, having used both this species and his indigenous *E.*

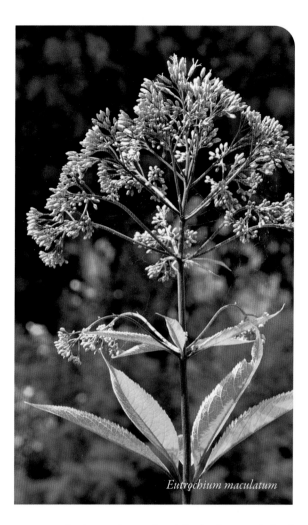

Eutrochium maculatum

serotinum for this condition, found that both species helped diabetes considerably, although he felt that the latter was the more effective of the two (Crellin and Philpott 1990a: 274).

The leaves have been utilized by various Native American tribes as a *vulnerary*. The Potawatomi of the Midwest have implemented the fresh leaves as a poultice for **burns** (Smith 1933: 52).

The decoction is made by boiling 20 grams of the root in 600 milliliters of water (Ody 1993: 138). Bass, in his appealing, down-home style, declared: "One quart of roots makes a gallon of medicine. The roots can be dried in the sun and stored in paper sacks. Boil one hour and strain it and keep it in the refrigerator or it will sour. ... If it don't turn your stomach, it is simple and safe" (Crellin and Philpott 1990a: 274). In view of the fact that the plant contains toxic pyrrolizidine alkaloids, however, it should not be used long term. (See further in Cautions, below.)

CAUTIONS

This plant should not be used in pregnancy or lactation or on a long-term basis. It should also not be given to young children or infants. ⫷

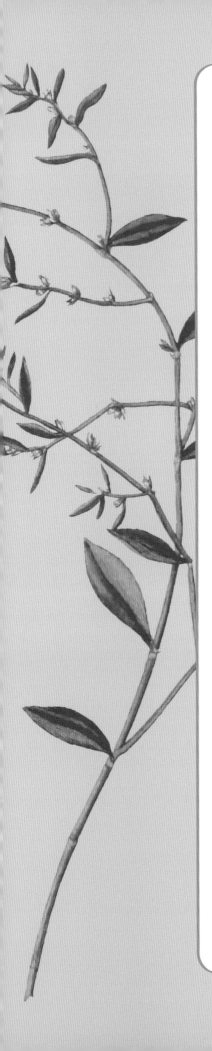

Knotweed

DESCRIPTION

Here we have a sprawling annual weed that reaches anywhere from 4 to 24 inches and is possessed of jointed stems marked by silvery or brown sheathes at the juncture points.

Knotweed's leaves are alternate, hairless, oblong, and pointed, both at their tip and at their base. They grow ½–1½ inches long. Each leaf has a prominent center vein.

The flowers, opening only on sunny days, are tiny and yellow, pink, or green. These give way to small, three-angled, reddish-brown seeds.

RANGE AND HABITAT

This is a cosmopolitan urban weed, found in hard-trampled areas such as the edges of parking lots, lawns, and sidewalks (including in between the slabs). It also thrives in dooryards and waste places.

MAJOR CONSTITUENTS

Knotweed contains polygonic acid; flavonoids (rutin, avicularin, quercetin, quercitrin, kaempferol, vitexin, isovitexin, delphinidin); hydroxycoumarins (umbelliferone, scopoletin); salicylic acid; plant acids (caffeic, chlorogenic); mucilage; and catechin. Nutrients include vitamin C and silicic acid.

FOOD

Eating raw knotweed can cause intestinal disturbances (Dobelis et al. 1986: 228), but it is edible once it is cooked. It is popular as such in Asia and was also at one time in Europe (Couplan 1998: 129). The seeds can be ground into flour.

HEALTH/MEDICINE

Knotweed was an esteemed herb of the ancients: back in the first century of our common era, the scholarly and skilled herbalist Dioscorides described this plant and its powers in detail, noting first that it "hath a binding, refrigerating faculty." He next went on to spotlight its usefulness for the **spitting of blood** and as a pessary for "ye womanish flux" and finally commented that a poultice of the leaves was used when there was "casting up of blood" (Dioscorides 1996: 4:4). The learned naturalist Pliny the Elder, a contemporary of Dioscorides, similarly related that the juice when taken with wine was capable of allaying **epistaxis** as well as **hemorrhage** in any part of the body (Pliny 1938 27:114–17). Celsus, writing about half a century later, alluded as well to knotweed's powerful *styptic* abilities (Celsus 1938: 5.1, 6.7.4). Then, too, the ancient physician Soranus even treated **uterine hemorrhage** with a knotgrass plaster or sometimes even with an actual injection of the juice (Jashemski 1999: 80).

The intervening centuries have verified that knotweed is indeed both a powerful *hemostat* and an *astringent*. Thus, owing to its demonstrable antihemorrhage effects, the Choctaw could imbibe a strong knotweed tea with the firm conviction that it would prevent miscarriage (Campbell and Roberts 1951: 286). Russian scientists have verified the herb's ability to stop uterine bleeding, and it is therefore part of official medicine in their country, with a commercially prepared liquid extract available (although only by prescription) (Zevin 1997: 93).

Knotweed has proven helpful for **diarrhea** and for its most severe form, **dysentery** (Lust 1974: 245; Willard 1992b: 148). Understandable, too, in view of its astringency, is that the tea has been recommended for **sore throat** and for **laryngitis** by the scientists composing German Commission E (Blumenthal 1998). The *PDR for Herbal Medicines* notes its traditional use as a hemostat, acknowledges its astringency, and further points out that it has been shown to inhibit the enzyme acetylcholinesterase, which is overactive in Alzheimer's disease (Fleming 1998).

Inflammation of the **mouth** and the **throat** is another indication for knotweed, according to the *PDR for Herbal Medicines*. A 1995 study confirmed the plant has anti-inflammatory properties, inhibiting both the cyclooxygenase pathway toward inflammation and exocytosis induced by platelet-activating-factor (PAF) (Tunón et al. 1995). Earlier research had likewise shown *anti-inflammatory* effects (Kresanek and Krejca 1989: 54). Interestingly, Dioscorides had long ago advocated its use for **gastric inflammation** (Dioscorides 1996: 4:4), and, centuries later, Ramah Navajo (Diné) in the western United States would use it similarly (Vestal 1952: 23).

Knotweed would seem, indeed, to be a good herb for the gastrointestinal tract in general. Pliny drew attention to its common implementation for **digestive ailments** (Pliny 1938: 27:114–17). Our herb has also been used in folk medicine for **cancer** of the stomach, breast, and kidneys (Duke 1985: 389).

Pliny held it to be effective for **colds** (Pliny 1938: 27:114–17), while the German Commission E of our present day holds it to be effective for **respiratory complaints**, including **bronchitis** (Blumenthal 1998). The *PDR for Herbal Medicines* lists its indications as "cough" and "bronchitis" and notes its traditional usage as an *anticatarrhal* (Fleming 1998). Knotweed's efficacy for pulmonary complaints may at least be partly due to its content of silicic acid, which strengthens connective tissue (Chevallier 1996: 251).

Knotweed was used in ancient Pompeii for **heart troubles.** In a fascinating continuity of tradition, it continues to be used for that complaint in the same region today (Jashemski 1999: 80). Other cultures in Europe have employed it to help reduce **hypertension** (Duke 1985: 389). Its success at lowering blood pressure seems to be due primarily to *vasorelaxant* properties (occurring via endothelium-dependent nitric oxide) identified in the plant (Yin et al. 2005).

A treasured *diuretic* (Kresanek and Krejca 1989: 54; Willard 1992b: 148), knotweed is best known by students of herbs as a *urinary* aid, especially as an herb capable of carrying away **urinary gravel** (Jackson 1873: 105; Kresanek and Krejca 1989: 148). Dioscorides, noting that it "moves

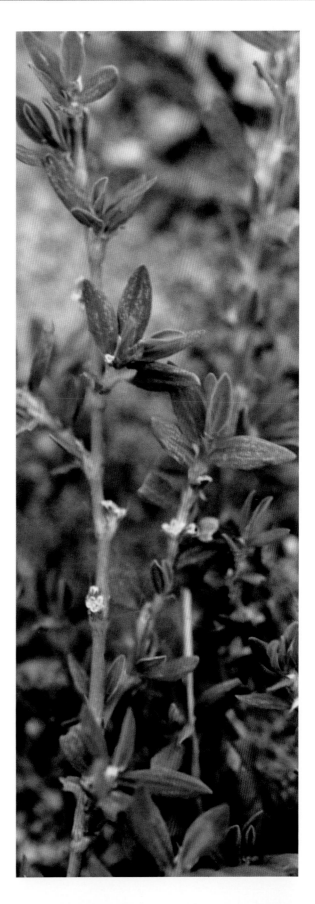

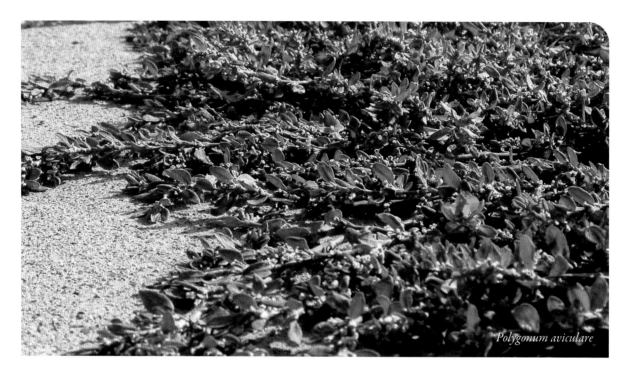
Polygonum aviculare

ye urine also manifestly," also highlighted its benefits for **strangury** (Dioscorides 1996: 4:4). William Cook, the noted Physiomedicalist physician, pointed out: "It acts rather efficiently upon the kidneys, relieving sudden suppression, with aching through the back and bladder" (Cook 1985). The Natura physician R. Swinburne Clymer noted, as well, that its "chief influence is on the bladder" and that it was regarded as a *lithotriptic* of last resort, often being combined with horsetail (*Equisetum* spp.) for best effect (Clymer 1973: 91).

Traditional Chinese Medicine (TCM) uses knotweed (under the name of *bian xu*) as a medicinal herb as well, paralleling some of the Western applications for this plant. TCM employs knotweed as a urinary aid (especially for painful or dribbling urine), as a hemostat (for a **bloody** or **mucoid vaginal discharge** as well as for **postpartum bleeding**), and as an astringent for **diarrhea** and for **dysentery** (Yanchi 1995: 106; Belanger 1997: 588). As to the latter affliction, Chinese research has established that knotweed is powerfully effective against **bacillary dysentery.** In one study involving 108 people who were afflicted with the condition and treated with a knotweed paste ingested daily, 104 recovered within five days (Chevallier 1996: 251). TCM also esteems knotweed for conditions such as intestinal worms, weeping eczema, fungal skin conditions, and certain kinds of jaundice (Yanchi 1995: 106; Belanger 1997: 588).

PERSONAL AND PROFESSIONAL USE

I've used knotweed myself for dysuria and have recommended it to clients in similar situations, as well as to those suffering from gastrointestinal inflammation, dysentery, bloody discharges of a passive nature, or cancer of the breast, stomach, or kidneys.

CAUTIONS

Contact dermatitis can occur in some persons who touch this plant. *Use in pregnancy or lactation is not advised.* ⤸

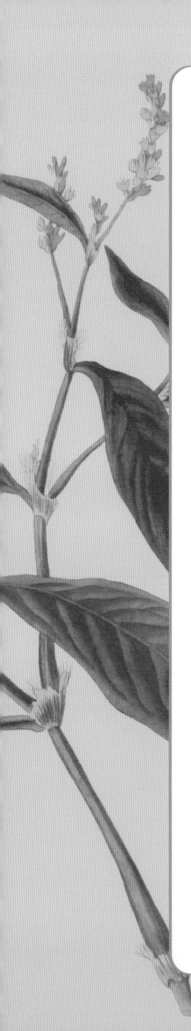

Lady's Thumb

Polygonum persicaria

DESCRIPTION

This perennial relative of both knotweed (see page 140) and smartweed (page 215) grows 6–30 inches tall and possesses a jointed stem that is reddish or pinkish hued.

The leaves of lady's thumb are lanceolate, 2–6 inches long, and marked by a dark, three-angled blotch in the middle of their blades (as if imprinted by a lady's thumb). In that this is a *Polygonum* species, papery sheaths occur at the leaf nodes—which, in this case, are fringed with short bristles.

The blossoms are white to pink to purple (often some of each color) and occur in terminal, elongate clusters that measure 1–2 inches long.

RANGE AND HABITAT

This interesting plant thrives throughout the Midwest in gardens, waste places, marsh edges, damp clearings, cultivated ground, and roadsides.

MAJOR CONSTITUENTS

Lady's thumb contains flavonoids (hyperin, meletin, kaempferol, isoquercitrin, and avicularin); chromones (including 5,7-dihydroxychromone); an essential oil; and an unidentified glycoside.

FOOD

Boiled for five or ten minutes, the young leaves are quite tasty, being somewhat reminiscent of spinach. Many wild-foods connoisseurs also add them to soups, stews, and casseroles.

HEALTH/MEDICINE

Lady's thumb is an esteemed *diuretic* and has a history of use by various Native American and other cultures for **gravel** (Foster and Duke 1990: 160) and for **scanty urine** (Angier 1978: 161). For these conditions, a teaspoonful is steeped in a cup of bubbling water and sipped cold during the day, to the tune of 1 or 2 cupfuls every twenty-four hours (Angier 1978: 161).

The plant is also *astringent* and has thus been implemented to treat **diarrhea**, **sores**, **ulcers**, and **aphthous sore mouth** (Rafinesque 1828–30: 2:66; Mockle 1955: 38). Its astringency probably also largely explains its folk-medicinal use for **eczema** (Potterton 1983: 18) and for **poison ivy rash** (Foster and Duke 1990: 160). It perhaps accounts, as well, for the longtime European and Ojibwe use for **gastric pain** (Mockle 1955: 38; Densmore 1974: 344; Foster and Duke 1990: 160). Lady's thumb has also been traditionally used for **jaundice** and for other **liver diseases** (Potterton 1983: 18; Silverman 1990: 75).

For ages, the plant has been appreciated as a *vulnerary* (Mockle 1955: 38). Here it has been poulticed onto **painful areas**, providing relief as an *anodyne* (Foster and Duke 1990: 160). A leaf tea has a long history of use as a foot soak for **rheumatism** (Potterton 1983: 18; Foster and Duke 1990: 160), including among the Iroquois, who

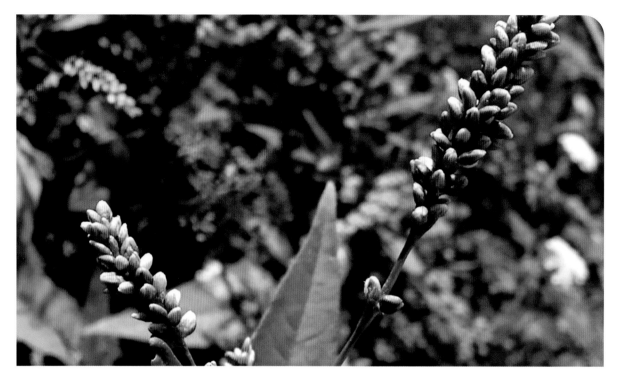

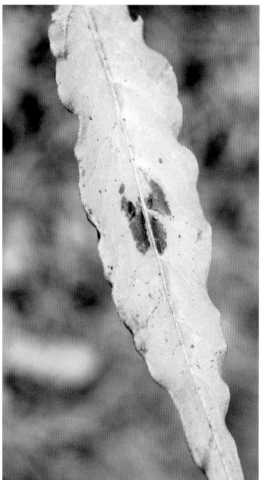

have boiled one plant in 1 gallon of water and then soaked their feet in it, thereafter bandaging them. On the next morning, the bandages are removed, and the entire process is repeated for that day (Herrick 1995: 144).

In Canada, there is a long-standing tradition of using this herb as an *anthelmintic* (Mockle 1955: 38). It has also been utilized by a variety of cultures for **cancer** (Hartwell 1970: 373). Various Native tribes found the plant helpful for **heart troubles** (Foster and Duke 1990: 160; Herrick 1995: 145), hence its alternative name of "heart's-ease." A mid-1950s study found it to be active against the tuberculosis organism in vitro (Fitzpatrick 1954: 530).

As for preparation and dosage, naturopath John Lust says to steep 1 teaspoon of the herb in 1 cup of water and then drink 1–2 cups a day (Lust 1974: 247).

PERSONAL AND PROFESSIONAL USE

I enjoy pointing out this plant, with its eye-catching "lady's thumb" imprint, to students when conducting wild-plant identification walks. However, I have not used it much in my herbal practice.

CAUTIONS

Raw lady's thumb possesses an acrid juice, which—though not as pronounced as some of its smartweed cousins—can irritate mucous membranes, such as the eyes, lips, mouth, and throat. A number of foragers have reported that the very young leaves seem to be free of this "smarting" nature, although I cannot confirm this and strongly advise against experimentation.

One should avoid rubbing one's eyes when harvesting, or otherwise handling, this plant. ⟪

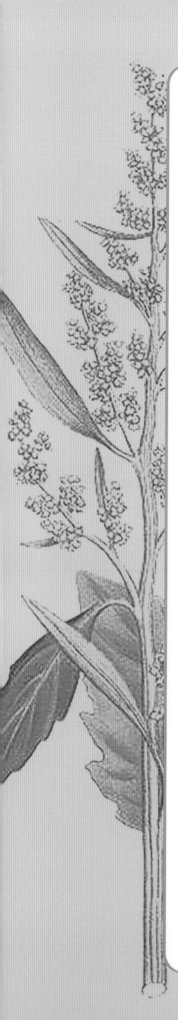

Lamb's Quarters

DESCRIPTION

Here we have an annual or perennial weedy plant, growing 1–5 feet tall (usually 1½–2½ feet), that produces ascending branches as it reaches maturity. Its stems are often red-streaked.

Lamb's quarters possesses alternate leaves, 1–4 inches long and marked by prominent, greenish-white center veins that sprout from long leafstalks. The young leaves are broad and triangular to diamond-shaped—much like a goose's foot (hence the alternative common name of goosefoot). They are blunt toothed to wavy edged and possessed of a mealy-white look to their undersides. This mealy whiteness also appears prominently on the top of the uppermost (newest) leaves, which look like they have been recently dusted with a fine, white powder. (The species name, *album*, meaning "white," is derived from this feature.) As the plant ages, the leaves—especially the upper ones—become more linear, and their edges smooth out. The uppermost leaves often become sessile at this time as well.

Many minute, sessile flowers appear in small, dense clusters arranged as spiked panicles at the ends of the stem and its branches and in the leaf axils. In late summer, these are replaced by papery fruits that encompass many small black seeds.

RANGE AND HABITAT

This is a cosmopolitan weed found throughout most of North America. Lamb's quarters prefers disturbed, well-worked soils, such as those of ill-kept gardens and lawns, waste places, roadsides, and grain fields.

MAJOR CONSTITUENTS

Lamb's quarter's contains oxalates, chenopodine (an alkaloid), ferulic acid, oleanolic acid, scopoletin, imperatorin, campesterol, stigmasterol, n-triacontanol, and ascaridole (in trace amounts). Nutrients include pro-vitamin A (11,600 imperial units per 100 grams), vitamin C (80 milligrams per 100 grams), thiamine, riboflavin, and niacin. A large amount of free-form amino acids are present as well. The roots contain polypodine B, ecdysteroids, and beta-ecdysone.

FOOD

Lamb's quarters was a staple of early humans' diets and was used quite extensively as a cultivated crop in Europe until just recently. This abundant weed is edible raw or when prepared as a potherb.

Many prefer to eat lamb's quarters raw as a trail nibble—especially when the leaves are young. Here the plant is quite a forager's dream, as one can clip off the upper few leaves and return a few days later to witness a new growth. (See the Cautions section, however, before endeavoring to pig out on pigweed!)

To prepare the plant as a potherb, it needs only to be boiled or steamed in salted water for seven to twelve minutes. (North Carolinians have always thrown off one or more waters in doing so, but most feel that this is not necessary.) The leaves lose bulk during cooking and so must be used in a large quantity in order to derive any substantial results.

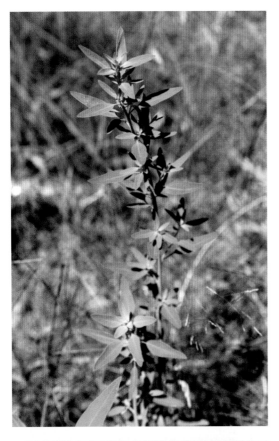

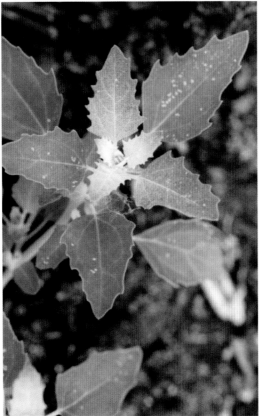

Nevertheless, one's efforts are rewarded: this is one of the tastiest of the weedy potherbs described in the present work! (I rank it only behind marsh marigold, page 148, and stinging nettle, page 226, as a wild-potherb delight.) In addition, lamb's quarters possesses a wide spectrum of vitamins and minerals. The Inuit cook the leaves with beans in order to offset the intestinal gas that would otherwise inevitably accrue when eating the latter.

The plant's leaves and stems even preserve well in the freezer. Simply blanch them for two minutes and then cool. Next, drain or dab dry. Finally, put them in freezer bags and then into the freezer.

The seeds also provide food and can be obtained by collecting the seedheads and then beating them against a rock to release their precious cargo. An incredible amount can be collected from each plant—at least fifty thousand seeds, and one authority counted seventy thousand on a single plant! They can then be boiled and made into mush or simply roasted. They can also be ground and made into a buckwheat-like meal for pancakes, biscuits, or bread. (Grinding is best done with a blender, as they tend to slip between grinder blades; alternatively, boil till soft, then crush, dry, and grind in a grinder.) The great French military leader Napoleon Bonaparte once even lived on bread made from these seeds when his cultivated food rations were low!

HEALTH/MEDICINE

This plant evidently possesses powerful *anti-inflammatory* (probably partly due to the scopoletin content) and/or *astringent* properties because a large variety of Native American tribes have used the bruised leaves as a poultice—or a tea made from them as a compress—for **burns** (including **sunburn**), **headache**, **wounds**, **inflamed limbs**, **piles**, **sore throat**, and **inflamed eyes** (Wyman and Harris 1951: 20; Herrick 1977: 316; Leighton 1985: 351; Asolkar et al. 1992: 196; EthnobDB). The Meskwaki (Fox) have even called upon a root infusion of lamb's quarters to deal with **urethral itching** (Smith 1928: 209).

This herb was also used by European settlers of California as a poultice for both **arthritis** and **rheumatism** (Westrich 1989: 99), while the juice obtained from the boiled greens was utilized to soothe a **toothache** (Westrich 1989: 99). The Mendocino of the same region have reverenced the larger and older leaves as being very helpful for a **stomachache** (Chestnut 1902: 346), while Iroquois out east have implemented a cold infusion of this herb to deal with **diarrhea**. Their manner of implementation was to steep a small bundle of the whole plant in 1 quart of water for five minutes, then allow the infusion to cool, and finally to drink it (Herrick 1977: 315).

On the other hand, other cultures, including the Chinese, the Sudanese, and the Spanish (EthnobDB), have coaxed *laxative* properties out of this plant—probably more so from its seeds. Lamb's quarters has also traditionally been used for **pinworms** (EthnobDB). Like its famed cousin, wormseed (*A. ambrosioides var. anthelminticum*), it contains ascaridole, a chemical that is deadly to parasites (the term even derives from a Latin word meaning "intestinal worm"!). Even though our species possesses this chemical in only trace amounts, unlike wormseed's huge quantity of it, its presence is undoubtedly a chief factor in lamb's quarters' time-honored *anthelmintic* reputation. A Pakistani scientific study published in 2007 demonstrated the herb's anthelmintic effects in vitro and in vivo (Jabbar et al. 2007).

A 2007 rabbit study found an extract from the seeds to be *contraceptive* in the sense of immobilizing sperm, so that intravaginal application blocked the establishment of pregnancy (Kumar et al. 2007).

Ethnobotanist Huron Smith informs us that the Potawatomi noticed that lamb's quarters possessed *antiscorbutic* properties and made a special point to include it in their diet (Smith 1933: 47). In view of the incredibly high vitamin C content since uncovered in this plant, their wisdom has been confirmed. Lamb's quarters also has a history of use in treating the skin condition known as **vitiligo**, which is currently thought to be due to dysfunction of the adrenal glands. Here, again, the plant's high content of vitamin C may be significant in that the adrenal glands store and use more of this vitamin than does any other part of the body.

Zulu tribes in Africa have put lamb's quarters to use in dealing with **enlarged spleen**, with **biliousness**, and with **liver problems** (Asolkar et al. 1992: 196). The Chinese have likewise used it for liver problems (EthnobDB).

Arabic peoples have a long tradition of using lamb's quarters for **tuberculosis** (EthnobDB). Interestingly, a 1954 American study confirmed that it inhibits a virulent human strain of tuberculosis (Fitzpatrick 1954: 530).

PERSONAL AND PROFESSIONAL USE

I have devoured quite a bit of lamb's quarters over the years and have really enjoyed the taste! I've also made mush out of the seeds.

CAUTIONS

Pregnant women should not consume the seeds of lamb's quarters, which can be abortive (Asolkar et al. 1992: 196).

Do not collect this plant in known high-nitrate soils or where cultivated crops that have been sprayed with herbicides flourish.

Do not eat regularly over a long period of time, as this herb contains oxalic acid in sufficient quantity to be harmful with extended use. Some serious poisonings occurred once in Europe when lamb's quarters was consumed in high amounts owing to a food shortage occurring as a result of a war (Cooper and Johnson 1988: 35). It is safe as an *occasional* trail nibble, in moderation, and the safety margin increases when it is cooked (which tends to break down the oxalic acid), allowing for periodic use as a small meal, if necessary, in this form. ⋘

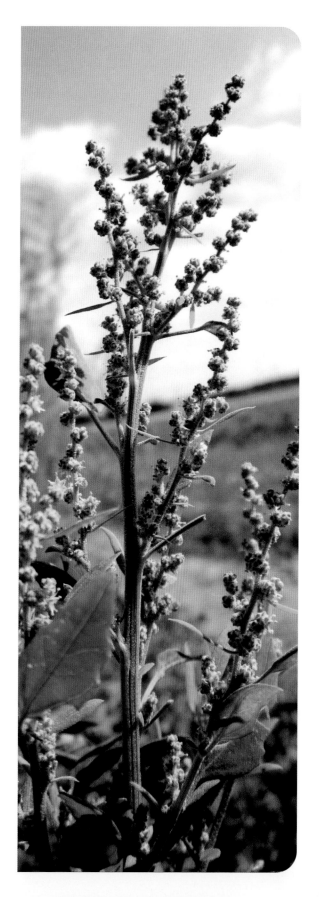

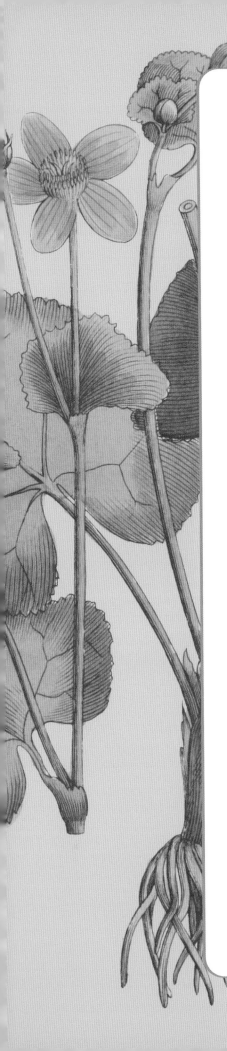

Marsh Marigold

DESCRIPTION

This interesting perennial plant is not a true marigold, contrary to what its name would suggest, but a buttercup instead. Growing to a height of 8–24 inches, it possesses a stem that is thick, stout, succulent, branching, and hollow—the latter feature enabling the leaves to ably float on the water (the favored habitat of this species).

The leaves are glossy, heart shaped to kidney shaped, wavy edged, and possessed of small, rounded teeth; altogether, as they are situated on the plant, they present a saucer-like appearance. They occur clustered at the base and scattered alternately along the stem. The latter leaves are smaller (3 inches across) than the former (5–6 inches across). Here a helpful identifier for this plant is the occurrence of a papery sheath where the leafstalks join the stem.

The gorgeous golden blossoms—composed not of true petals but of five to seven sepals—emerge in May, often opening and closing with the appearance and disappearance of the sun. They resemble those of their fellow buttercups but are larger, being approximately 1–2 inches across.

RANGE AND HABITAT

Marsh marigold occurs throughout the northern two-thirds of the United States, including in at least 75 percent of counties in the Midwest and in Labrador, Newfoundland, and adjacent areas up to the Arctic Circle. Its preferred habitat is in, or very near, water—swamps, marshes, ditches, streams, and ponds.

SEASONAL AVAILABILITY

The blossoming plants are limited to May in the Midwest, but leaves can be harvested for a month or so afterward (if having been positively identified earlier, in their flowering stage).

MAJOR CONSTITUENTS

Marsh marigold contains triterpenoid saponins (including hederagenin, hederagenic acid, and oleanolic acid); the glycoside ranunculin; coumarins; beta-sitosterol; triterpene lactones (palustrolide, epicaltholide, and caltholide); very small quantities of isoquinoline alkaloids; and the pigment calthaxanthin.

FOOD

Although marsh marigold contains a glycoside that makes it impossible to eat raw (it could blister the mouth badly), this principle dissipates at 180 degrees Fahrenheit, so the plant can be used as a potherb by drying and/or boiling. Ideally, one should gather the stem and the leaves before the flowers open, although very shortly after flowering is allowable. These plant parts *must* be boiled, in several (three or more) changes of water— the entire boiling time should be at least twenty to thirty minutes, the lower time for younger plant parts and the higher time for segments from an already flowered plant. Unfortunately, the whole process is very difficult to time out just right. As overcooked plants are tasteless, and undercooked ones leave a sting in the throat, first-time efforts are often frustrating.

This, then, is my method: I get two pots and fill them with water. I then turn on the burner under one to start it boiling. Two to three minutes later, I turn on the burner under the other one. When the first pot is boiling, I immerse the plant parts therein. About two to three minutes after the water in the first pot has returned to a boil, I transfer the plant contents to my second, now boiling, pot. Immediately, I pour out the liquid of the first pot into the sink under running water, then quickly rinse out this pot, refill it with clean water, and put it back on the burner. As soon as it is boiling, I transfer the plant contents from the second pot into this one and finish cooking here for the remainder of the boiling period (based on the age of the plant, as mentioned above).

Marsh marigold lends itself to a variety of recipes, some of which can be gleaned from the better foraging manuals. However, I prefer the plant simply boiled as above, topped with a dab of butter and some sea salt.

Not only is this wetland herb quite tasty when properly cooked, but it is high in vitamins and in iron.

HEALTH/MEDICINE

Marsh marigold has been extensively used in folk medicine for a long time. However, its use has not been entirely without risk (see Cautions), and other herbal aids can often substitute at less of a risk. Presented below, however, is a summary of some of its traditional applications.

First of all, *Caltha palustris* has been used in folk medicine for genitourinary problems, primarily for **dysmenorrhea** (Bhandari et al. 1987: 98) and for **urine stoppage**—the latter by the Midwest's Ojibwe, who have implemented the leaves and the stem (Densmore 1974: 348).

Secondly, it has been utilized as a respiratory aid. Herbalists of both yesterday and today have found that marsh marigold, properly prepared, can serve as a useful aid for **bronchial** or **sinus infections** (Moore 1979: 106; Bhandari et al. 1987: 98). The Ojibwe, as one example, have greatly appreciated a decoction of the roots for its *expectorant* ability (Densmore 1974: 340–41; Foster and Duke 1990: 88). They have also combined a *Caltha* tea with maple sugar to form a **cough** syrup that was popular among colonists (Foster and Duke 1990: 88). Finally, they employed a poultice of the root—dried, powdered, and moistened—for application to **scrofula** (tuberculosis) sores (Densmore 1974: 354).

Thirdly, marsh marigold would appear to exert *antispasmodic* effects. Turkish folk medicine has also long employed the plant for **spasms** (EthnobDB). It may even be possessed of *anticonvulsive* potential: M. Grieve relates how that possibility came to the fore in quoting William Withering, the famed eighteenth-century physician who (re)discovered digitalis, as follows: "On a large quantity of the flowers of [this

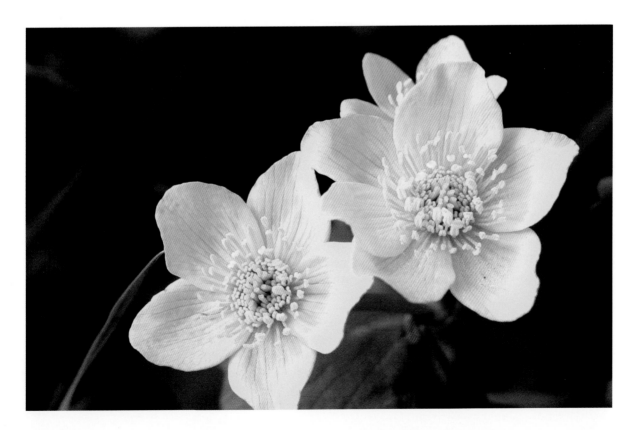

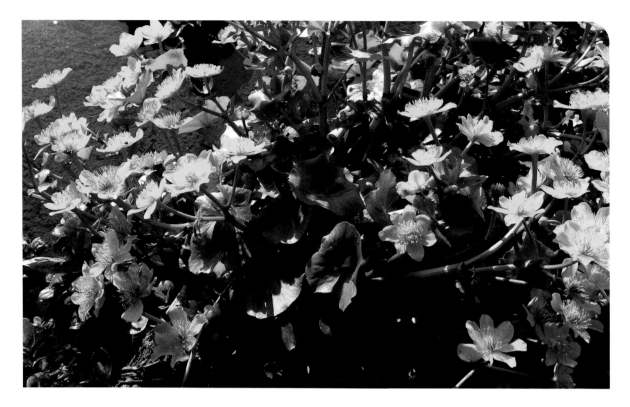

plant] being put into the bedroom of a girl who had been subject to fits, the fits ceased ... it would appear that medicinal properties may be evolved in the gaseous exhalations of plants and flowers" (Grieve 1971: 2:519). These anticonvulsive effects have been sought through the imbibing of an infusion of the dried flowers. Here, although nothing as dramatic as Withering's aromatherapeutic experience has been recorded, some positive results have been noted (North 1967: 117; Jordan 1976: 147).

Fourthly, a warmed leaf poultice has been carefully applied and watched, by skilled herbalists, as a counterirritant for **rheumatism** and for **facial paralysis** (Moore 1979: 106; Westrich 1989: 81).

Fifthly, a drop of the acrid juice onto a **wart**, applied once daily, has been an old folk remedy to rid such an unsightly growth (Gibbons 1970: 141–42; Dobelis et al. 1986: 245).

Finally, saponins isolated from marsh marigold have been found to be potent *molluscicides* (Bhandari et al. 1987: 99), suggesting that the plant may prove useful for **snail infestations**, which are responsible for serious and widespread disease in developing nations.

PERSONAL AND PROFESSIONAL USE

The sheer beauty of a wetland filled with blooming marsh marigold plants is difficult, if not impossible, to describe. I can say that it is a sight that I never fail to enjoy, year after year, each and every spring!

I can also say that properly cooked marsh marigold is my all-time favorite potherb.

CAUTIONS

This herb is reportedly toxic if used raw, capable of producing mucosal blistering. It used to be felt that helleborin, a cardioactive glycoside found in the related genus, *Helleborus* (which is in the same family as *Caltha*), was the principle responsible for marsh marigold's blistering effects. Indeed, R. N. Chopra reported it as found in the roots of the present plant, along with veratrin (Chopra et al. 1956: 47). But research since that time (Bruni et al. 1986) has revealed that the heavy-handed culprit is actually protoanemonin, an irritant oil formed by enzymatic action from ranunculin, a glycoside present in marsh marigold and in more toxic members of the buttercup family. The transformation to protoanemonin is initiated when the plant is damaged in any fashion, such as by foraging or through ingestion. Since protoanemonin poisoning is not a pleasant thing to experience, cooking plants carefully per the instructions provided on page 149 is strongly advised. Both cooking and drying destroy the toxic irritant principle contained in this plant (by converting the protoanemonin to innocuous anemonin). In view of this, some have employed a tea made from the fully dried plant in order to benefit from one or more of the therapeutic benefits listed above. But even this is not without its hazards: Michael Moore cautions that any such tea should comprise no more than a scant teaspoon of the dried herb per cup of water and that significant quantities should not be drunk nor should smaller quantities be imbibed for more than a few days, since kidney or liver inflammation could accrue to some individuals due to the residual acridity (Moore 1979: 106). ⤺

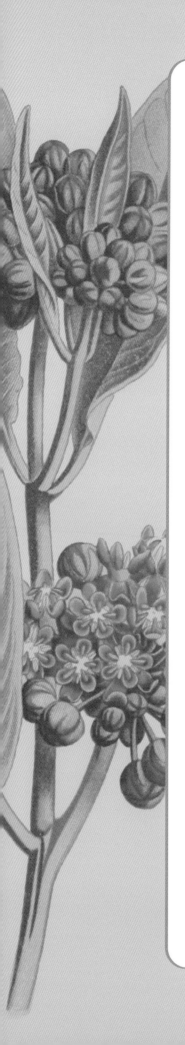

Milkweed

Asclepias syriaca

DESCRIPTION

Milkweed is a native perennial that can reach a height of 5 feet but usually tops off at 2–3 feet. The stem is stout, erect, and hairy and tends not to branch.

The plant's fleshy, dark-green leaves are opposite, oblong, smooth edged, and nearly sessile. They possess a conspicuous midrib and are a bit hairy. In length, they grow anywhere from 4 to 10 inches, while their width is 2–4 inches.

The gorgeous, pleasantly scented, lilac-colored flowers are arranged in dense umbels on the upper one-third of the plant—at the tip of the stem as well as on stalks arising from the leaf axils. There are 25–140 flowers in a cluster. Individual blossoms have five reflexed petals.

The eventual fruits are large, warty pods that grow to 5 inches. They finally split along one side, revealing their silky seeds, which are then scattered hither and thither by the wind.

Milkweed is, of course, the host plant to the lovely monarch butterfly and to its attractive striped larva, the latter of which metamorphoses into the former via a striking green chrysalis dotted with gold that can sometimes be found hanging from this plant.

RANGE AND HABITAT

This conspicuous plant can be found in dry, sunny, open places—prairies, railroad embankments, meadows, roadsides, old fields, pastures, vacant lots, woodland margins, and the like. Recent evidence has revealed that it is losing its habitat, especially in farm fields.

MAJOR CONSTITUENTS

Milkweed contains polyphenols, cinnamic acid, asclepain (a proteolytic enzyme in the latex), caoutchouc (also in the latex), and cardioactive glycosides.

FOOD

Milkweed yields some mighty good repasts, with one or another of its succession of structures becoming available as food until the end of the summer. The initial culinary possibilities arrive with the young, still-unfurled shoots (i.e., with the leaves still largely clasping the stem), which can be hand-rubbed to remove their natal wool and then cut and cooked like asparagus, in two waters. Even when the leaves are fully opened, many wild-food enthusiasts urge that the topmost ones can still be gathered and cooked.

Once the grayish-green flower-bud clusters appear and are about 1 inch across, they can be harvested and cooked like broccoli (see below). They can also be blanched and frozen for use during the winter months. As for the eventual blossoms, when the Swedish botanist Peter Kalm was traveling in North America and recording observations on its plants, he observed that "the French in Canada make a sugar of the flowers, which for that purpose are gathered in the morning when they are covered with dew. This dew is pressed out, and by boiling yields a very good brown, palatable sugar" (Kalm 1966: 387).

In late summer, the warty seedpods, while still young—up to 1½ inches long and firm to the touch, not elastic, as they will eventually become when they develop their silk-ridden seeds—can be boiled in salted water to which a pinch of baking soda has been added (see below). The texture and taste of the finished product is reminiscent of okra. If cooked instead with meat, these pods will tenderize it due to their enzyme content. (Here the Sioux [Oceti Sakowin] capitalized on the phenomenon by cooking the pods with buffalo meat.)

Numerous other Native American tribes relished one or all three of the above plant parts for food (Kindscher 1987: 56–57). A bitterness that may hint of a subtoxic element in the sap occurs in plants in the northeastern United States but does not seem to be much of a problem here in the Midwest—probably because, as Wisconsin forager Sam Thayer opines, our milkweed does not interbreed with other closely related species, since such are not common to our area (Thayer 2001). Yet traditional wisdom on the part of wild-foods connoisseurs has urged that the leaves and pods always be cooked in at least three waters and that the first bath (never from a cold-water start, but always from already boiling water) should last at least four minutes before the water is changed. The second and third baths are allowed to go only one minute each or until the water has returned to a boil after the pods have been placed therein. The final boiling is done for about ten to fifteen minutes. The buds, however, may be cooked in three waters in quicker succession—that is, for only seven minutes total (the first bath for two minutes, the second bath for one, and the last in salted water for about four minutes).

HEALTH/MEDICINE

This native plant has a long tradition of usage in our nation as a medicine and was even listed in the *United States Pharmacopeia* from 1820 to 1863. It is probably best known to the casual herbal student of today as a treatment for **warts**, on which its milky juice has been rubbed by many, including the Rappahannock, Iroquois, Catawba, and Cherokee tribes (Speck 1942: 30, 32; Hamel and Chiltoskey 1975: 44; Herrick 1995: 199). Some of these tribes have also implemented it for **ringworm** (Speck 1942: 30, 32). Others, including residents of the Appalachian region (Bolyard 1981: 45; Crellin and Philpott 1990b: 251n64), have used it for **poison ivy rash**. (Here the application could be painful, although it was also often successful.)

In one of his popular books on wild plants, naturalist and herbalist Tom Brown Jr. relates his interesting experiences with all three of the aforementioned applications, except that his fungal malady tested was **athlete's foot** and not ringworm. (Appalachian folk medicine, too, has traditionally used it for sores and cracks between the toes: Bolyard 1981: 45.) For athlete's foot and for poison ivy rash, Brown informs us that he breaks up the stems into cold water, strains them out, and then uses the white liquid as a wash, leaving it on for a few moments and then rinsing it off (Brown 1985: 137–38). For warts, he relates that, as a lad, he applied the juice to a wart twice a day for seven days, in accord with his mentor's instructions, and obtained successful results, although it took a whole week for the wart to dry up and fall off. This age-old treatment for warts may be effective because the

juice contains the proteolytic enzyme asclepain—which, as former US Department of Agriculture consultant James Duke points out, might serve not only to soften the warts but perhaps to inhibit the virus as well (Duke 1997: 453–54; cf. Moore 1979: 106).

Milkweed has a good reputation as an *expectorant* (Grieve 1971: 1:64–65), being *anticatarrhal* (Mockle 1955: 74). Thus, venerated Southwest American herbalist Michael Moore found that it softened bronchial mucus and even dilated the bronchioles a bit (Moore 1979: 106). Early American physicians even used powdered milkweed roots as an **asthma** remedy. For example, one physician from the early 1800s deemed it *expectorant* and said that it was quite useful in asthma and in **catarrhal infections of the lungs** (Clapp 1852: 847). The early American botanical scholar Constantine Rafinesque wrote that it also inhibited the **pain** of asthma, thus serving effectively as an *anodyne* (Rafinesque 1828–30: 1:76). As to preparation and dosage, Moore wrote of using a decoction made by boiling a teaspoon of the chopped root in a cup of water that was then drunk hot, but he warned that anything above this amount could induce nausea (Moore 1979: 106). Modern British herbalist Mary Carse finds a hot infusion of the flowers to be most effective for the respiratory problems described above (Carse 1989: 131). She gathers these blossoms when dewy in the morning and then boils them down into a syrup, which she then strains and uses for a **cough** (Carse 1989: 131).

Our herb is also a celebrated *diuretic* (Rafinesque 1828–30: 1:76; Gunn 1859–61: 829), increasing both the volume and the solids of urine (Millspaugh 1974: 134). It has thus been used by various Native American tribes for kidney troubles, including by the Natchez for **Bright's disease**. Here, interestingly, it was required that any patient under treatment not ingest any salt (Swanton 1928: 667). The treatment itself entailed cutting the root into small pieces and then making a tea, of which three swallows were drunk three times a day (Taylor 1940: 52). The Cherokee have valued it for urinary **gravel** (Hamel and Chiltoskey 1975: 44). Mary Carse finds it to be soothing to the genitourinary tract, analgesic to a backache caused by kidney problems, and even helpful for **gallstones** (Carse 1989: 131). Michael Moore noted that it is of especial aid in chronic kidney weakness typified by a slight, nonspecific ache in the middle back that is most noticeable in the morning (Moore 1979: 106). Both Carse and Moore stressed that it is best used as an infusion for the kidney problems (Moore 1979: 106; Carse 1989: 131). Moore suggested that 1 tablespoon of the chopped root be boiled in 1 pint of water and then ½ cup of the decoction be drunk four times a day (Moore 1979: 106). Carse says to use 1 teaspoon of the powdered root in 1 cup of boiling water and then to drink ½ cup, cold, three times a day for gallstones or for **edema**; she warns, however, that the tea is too risky for children, owing to a possible toxic potential

(Carse 1989: 131). Early American physician John C. Gunn said to take ½ pound of the dried root, bruise it, decoct it in 6 quarts of water, and then boil the mess down to 2 quarts, thereafter taking ½ teacupful of the liquid three to four times a day (Gunn 1859–61: 829).

Milkweed's diuretic effect, in combination with the *cardiotonic* effect produced by its cardioactive glycosides, has yielded use of the root tea for **dropsy**—both by various Native tribes (Hamel and Chiltoskey 1975: 44; Lewis and Elvin-Lewis 1977: 193) and by early-American physicians (Rafinesque 1828–30: 1:76; Gunn 1859–61: 829). Such a diuretic effect, combined with a demonstrable *diaphoretic* action (Millspaugh 1974: 134; Hutchens 1991: 196), has likewise proven useful for **rheumatism** (Johnson 1884: 230–31; Hutchens 1991: 196).

This meadow-loving plant has also been used by the Midwest's Ojibwe as a *galactagogue* (Densmore 1974: 360). Early American healers implemented it as an *emmenagogue* (Gunn 1859–61: 829). Various Native tribes, including the Ojibwe and the Mohawk, have even used it as a female *contraceptive* (Rousseau 1945a: 59; Densmore 1974: 320).

Yet there's more: milkweed leaves have been used as a *vermifuge* by the Mohegan (Tantaquidgeon 1972: 128–29), the Natchez have implemented the same for **syphilis** (Swanton 1928: 667), and the Cherokee have drunk a tea made from the roots for various **venereal diseases** (Hamel and Chiltoskey 1975: 44).

PERSONAL AND PROFESSIONAL USE

Since my teen years, I've enjoyed cooking and eating milkweed flower buds and seedpods.

I've also long held a special fascination for monarch butterfly larvae and for the many other tiny creatures that feed, or live, on the milkweed plant (such as milkweed beetles, tussock moth larvae, aphids). When my children were small, we used to enjoy watching these creatures together. Now that I have grandchildren, I am able to share this delight with them as well!

In my integrative natural-therapies clinic, my recommendations to clients to use milkweed's latex on warts has generally yielded good results as long as they have followed my directions to apply the *fresh* latex to their warts *three* times a day for *ten* days.

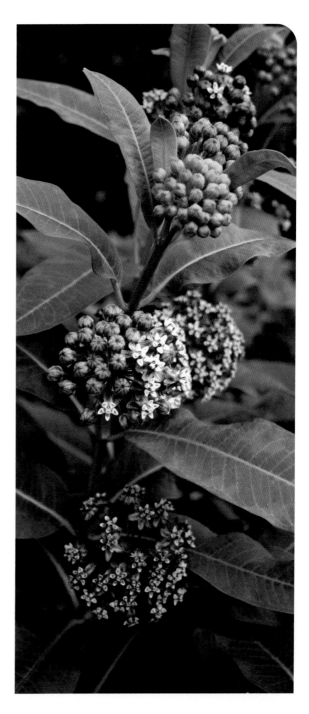

CAUTIONS

Don't confuse milkweed with the similar-looking dogbane (*Apocynum androsaemifolium*), a toxic plant. When both plants are mature, they are easily distinguished: at this stage, dogbane, unlike milkweed, has a branching stem and it also contains tiny white bell-shaped flowers that appear in cymes rather than in umbels as with milkweed. When young, however, the two plants closely resemble each other. The distinguishing features at this stage are as follows: milkweed has hairy stems (which, however, can only be seen under magnification) and a very prominent marginal vein on the leaf; dogbane's stems are smooth, tough, thinner than milkweed's, and often red-tinged. Thayer notes that dogbane's leaves squeak when rubbed together, but milkweed's do not.

Therapeutic use of milkweed would most wisely be done under the supervision of an experienced herbal professional in that the extent and the impact of cardioactive glycosides in milkweed has not as yet been fully determined. ⪡

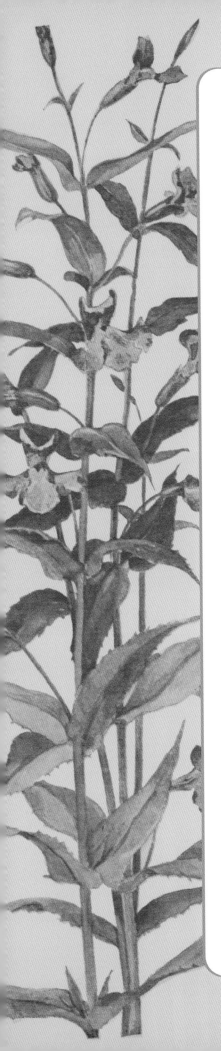

Monkey-Flower

Mimulus ringens, M. glabratus

DESCRIPTION

This pretty plant springs up to a height of 1–4 feet. Its opposite leaves lack a stalk and, in fact, actually clasp the stem. Coarsely toothed, they are oblong to lanceolate and grow 2–4 inches long.

Several purplish blossoms can be found on slender stalks growing from the leaf axils. These flowers, which have four stamens, are irregular and possessed of two lips: the upper lip is erect and has two lobes, while the lower lip is puffy and three-lobed, displaying two yellow spots on its inside portion. The corolla structure, viewed in its entirety, gives the impression of a monkey's face—ergo the plant's common name.

RANGE AND HABITAT

Monkey-flower can be found growing in open, wet places such as on streambanks and lakeshores and in ditches, marshes, and wet meadows. Its range is throughout much of the Midwest, less commonly so in the far western portion.

FOOD

There are over 150 species of *Mimulus* worldwide, and a number of these have been utilized for food. Most commonly, the leaves are eaten, either as a trail nibble or as an ingredient in salads. It is usually agreed that they taste best if gathered before the plant flowers, although monkey-flower can be difficult to identify at this point in time.

The leaves of our two species are edible. My opinion is that they have a strong, but not unpleasant, taste. However, a species of the western states, *M. guttatus* (yellow monkey-flower), is by far the most popular food species of *Mimulus* in the United States and it has been especially appreciated as a salad ingredient by the Native and non-Native inhabitants of the Rocky Mountain region (Coffey 1993: 217). Its leaves have a salty taste, and therefore several Native tribes have used them in recipes to enhance the dish's overall flavor. On certain occasions, too, the leaves have been torched and the ash used directly as a salt (Strike and Roeder 1994: 92). Yellow monkey-flower's stems and leaves are also enjoyed as a steamed potherb, often being added to soups or to casseroles (Schofield Eaton 1989: 201).

HEALTH/MEDICINE

Long appreciated as a *vulnerary*, the bruised or chewed leaves and stems of various *Mimulus* spp. can be applied as a poultice to minor wounds such as **bites**, **cuts**, and **scratches** (Schofield Eaton 1989: 202), as the Maidu have done (Strike and Roeder 1994: 92–93). The effects here may be due to *astringent* properties evidently possessed by this plant, in that other Native tribes have found *Mimulus* useful for **diarrhea**, **hemorrhage**, and as a wash for **sore eyes** (Strike and Roeder 1994: 92–93).

The roots of *M. ringens* are highly esteemed by the Iroquois, who have used them as part of a compound infusion for **epilepsy** and as a wash to counteract **poison** (Herrick 1977: 435).

The Costanoan have treated **urinary problems** with an infusion of a species not found in the Midwest, *M. aurantiacus* (Bocek 1984: 253; Strike and Roeder 1994: 92–93). A decoction of its leaves and flowers has been esteemed by the Tubatulabal for dealing with **stomach discomforts**, while the Maidu have used such to treat **nervous disorders**

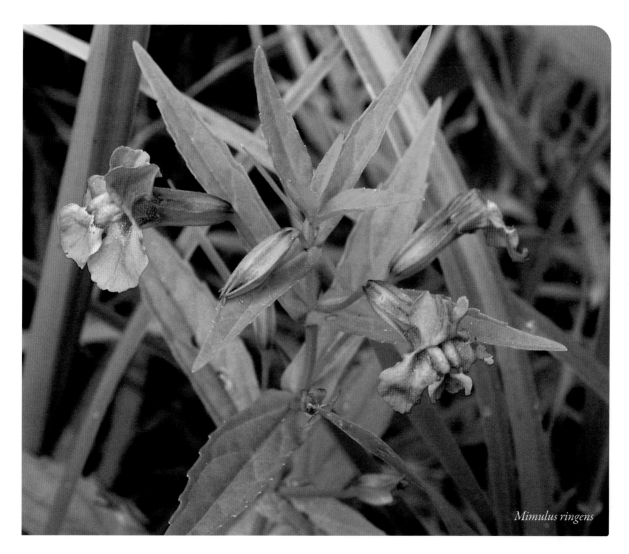

Mimulus ringens

(Strike and Roeder 1994: 92–93). The latter have also found monkey-flower helpful to reduce a **fever** (Strike and Roeder 1994: 92–93).

Mimulus guttatus flower essence is used in flower-essence therapy to embolden persons who have a fear of something known (as opposed to a fear of something unknown, for which aspen, *Populus tremula*, is used). This could be a person, a place, or a situation—such as a social scenario or a trip to the dentist—but it is a fear that is easily named.

PERSONAL AND PROFESSIONAL USE

I look forward to finding this plant each summer to add some taste variety to my wild-foods outings but also simply to admire its beauty, as it is a very pretty plant.

I've recommended *Mimulus guttatus* flower essence to clients on a number of occasions, always with excellent results. It truly does embolden them to overcome their fear of known things and to stand up for themselves! ⧏

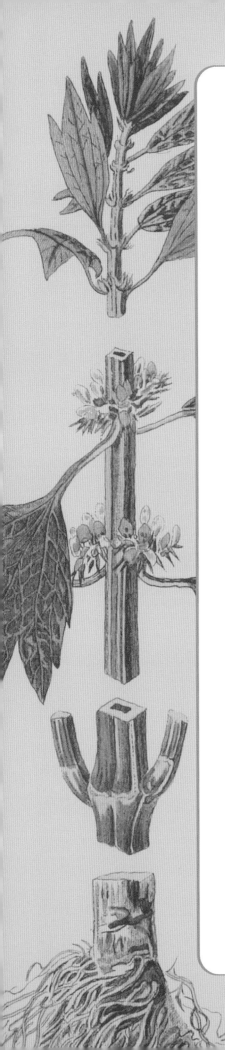

Motherwort

Leonurus cardiaca

DESCRIPTION

Here we have a sparsely branched perennial herb growing 2–4 feet tall. As a member of the mint family, it possesses that family's characteristic square stem.

As also do all mints, it bears opposite leaves, which in this case are noticeably held out quite stiffly. These leaves are long stalked and toothed. Unlike those of other mints, however, they are deeply cut (lobed). While the stem leaves have three pointed lobes, the lower leaves are maple-like—that is, they possess three to five lobes, with each one growing up to 4 inches long. Unlike other mints, too, motherwort lacks a "minty" scent.

Lilac to pale-lavender flowers occur in spiny clusters situated at leaf axils along the stem. (They are spiny because the sepals are sharp tipped.) Each flower is two-lipped, with a fuzzy upper lip.

RANGE AND HABITAT

Motherwort occurs throughout most of North America and entirely throughout the Midwest. It can be found growing in fields, waste places, fencerows, trailsides, and old homesteads.

MAJOR CONSTITUENTS

Motherwort contains alkaloids (leonurinine, leonurine, leonuridine, turicine, betonicine, stachydrine); iridoid glycosides (including leonurid [ajugoside]); cardiac glycosides (bufanolides); essential oil (including carophyllene, alpha-humulene, alpha-pinene, beta-pinene, limonene, linalool, and marrubiin); resin; flavonoids (genkwanin, hyperoside, kaempferol, apigenin, quercetin, quercitrin, rutin, and isoquercitrin); organic acids (malic and citric); oleanolic, caffeic, chlorogenic, and ursolic acid; verbascoside; sterols; pseudotannins (catechin, pyrogallol); and tannic acid. Nutrients include pro-vitamin A and vitamins C and E and choline.

HEALTH/MEDICINE

Motherwort is perhaps best known as an *emmenagogue* (Ody 1993: 74; Willard 1993: 287), helping to alleviate **menstrual pains** (Ody 1993: 64) and being indicated primarily when the flow is scanty due to cold and where there is irritability and unrest, sometimes accompanied by pelvic or lumbar pain as well (Moore 1994b: 13.2). The Eclectic physician Finley Ellingwood noted that his predecessor John King had "regarded motherwort as superior to all other remedies in suppression of the lochia," adding that he himself "had used it with excellent results" (Ellingwood 1983: 483). Its emmenagogue activity is explained by the content of an alkaloid, leonurine, named after its genus (*Leonurus*), which has been shown to encourage uterine contraction (Zhang et al. 2018).

Traditional Chinese Medicine also finds the related Asian species *Leonurus heterophyllus* of value for dysmenorrhea and for **amenorrhea** caused by impeded blood circulation (Yanchi 1995: 119). Motherwort can often relieve a menstrual headache, with one authority advising 8–15 drops of the tincture every three hours during an attack and otherwise three times a day as a preventive. This is advised in conjunction with a tincture of partridgeberry (*Mitchella repens*), dosed identically (Clymer 1973: 188). Motherwort has also proven its mettle as a partus preparator during the last couple weeks of pregnancy (used two to three times a day), in which capacity, owing to its alkaloidal content, it tones the uterus so that it can achieve coordinated contractions during labor (Kong et al. 1976; Mowrey 1986: 138; Mabey et al. 1988: 68; McIntyre 1995: 97; Newall et al. 1996: 197).

This striking plant is also one of the outstanding *nervine* herbs available to herbalists, and one I advise quite a bit for family, friends, and clients. First, it is somewhat helpful for **nerve pain**, as occurs in **sciatica** (Clymer 1973: 97) and in **shingles** (McQuade-Crawford 1996: 161). Secondly, like skullcap (*Scutellaria* spp.—see page 212), it is effective for helping to obviate **nervousness** and **anxiety**, especially when associated with disturbed sleep, feeble digestion, debility, heart problems (see below), or any of the conditions described above (Ellingwood 1983: 483). In fact, both the Cherokee and the Iroquois have used it for nervous complaints (Rousseau 1945b: 98; Hamel and Chiltoskey 1975: 45), while famed British herbalist Nicholas Culpeper observed: "There is no better herb to take melancholy vapours from the heart, to strengthen it, and make a merry, cheerful blithe soul than this herb" (Culpeper 1983). Its leonurine has even demonstrated nervous-system relaxant effects (Yeung et al. 1977).

Then, too, motherwort can also—sometimes remarkably—resolve menopausal **hot flashes**, especially when such are associated with nervous tension and palpitations (McQuade-Crawford 1996: 161). In fact, as to **palpitations**, our herb is probably the best one on the planet for these.

As one example, motherwort is commonly used by herbalists for **hyperthyroidism**, helping to stabilize the **tachycardia** occurring with this condition; it is often combined with lemon balm (*Melissa officinalis*) and bugleweed (*Lycopus* spp.—see page 52) to treat the disorder from all angles, the latter two herbs serving to lower production of thyroid hormones. Our herb is even approved for this use in the *German Commission E Monographs*, prepared by German scientists associated with the governmental organization in that nation that is the equivalent of our FDA (Blumenthal 1998).

Motherwort's effects on palpitations are accomplished via two pathways: the nervous system and the cardiovascular system. In the first regard, the German phytotherapist-physician Rudolf Fritz Weiss commented: "My own investigations have shown that there is indeed a medicinal action, mainly for functional heart complaints due to autonomic imbalance. It appears to be predominantly sedative, similar to valerian. It is necessary, however, to take the drug for a long period, over months" (Weiss 1988: 186). Secondly, motherwort serves as a *cardiotonic*, and as such it is indicated for **cardiac debility** (Hyde et al. 1976–79: 1:133). Although there was little scientific validation of the herb's cardiotonic effects in the twentieth century, several twenty-first-century studies have verified beneficial effects on the heart. In a paper published in 2014, Lithuanian scientists found that motherwort supported cardiac

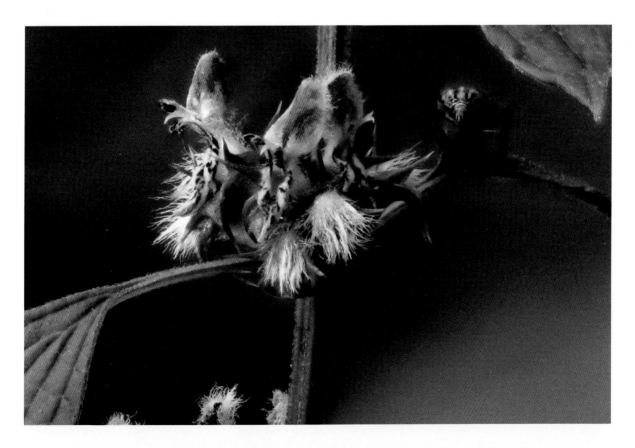

mitochondria, which generates adenosine triphosphate, or ATP (energy currency), for cardiac function (Bernatoniene et al. 2014). A study by the Clinic for Cardiac Surgery at the University of Leipzig found beneficial effects from motherwort on cardiac ion currents (Ritter et al. 2010). Then, in a clinical trial, when a motherwort oil extract was given to fifty patients with arterial hypertension and accompanying anxiety and sleep disorders for a period of twenty-eight days, positive effects were observed in 88 percent of the patients in all three of these complaints (Shikov et al. 2011). Finally, several studies have demonstrated that motherwort exerts an antiadhesion effect on *Staphylococcus aureus* in the context of **infective endocarditis** (Micota et al. 2014; Sadowska et al. 2019).

Chinese studies with rats have shown that the related *L. heterophyllus* relaxes pulsating myocardial cells, improves circulation (both cardiac circulation and microcirculation), and inhibits platelet aggregation, thus serving several vital functions that stymie potential situations that can lead to **heart attacks** (Zhang et al. 1982: 267; Xia 1983). Another Chinese study found that *L. heterophyllus* prevented **strokes** in animals (Kuang et al. 1988). Additional Chinese research with animals found that the plant decreased not only platelet aggregation but blood viscosity and the volume of fibrinogen in the blood (Chang and Li 1986; Zou 1989).

Our herb has also been found to help alleviate **albumin in the urine** (Willard 1993: 288). It would seem to eliminate congestive material in general, thus even proving of aid for a condition such as **rheumatism** (Clymer 1973: 97). A demonstrated *anti-inflammatory* effect may also contribute to motherwort's assist for rheumatism (Fetrow and Avila 1999: 440).

A study conducted in the early 1990s demonstrated *virucidal* activity for this herb: an aqueous extract was shown to inactivate tick-borne encephalitis (TBE) almost completely in vitro, as well as in vivo with mice. Such a tea both increased survival rate and prolonged average longevity (Fokina et al. 1991).

Traditional Chinese Medicine uses not only the plant (for the heart and for the uterus: Holmes 1997–98: 2:572–73), but also the seed, which is said to brighten the vision and is even used to help heal **conjunctivitis** (Ziyin and Zelin 1996: 135; Holmes 1997–98: 2:572).

PERSONAL AND PROFESSIONAL USE

This is the first plant to which I turn for clients with hypomenorrhea or amenorrhea, functional heart complaints, or the tachycardia of hyperthyroidism. With the latter complaint, I use it in conjunction with immune modulators, such as bugleweed (page 52) and self-heal (page 201), if the hyperthyroidism is autoimmune, as in Graves' disease. I also combine it with schizandra (*Schisandra chinensis*) berry for stool incontinence due to nervousness.

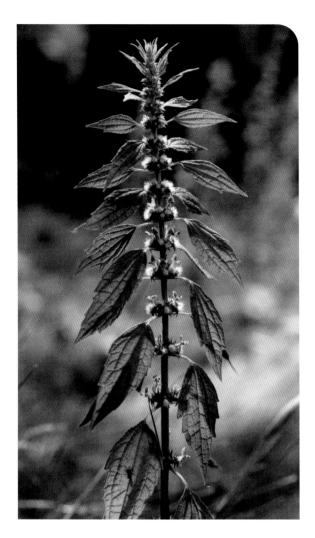

I had an amazing experience with motherwort that I will never forget: I was leading some of my students on a wild-plant walk when one of them veered off toward a nearby riverbank, having felt drawn there. Wondering where she was, two of the other students and I turned to catch sight of her by the riverbank, holding her arms above and around some motherwort plants. Suddenly, a glow enveloped both her and the plants! "Did you see what I just saw?" I asked the two students next to me. "Uh-huh," they both answered in unison, as their jaws proceeded to drop!

CAUTIONS

Some persons can develop contact dermatitis from touching this plant, and the effect will flare with sunlight.

Motherwort *should not be used during pregnancy* due to its emmenagogue and parturitive effects. Also, it should be avoided during menstruation if the flow is heavy (menorrhagia).

Motherwort should be used with caution and under professional supervision when there is simultaneous use of either anticoagulants or digitaloids. ⧗

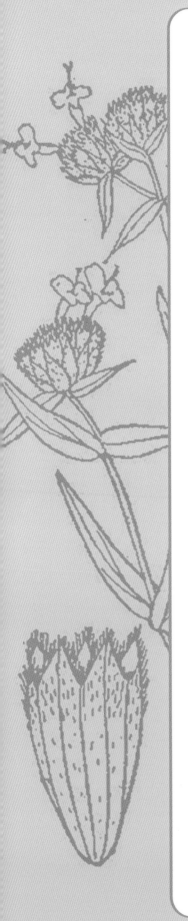

Mountain Mint

Pycnanthemum virginianum

DESCRIPTION

Possessed of a powerful minty fragrance, this plant grows 1–3 feet high. Like all mints, it has a square stem, which in this case is blanketed with many tiny hairs.

Growing to 3 inches long, the opposite leaves are lanceolate to ovate, rounded at their base, and whitish on their underside. The uppermost leaves often look as though they have been dusted with talc. The leaves are toothless and nearly sessile on our *Pycnanthemum virginianum*, while they are noticeably toothed and stalked on species outside the Midwest.

The many small flowers, white to lavender, are two-lipped (the upper lip being single-lobed, but the lower lip being three-lobed and spotted with purple) and appear in dense, flat-topped clusters. These cymes appear in the leaf axils or terminally on the stem and its branches. They are cupped underneath with hoary bracts.

RANGE AND HABITAT

Mountain mint can be found on streambanks and in open woods, thickets, wet meadows, and moist prairies. It thrives in the lower three-quarters of the Midwest.

MAJOR CONSTITUENTS

Mountain mint contains an essential oil consisting of pulegone, carvacrol (approximately 25 percent or more), geraniol, limonene, and other terpenes.

FOOD

The dried leaves make a pleasant tasting tea as well as one darn good mint julep! There are a variety of opinions on how to best prepare the latter: Anne Marie Stewart and Leon Kronoff suggest gathering about ⅓ cup of fresh leaves and putting them in a blender, at low speed, with 6 tablespoons of sugar (as a health nut, I would skip the sugar). Next, they advise adding 2 cups of shaved ice and 8 ounces of bourbon and then blending again—but this time at high speed, until the mess attains a soft-frozen consistency (Stewart and Kronoff 1975: 131). Others would crush the leaves and drench them with the bourbon, then steep the mess for several hours to several days, and then finally strain it and serve it over shaved ice (Phillips 1979: 142). Either way, it's hard to go wrong: this drink is as good as its reputation!

HEALTH/MEDICINE

Mountain mint has been appreciated as a treatment for **colds** by many peoples, including the Cherokee, who have also poulticed the plant's leaves onto the head of a person suffering from a **headache** (Hamel and Chiltoskey 1975: 45). The Lakota, meanwhile, have implemented the herb to deal with a bad **cough** (Rogers 1980: 50).

Mountain mint has been much appreciated by both the Cherokee and the Ojibwe to break a fever (Densmore 1974: 354; Hamel and Chiltoskey 1975: 45). Such an effect is perhaps achieved because, as the *United States Dispensatory* noted, "its hot infusion is diaphoretic" (Wood et al. 1926: 1441).

Like most mints, *Pycnanthemum* is a valuable *carminative* and was appreciated as such by the Cherokee (Hamel and Chiltoskey 1975: 45). This, in fact, remains its most oft-used application today—to dispel gas in the intestines.

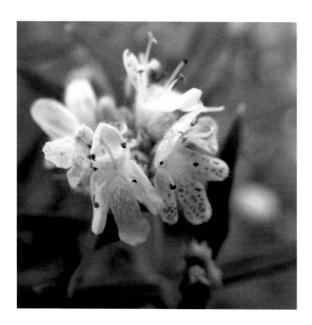

The Cherokee also found that a tea of mountain mint's leaves was useful for **heart trouble** (Hamel and Chiltoskey 1975: 45). Our own area's Meskwaki (Fox) have advised a tea of this plant for those who were "all run down" (Smith 1928: 226). In perhaps a related use, the plant was used as a *stimulant* by early American physicians and folk healers (Smythe 1903; Burlage 1969: 94).

Like most other mints—including catnip (see page 69), horsemint (page 132), and motherwort (page 156)—mountain mint has a history of use as an **emmenagogue** (Smythe 1903; Burlage 1969: 94; Foster and Duke 1990: 68). The Cherokee also had a specific application for males: such ones with an **inflamed penis** would soak the organ in a receptacle filled with a tea of this plant (Hamel and Chiltoskey 1975: 45).

A final application is also worth mentioning: James Duke, a former USDA consultant and prolific author on herbal medicine, finds mountain mint to be an excellent topical mosquito *repellant* (Duke 1997: 291). Such an application has even been scientifically evidenced for a related mint, catnip (see page 69).

PERSONAL AND PROFESSIONAL USE

This plant is not typically available on the herb market, and I know of only two, small stands in the wild, so I have not had opportunity to use it much for clients. I do very much enjoy the aroma of the plants when I encounter it, however. Occasionally, too, I chew some of the leaves and apply them to my skin when the skeeters are exceptionally troublesome.

CAUTIONS

Most mints are *contraindicated in pregnancy*, and this one is no exception, owing to its content of both pulegone and carvacrol. ⬿

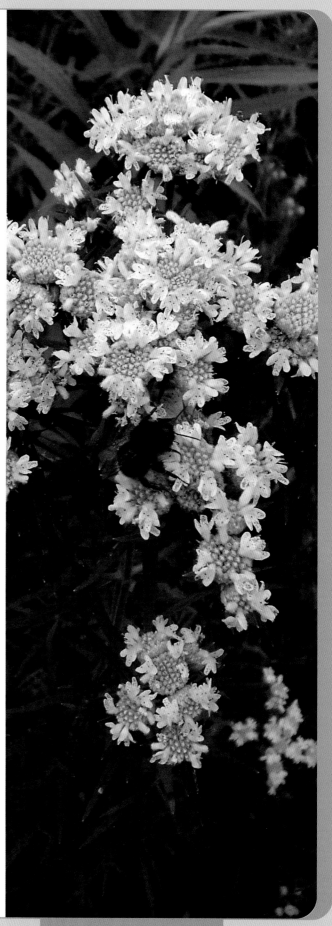

mountain mint

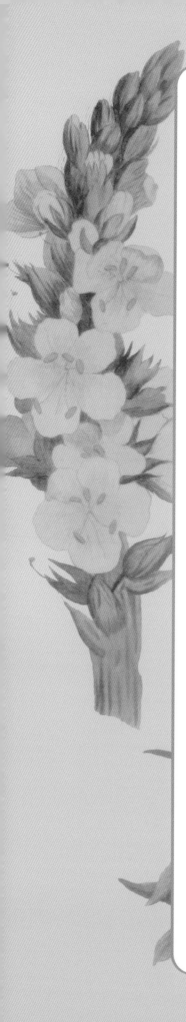

Mullein

DESCRIPTION

Here we have a striking biennial, sometimes reaching a height of 10 feet!

At the beginning of its existence, this plant's large (up to 19 inches long and 5 inches wide!), hairy (even velvet-like) leaves form a rosette that is difficult to mistake in that stage. Come winter, the rosette survives or dies back under the snow. But next spring, the plant begins to shoot up a tall center stem (4–10 feet!) topped by a club-like spike bearing many flowers. Its full height is reached by late summer, and the stalk persists throughout the winter.

The stem is round, fibrous, and sometimes winged, and it tends to branch toward the top. It contains a white pith. The club head is clustered with small yellow to yellow-orange five-petaled flowers (½–1 inch), which open only randomly, so that one inevitably finds the spike to possess a patchy appearance (part green with unopened flowers and part yellow with opened blossoms).

Leaves of the second-year plants occur clustered at the base and along the stem, often tapering into the stem toward the top. They are large, ovate, and densely covered with the fine, bristly hairs characterizing the basal leaves.

The plant ingeniously retains moisture in the dry, sunny environments in which it thrives, trapping rainwater with the hairs on its upper leaves and then dripping that down to the lower leaves.

RANGE AND HABITAT

You will find this tall weed springing up on the edges of highways, in fields, and in wasteland throughout the United States and southern Canada. In fact, wherever it is open and dry, you will probably find mullein! It can be found throughout the Midwest (although less so in the northern one-third of the region).

MAJOR CONSTITUENTS

The leaves contain iridoids (aucubin, catalpol); coumarins; flavonoids (verbascoside, hesperidin, rutin, apigenin, luteolin); triterpenoid saponins (verbascosaponin); traces of essential oil; sterones; rotenone; caffeic acid derivatives; amaroid; resin; mucilage; tannins; malic acid; phosphoric acid; and calcium phosphate. Nutrients include vitamins (pro-vitamin A, B-complex, and C) as well as calcium, chromium, iron, magnesium, manganese, sodium, sulfur, silica, and selenium. The root contains sugars (raffinose, verbascose, stachyose, pentose, and sucrose). The flower contains thapsic acid, arabinose, galactose, and uronic acids. The seed contains fatty acids (linoleic, oleic, palmitic) and beta-sitosterol.

FOOD

Mullein's velvety leaves, when properly dried, make a marvelous-tasting tea. The leaves themselves should not be consumed, either raw or cooked, since they contain both irritating stinging hairs and high amounts of aluminum. Steeping them is regarded as safe, since minerals are not easily transported into an infusion unless it is left to steep for many hours. However, the infusion needs to be strained through a coffee filter to trap the irritating hairs.

Some people enjoy nibbling on the little yellow flowers, sucking the juice out of them. Yet one should always discard the mildly toxic seeds.

HEALTH/MEDICINE

There are few herbs in my healing arsenal that I utilize more frequently than mullein! This versatile herb, listed in the *National Formulary* from 1916 to 1936, is both an *astringent* and a *demulcent* (the latter owing to its content of mucilage). In accord with these physiological effects, the late-first-century naturalist Pliny the Elder noted mullein's popular use for **diarrhea** (Pliny 1938: 26:44), while his herbalist contemporary Dioscorides described its use for "fluxes of the belly" (Dioscorides 1996: 4:104). Mullein has been recognized by twenty-first-century herbalists as one of the herbs of choice to treat adult diarrhea (Shook 1978: 195). Herbalist Mary Carse recommends it even over the most renowned botanical for this affliction, blackberry root and leaves, urging one to switch to blackberry only if mullein doesn't work (Carse 1989: 135). The herb is often helpful, as well, for another intestinal condition with which some persons are afflicted: **colitis** (Keville and Szolkowski 1991: 202). I have seen it work wonders for this condition, although it is not a cure.

Mullein's astringency further explains the traditional application of a strained infusion of the leaves to soothe both **laryngitis** and **sore throat.** Its most famous application for the respiratory tract, however, has been as an *expectorant* (Blumenthal 1998), its success here owing to a reflex action arising from an irritation of the gastrointestinal mucosa by its saponins. This is accompanied by an improvement in the tone of mucous membranes so that production of fluids is increased and therefore a cough is made more productive (Hoffmann 1986: 210; Fetrow and Avila 1999: 444). The German physician-phytotherapist Rudolf Fritz Weiss held mullein to be one of the best botanicals to treat **chronic bronchitis** (Weiss 1988: 198). It is specific in herbal therapy for a tight, hacking, dry, and nonproductive **cough**, not only when found in viral afflictions but also when finding form as a smoker's cough or a nervous cough (Moore 1994b: 15.2)—or, as Dioscorides would have it, simply an "old cough" (Dioscorides 1996: 4:104). The cough may also be worse when lying down (Moore 1994b: 4.5). The Catawba have even boiled the root to make into a syrup to help alleviate children's **croup** (Speck 1937: 190).

Those with **asthma** often find some relief from steam treatment with mullein and from drinking the tea. Steam application for asthma has been practiced by the Micmac (Lacey 1993: 35), while the Mohegan and Penobscot have smoked the leaves for same (Speck 1917: 310; Tantaquidgeon 1928: 265; Smith 1933: 83; Lewis and Elvin-Lewis 1977: 299–300). Interestingly, a very large variety of Native American tribes have used mullein leaves for troubles in the lungs or chest (Moerman 1986: 1:505–6).

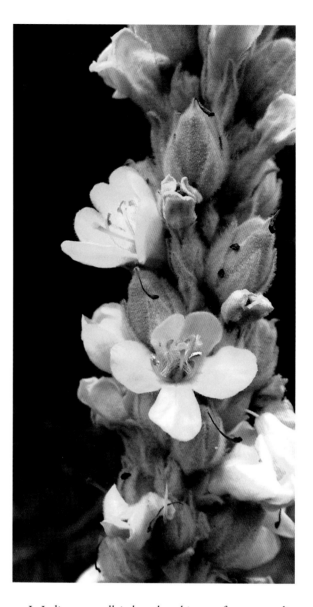

In India, too, mullein has a long history of use as a medicinal plant for pulmonary and other afflictions. In fact, in this area of the world, fresh mullein leaves have been boiled in milk and the resultant drink imbibed for **tuberculosis**, often with excellent results! This success was shared on the American continent by the early settlers (Lewis and Elvin-Lewis 1977: 299–308) as well as by the Iroquois and the Salish (Teit 1928: 293; Herrick 1977: 432). In fact, the scientific name of the family to which the mullein weed belongs, Scrophulariaceae, is related to **scrofula**, an old term for chronic swollen lymph nodes eventually identified as a form of tuberculosis. In harmony with this, in the early 1950s, a virologist who tested the effects of about three hundred different plants on a virulent human strain of the tuberculosis bacterium found that mullein was one of seventy-two plant extracts that yielded complete inhibition of growth at a dilution of 1:40—a significant ratio (Fitzpatrick 1954: 531).

There are several possible reasons for its efficacy in this regard, but nobody knows yet for sure just why it helps. However, the plant has for some time been known to possess *antimicrobial* properties, and studies have shown pronounced activity against *Bacillus cereus* and *Trichomonas vaginalis* (Fakhrieh-Kashan et al. 2018; Mahdavi et al. 2019). Its iridoid glycoside, aucubin, is definitely *antiseptic*. In the opinion of some, another of its chemicals, verbascose, may at least partly account for its action against tuberculosis, while the plant's saponins may help disinfect the lungs (Heinerman 1979: 158; Lepore 1988: 181). The flavonoids and the tannins may also play a hand. The flower has been shown to possess *antiviral* action in vitro against herpes-family viruses and influenza A and B (Slagowska et al. 1987; Zgórniak-Nowosielska et al. 1991; McCutcheon et al. 1995). Then, too, the leaves have long been used for **swollen lymph nodes** (Carse 1989: 135; Willard 1993: 188). The Cherokee have poulticed scalded leaves onto swollen nodes and also placed them around the neck for **mumps** (Hamel and Chiltoskey 1975: 45), while the Iroquois have preferred a smashed bunch of leaves as a poultice for this latter affliction (Herrick 1995: 216).

Mullein is appreciated by many as an aid to ear health. The Iroquois, for one example, have applied a poultice of heated leaves to an **aching ear** (Herrick 1977: 432). Likewise, a renowned use of the flowers is as the main ingredient in an old earache remedy: the flowers are combined with olive oil and then sun-treated (either by direct sunlight or by strong window-filtered sunlight) for a few days to produce a concentrated bottle of oil. After being carefully strained through cheesecloth, this is stored in a cupboard, to be brought out as needed and used with an ear dropper. (Herbalist Michael Moore pointed out that setting the mixture on one's basement water heater for several weeks would accomplish the same task: Moore 1979: 113.) It appears to take the edge off of the pain, as two studies have suggested (Sarrell et al. 2001; Sarrell et al. 2003). Charles Millspaugh observed that the same oil can be applied to **hemorrhoids**, with excellent results (Millspaugh 1974: 432).

Indeed, mullein flower definitely possesses mild *anodyne/analgesic* ability, making it somewhat useful for acute or chronic **pain** of almost any kind. The great herbal physician Edward E. Shook once called mullein "the only herb known to man that has remarkable narcotic properties without being poisonous. It is the great pain killer and nervous soporific, calming and quieting all inflamed and irritated nerves" (Shook 1978: 199). Here the first-century herbalist Dioscorides found mullein helpful for **eye inflammation**, for **toothache**, and for **scorpion stings** (Dioscorides 1996: 4:104). Centuries later, the Iroquois would moisten the heated leaf with vinegar and poultice it onto the face of a person afflicted with a toothache. One modern herbalist finds it particularly valuable for the pain

of **sciatica** (Donson 1982: 85). America's Eclectic physicians appreciated that mullein was "mildly nervine, controlling irritation, and favoring sleep" (Felter and Lloyd 1898). The flower tea is especially useful as a *sedative* for **insomniacs** (de Bairacli Levy 1974: 101).

Mullein has especially been used as a local application to **sprains**, **bruises**, and various other **injuries**, including by Native American tribes as diverse as the Catawba, the Iroquois, the Malecite, and the Lenape (Delaware; Oklahoma) (Speck 1937: 190; Tantaquidgeon 1942: 66, 82; Mechling 1959: 246; Herrick 1995: 215–16). The Canada Lenape (Delaware) have used a crushed mullein-leaf poultice for **swellings** (Tantaquidgeon 1972: 108). The Rappahannock have used two different applications for sprains and for swellings: for the former, they have boiled leaves in a gallon of water until 3 pints remain, then rubbed it on the swelling; for sprains, they have simply applied boiled leaves as hot as the person can stand it (Speck 1942: 28). For swellings and for **abscesses**, the Iroquois have cut a piece of leaf the size of the problem area and applied it just when it is about to open (Herrick 1995: 215). When the swelling is related to an injury, however, they have often instead boiled a plant in water, then mashed the warm leaves and tied them on the swelling as a poultice. Finally, they have imbibed what was left of the decoction (Herrick 1995: 216).

Richard Mabey suggests that mullein-flower oil also be applied to **rheumatic joints** (Mabey et al. 1988: 113). Likewise, Alexandra Donson gives mullein reverential inclusion in her informative tome on therapeutic herbs for **arthritis** and **rheumatism** (Donson 1982: 85). Appalachian folk medicine has long appreciated mullein tea and leaf poultices for both conditions as well (Bolyard 1981: 133). Then, too, many have found that a warm leaf poultice on the big toe is most helpful for the excruciating pain of **gout** (Morton 1974: 156; Bolyard 1981: 134). Indeed, lab tests have shown this common weed to possess some *anti-inflammatory* effects: its glycoside, verbascoside, even inhibits 5-lipoxygenase, the enzyme responsible for the formation of inflammatory leukotrienes (Dobelis et al. 1986: 259; Fetrow and Avila 1999: 444).

Because the herb is revered as having an affinity to hollow, boggy body structures (Landis 1997: 189), its main effect is seen with the lungs (as noted previously) and with the **bladder**, where it acts to support the structure. Thus, a traditional remedy for **urinary obstruction** has been an infusion of mullein, cleavers (see page 86), and the leaves of wild strawberry (page 273) (Bolyard 1981: 134). The Eclectic physicians treasured the herb for "urinary irritation with painful micturition," finding it most "useful in allaying the acidity of urine which is present in many diseases" (Felter and Lloyd 1898). The herb's mucilage, tannin, and other anti-inflammatory principles make it invaluable for **cystitis** and for **urinary tract infections** (Mabey et al. 1988: 113).

Southwest American herbalist Michael Moore explained that steeping ¼ teaspoon of the crushed root in ¼ cup of water and then taking some of this tea before retiring will strengthen the bladder, helping to alleviate **bedwetting** (Moore 1979: 113). Furthermore, herbalist David Winston has found the root to be most helpful for facial nerve pain such as occurs with **Bell's palsy**, **trigeminal neuralgia**, and the like (Winston 1999: 46).

UTILITARIAN USES

A utilitarian use for mullein is to employ the dead or dying club heads as torches, a use often put to them by Native Americans. The stem can also be used as the key element in what outdoor enthusiasts call a fire hand drill, a device constructed out of outdoor materials to initiate a spark for tinder (Brown 1985: 147).

PERSONAL AND PROFESSIONAL USE

Mullein-leaf infusion is one of my favorite herb infusions for taste. I use it quite a bit during cold and flu season.

In my clinical practice, I have used the leaf quite extensively as an expectorant and have found it to be quite reliable. In this regard, I not only advise drinking the tea but, for nasal or sinus congestion, inhaling the vapor from a freshly steeped tea as well. (I've actually made a number of converts to herbal medicine with this simple procedure.)

I've also advised use of the root on many an occasion to strengthen the bladder when there is nocturia (nighttime urinary urgency) or stress incontinence (bladder leakage upon coughing or sneezing or from some other stressor). It's a spectacular remedy for this, with the only caveat being that it can sometimes worsen constipation in those so afflicted. It does not seem to constipate persons who are regular, however.

I've had many an occasion to recommend mullein-flower oil as an application to the outer ear canal to loosen wax and to reduce inflammation in the ear, always with noticeably good results.

I appreciate mullein so much that I featured a photo that I took of it on the cover of another book I wrote about herbs, *300 Herbs*, published in 2003.

CAUTIONS

Because the hairs on the leaves collect not only moisture for the plant's survival in its arid habitat but inadvertently also dust, pollutants, and the like, the leaves should be rinsed and shaken dry before being dried for tea. Of course, too, they should not be collected from any area where there are known pollutants (such as from a roadside).

A tea made from the leaf or flower must be carefully strained because these fine hairs will otherwise irritate the throat. This is best accomplished by pouring the tea through a paper coffee filter. ‹‹‹

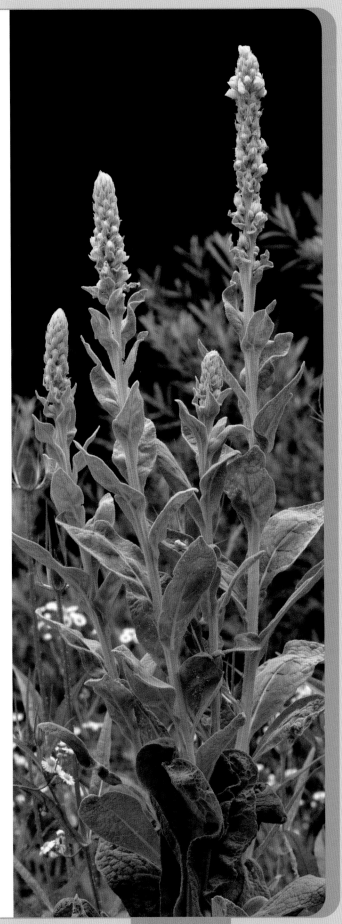

mullein

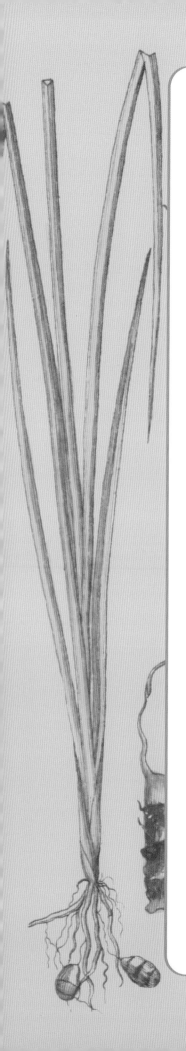

Nutgrass

CHUFA; NUTSEDGE; UMBRELLA SEDGE

Cyperus spp.

DESCRIPTION

This is a perennial herb with a triangular, smooth, unbranched stem. When flowering, it can reach a height of 3 feet, but it usually tops off at 1–2 feet.

The leaves are grass-like, light green, rough edged, and possessed of a prominent midrib. The basal ones rise about 6 inches from the ground but can grow as high as the plant's flower cluster (see below). Two to six smaller leaves form an involucre just below the flower cluster. Occasionally, stem leaves can be found at the nodes between these two groups of leaves.

Flowers are contained in an umbel, resembling an inverted umbrella (thus the alternative common name of umbrella sedge). They are composed of five or six rays that, in turn, are subdivided. (The overall appearance is that of straw-colored spikelets, flattened on the top.) The eventual fruits are small, yellowish triangular nutlets.

This plant is both known and named for its dark, round, ½-inch-long tubers, which are born from scaly, underground stems. These contain a milky juice.

Several species occur in the Midwest, including the following:

Cyperus esculentus (chufa, yellow nutgrass) grows 6–30 inches tall. It has a yellowish-green stem and bears yellow to yellowish-brown flowers. Its subtending bracts are longer that its inflorescence.

C. odoratus (fragrant nutgrass) is similar, but, as its name implies, it is *fragrant*.

C. rotundus (purple nutsedge, coco grass), a species native to the Eurasian continent as well as thriving in the southwestern United States and Mexico, has popped up in a lone Minnesota county. It has purplish flowers shorter than its subtending bracts, and its tubers possess scales that are shiny and red.

RANGE AND HABITAT

Nutgrass thrives in moist and sandy fields, roadsides, lakesides, and streambanks. It can be found in the southern three-fourths of the Midwest.

MAJOR CONSTITUENTS

The tuber contains a potent essential oil (consisting of carophyllene, p-Cymol, camphene, cyperene, limonene, and other terpenes). It also contains a fixed oil, alkaloids, glycosides, phenols, steroids, flavonoids, sesquiterpenoids, protein, calcium, and starch.

FOOD

Nutgrass tubers, which taste like sweet nuts, as the name implies, have been used by many cultures throughout history and have even been found in Egyptian tombs dating back as far as 2400 BCE!

The tubers of our yellow nutgrass, or chufa—note the species name, *esculentus*, referring to the esculent potential of the species—must usually be dug from the ground and not merely pulled, as otherwise they tend to break off and remain in the soil. Once secured, they need to be peeled of their dry, tough rind. At this point, they can be eaten raw or tossed into salads.

A delicious milky drink can be made by soaking the tubers in water for two days and then mashing them in fresh water, adding sweetener, and straining out the solid matter. The measurements used in this recipe are ½ pound of tubers to 4 cups of water, but that is for the cultivated variety, and it is doubtful that today's forager could round up ½ pound of tubers in an outing. Therefore, one could scale this ratio according to what one has actually collected: for example, 2 ounces of mashed tubers would be mixed with 8 fluid ounces of water.

The tubers can also be steamed or roasted till dark brown and then peeled and consumed. Alternatively, they can be roasted, ground, and brewed as a coffee substitute (about 1 tablespoon to 1 cup of water) or used as flour. The roasting must be done in a slow oven with the door left slightly ajar to let moisture escape; otherwise the tubers will not become brittle enough to grind.

The base of the stem can also be cut free and eaten raw and is quite tasty. These "hearts" can alternatively be tossed into stews. Nutgrass seeds can also be collected, dried, ground, and used as flour.

HEALTH/MEDICINE

The Paiute have poulticed both the smashed tuber of *Cyperus esculentus* and tobacco leaves onto **athlete's foot** (Clarke 1977: 162). Success here was probably due to nutgrass's essential oil, in that such oils are often antifungal to a marked degree. A rat study published in 2017 showed significant hepatoprotective activity on the part of this species (Onuoha et al. 2017). Wild-foods pioneer Euell Gibbons considered this species' tuber to be a superb nutritive vegetable and quite helpful to digestive function as well (Gibbons 1970: 264). The tuber of *C. odoratus* also has *stomachic* properties (Porcher 1849: 850–51; Potterton 1983: 82), while *C. rotundus* is usually reverenced as a superb *hepatic* herb (Landis 1997: 335). Twentieth-century scientific research found the latter to exert *anti-inflammatory*, *antipyretic*, and *analgesic* activities (Gupta et al. 1971: 76), while twenty-first-century studies have additionally found *anthelmintic*, *antiallergic*, *antiarthritic*, *anticandida*, *anticariogenic*, *anticonvulsant*, *antidiarrheal*, *antiemetic*, *antihyperglycemic*, *antihypertensive*, *antimalarial*, *antiobesity*, *antioxidant*, *antiplatelet*, *antiulcer*, *antiviral*, *cardioprotective*, *cytoprotective*, *cytotoxic*, *gastroprotective*, *hepatoprotective*, *neuroprotective*, *ovicidal*, *larvicidal*, and *wound-healing* activities (Kamala et al. 2018). (I had to stretch my arm and shake my hand after typing all of those!)

The famed European herbalist Nicholas Culpeper extolled the *carminative* virtues of the native European perennial, *C. longus* (sweet cyperus) and also remarked that it was a *diuretic* (Potterton 1983: 82). This species, however, does not occur in the Midwest. Neither does *C. articulatus*, which is a *vermifuge*, according to the early American physician Francis Porcher (Porcher 1849: 850). However, it would

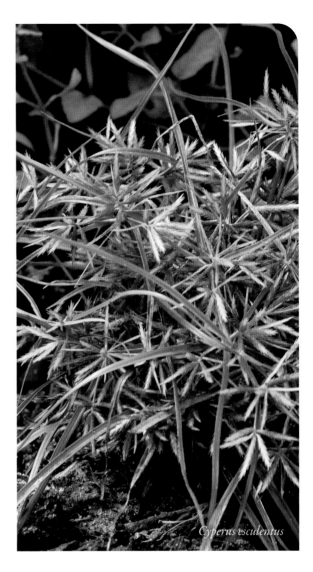

Cyperus esculentus

not be surprising if the various species of *Cyperus* shared all of the physiological effects outlined above, owing to their common possession of essential oil.

PERSONAL AND PROFESSIONAL USE

I have found *C. rotundus* rhizome to be a most useful application for depression related to liver congestion. For this complaint, I usually recommend the tea, owing to its very pleasant aroma and taste. (One of my clients who used it in this form said that it tasted "Christmassy." Indeed, to me it smells like eggnog, a drink long associated with Christmas.) The tincture works well here, also.

Then, too, I will often include a tincture or a tea of nutgrass in a custom-crafted formula for menstrual cramps, abdominal bloating, nausea, or muscle spasms.

CAUTIONS

Owing to nutgrass's *emmenagogue* properties, it *should not be used during pregnancy.*

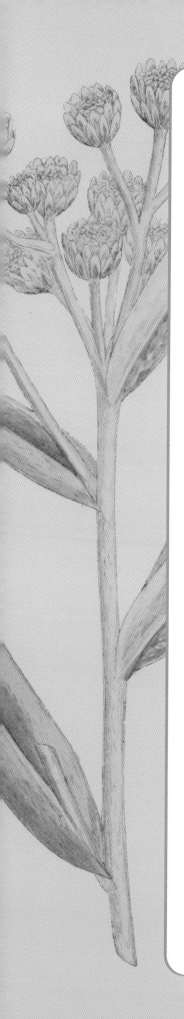

Pearly Everlasting

COTTONWEED; INDIAN POSY; LIFE EVERLASTING

Anaphalis margaritacea

DESCRIPTION

Pearly everlasting is a native perennial growing 1–3 feet tall with an erect stem that branches at the top. The entire plant is covered with a loose cottony substance and bears an unusual, musky sort of scent.

The many alternate, sessile, smooth-edged leaves are linear to lanceolate, 3–5 inches long, and often curled. Their surfaces are greenish white, while their undersides are more whitish.

The dioecious (male and female) blossoms are golden, globe-shaped disk flowers, about ¼ inch wide. Resting in stiff, shiny, pearly-white bracts, they are arranged as compound corymbs.

RANGE AND HABITAT

This plant thrives in sunny and dry areas such as pastures, roadsides, waste places, and old fields. It grows in northeastern Minnesota and in adjacent parts of Wisconsin.

SEASONAL AVAILABILITY

The flower heads—which ideally should be gathered while still compacted—are available in late summer.

MAJOR CONSTITUENTS

Pearly everlasting contains essential oil (which includes anaphalin, a monoterpene), resin, a phytosterol, flavones, tannins, transdehydromatricariaester, tridecapentain-en, and 5-chlor-2-5,6-dihydro-2h-pyran.

HEALTH/MEDICINE

One of this herb's alternative common names, life everlasting, derives from the plant's ability to survive for up to a year after being picked, so that this plant is quite popular in floral arrangements. This unusual "survival" aspect of the plant, however, has been thought to carry over to humans (and to animals) who use the plant, in the sense of imparting *vitality* and *longevity* to these creatures. Thus, the Northern Cheyenne of Montana rubbed the dried and powdered flower bundles all over their arms and legs before going into battle so as to ensure strength and vitality in warfare. They also applied it topically to their horses for the same reason (Grinnell 1905: 42; Grinnell 1972: 187; Hart 1981: 18).

However, the plant's most celebrated and oft-utilized activity is its *astringency*. Here, it is sometimes utilized topically for **burns**, especially in Quebec folk medicine (Coffey 1993: 240) and among the Tête de Boule (Raymond 1945: 119). The exact manner of how they prepared and applied the plant is not, at present, known. However, Michael Moore, an herbalist who practiced in the American Southwest in the latter half of the twentieth century, recommended simmering the dried flower heads briefly in a small portion of water, then cooling them to lukewarm temperature, then applying them to the burn, and, finally, covering them with a moist cloth (Moore 1993: 19).

Diarrhea and **bowel hemorrhage** have likewise been treated with this powerfully scented herb (Rafinesque 1828–30: 2:224; Felter and Lloyd 1898; Grieve 1971: 2:477;

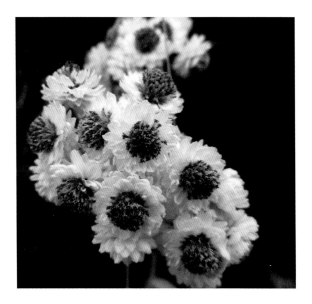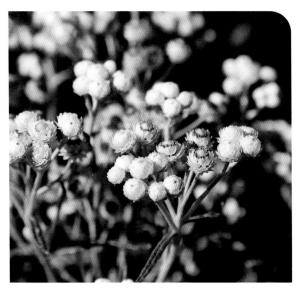

Millspaugh 1974: 89; Herrick 1995: 22). Then, too, the application of a decoction of pearly everlasting to **hemorrhoids**, a procedure popular among certain Native American tribes (Lewis and Elvin-Lewis 1977: 293), has brought soothing relief to many. An infusion has also long been traditional as a swish for **mouth sores** and as a gargle for **sore throat** (Callegari and Durand 1977: 14). The Iroquois have appreciated an infusion of the plant as a wash for **sore eyes** (Herrick 1995: 228). Tannins in the plant are, no doubt, at least partly responsible for the efficacy of the above-listed applications.

Bruises have also yielded to topical application, as older editions of the *United States Dispensatory* noted (cf. Felter and Lloyd 1898; Grieve 1971: 2:477). The preferred manner of implementation here has been a compress made from an infusion of the plant. The early-nineteenth-century botanical authority Constantine Rafinesque wrote that pearly everlasting was also helpful when used as a wash for "tumors, contusions, [and] sprains" (Rafinesque 1828–30: 2:224; cf. Millspaugh 1974: 89). Canada's Kwakiutl, too, have long esteemed the topical application of pearly everlasting for **swellings** (EthnobDB). It appears, then, that the plant exerts some *anti-inflammatory* effects in addition to the astringent properties highlighted earlier (Moore 1993: 19). Its use by modern herbalists for **allergic asthma**, as well as for **swollen mucous membranes** in general—where it effectively decreases **edema**—reinforces this conclusion (Moore 1993: 19).

Because this plant has *laryngeal* and *expectorant* effects (Chai 1978: 70), it has traditionally been implemented for **pulmonary catarrh**, as was noted in the *US Dispensatory* for 1942 (cf. Grieve 1971: 2:477). The Cherokee have appreciated this application, drinking a tea of the plant—or even smoking it—to achieve the desired effects (Hamel and Chiltoskey 1975: 48). They have done the same to alleviate **bronchial coughs** (Hamel and Chiltoskey 1975: 48). The

Montagnais have used it, by way of decoction, for **coughs** and for **tuberculosis** (Speck 1915: 314). The Mohegan have used an infusion of pearly everlasting for **colds** (Tantaquidgeon 1928: 265). The Native peoples of Baja California Sur use it as a component in a compound infusion for coughs, colds, and bronchitis, in which case it is taken before retiring, to enable sound sleep (Kay 1996: 153). For **asthma**, the Mohawk have combined an infusion of pearly everlasting flowers with a decoction of mullein (*Verbascum thapsus*) root (see page 161) (Rousseu 1945a: 63).

This plant has been used by the Native peoples of Baja California Sur for **fever** (Kay 1996: 153). The Thompson have used a decoction of pearly everlasting root for **rheumatic fever** (Turner et al. 1990: 50). Energetically, it is thought to be a *cooling* and *drying* herb, indicated when the tongue is red tipped and moist (Moore 1993: 19).

Steam inhaled from *Anaphalis* tea splashed onto hot rocks has been appreciated by the Cherokee as a cure for certain forms of **headache** and also for **blindness** caused by intense sunlight (Hamel and Chiltoskey 1975: 48). Washington's Quileute have likewise steamed tribe members afflicted with **rheumatism** (Gunther 1973: 48). Our own area's Ojibwe have used a steam of the plant—after powdering it and sprinkling it on live coals—to ease **paralysis**, often in combination with a steam of wild mint, *Mentha arvensis* (see page 264) (Smith 1932: 362; Densmore 1974: 362–63).

As a point aside, I can personally appreciate why the wild mint might have been added, since pearly everlasting smells (and tastes) terrible! I, therefore, only use it personally when absolutely necessary and then only in combination with other herbs so as to dull the taste as much as possible.

In view of the horrific smell and taste, I don't find it surprising that this herb also has some *vermifuge* properties, as Rafinesque pointed out (Rafinesque 1828–30: 2:224). ⫷

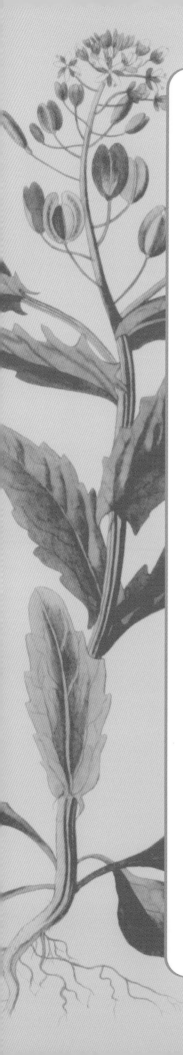

Pennycress

Thlaspi arvense

DESCRIPTION

Pennycress is an annual herb with a smooth stem that grows 6–24 inches tall.

This plant has both basal leaves and stem leaves. The former begin as a rosette of lanceolate, coarsely toothed blades that eventually reach a length of 4 inches. When the stem shoots up, it begins to show alternate, wavy-edged leaves that grow 1½–2½ inches long. These are sessile and, in fact, actually clasp the stem.

Flowers are four-petaled, as is typical of the mustard family to which this weed belongs. They are also white and ¼ inch wide and appear in short, spiked clusters that reach a length of 1–2 inches.

The striking seedpods (fruits) are round and look like pennies, and thus the plant's common name. They are papery, deeply notched at the tip, and filled with tiny black seeds. Initially, they are green, but they eventually become tan.

RANGE AND HABITAT

This plant grows throughout the Midwest in dry, sunny places such as old fields, waste places, gardens, and roadsides.

MAJOR CONSTITUENTS

Pennycress contains a glycoside (sinigroside) and an irritant oil (allyl isothiocyanate). Nutrients include a substantial quantity of vitamin C.

FOOD

The Cherokee have eaten the leaves of this plant as a food. Having munched on pennycress leaves several times myself, I can testify that the taste, while strong, is not particularly bad, especially if mixed with other greens so as to make a salad. The smell, however, is quite unpleasant and gives rise to the plant's alternative common name of stinkweed!

The seedpods can be dried, ground, and used as a pepper substitute. As such, they can also be mixed with olive oil and white vinegar to make a tasty salad dressing (Medve and Medve 1990: 61).

HEALTH/MEDICINE

Pennycress was an important ingredient in theriac, the famed antidote to poison whose formula was said to have been developed by Mithridates IV Eupator, king of Pontus in the first century BCE, who is said to have made himself invulnerable to poison by taking increasingly large doses of the concoction. A century later, the Roman naturalist Pliny the Elder would note, in his *Natural History*, that the most important medicinal applications of the plant were "for the groin, all kinds of gatherings, and wounds" (Pliny 1938: 27:114).

Centuries later, when the Iroquois experienced a **sore throat**, they would make an infusion out of this plant in order to gargle it and to drink it (Herrick 1977: 341; Herrick 1995: 155).

Traditional Chinese Medicine has long used this herb, called *bai jiang cao* in that system, for "toxic heat" conditions such as **insect bites and stings**, **hemoptysis**, and **acute infections** such as **abscesses**, **mastitis**, **mumps**, and even **appendicitis** (Belanger 1997).

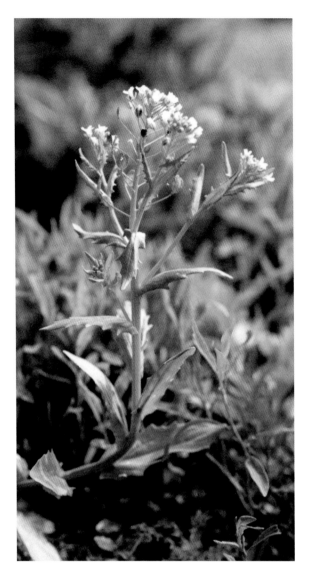

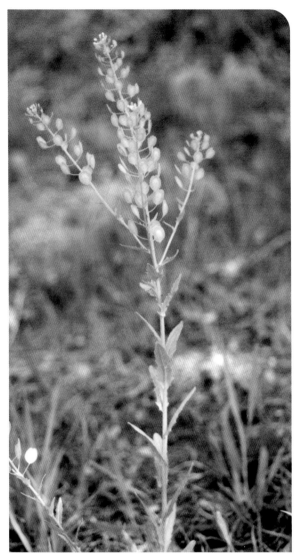

The Ramah Navajo (Diné) have used the related *Thlaspi fendleri* as a cold infusion for **itch**—both as a tea and as a lotion (Vestal 1952: 29).

PERSONAL AND PROFESSIONAL USE

I have found this plant to be very useful as a formula ingredient for acute reproductive infections or conditions such as acutely swollen inguinal lymph nodes, orchitis, endometritis, cervicitis, peritoneal cancer, and even premenstrual flareups of endometriosis. The bulk herb is available from some Chinese medicine suppliers, but I prefer to wildcraft it because it has been scientifically demonstrated that this herb draws industrial toxins to it like a magnet, and I have no way of knowing how close the marketed herb may have grown to industrial pollution in China—something that, unfortunately, is quite rampant in that nation.

CAUTIONS

It is thought that this plant has toxic potential, as cattle have been poisoned from grazing on it. Such poisoning, however, may simply have resulted from the fact that this herb draws industrial toxins to it, as mentioned above—to the extent that it has even been used in environmental science as a pollution indicator! Hence, this plant should never be gathered for food or medicine if found growing in the proximity of a source of pollution.

Traditional Chinese Medicine points to dizziness and nausea as possible side effects from using this plant.

James Duke, a former economic botanist with the US Department of Agriculture, cautions that internal bleeding could potentially result from overconsumption of pennycress.

Pennycress should not be taken during either pregnancy or lactation. ⬿

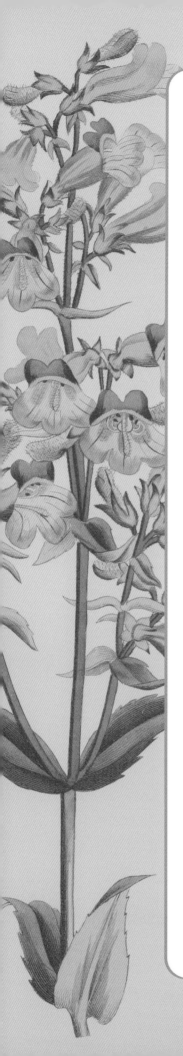

Penstemon

Penstemon grandiflorus, P. gracilis

DESCRIPTION

Penstemon is a very lovely native perennial. The major species, *Penstemon grandiflorus* (large-flowered penstemon, large-flowered beard-tongue), reaches a height of 2–4 feet, while *P. gracilis* (slender penstemon, lilac-flowered beard-tongue) tops off at only 6–18 inches.

The leaves of both species are opposite, 1–3 inches long, and short stalked (often even clasping the stem). Those of *P. grandiflorus* are egg shaped, smooth edged, waxy, thick, leathery, and bluish green, whereas those of *P. gracilis* are narrow and toothed.

Two to six flowers appear just above the stem's upper leaf node. The large-flowered penstemon is so named because its gorgeous bell-shaped lavender blossoms reach a length of about 2 inches, whereas the smaller species bears flowers growing to about ¾ inch. The blossoms of both species flare at their ends into two upper lobes and three lower lobes. They each possess five stamens, one of which is sterile and somewhat hairy at the tip, giving rise to the alternative common name of beard-tongue.

So striking is the large-flowered penstemon with its lilac colored flowers and its bluish sheen that it never fails to catch the eye, even when nestled among dozens of other flowering plants in a field or meadow. Truly, it is beauty personified!

RANGE AND HABITAT

Penstemon grows in sandy soil in locales such as fields, prairies, and thickets. Both species tend to grow in the middle latitudes of the Midwest, being less common in Wisconsin and in other areas of our region.

MAJOR CONSTITUENTS

Penstemon contains cardioactive glycosides such as gitoxin, lanatoside B, and acetyldigitoxin.

HEALTH/MEDICINE

"Penstemon in, pain out!" might likely have been a slogan of many Native American tribes. The Navajo (Diné), for instance, discovered that the plant is invaluable for **toothache** (Wyman and Harris 1951: 42–43; Hocking 1956: 162). To relieve a **stomachache**, the Kiowa found a decoction of penstemon roots to do the trick (Vestal and Schultes 1939: 51). Our own region's Dakota likewise discovered an *analgesic* application for the boiled roots, using the decoction for **pains in the chest** (Kindscher 1992: 267). (If these were angina pains, then the plant's cardioactive glycosides may well have been a factor in offsetting them.)

Then, too, various tribes of the southwestern United States have used penstemon as a *vulnerary*, especially for **burns**, **wounds**, and **bites** (Wyman and Harris 1951: 42–43; Hocking 1956: 162). The Navajo (Diné) have even combined penstemon flowers with the blossoms of a *Castilleja* species to produce an infusion for topical use on **centipede bites** (Weiner 1980: 33). California's Costanoan have implemented the western species, *P. centranthifolius*, as a poultice for **deep**, **infected sores** (Bocek 1984: 254). A modern application discussed by LoLo Westrich in her book *California Herbal Remedies*

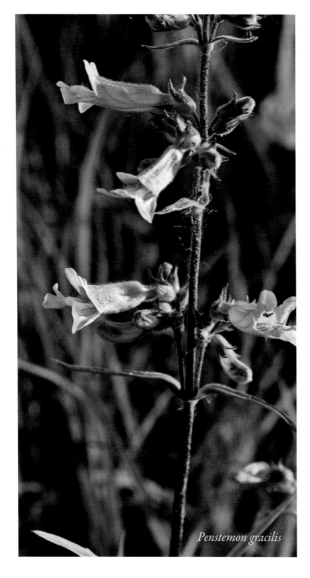

Penstemon gracilis

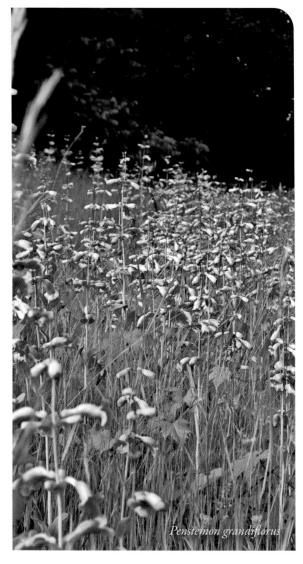

Penstemon grandiflorus

is to mash or blend a *Penstemon* species and then mix it with olive oil as an external application for **chapped hands**, **rashes**, and **cold sores** (Westrich 1989: 97). In this regard, Southwest American herbalist Michael Moore proffered an excellent recipe for a penstemon salve for **skin** and **external mucous-membrane irritation** or **inflammation**: he said to pulp penstemon (via a hand mill, blender, food processor, or juicer) and then combine it with equal amounts of a base oil—such as almond, apricot kernel, or olive—thereafter setting the concoction in a warm place for a week. When that time has elapsed, strain or express it through a cloth, add some beeswax, and then warm the combination till the wax melts. Finally, transfer the mess into a wide-mouthed pot, stir it, and allow it to set (Moore 1979: 123–24).

The astute reader may recall that this sort of salve preparation is reminiscent of a mullein-oil preparation mentioned under that plant's profile (see page 161). This is not surprising in that penstemon is so closely related to mullein that the two plants would only naturally have similar uses via similar preparations! In fact, a careful look at penstemon's applications as outlined here will remind one closely of the spectrum of mullein's uses. Both plants are said to exert *anti-inflammatory*, *analgesic*, and *antimicrobial* effects.

CAUTIONS
Penstemon is a member of the same family as foxglove, and thus caution should be exercised in its use owing to possible poisoning from cardioactive glycosides. These are most concentrated in the flowers, though even there, they occur in a much lower concentration than they do in foxglove. ⋘

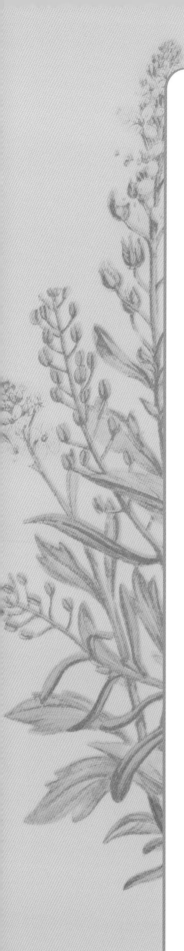

Peppergrass

POOR MAN'S PEPPER; PEPPERCRESS; VIRGINIA PEPPERWEED

Lepidium densiflorum, L. virginicum

DESCRIPTION

Peppergrass—represented in the Midwest by two species, *Lepidium densiflorum* and *L. virginicum*—is one of several "cresses" to be found here, distinguished from the cow (or field) cress, *L. campestre*, and two introduced species, *L. perfoliatum* and *L. sativum*. (The latter is the popular cultivated salad ingredient known as garden cress.) It should also be distinguished from field pennycress (stinkweed), *Thlaspi arvense* (see page 169), which has penny-sized seedpods, four times as large as those of peppergrass!

This is either an annual or a biennial herb. It can grow to 1½ feet high but is usually recognized in the spring when it is one of the few weeds up and running and about 3–6 inches high.

Peppergrass starts as a basal rosette of deeply cut (lobed) leaves, which are about 2 inches long and possessed of double-toothed margins. The terminal lobe is noticeably larger than the side lobes. The eventual stem leaves are smaller, narrower, willow-like, pointed at their tips, and only slightly toothed. They taper to a very short leafstalk or simply clasp the stem and appear one at a node, alternating up along the stem. One feature distinguishing *L. densiflorum* (green-flower pepperweed) from *L. virginicum* (Virginia pepperweed) is that the leaves of the former are slightly pubescent, whereas those of the latter appear to be without hairs (the hairs are there, but they are so small as to not be visible to the human eye).

Inflorescence is in the form of narrow, elongate clusters of small white or green flowers consisting of four petals and four sepals (characteristic of the mustard family to which this plant belongs) appearing at the tips of the stem and of the branches. In *L. densiflorum*, the flowers are more greenish than whitish, and the petals are shorter than the sepals (sometimes the former are even entirely absent). In *L. virginicum*, the flowers are more whitish than greenish, and the petals are as long as, or longer than, the sepals.

Like some other plants bearing terminal racemes, peppergrass frequently has both flowers and fruits growing at the same time, with the fruits appearing the lowest on the branches. These take the form of flattened, orbicular seedpods, 2½–4 millimeters wide, shallowly notched at their apex, and slightly winged. Each pod contains only two seeds.

RANGE AND HABITAT

This is a cosmopolitan weed, growing throughout the United States and southern Canada. It inhabits vacant lots, fields, and trailsides.

MAJOR CONSTITUENTS

Peppergrass contains glucosinolate compounds and nutrients that include extremely high amounts of pro-vitamin A and vitamin C, vitamin E, and some B vitamins.

FOOD

The pungent seedpods of this plant are renowned as yielding the "poor man's pepper," as its alternative common name indicates. These are excellent in camp stews, added toward the end. The pods can also be chopped and mixed with vinegar and salt and used as a

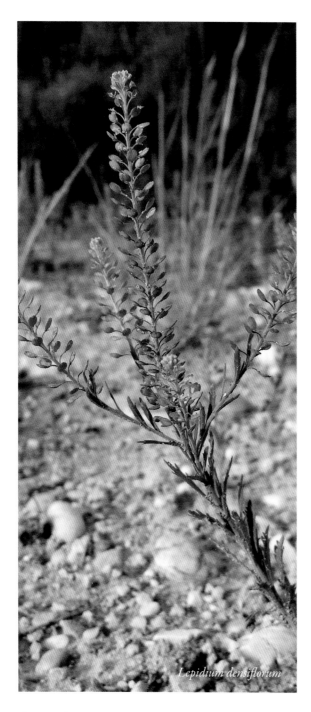

Lepidium densiflorum

HEALTH/MEDICINE

Early American physicians and healers found peppergrass to exert *antiscorbutic*, *deobstruent*, and *stimulant* effects, using it to treat **scurvy** and **skin problems**. The latter application gained considerable popularity (Clapp 1852: 739ff.), especially in the respect that this plant was highly regarded as a treatment for **poison ivy rash**, a use pioneered by the Menomini, Maidu, and other Native tribes, all of whom have implemented a wash made from an infusion of the plant, or sometimes simply the bruised plant itself, as a poultice (Smith 1923: 33; Strike and Roeder 1994: 81). Then, too, the Cherokee implemented a bruised-peppergrass poultice to quickly draw out a **blister** (Hamel and Chiltoskey 1975: 48). The Keres and other western tribes even rubbed the crushed plant onto **sunburn** (Swank 1932: 51).

Early American physicians also discovered that the plant was possessed of *diuretic* activity, so it was implemented to help treat **dropsy** (Clapp 1852: 739ff.). Likewise, the Lakota have utilized a peppergrass infusion for **kidney problems** (Rogers 1980: 41). Traditional Chinese Medicine uses seeds of the related species, *Lepidium apetalum*, for **water retention** in the **chest** or **abdomen** (Reid 1992: 140).

Peppergrass has also been used to treat **inhibited sexual desire** (thus adding a little "pepper" to one's love life!). The Lumbee have used it most effectively in this regard (Croom 1983: 83–84), and some herbalists since then have taken the cue. A related species, *Lepidium meyenii* (maca), has traditionally been used in Peru for the same purpose and has accumulated a number of animal studies and clinical trials in verification of such a libido-stimulating effect, especially when used at a dosage of 3,000 milligrams a day (Zheng 2000; Cicero et al. 2001; Gonzales et al. 2002; Dording et al. 2008; Stone et al. 2009; Zenico et al. 2009).

While the libido-stimulating effect of our indigenous peppergrass may be due to stimulant effects produced by the plant (Crellin and Philpott 1990a: 333), which might also explain its reputation as a reducing aid for **obesity** (an application that was made popular by the Mahuna: Romero 1954: 66), the above-cited research on maca pointing toward *adaptogenic* effects leads one to conclude that its American relative may well produce those same effects. Yet, to date, the two North American species have been almost entirely ignored by the scientific community—something that, sadly, is typically the case with plants growing wild in North America.

In yet another of its many and varied applications, peppergrass has been used in white folk medicine (Crellin and Philpott 1990a: 333) and among the Cahuilla and Maidu of California (Strike and Roeder 1994: 81) as a shampoo ingredient to offset **hair loss.** There may be an as-yet-unidentified regenerative effect here, since the related species *L. sativum* has been shown to rapidly heal **broken bones** (Ahsan et al. 1989; Juma 2007: 23) in line with traditional Arab use (Ageel

dressing for wild game. The seeds have been parched and ground into mush by Native American tribes in California (Strike and Roeder 1994: 81).

The leaves are typically mixed with other greens to create salads. The explorers Lewis and Clark, in their famed cross-country expedition, came across what they described as a "sand-bar extending several miles, which renders navigation difficult, and a small creek called Sand Creek on the south, where we stopped for dinner, and gathered wild cresses or tongue-grass" (from their official journal).

et al. 1989) and since a quick rub of our native *Lepidium* has been used to heal the skin from sunburn (despite the mustard family's reputation for being rubefacient!), as described above.

The herb evidently has a healing effect on the respiratory system as well, no doubt due to its pungency and/or vitamin C content, if not also owing to other factors. Thus, the Cherokee have used a peppergrass poultice to help heal **croup** (Hamel and Chiltoskey 1975: 48). Early-nineteenth-century American physician Asahel Clapp noted that it was commonly used in his time for **chronic coughs** and that it possessed *expectorant* effects (Clapp 1852: 739). A compound infusion inclusive of this plant has even been implemented by the Houma to help manage **tuberculosis** (Speck 1941: 64). Traditional Chinese Medicine uses the related species *L. apetalum* as an expectorant as well (Reid 1992: 140).

In the highlands of Chiapas, Mexico, peppergrass has traditionally been used for **diarrhea** and for its more severe form, **dysentery**. Interestingly here, a 2003 scientific study found that a crude extract from peppergrass's roots exerted *antiprotozoal* activity against *Entamoeba histolytica* trophozoites, one of several pathogens that can cause these conditions. Further research found that the plant's content of benzyl glucosinolate was the active agent in this regard (Calzada et al. 2003).

Finally, the Isleta found that chewing several peppergrass leaves dissipated certain types of **headache** (Jones 1931: 34).

PERSONAL AND PROFESSIONAL USE

I recommend the use of the fresh herb, available as the related species *Lepidium sativum* at some supermarkets in my area, as a salad or sandwich ingredient for persons possessed of low bone density (osteopenia or osteoporosis) or to accelerate the healing of broken bones. I also tend to add a tincture of the wildcrafted herb to formulas for clients afflicted with low libido, pulmonary or bronchial congestion, or obesity—especially if two or three of these conditions overlap.

CAUTIONS

The infusion can be emetic. Also, one should exercise caution in applying any member of the mustard family to the skin, as irritation, redness, or blistering may occur—especially if left on for too long a period of time. ⤸

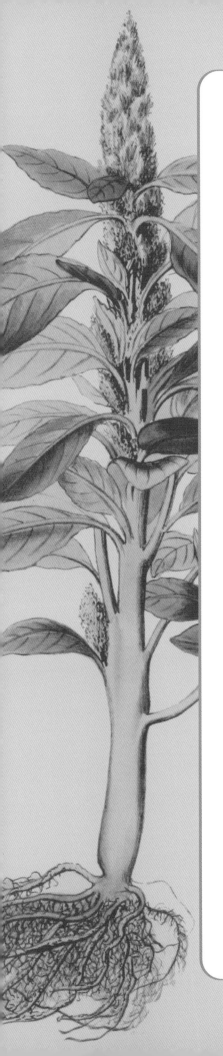

Pigweed

RED AMARANTH; REDROOT PIGWEED

Amaranthus retroflexus

DESCRIPTION
Pigweed is a coarse, stout-stemmed annual plant that can grow to 6 feet but usually tops off at 2–4 feet. Older plants have a red root and often red (or red-striped) stems as well.

The dull-green leaves are long stalked, egg shaped to lanceolate, long pointed, prominently veined, and possessed of wavy margins. They commonly grow 2–4 inches long (although they can reach as much as 10 inches!) and alternate along the stalk. Quite often, at least some of them are tinged with red.

The greenish flowers are densely crowded into spikes that appear at the tip of the stem and on short stalks from the leaf axils. They are usually dioecious—that is, possessed of male and female flowers on separate plants. (Occasionally, both sexes can be found on the same plant.) The eventual fruits are flattened and possessed of small, shiny black seeds to the tune of over one hundred thousand per plant!

RANGE AND HABITAT
This weed is sparsely scattered throughout the Midwest, growing in wasteland and especially on cultivated ground or in areas with livestock (as it prefers manured soils).

MAJOR CONSTITUENTS
Pigweed contains saponins and mucilage. Nutrients include pro-vitamin A, vitamin C (80 milligrams per 100 grams), and iron (3.9 milligrams per 100 grams).

FOOD
The young, tender leaves and stalks (from plants less than 6 inches tall) can sparingly be added to salads. They can also be prepared as a potherb, boiled like spinach for ten to twenty minutes.

The plentiful seeds can be boiled into mush (two parts water to one part seeds, cooked until the water is absorbed) or ground into meal and thereafter used half and half with wheat flour or cornmeal in pancakes and other recipes. Before being ground, however, they are best roasted for one to one and a half hours in the oven at 350 degrees Fahrenheit, stirred every so often.

HEALTH/MEDICINE
Although pigweed is revered as a wild food, its medicinal uses are little known. However, it possesses some very useful properties in this regard. First, it is *astringent* (Lust 1974: 95; Chai 1978: 69), making it useful for **sore throat** and **diarrhea** and as a douche for **leukorrhea** (Krochmal and Krochmal 1973: 35; Lust 1974: 95; Chai 1978: 69). Secondly, it is *hemostatic*, primarily due to its astringency (Lust 1974: 95; Chai 1978: 69), and thus has a cherished reputation for halting external **bleeding** (Lust 1974: 95; Chai 1978: 69) as well as curtailing both **bowel hemorrhage** and **menorrhagia** (Krochmal and Krochmal 1973: 35; Lust 1974: 95; Angier 1978: 34–35).

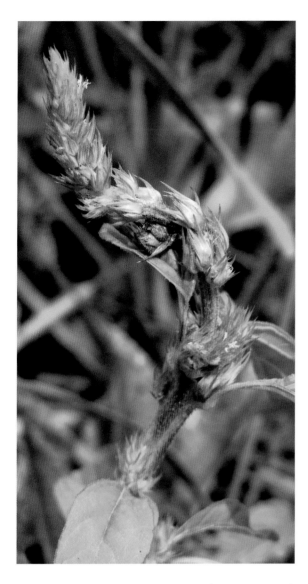

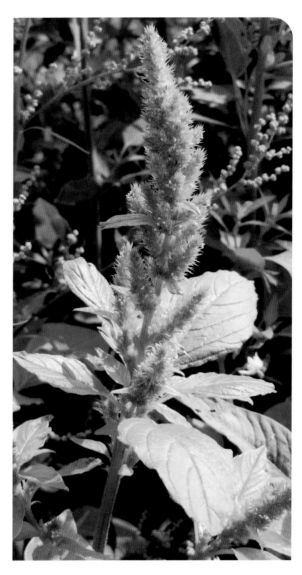

The plant is also a valuable *alterative* (Tierra 1988: 339). Externally, it has been used as a wash for **ulcers** (Stuart 1982: 23), **hives**, **eczema**, and **psoriasis** (Krochmal and Krochmal 1973: 35; Angier 1978: 34–35; Stuart 1982: 23). Efficacy with these conditions must at least be partly due to the plant's high concentration of saponins, which possess verified *disinfectant* effects.

As to the form and amount of use for medicinal purposes, naturopath John Lust lists a tincture dosage of ½–1 teaspoon. To make an infusion instead, he suggests steeping 1 teaspoon of the crushed leaves in 1 cup of boiled water (Lust 1974: 95).

PERSONAL AND PROFESSIONAL USE

I've eaten pigweed once or twice and did not find it to be unpleasant. Medicinally, I had the opportunity to implement its astringent properties on one occasion when on a nature excursion but otherwise have had little experience with this plant.

CAUTIONS

Plants growing in cultivated areas or western soils can accumulate potentially dangerous amounts of nitrates. 🌿

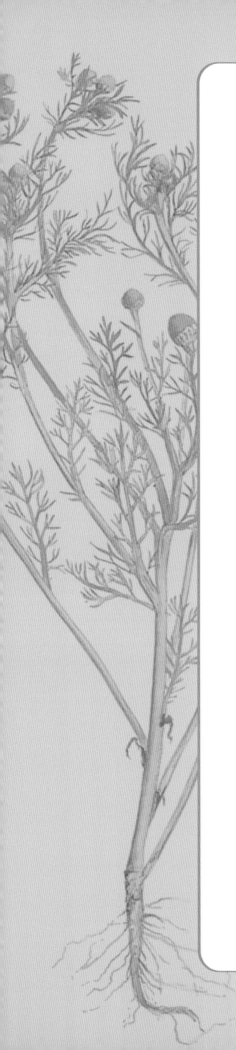

Pineapple-Weed

DISC MAYWEED; WILD CHAMOMILE

Matricaria discoidea [alternatively, *Matricaria matricarioides; Chamomilla suaveolens*]

DESCRIPTION
This is a shrimpy annual weed (2–6 inches tall) that is closely related to chamomile (*Matricaria recutita*) and is often even referred to as wild chamomile. Sprawling and branching in appearance, it is possessed of alternate, finely dissected leaves that grow ½–2 inches long. (They look a lot like those of parsley but are even thinner.)

Small (¼-inch-wide), spherical, yellow-green flower heads appear at the tip of the stem and of its branches, each composed of many tiny, tubular disk flowers but lacking ray flowers. This is in marked contrast to chamomile, which possesses white ray flowers.

Dry fruits, or achenes, begin to develop from the flower heads in late summer, each containing only a solitary seed. The fruits are tan to gray in color.

RANGE AND HABITAT
This is an almost cosmopolitan weed in North America, growing everywhere on this continent except for the upper one-third of Canada. Naturalized from either the western United States or, as some allege, northeast Asia, it is now a common urban weed, growing between sidewalk slabs, at the edges of driveways, and on roadsides. It can also be found at the edges of fields and paths, in barnyards, on railroad embankments, and in various, so-called waste places.

MAJOR CONSTITUENTS
Pineapple-weed contains helaniol (a triterpene alcohol); coumarins; dicaffeolylquinic acid; chlorogenic acid; a large variety of flavonoids and other glycosides (ferulic acid glycoside, quercetin galactoside, apigenin acetylglucoside, malonylapigenin glucoside, luteolin glycoside, quercetin glycoside, apigenin glycoside), and an essential oil with (E)-beta-farnesene as its major component.

FOOD
The flower heads can be infused to make a pleasant pineapple-scented tea.

HEALTH/MEDICINE
This herb has unfortunately been far overshadowed by its cousin, chamomile, and thus is vastly underutilized by today's herbalists. However, it has most of chamomile's valuable properties—plus a few more!—and is much more readily available in that it is a common weed. The significance of this may be gauged by the fact that chamomile suffers greatly in potency when dried for any length of time, as is typically the case when it is procured from commercial sources.

While little used by white healers of today, pineapple-weed has a protracted history of use by Native tribes, especially those of Alaska and of Canada's northern territories, many of whom still treasure it as an important item in their materia medica. The Dena'ina Athabascan boil the herb and give a cup of the tea to mothers after childbirth as well as a few drops to the newborns, feeling that this herb "cleans them both out and helps the mother's milk to start" (Kari 1977). This *galactagogue* effect is also appreciated

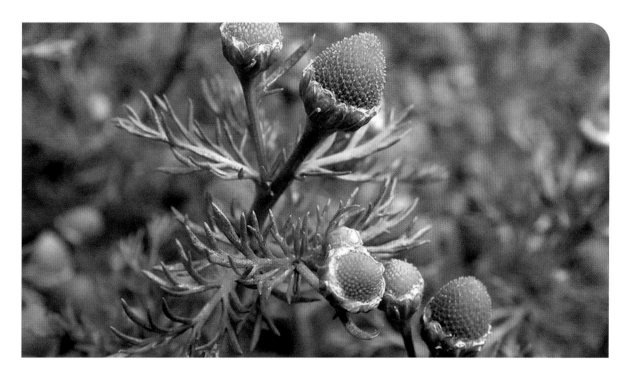

by Native Americans living in the vicinity of Port Graham, Alaska (Schofield Eaton 1989: 304). Then, too, Aleut elders drink pineapple-weed tea to offset **stomach upset** and **colic** (Smith 1973). The Kuskokwagmiut imbibe it for **indigestion** (Oswalt 1957: 22–23).

These *stomachic* and *carminative* effects are the herb's most celebrated uses and have been widely implemented by Native American tribes as well. Thus, California's Cahuilla and Diegueño found the plant to be of great aid for both **colic** and **diarrhea** (Westrich 1989: 101; Strike and Roeder 1994: 91). The Salish have used pineapple-weed for the same discomforts (Shemluck 1982: 341), while the Costanoan and Kuskokwagmiut have used it for **stomach pain** and for **indigestion** (Oswalt 1957: 22–23; Bocek 1984). The Maidu have appreciated an infusion of the flowers for **gastrointestinal cramps** and a decoction of the leaves and flowers for **diarrhea** (Strike and Roeder 1994: 91).

This plant is also a pretty good *emmenagogue*, thus proving helpful for **menstrual cramps**—perhaps its chemical helaniol, shown to exert anti-inflammatory effects, is of aid here (Akihisa et al. 1996)**.** It can also sometimes deliver a **retained placenta**. The Flathead (Salish) and Diegueño came to appreciate both assists (Shemluck 1982: 341; Strike and Roeder 1994: 91). It is a fair *febrifuge*, too, for which application the Maidu, Costanoan, and Coast Miwok have used it (Strike and Roeder 1994: 91). The Diegueño have also tapped in to its *antipyretic* powers, reserving a simple flower tea for youngsters but a whole-plant infusion for adults (Strike and Roeder 1994: 91). (This distinction may simply have been owing to patient compliance, because the flowers are sweet and pleasant to the taste, but the leaves are somewhat bitter.)

Finally, the celebrated European phytotherapist Rudolf Fritz Weiss noted, in his opus on botanical medicine (Weiss 1988: 122–24), that pineapple-weed flowers have been clinically verified as possessing powerful *vermifuge* properties. He had been especially impressed here by the work of the French phytotherapist Henri LeClerc, who had confirmed vermifuge effects in worm-infested soldiers. Weiss's own observation was that it was most effective with **threadworms** but that **roundworms** and **whipworms** are also susceptible to its effects as long as the remedy is continued for an extended period of time. In a similar vein, the Flathead (Salish) found this herb to be a good **insect repellant** (Shemluck 1982: 342).

PERSONAL AND PROFESSIONAL USE

Pineapple-weed is the first herb I turn to for many of the gastrointestinal problems listed here—especially for indigestion from emotional wrestling, as can occur in irritable bowel syndrome or simply from acute stress situations—in that I have found it to be quite dependable. It is not readily available on the herb market, however, necessitating that I wildcraft it. I've also rubbed it on my skin and clothes in an effort to dissuade insect attacks when out of doors, finding that it helps a bit.

CAUTIONS

This plant *should not be used during pregnancy*, owing to its content of helaniol, a chemical responsible for its vermifuge effect, and owing to its expulsive effects on the placenta. ⧏⧏

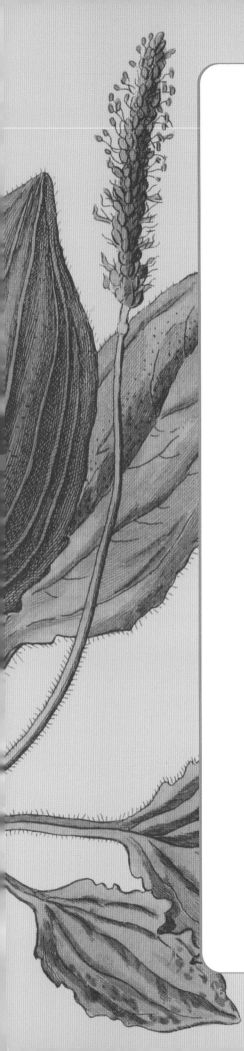

Plantain

SOLDIER'S WOUNDWORT; WAYBREAD

Plantago major

DESCRIPTION

This is a perennial plant with a short rootstock growing 4–20 inches high.

The herb starts as a basal cluster of bright-green, spade-like leaves that are smooth edged, finely haired, and blatantly veined in parallel fashion—a total of seven veins running down the length of the leaf. Each leaf bears a thick petiole that is about as long as the blade.

Eventually, a tall and leafless center stalk forms, bearing a flower spire. This whole structure can reach 8 inches.

The greenish-white flowers, small and inconspicuous, are arranged on the top portion of the stalk in a tightly clustered fashion, so that the entire structure gives the impression of a long pipe cleaner.

In autumn, the flowers transform into fruits (seedpods), each bearing twelve to eighteen seeds that are very tiny and angular.

RANGE AND HABITAT

Plantain is a cosmopolitan weed—it occurs throughout the United States and Canada and in most other parts of the world. Originating in the Old World, it was inadvertently brought to the Americas by the settlers. Its preferred habitat is ill-kept lawns, roadsides, in between sidewalk slabs, pastures, cultivated fields, waste places, edges of parking lots, and wherever people tend to walk! During the American colonial era, the Native Americans called it "white man's foot" because it seemed to pop up wherever the white man proceeded to tread.

MAJOR CONSTITUENTS

Plantain contains iridoid glycosides (aucubin, catalpol); flavonoids (apigenin, luteolin, baicalein, plantagoside, scutellarin, hispidulin, nepitrin, homoplantaginin, aucuboside); phenolic (hydroxycinnamic) acids (salicylic, rubichloric [asperuloside], vanillic, syringic, caffeic, ursolic, *p*-coumaric, chlorogenic, neochlorogenic); oleanolic acid; planteolic acid; organic acids (citric, fumaric); unsaturated fatty acids (linoleic, linolenic); amino acids; enzymes; allantoin; mucilage; and tannins. Nutrients include goodly amounts of pro-vitamin A and vitamins C and K and the minerals zinc, potassium, and silica.

FOOD

I enjoy young, raw plantain leaves in salads. (They can also be munched "as is" but possess a strong taste that is best offset by mixing them with other greens.) This common broadleaf also makes a good cooked vegetable. Here, the leaves are usually soaked in salted water for a few minutes and then boiled or steamed for anywhere from three to fifteen minutes, depending upon whether you like them crispy or tender, in very little water (just enough to cover them). They can then be eaten as is or combined with cheese or lemon juice in a variety of dishes. Alternatively, one can simply chop the leaves and add them to omelets, casseroles, and stews. The master wild-foods forager Euell Gibbons once told of a couple he knew who blended, cooked, and strained plantain to feed to their infant child, owing to the fact that the plant is so rich in nourishing factors (Gibbons 1971: 163).

HEALTH/MEDICINE

Plantain's *cooling* and *drying* energies allow it to be used in such multifarious ways that a profile such as this one could only begin to scratch the surface. However, let's try.

First, we should note that plantain's medicinal wonders have been venerated from antiquity: Dioscorides, a first-century herbalist who may have been a medical officer under Nero or Claudius, noted that plantain had a "drying, binding facultie" (Dioscorides 1996: 2:153) and went on to attest to its uses, time honored even then, for **sores** or **ulcers** (including **canker sores**) and **bleeding**, especially of the **gums** and the bowel (**flux**). Celsus, a medical practitioner or educator who lived about the same time, said that if "bleeding comes from the throat, or from more internal parts ... the patient should sip ... plantain ... juice" (Celsus 1938: 2.4–7). Several chemicals in the plant may be responsible for its renowned hemostatic property, including the significant amount of vitamin K (37 milligrams per gram in dried, June-gathered leaves), the saturated primary alcohols, the caffeic acid derivatives (at least one of which is hypotensive), and/or the flavonoids (Samuelsen 2000).

The plant is a fine *astringent*, which might contribute to the uses explicated by these ancient herbalists. Such astringency might also at least partly elucidate plantain's likewise time-honored application for **sore nipples** (Krochmal and Krochmal 1973: 172; Bolyard 1981: 113) and for **hemorrhoids**, the latter use being highly recommended in the *British Herbal Pharmacopoeia* (Hyde et al. 1976–79: 1:163). For hemorrhoids, American herbalist Susun Weed prefers a combination of plantain and yarrow (*Achillea millefolium*—see page 282) in ointment form, which she has found efficacious both for offsetting the pain of the hemorrhoids and for shrinking them (Weed 1986: 32).

Astringency would seem at least partly to explain the tradition of using plantain leaves and roots for **diarrhea** (de Bairacli Levy 1974: 112). In the first century, Celsus even advised the use of plantain in combination with blackberry fruit, another highly astringent botanical, to help arrest **dysentery** (Celsus 1938: 4.23). Bearing in mind that one common cause of dysentery is infection with *Giardia*, it is of interest that a 1994 in vitro study found that plantain proved superior to tinidazol, a drug typically used for this infection, in killing the organism (Ponce-Macotela et al. 1994).

The Eclectics cherished plantain for "diseases of the gastrointestinal mucous surfaces, when there are pinching or colicky pains" (Thomas 1907: 1009). Concordantly, the Russian Ministry of Health has recommended plantain for treating chronic **colitis** (Hutchens 1991: 221; Zevin 1997: 119). In modern Pompei, where this application is also appreciated, five leaves are heated in ½–⅓ liter of water, and this tisane is drunk throughout the day (Jashemski 1999: 78). Extensive clinical experience in Russia has revealed that the plant is also invaluable for **gastric inflammation** (Hutchens

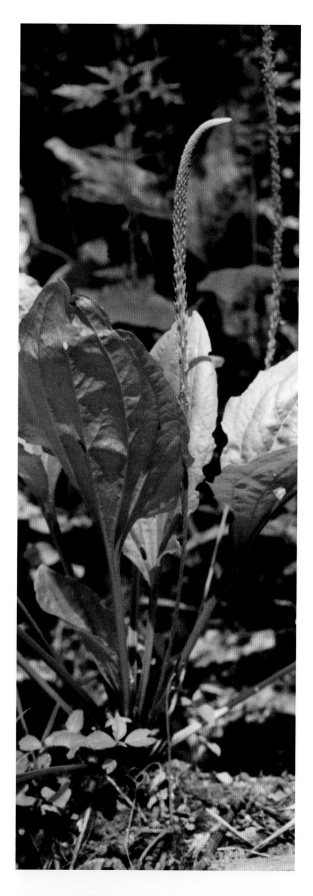

1991: 221), probably at least partly because the herb's proteolytic enzymes act as a mild vasoconstrictor (Moore 1979: 129; Ody 1993: 86). Most significantly, however, a Romanian study published in 1990 found that a polyholozidic fraction extracted from the leaves and seeds exhibited a "statistically significant gastro-protective action ... in two experimental models" (Hriscu et al. 1990). Not surprisingly, then, plantain has also long been a revered aid for **ulcers** in the stomach and on the surface of the body, especially the juice (Moore 1979: 129), which application has been used by some of the native peoples of North America (Lacey 1993: 90).

Another traditional application of the juice, tea, or tincture has been as a topical treatment for **aching teeth** (de Bairacli Levy 1974: 112; Brown 1985: 174). British herbalist Mary Carse even recommends drops of the strong decoction in **tooth cavities** until they can be professionally repaired (Carse 1989: 143). Further on this, an early American physician once wrote to another physician about the amazing benefits of the fibrous strings in the herb's leafstalk and how they can actually vanquish the pain of a carious tooth if placed in the ear on the same side as the aching molar (Millspaugh 1974: 420; Lewis and Elvin-Lewis 1977). The Eclectic physician Finley Ellingwood was likewise enamored of plantain's application for dental pain, noting here: "The juice on a piece of cotton applied to a tooth cavity, or to the sensitive pulp, has immediately controlled intractable cases of toothache" (Ellingwood 1983).

A swish of the tea or diluted tincture is also most welcome for **sore** or **inflamed gums** or **mouth**, and this treatment is even endorsed by the scientists who authored the German *Commission E Monographs* (Blumenthal 1998). I have found it to be especially appreciated by those suffering from oral inflammation due to **carrageenan sensitivity**—a largely unknown but important problem in modern society caused by greedy food industrialists tampering with nature in order to make the cheapest possible food stabilizer regardless of the harm to human health that it might entail. What is involved here is that the food industry takes the seaweed known as irish moss (*Chondrus crispus*) and changes its molecular weight to create the stabilizer carrageenan, which is added to creamy foods and sauces to give them body and to maintain a consistent, lump-free smoothness. What the food industry doesn't tell us is that the same product is used in scientific laboratories to inflame rat paws so that anti-inflammatory medicines can be tested against the swelled appendages! People with disturbed beneficial intestinal microflora (especially *Lactobacillus* and *Bifidus* spp.) seem to be especially sensitive to its inflammatory potential (Murray and Pizzorno 1998: 593). A few researchers even suspect carrageenan as being a causative or contributing factor to inflammatory bowel disease (Crohn's disease and ulcerative colitis) (Murray and Pizzorno 1998: 593). Interestingly, a lab study has found plantain to inhibit carrageenan-induced inflammation in rat paws (Shipochliev et al. 1981; Mascolo et al. 1987). More recently, both an aqueous extract and an ethanolic extract of freeze-dried plantain was found to exert powerful *anti-inflammatory* action against an oral epithelial cell line (H400) (Zubair et al. 2018).

Not surprisingly, such an anti-inflammatory effect for plantain has also otherwise been well demonstrated (Lambev et al. 1981; Murai et al. 1995; Guillén et al. 1997). The action appears to be due to a combination of the plant's iridoids, flavonoids, and hydroxycinnamic acids (Maksyutina 1971a; Maksyutina 1971b; Shipochliev et al. 1981; Mascolo et al. 1987; Bruneton 1995: 100; Ringbom et al. 1998; Herold et al. 2003). Its soothing aid as an eyewash for **sore eyes** may also stem from this property, as well as from the plant's astringency: Pliny the Elder had noted the tradition of droppering a cooled infusion into the eyes for **ophthalmia** (Pliny 1938: 25:91). In the modern European tradition, a compress of a plantain infusion has been used for both **blepharitis** and **conjunctivitis** (de Bairacli Levy 1974: 112; Stuart 1982: 114). It is also widely used in both Central and South America for **eye infections** (Samuelsen 2000).

As to other inflammatory conditions, numerous peoples have long praised the relief obtained by binding the leaves to the soles of **aching feet** after a long walk (Kay 1996: 216), a use that I have employed on several occasions so that I can add my own positive testimony. Native tribes such as the Algonquin, Flambeau Ojibwe, and Canada's Lenape (Delaware) found that the crushed leaves rapidly healed **bruises** when applied topically (Tantaquidgeon 1972: 108). Several other tribes implemented the crushed leaves or the juice for **swellings**, **cuts**, and **sores** (Tantaquidgeon 1972: 108; Train 1988: 80; Herrick 1995: 211). Indeed, plantain's most famous use has certainly been as a **wound** herb, not only because of its ability to curtail the flow of blood (as delineated above) but also because of its ability to regenerate the damaged tissue and also to disinfect the wound.

As to wound repair, several studies have finally been done to affirm this activity. In the first one, conducted by a Brazilian university's Lab of Tissue Processing, the topical use of plantain on wounds in mice was compared with a commercial ointment typically used in modern Brazilian medicine for wounds, with the result that the plantain application reduced wound size as quickly as the control ointment, but by the ninth day had induced neoepithelial formation and by the fifteenth day had closed the wound, neither of which transpired with the control ointment (Thomé et al. 2012). In the second study, performed at the Swedish University of Agricultural Sciences, the fresh leaf (by way of both a tincture and an aqueous extract) increased the proliferation and the migration of oral epithelial cells in a scratch test compared to a negative control (Zubair et al. 2012). A follow-up study by the same lead author found both an aqueous extract and an ethanol extract to stimulate wound healing in porcine skin (Zubair et al. 2016), while a 2019 study published in the *World Journal of Plastic Surgery* found a combination of plantain and aloe vera to enhance wound healing in full-thickness skin wounds by enhancing fibroblast proliferation, collagen bundle synthesis, and revascularization (Ashkani-Esfahani et al. 2019).

As to disinfectant activity, the fresh plant, crushed to activate its enzymes, has been shown to exert a moderate degree of antibacterial activity, specifically against both *Bacillus subtilis* and *Staphylococcus aureus*, which has been largely attributed to its two iridoid glycosides, aucubin and catalpol (Lin et al. 1972; Tarle 1981; Cáceres et al. 1991; Holetz et al. 2002). Antioxidant activity seems to play a large role in this antibiotic activity (Bol'shavoka 1998). Yet, because the enzymatic action is nullified by heat, use of the herb in its raw state or as a cold infusion or as a tincture of the fresh herb is necessary to achieve the antimicrobial effect (Blumenthal et al. 2000: 309). Thus, too, in a test-tube study conducted in the 1950s, a cold infusion of plantain made from a forty-eight-hour sample yielded moderate effects against a virulent human tuberculosis organism, the roots being more active than the leaves (Fitzpatrick 1954: 530). This calls to mind Pliny the Elder's report that plantain, eaten as a food or the juice when drunk, favorably affected the course of tuberculosis, especially in combating the **wasting** aspect of this disease (Pliny 1938: 26:68).

Through mechanisms not as yet entirely understood, plantain serves as an *antitoxin* par excellence, proving capable of drawing out or neutralizing the poison or infection involved in **wounds**, **boils**, **bites**, **stings**, **infected cuts**, **abscesses**, **blood poisoning**, and **poison ivy rash** (de Bairacli Levy 1974: 112). The mysterious "drawing" power possessed by this lowly weed is so powerful that the Ponca even found that applying heated leaves to **thorns** or **splinters in the foot** could easily remove them (Gilmore 1991: 63). Pliny the Elder further underscored this power by relating that plantain could be used topically on **carbuncles** to make them burst and that for **shingles**, "plantain is thought to be the sovereign remedy, if it is incorporated with fuller's earth [itself possessed of great 'drawing' power]" (Pliny 1938: 26:72). There may be *nervine* effects involved with the application for shingles as well, since Alma Hutchens relates that she has experienced good success in using 2–5 drops of plantain tincture every ten minutes to dull the pain of **neuralgia** (Hutchens 1991: 219).

There is so much information relative to plantain's use for these toxic conditions that we would do well to consider the applications for each of them separately.

First, then, as to **boils**, Appalachian folk medicine has long implemented wilted or bruised plantain leaves to bring these nasty, painful afflictions to a head (Bolyard 1981: 112). It has often been observed by persons so afflicted that such a poultice will cause the core to be expelled in a mere twelve to thirty-six hours!

Secondly, as to **infected cuts**, **abscesses**, and **blood poisoning**, a number of Native American tribes found plantain to be a godsend for these conditions (Train et al. 1988: 79; Herrick 1995: 211). Ethnobotanist Huron Smith, in a 1930s study of the Ojibwe, related that he himself "cured a badly swollen and lacerated hand, which swelled to three times its normal size, probably because dirt from a sewer was ground into it, with the simple leaf bound upon the hand" (Smith 1932: 381). Herbalist Rosemary Gladstar has testified that plantain poultices and tea taken internally saved a friend who was badly wounded and blood-poisoned from a wilderness emergency (Schofield Eaton 1989: 308). Such instances are not atypical, as two clients of mine could well testify: One was a man who had a tennis-ball-sized abscess in his mouth and was having no luck with penicillin, so he was in great desperation owing to his pain and discomfort. Another was a young woman with a swelling just about the same size. Plantain tincture, applied repeatedly as a compress, fixed them both up just fine, to their utter amazement. Although I have witnessed plantain's successes now with a good number of clients, family members, and friends over the years, I am still amazed at the astonishing results that it can obtain. This is one incredible herb!

Third, as to bites and stings, numerous Native American tribes—such as the Algonquian, Cherokee, Flambeau Ojibwe, and Mohegan—used the rough, lower undersides of fresh plantain leaves to draw out the poison from the **bites** of **snakes** and **insects** (Speck 1917: 319; Smith 1932: 380; Tantaquidgeon 1972: 74; Hamel and Chiltoskey 1975: 50). This application, as well as the use of a poultice of wilted plantain leaves for same, was widespread among both Native Americans and European settlers. The Cherokee have also treated **yellowjacket stings** with such a poultice (Hamel and Chiltoskey 1975: 50). Ethnobotanist Frances Densmore even described, in some detail, an incident wherein an Ojibwe man saved his snakebitten wife from certain death with a moistened plantain-root poultice (Densmore 1974: 353). Then, too, in the year 1750, the South Carolina legislature even purchased a snakebite recipe consisting chiefly of plantain roots from a black slave (Millspaugh 1974: 420; Crellin and Philpott 1990a: 345).

The Iroquois have ground up plantain leaves and applied them to **spider bites** (Herrick 1995: 210), as have the Mohegan and the Mahuna (Romero 1954; Tantaquidgeon 1972). Even the bites of poisonous spiders have been brought to nothing with this amazing plant—such as, for example, those of the violin (brown recluse) spiders. In a 1997 issue of *Medical Herbalism*, herbalist Sasha Daucus related her experiences in treating bites from these spiders with fresh plantain-leaf poultices. In one instance, her client, presenting with an initially small and itchy bite that in ten days had developed into a nasty open gash, received an overnight plantain poultice and on the very next day went on to expel a tiny black core from the wound, thereafter healing rapidly (Daucus 1997). This is not surprising in view of plantain's "drawing power" and what we saw above relative to a plantain poultice often causing the core of a boil to pop out. Daucus explains that her favorite method of application is to advise her arachnid-attacked clients to pick a fresh leaf and then to rinse it, chew it, and apply it as a poultice. She also allows a plantain oil (made from the dried leaf soaked in olive oil, one part leaf to two parts oil) to be used when fresh plantain leaf is unavailable, such as during the winter.

My own experience in using plantain on **mosquito bites** is similar: I have found that chewing a leaf and then rubbing it thoroughly into the bites works rapidly to negate both the toxin and the itch, although applying the tincture works just fine, too. The quick results (in one to five minutes) that one experiences can truly be awe-inspiring: what has kept one awake for hours quickly quiets down and permits a restful sleep for the remainder of the night. Although I don't like to make guarantees, I can pretty much assure you that every outdoor enthusiast with whom you share this remedy will never stop thanking you!

Third, as to **poison ivy rash**: Appalachian folk medicine has tracked good success with a poultice of plantain leaves (Bolyard 1981: 112), as the late, great Alabama herbalist Tommie Bass found to be the case (Crellin and Philpott 1990b: 152). My own experience with clients has likewise been most satisfying and successful—I have had about three dozen cases that I can remember, and in most of them I advised wrapping the rashy areas in either a poultice of the crushed, fresh leaves or a gauze compress of the cooled infusion, which quickly thwarted the itching and dried up the rash. (I myself am among the 15–20 percent of the populace that is immune to poison ivy—quite fortunate, given the fact that I am often forced to tramp through so much of this stuff in my wilderness wanderings.) A physician's report published in a widely known and respected medical journal also described the successful use of plantain leaf to permanently relieve the terrible itching associated with this condition in ten people among his family and friends who had contracted the rash (Duckett 1980).

Not only poison ivy rash and mosquito bites, however, but almost every kind of **itching** yields to the power of plantain, something that I have witnessed often and that Bass also found to be true (Crellin and Philpott 1990a: 345f; Crellin and Philpott 1990b: 152). Susun Weed thus understandably advises a plantain salve for **diaper rash** (Weed 1986: 112), something that I have recommended, to good effect, on numerous occasions. Her remedy for baby's **thrush** is another winner, which is to soak plantain seeds overnight, skim off the slime appearing on top of the water in the morning, and then apply this goo to the affected

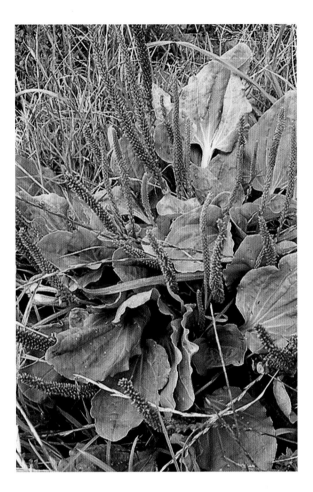

areas (Weed 1986: 110). For toddlers, the British tradition advises that 1 ounce (28 grams) of seeds be boiled in 1½ pints (852 milliliters) of water until 1 pint of fluid remains and then the solution cooled and a tablespoonful given to the thrush-afflicted youngsters (Potterton 1983). It is of interest here that three in vitro studies have found that plantain manifests *antifungal* activity against *Candida albicans*, with one of these (Sharma et al. 2016) examining use of the herb in the oral cavity and finding it comparable to standard pharmaceutical fungal agents (Holetz et al. 2002; Sharma et al. 2016; Shirley et al. 2017).

A proven *diuretic* as well (Doan et al. 1992), used as such by both Europeans (Hyde et al. 1976–79: 1:163) and Native Americans (Mayes and Lacy 1989: 82), plantain has been greatly treasured for **urinary gravel**, **urinary tract infections**, **cystitis** (especially when accompanied by hematuria), **urethritis**, **prostatitis**, and various other **urinary complaints** (Hamel and Chiltoskey 1975: 50; Hyde et al. 1976–79: 1:163; Moore 1979: 129; Green 1991: 235, 244; McIntyre 1995: 217). The Eclectics treasured it especially for conditions such as **dysuria**, **hematuria**, and the **enuresis** of children when due to a relaxed sphincter of the bladder and a consequent copious discharge of clear urine, which indications have been followed by British herbalists influenced by these physicians (Felter and

Lloyd 1898; Felter 1922; Harper-Shove 1938). It has also been utilized by herbalists for **interstitial cystitis** (Tilgner 2000).

The diuretic effects no doubt contribute to its legendary aid for both **gout** and **rheumatism**, especially since plantain's aucubin has been experimentally shown to be contributory toward uric acid excretion (Wren 1988: 311). Possibly the diuretic effect contributes somewhat to plantain's time-honored efficacy for **obesity** as well, although Russian research has found the polyphenols in the leaves to be the largest contributing factor (Maksyutina et al. 1978).

Many have appreciated plantain's aid for **coughs** (Millspaugh 1974: 420). It is a wonderful *expectorant*, owing chiefly to its content of saponins (McIntyre 1995: 217). This wonderful herb is also strongly *anticatarrhal* (Blumenthal 1998) and thus useful for **catarrhal congestion in the middle ear**, **ear infections**, and **sinus problems** involving static catarrh (McIntyre 1995: 217). Clinical trials conducted by Eastern European scientists even found that a plantain preparation significantly reduced the coughing, wheezing, irritation, and pain of **chronic bronchitis**. In one of these trials, "a rapid effect on subjective complaints and objective findings was obtained in 80 per cent" of the twenty-five patients studied over a period of one month (Matev et al. 1982; cf. Koichev 1983).

Plantain has long been used in Bulgaria to treat **cancer of the spleen** (Hutchens 1973: 346). Interestingly, scientific research conducted in the late 1980s revealed that when the herb's polyphenol complex (designated as plantastine) was introduced into the diet of rats, it proved capable of *cutting in half* the tumor yield chemically induced in the rats by the authors of the study as well as reducing the toxic damage to their livers as a consequence of the carcinogenic drugs (Karpilovskaia et al. 1989). A study conducted a few years later by the Federal University of São Paulo in Brazil found that intracellular fluid of plantain injected subcutaneously into female breeding mice largely prevented the formation of breast cancer in the rodents. While the malignancy occurred in 93.3 percent of the controls, it appeared in only 18.2 percent of the plantain-treated mice! (Lithander 1992) Twenty-first-century research has demonstrated additional *antitumoral* and *antineoplastic* cell-transformation effects and has shown that plantain exerts profound beneficial effects on the immune system (Gomez-Flores et al. 2000; Chiang et al. 2003: 225; Ozaslan et al. 2007; Choi 2012; Kartini et al. 2017).

Plantain has also been shown to be *hepatoprotective* (Chang and Yun 1985: 269; Hussan et al. 2015). Not surprisingly, then, herbalists in both the West and the East esteem the use of this herb, taken by way of infusion, for **viral hepatitis.** Taiwanese research has established that it does possess antiviral activity, attributed to its content of caffeic acid (Chiang et al. 2002; Chiang et al. 2003). It has also been shown to be *renoprotective* when used with the chemotherapy drugs cisplatin and doxorubicin (Parhizgar et al. 2016; Entezari Heravi et al. 2018; Naji et al. 2018).

PERSONAL AND PROFESSIONAL USE

The numerous ways in which I have used this most versatile herb—both personally and professionally—can be gleaned from a thorough reading of the preceding text, for I have implemented practically every one of the applications enumerated and almost always with remarkably successful results.

CAUTIONS

The seeds, and probably the plant as well, should not be used by those with allergies to psyllium (*Plantago psyllium*), a related species. ⬳

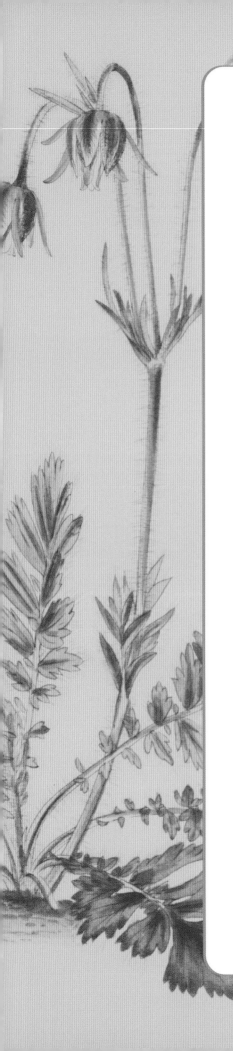

Prairie Smoke

TORCH FLOWER; LONG-PLUMED AVENS;
OLD MAN'S WHISKERS; THREE-FLOWERED AVENS

Geum triflorum

DESCRIPTION

This is a perennial herb that grows 6–16 inches high and thrives in large colonies owing to proliferation from its creeping underground stems. The plant's aerial stem is upright, soft, and hairy.

Prairie smoke possesses both basal leaves and stem leaves. The former are fern-like, being pinnately compound and consisting of seven to nineteen leaflets that grow to 9 inches long, with the largest ones growing toward the tip of the leaf. The stem leaves are few—often consisting of only one pair—and situated near the middle of the stem. They are much smaller in length than the basal leaves, being only ¾–1 inch long.

Urn-shaped russet-pink to russet-purple flowers appear in the spring, consisting of five petals and five calyx lobes. These blossoms are situated in groups of three at the ends of leaning stems, where they present a nodding appearance.

The fruits, which replace the flowers by as early as the beginning of summer, are seed-like in form and tipped with prominent, plume-like hairs, giving the appearance of a feather duster. (The plant's common name of prairie smoke derives from their striking form.)

RANGE AND HABITAT

Prairie smoke thrives in prairies, rocky hillsides, and open woodlands. It can be found in the eastern two-thirds of the United States (mainly in the northern half) and into most of Canada. In the Midwest, it thrives in the southern, central, and western portions of Minnesota.

MAJOR CONSTITUENTS

Prairie smoke contains gein, a phenolic glycoside.

FOOD

After a long, cold winter devoid of fresh vegetables, Native American tribes anxiously awaited the appearance of prairie smoke's fern-like leaves in the spring, since it was one of the first edible plants to burst forth at this time. They then gathered, cooked, and relished the pleasant-tasting, bright-pink rhizomes (Scully 1970: 11). The Thompson and some other tribes also made a tea from the plant's rhizomes to drink for taste (Ward-Harris 1983). Ethnobotanist Virginia Scully made note of its pleasant taste and even compared it to sassafras tea (Scully 1970: 11).

Likewise, an acidic, astringent, and quasi-chocolate-tasting beverage can be made from the fresh or dried roots of a related species, *Geum rivale*, the water avens (also called purple avens), which also appears in the Midwest. Here, the root stalk is cut into pieces and boiled (Harrington 1967: 360). It is felt by many that the taste of this tea is most agreeable when prepared from the spring- or autumn-gathered roots.

HEALTH/MEDICINE

Medicinal uses of prairie smoke relate chiefly to its *astringent* properties. (The related *G. rivale* was listed in the *United States Pharmacopeia* from 1820 to 1882 as an astringent.) The Blackfoot have utilized these astringent properties by preparing a decoction of the plant's roots to bathe **sore or inflamed eyes** (McClintock 1923: 321; Goodchild 1984: 143), swish in the mouth for **canker sores** (Hellson and Gadd 1974: 66), or gargle for **sore throat** (Hellson and Gadd 1974: 66; Goodchild 1984: 136).

Members of this tribe have also mixed the root with grease and applied the combo to **blisters**, **sores**, **rashes**, and flesh **wounds** (McClintock 1923: 321; Hellson and Gadd 1974: 275). Similarly, the Thompson have bathed **body aches** and **pains** with a wash made from the rhizomes as well as used such by way of steam treatment (Steedman 1928: 466; Turner et al. 1990: 48). A tea of the plant's aerial portions has been used by the Blackfoot as a *tonic* (McClintock 1923: 321; Hellson and Gadd 1974: 72; EthnobDB). The Thompson have also valued *G. triflorum* as a tonic but preferred a decoction of the roots to the aerial portions (Turner et al. 1990: 44). The Midwest's Ojibwe have used a compound decoction of the root for **indigestion** and even chewed the roots themselves before undergoing feats of endurance (Densmore 1974: 342ff).

The Flathead (Salish) have appreciated prairie smoke for **chills**, while the Blackfoot have esteemed it for a bad **cough** (McClintock 1923: 321; Hellson and Gadd 1974: 72; EthnobDB).

The related yellow avens (*G. aleppicum*) and large-leaved yellow avens (*G. macrophyllum*), both found in the Midwest, closely resemble *G. triflorum* in their properties and applications, although they are somewhat different in

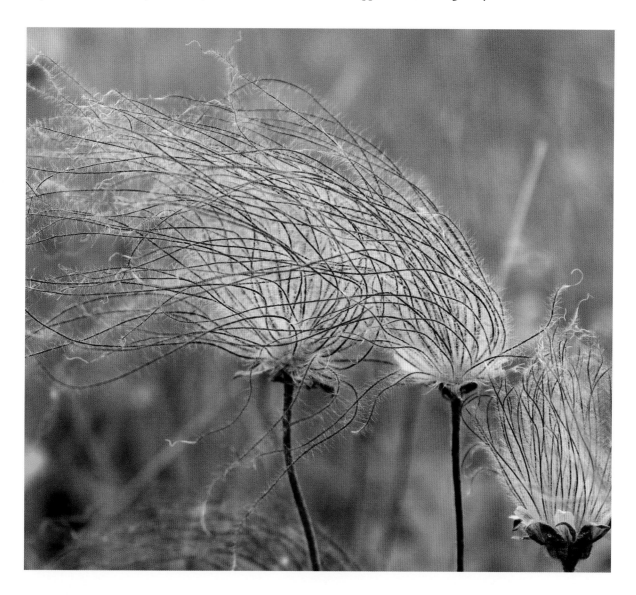

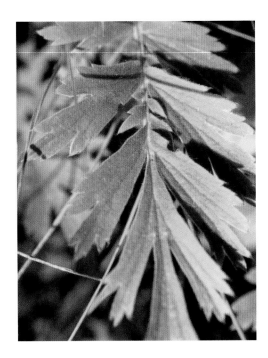

appearance—possessing, as their respective common names suggest, yellow blossoms. As to healing applications of these species, the former's roots have been boiled by the Ojibwe to make a weak decoction that has been drunk for **cough** and for **soreness in the chest** (Hoffman 1891: 200), while the latter has been utilized by the Snohomish and Quileute as a poultice for **boils** (Gunther 1973: 37). The Bella Coola have likewise applied the latter's leaves to boils after chewing or bruising them (Smith 1929: 59). The Quileute also poulticed this species' leaves onto **open cuts** and chewed them to facilitate labor (as a *parturient*) (Gunther 1973: 37). As to another gynecological use, the Chehalis have steeped *G. aleppicum*'s leaves to make a tea to drink as a *contraceptive* (Gunther 1973: 37).

The Thompson discovered that a decoction of this species' root was a godsend for serious rash-causing diseases such as **smallpox**, **measles**, and **chicken pox** (Steedman 1928: 507). Smallpox took a heavy toll among many Native communities; but according to anthropologists James Teit and Elsie V. Steedman, who studied the Thompson in depth, none among this tribe who faithfully imbibed this beverage died during the final smallpox epidemic that swept through North America, which otherwise took a massive toll (Steedman 1928: 476).

PERSONAL AND PROFESSIONAL USE

My chief appreciation for prairie smoke lies in its great beauty. Watching these plants swaying in the breeze is a breathtaking sight! ᴗ᷾

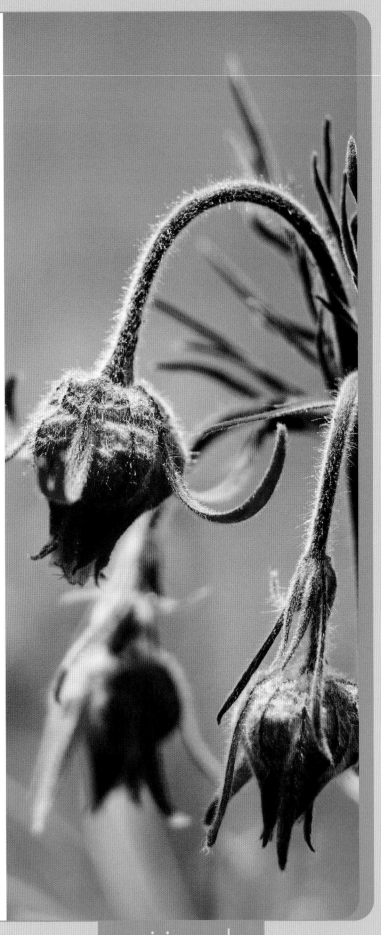

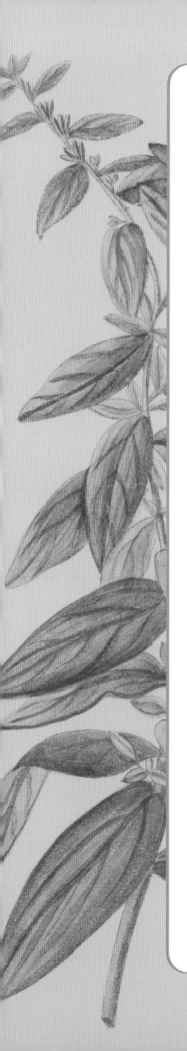

Puccoon

GROMWELL; INDIAN PAINT; STONE SEED

Lithospermum spp.

DESCRIPTION

Puccoon is a native perennial sporting gorgeous yellow blossoms and thin leaves. It grows 4–20 inches tall. Several species are found in the Midwest, including the following:

Lithospermum canescens (hoary puccoon) has several erect green stems covered with soft white hairs. It has alternate, lanceolate, mostly sessile leaves, about 1 inch long, growing only on the upper part of the stem. The corolla is orange-yellow and tubular, with five flaring lobes. This species is possessed of a thick red root.

L. caroliniense (hairy puccoon, Carolina puccoon) has an orange-yellow corolla. Its stems and leaves are rough to the touch, being covered with stiff, spreading hairs—longer than in *L. canescens*, above. Its roots are black, not red, as in the above species.

L. incisum (narrow-leaved puccoon) has a lemon-yellow corolla with fringing on the margins of its petals. The surface of its leaves is covered with stiff hairs that lie flat. As the common name implies, the leaves of this species are narrower than those of others.

L. latifolium (American gromwell) has ovate to ovate-lanceolate leaves that are 2–5 inches long and 1–2 inches wide.

RANGE AND HABITAT

Puccoon thrives in fields, prairies, and dry, open woods. The various species occur throughout most of the Midwest, except rarely in the northern counties.

SEASONAL AVAILABILITY

This plant is gathered in late spring or early summer when flowering.

MAJOR CONSTITUENTS

Puccoon contains lithospermic acid; shikonin; caffeic, chlorogenic and ellagic acids; tannins; mucilage; and resin.

FOOD

The narrow-leaved puccoon has been utilized by several Native American tribes as food. The Okanogan of British Columbia have relished the plant as a potherb. The Blackfoot and Thompson have boiled or roasted the roots and feasted on them. The Shoshone have enjoyed sipping on a tea made from the roots.

HEALTH/MEDICINE

In 1612, Captain John Smith wrote of *L. canescens* that it had a small root "which being dried and beat in powder turneth red; and this they [the Native tribes of the region] use for swelling, aches, anointing their joints, painting their heads and garments" (cited in Coffey 1993: 191). The Midwest's Menomini have also used this species, including it in a compound infusion to offset **convulsions** (Densmore 1932: 128). Other tribes have used a tea of this species as a wash for **fever** with **spasms** (Foster and Duke 1990: 136).

The Lakota have reduced the black-skinned roots of the hairy puccoon (*L. carolinense*) to a powder and used it on **chest wounds**, including those made by bullets (Munson 1981: 236). The Cheyenne found that rubbing the powdered plant of the narrow-leaved puccoon (*L. incisum*) onto **paralyzed body parts** seemed to help renew them, causing a prickly sensation (Grinnell 1905). (Alternatively, they have utilized the chewed, green plant.) They also chewed this species and spit it onto the faces of drowsy persons in order to keep them awake! (Grinnell 1972: 185; Hart 1981: 15)

Narrow-leaved puccoon has been implemented by the Hopi for **hemorrhages** (Colton 1974: 331) and by the Sioux (Oceti Sakowin) and Teton for **lung hemorrhages** in particular (Densmore 1918: 269; Munson 1981: 236). The Ramah Navajo (Diné) found it helpful for both **coughs** and **colds** (Elmore 1944: 71, 96) and also pulverized the roots and seeds to use as an eyewash (Vestal 1952: 41). They have further employed a decoction of the roots to use as a compress on the **sore umbilicus** of a new mother or of her baby (Elmore 1944: 71). The Zuni have appreciated narrow-leaved puccoon for **swellings**, **sore throat**, **abrasions**, **skin infections**, and **kidney problems** (Stevenson 1915: 56; Camazine and Bye 1980: 374).

L. incisum is one of two species of puccoon that has been used by Native tribes as an *oral contraceptive*. Here it was the herb of choice of the Navajo (Diné) (Hocking 1956: 161), whereas *L. ruderale*, stoneseed (flourishing in states west of the Midwest), was the species employed by tribes of the Nevada region (Vogel 1970: 242–43). The latter has been tested and found to be contraceptive in animals, suspected by the authors of one study to inhibit gonadotrophins in the ovaries (Winterhoff et al. 1988; cf. Vogel 1970: 242–43). Likewise, the European puccoon (*L. arvense*) has been used as an oral contraceptive, as it suppresses the menstrual cycle (Trease and Evans 1973: 364). Unfortunately, however, puccoon seems to inhibit hormonal production by the thyroid gland as well as some of the other endocrine glands (Hartenstein and Mueller 1961; Breneman et al. 1996), which for most persons would be detrimental to homeostasis.

PERSONAL AND PROFESSIONAL USE

While I've never used this plant for food or for medicine, I very much treasure its beauty. I know several meadows where it grows amidst other beauties, such as butterfly-weed (see page 66), penstemon (page 171), spiderwort (page 223), and fragrant giant hyssop (page 120), and I frequent these locations often to meditate, to pray, and to rest.

CAUTIONS

Puccoon is contraindicated with hypothyroidism, pregnancy, and lactation. ⤶

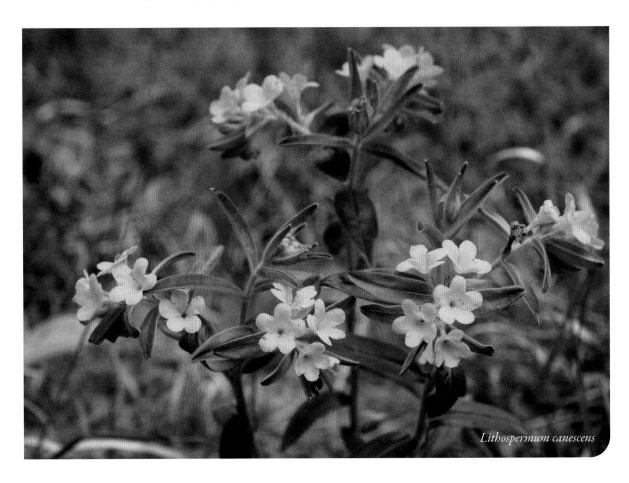

Lithospermum canescens

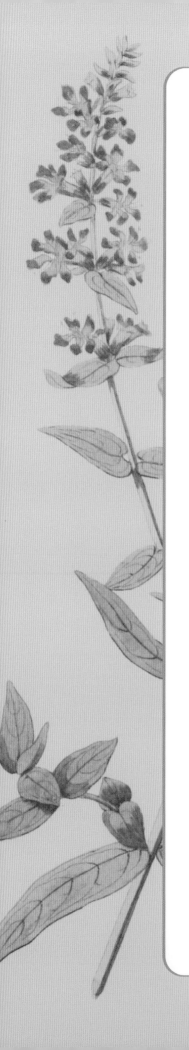

Purple Loosestrife

Lythrum salicaria

DESCRIPTION

This is a common, tall-spiked perennial import from Europe, possessed of a stout stem and growing 2–5 feet tall.

Its leaves are situated either oppositely or whorled in threes and are narrow and lance shaped.

Flowers appear clustered on long wands on the top half of the stem. They are ½– ¾ inch wide and rose to purple in color. Generally six crinkled petals (occasionally five, rarely four) are seen upon investigation.

RANGE AND HABITAT

Purple loosestrife is found in swamps, in marshes, on the borders of ponds, in ditches, and in wet meadows—often in large colonies. Its range is from southern Canada into the northern United States. It is practically ubiquitous in the Midwest, despite concerted efforts to control it. The plant can become a menace to others, which it tends to crowd out owing to its habit of growing in dense colonies. This ricochets further into the animal kingdom in that the diverse vegetable food-chain needed by many animals is thereby threatened.

MAJOR CONSTITUENTS

Purple loosestrife contains tannic acid, gallotanic acid, ellagic acid, anthocyanins, orientin, vitexin, pectin, beta-sitosterol, chlorogenic acid, salicarin, resin, phthalides (phthalates), and *p*-coumaric acid. Nutrients include pro-vitamin A and calcium (but as unusable oxalate).

HEALTH/MEDICINE

Purple loosestrife's traditional use as a **burn** remedy has been confirmed by chemical analysis, which reveals not only a high amount of tannin but also the presence of the related ellagic acid. The presence of these chemicals also explains the plant's time-honored use as an *astringent* for **mouth sores**, **sore throats**, and—in combination with the pectin present—**diarrhea**, its most renowned application (Bruneton 1995: 329). (The folk medicine of both Spain and Turkey has long relied upon this plant as an *antidiarrheal*: EthnobDB.) Undoubtedly, too, the tannins are largely behind the plant's traditional use as a wash or douche for **leukorrhea** (Tierra 1988: 339), its topical application to **sores** or **ulcers**, and its implementation as an eyewash for **sore eyes**, including **ophthalmia** (Tierra 1988: 339).

Further as to the eyes, herbalist Peter Holmes finds *Lythrum* useful for **vision impairment** or **disturbances**, particularly **blurred vision** and especially as it relates to the Traditional Chinese Medicine syndrome known as "kidney *qi* stagnation," which is characterized also by skin rashes, malaise, and painful, dark urination (Holmes 1997–98: 2:649).

Because it possesses strong *hemostatic/styptic* properties—the genus name, *Lythrum*, even derives from a Greek word for blood, in recognition of this physiological function—the plant will rapidly stop **bleeding**, including, most famously, **uterine bleeding** (Stuart 1982: 89; Holmes 1997–98: 2:648).

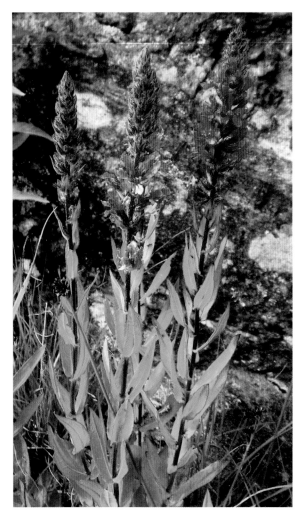

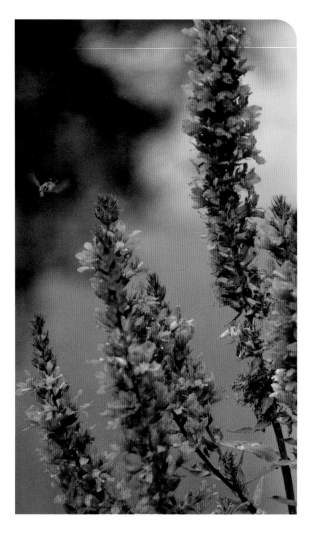

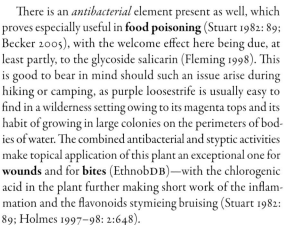

There is an *antibacterial* element present as well, which proves especially useful in **food poisoning** (Stuart 1982: 89; Becker 2005), with the welcome effect here being due, at least partly, to the glycoside salicarin (Fleming 1998). This is good to bear in mind should such an issue arise during hiking or camping, as purple loosestrife is usually easy to find in a wilderness setting owing to its magenta tops and its habit of growing in large colonies on the perimeters of bodies of water. The combined antibacterial and styptic activities make topical application of this plant an exceptional one for **wounds** and for **bites** (EthnobDB)—with the chlorogenic acid in the plant further making short work of the inflammation and the flavonoids stymieing bruising (Stuart 1982: 89; Holmes 1997–98: 2:648).

The anthocyanin-rich flowering tops are official medicine in the French *Pharmacopoeia*, tenth edition. French herbalists use them to heal **piles** and **venous insufficiency** (Bruneton 1995: 329). This application is also utilized in both Turkey and Iraq (EthnobDB).

A series of animal studies conducted in the 1980s (using rabbits, mice, and rats) found an extract from this plant to be powerfully *hypoglycemic*, markedly reducing blood-sugar levels in the various creatures tested (Torres and Suarez 1980; Lamela et al. 1985; Lamela et al. 1986). This, of course, suggests a possible application in **diabetes**.

PERSONAL AND PROFESSIONAL USE

I have used the flowers as a source of anthocyanosides to improve my terrible night vision, especially when I have run out of my capsules of bilberry (*Vaccinium myrtillus*), the herb that is highly touted for this purpose in modern Western herbalism. They seem to work just as well, but the price comparison is the real clincher: over $20 for a bottle of bilberry capsules, while the purple loosestrife blossoms are plentiful and free!

I once used the crushed leaves of this plant as a poultice to stem the blood from a cut.

CAUTIONS

Because the body of this plant contains calcium oxalate and is also very rich in tannins, it should not be used internally on a regular basis. ⤎

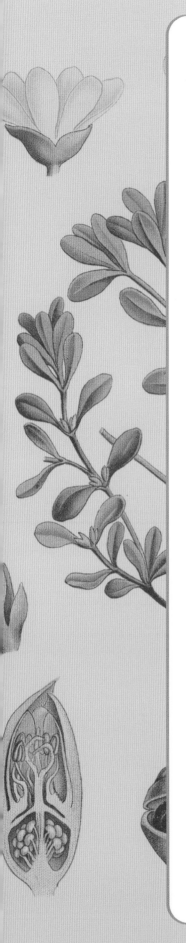

Purslane

DESCRIPTION

Purslane is an annual weed with a sprawling or a trailing inclination. The stems are smooth and red or pink-flesh-colored. The branches allow this weed to reach a length of 12 inches, whereby it carpets the ground like a dense mat.

The inch-long leaves are teardrop to paddle shaped, being noticeably widest at their tips. They are thick and succulent—almost rubbery. They occur most commonly in groups of five and sometimes display a purplish tint.

The small yellow flowers are borne singly in leaf axils or at the stem tips. They each possess five petals and open only on sunny mornings. Tiny black seeds are scattered throughout the plant, contained in capsules resembling flower buds.

RANGE AND HABITAT

This is a ubiquitous weed that is common to gardens, waste places, edges of driveways, and eroded areas throughout the Midwest.

MAJOR CONSTITUENTS

Purslane contains norepinephrine; dopa; cyclopoda alkaloids (oleracein A, B, C, D, and E); triterpenoids of the beta-amyrin type; sterols; caffeic acid; organic acids (malic, citric, oxalic); flavonoids (kaempferol, myricetin, luteolin, apigenin, quercetin, genistein, genistin); monoterpenes (portuloside A and B); portulene (a diterpene); glutathione; catechol; bergapten (5-methoxypsoralen); melatonin; phosphatidylcholine; and phosphatidylserine. Nutrients include free-form amino acids, omega-3 fatty acids in goodly amounts, high amounts of pro-vitamin A (one sample was tested at a whopping 8,300 imperial units per 100 grans!), folic acid, niacin, pyridoxine, riboflavin, vitamin C (26 milligrams per 100 grams), vitamin E (as alpha-tocopherol), and minerals such as iron (3.5 milligrams per 100 grams), lithium, potassium (494 milligrams per 100 grams!), sodium (45 milligrams per 100 grams), calcium (65 milligrams per 100 grams), and magnesium (at nearly 2 percent of the plant's dry weight).

FOOD

Because of its low-lying form, this plant is often gritty and should therefore be washed before being prepared for consumption. Thereafter, it can be boiled in salted water for three to ten minutes.

In view of its salty and oily taste, it is delicious eaten just as it comes out of the pot, with no additions being necessary. However, it is even more scrumptious served with crumbled bacon or mixed into casseroles or stews! What is more, it can be blanched for two minutes and then frozen for future use. Who could ask for more?

The seeds can be ground into meal and mixed with wheat flour to make breadstuffs or can be boiled and made into porridge.

HEALTH/MEDICINE

Purslane has been appreciated by various cultures as a valuable *vulnerary* for **bee stings**, **sores**, **swellings**, and **snakebite** (EthnobDB). The Iroquois have poulticed the plant

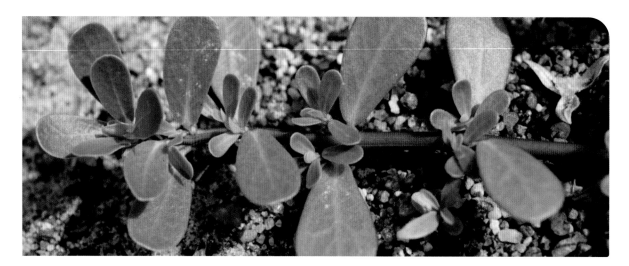

onto both **burns** and **bruises** (Herrick 1995: 143), and it has also been poulticed onto **boils** and **erysipelas** (de Bairacli Levy 1974: 115–17; Tierra 1988: 199; Reid 1993: 102). In harmony with these traditional uses, a scientific study published in 2000 confirmed that a tincture of the aerial parts (dried leaves and stem) demonstrated marked *anti-inflammatory* and *analgesic* effects when used topically (Chan et al. 2000), and a 2004 study revealed that topical purslane accelerated wound healing by decreasing the surface area of the wound and by increasing tensile strength (Rashed et al. 2003: 131).

In the 1990s, former US Department of Agriculture scientist James Duke noted that purslane's chemical profile might lend it for use in helping to prevent or offset **asthma** and **heart disease** (Duke 1997: 67, 247). Scientific research has confirmed these suspicions: two different studies published in 2012 showed anti-inflammatory effects in vascular endothelial cells (Lee et al. 2012a; Lee et al. 2012b), while a study published in 2004 revealed that purslane manifests *bronchodilating* effects (Malek et al. 2004). This latter study and several others have been collated and reviewed by a team of medical scientists from Iran, who found that purslane extracts decrease inflammatory cytokines and chemokines, promote antioxidant activity, and relax tracheal smooth muscle (Khazdair et al. 2019).

In the 1890s, Parke-Davis marketed a fluid extract of the herb, noting that it was *diuretic* and indicated for "chronic catarrhal affections of the genitourinary tract" (Crellin and Philpott 1990a: 363). Modern scientific studies have also confirmed this application: a 2012 study revealed that purslane ameliorates **diabetic nephropathy** by means of suppressing both fibrosis and inflammation in the kidneys (Lee 2012).

Since ancient Roman times, the seeds have been esteemed as a *vermifuge*. Clinical studies in China have verified that the juice is active against **hookworm infestation**, while other studies there and elsewhere have suggested that purslane exerts vermifuge, *antibiotic*, and *antifungal* effects (Chevallier 1996: 253; Oh et al. 2000; Quinlan et

al. 2002). A randomized, double-blind, placebo-controlled trial found that purslane, taken orally, eliminated or dramatically improved **lichen planus** in 83 percent of thirty-seven volunteers studied over a period of three months, while only 17 percent in the control group experienced some mild improvement. Such studies might at least partly explain purslane's historically observed efficacy in helping to heal dysentery, boils, and erysipelas (Agha-Hosseini et al. 2010).

Yet other studies have shown positive effects with conditions such as **diabetes** (Shen and Lu 2003; El-Sayed 2011; Lee 2012; Lee et al. 2012b) and **candidiasis** (Soliman et al. 2017). In an in vitro study, purslane has also shown remarkable activity against **hepatitis C** (Noreen et al. 2015), a horrible disease that has shown stubborn resistance to most natural agents, while the few pharmaceutical agents for this condition can lead to very harmful side effects. Purslane is also being investigated relative to several types of **cancer** (glioblastoma and breast cancer) and has manifested cytotoxicity or other mechanisms of attack against these dreaded diseases (Nile et al. 2017; Baradaran et al. 2019).

The fact that purslane actually contains both dopa (the precursor to dopamine) and norepinephrine (Feng et al. 1961; Chen et al. 2003) suggests possible application in neurological conditions wherein norepinephrine and/or dopamine is deficient, such as Parkinson's disease for the latter. However, any therapeutic benefits in these regards remain to be clinically demonstrated. Still, a couple of studies using purslane extracts in animal models of Parkinson's disease have shown great promise (Martins et al. 2016; Truong et al. 2019).

PERSONAL AND PROFESSIONAL USE
I really enjoy eating cooked purslane leaves, especially when they are mixed with bacon chips!

CAUTIONS
Purslane should not be used medicinally during pregnancy. ⤙⤙

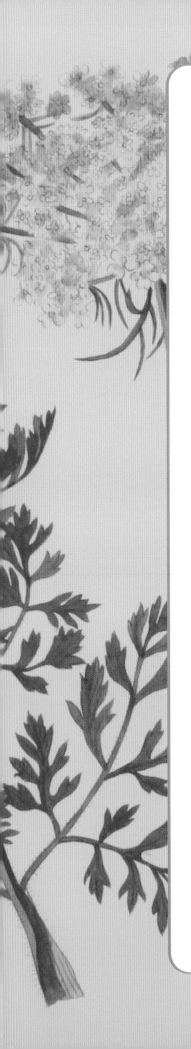

Queen Anne's Lace

WILD CARROT; BIRD'S NEST

Daucus carota, ssp. *carota*

DESCRIPTION

This is a biennial growing to 6 feet tall (2–3 feet being average). It is possessed of a hairy stem and a carrot-scented white root.

Queen Anne's lace first sees the light of day as a basal rosette of compound and finely divided leaves (much like those of a fern), at which stage it sometimes exudes a carrot-like scent when crushed. A hairy, branching stem appears in the second year, sporting alternate and dissected leaves.

Small white flowers eventually form in flat-topped clusters (compound umbels), about 3–5 inches wide, at the top of the plant. There is often a tiny, solitary flower in the center of the cluster that is colored reddish brown to dark purple—an important identifier distinguishing this plant from some toxic lookalikes (see Cautions). The umbels reside on stiff, feathery, three-forked bracts resembling a collar.

Once fruits replace the flowers, the umbel's branches begin to curve upward, presenting the appearance of a hollow cup or a nest (giving rise to the plant's alternative common name of bird's nest).

RANGE AND HABITAT

Queen Anne's lace is a cosmopolitan weed that flourishes in dry, open areas—sandy soil, waste places, disturbed ground, roadsides, open woods, fields, and meadows.

MAJOR CONSTITUENTS

The leafage contains an essential oil (inclusive of terpinen-4-ol, limonene, geraniol, carophyllene, carotol, daucol, asarone, pinene); the alkaloid daucine; glycosides; flavonoids (luteolin, apigenin, kaempferol, chrysin, quercetin); porphyrins; and coumarins. The seeds contain an essential oil and are high in myristicin, as well as in nutrients such as fatty acids (oleic, linolenic, butyric, palmitic) and potassium. The root contains nutrients such as thiamine, riboflavin, choline, and vitamin C. It is debatable whether beta-carotene, which occurs in the domesticated carrot, is present in the wild species or at least in all samples.

FOOD

The whitish first-year roots, if gathered in late fall—or, even more preferably, in the following spring before the flower stalk emerges—are passable as survival food but are best mixed into "wild" stews and casseroles instead of being eaten by themselves. Note that they possess a woody core, which must be discarded before they are consumed.

Peeled young flower stalks are also edible. They are crisp and peppery when eaten raw. They can also be boiled in salted water for about ten minutes.

HEALTH/MEDICINE

Queen Anne's lace is detailed in the *British Herbal Pharmacopoeia,* and it was listed in the *United States Pharmacopeia* from 1820 to 1882 as a *stimulant, menstrual excitant,* and *diuretic.* The effect upon menstruation would seem to accrue primarily from the seeds, which are *warming* and *stimulating.* Such effects might also elucidate the

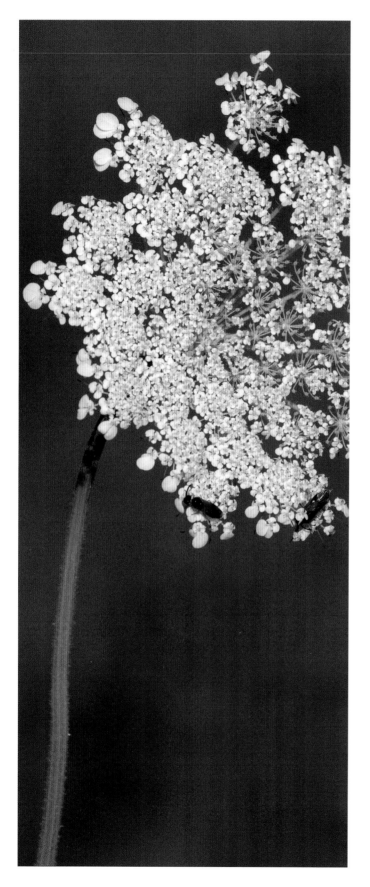

Lumbee use of the plant as a compress applied to the chest of a young child afflicted with a **chest cold** or **pneumonia** (Croom 1983: 56). As to the *diuretic* effect also listed in the *US Pharmacopeia*, nineteenth-century physician and plant scientist Asahel Clapp wrote: "An infusion of the seeds or the roots and leaves is an excellent diuretic. Thatcher, Chapman, Eberle speak very favorably of the efficacy" (Clapp 1852: 777). So did celebrated seventeenth-century herbalist Nicholas Culpeper, who wrote that wild carrot "provoketh urine … and helpeth to break and expel stones" (Culpeper 1983: 38–39).

Because such an effect would also promote excretion of uric acid, Queen Anne's lace has likewise historically been deemed effective for both **gout** and **rheumatism** (Crellin and Philpott 1990b: 135; Newall et al. 1996: 264–65). In addition, it has served as a traditional *antiseptic* and diuretic for the treatment of both **cystitis** and **prostatitis**, proving especially helpful in relieving the pain of the associated **strangury** (Johnson 1884: 152) and even for the very **stoppage of urine**, as the Iroquois discovered (Herrick 1995: 195). Queen Anne's lace has also traditionally been used for the type of **dropsy** associated with heart conditions, and here it is of significance that cardiovascular effects have been observed for this plant in animal models (Gilani et al. 1994), including a reduction of heart rate and blood pressure (Fetrow and Avila 1999: 534). Finally, Alabama herbalist Tommie Bass heartily utilized the diuretic aspect of wild-carrot tops (not seeds per se) as part of his famous "[weight]-reducing program" but felt that while it "works on the same system [as do] water tablets," it nevertheless "works through the pores" (Crellin and Philpott 1990b: 120). Scientists, however, have suggested rather that the diuretic effect is probably due to the chemical terpinen-4-ol, which seems to stimulate diuresis through renal irritation (Newall et al. 1996: 264–65).

A tea from the seeds has historically been used for **flatulence**. In early America, physician and plant scientist Francis Porcher noted the frequent use of the root for "spasmodic vomiting, flatulent colic, and nervous headaches" (Porcher 1869). The primary factor here seems to be an *antispasmodic* effect that the seeds have on smooth muscle, probably owing to their essential oil. Such an effect has been experimentally verified and likened to that of papaverine, although deemed weaker (Gambhir et al. 1979; Dobelis 1986: 279).

The blossoms, when picked at full bloom, have been steeped as a tea by the Mohegan and the Oklahoma Lenape (Delaware) for use in **diabetes** (Tantaquidgeon 1972: 118–19, 130–31). Queen Anne's lace has also traditionally been used for **jaundice** and for other **liver disorders**. *Hepatoprotective* activity has been observed in animal studies implementing the potent liver toxin carbon tetrachloride (Handa et al. 1986; Bishayee et al. 1995).

A useful *vulnerary*, Queen Anne's lace has been poulticed onto both **bruises** and **cuts.** The Cherokee have bathed **swellings** with a tea made from its leafage (Hamel and Chiltoskey 1975: 51).

A very limited *antifungal* activity has been observed and related to the essential oil, though it was active against only one organism—*Botrytis cinerea*—out of nine tested (Guérin and Reveillere 1985). Then, too, the seeds have historically been held to be a valuable *anthelmintic*.

The seeds are usually used by way of infusion, with ⅓–1 teaspoon (maximum) added to 8–16 ounces of water and then infused (or gently simmered) for fifteen to thirty minutes, with such being drunk at a dose of ½–1 cup for a maximum of three times a day, or simply for flatulence as a single serving after a meal (Carse 1989: 164, 174; Hutchens 1991: 299–300). The aerial portions, which Bass says should be gathered in June just before they open their blossoms (Crellin and Philpott 1990b: 135), have usually been implemented to the tune of 1 teaspoon per cup—or, as Bass says, "a big handful makes a quart of tea" (Crellin and Philpott 1990b: 135)—steeped for fifteen minutes and then drunk up to three times a day.

PERSONAL AND PROFESSIONAL USE

I have found that a tincture of the seeds is an excellent carminative for stubborn flatulence, although I prefer the seeds of cow-parsnip (see page 91) or the dried fruits of prickly ash (*Xanthoxylum* [alternatively, *Zanthoxylum*] *americanum*) for that purpose, should either of the latter two be available. All three of these remedies are difficult to find on the herb market nowadays, necessitating that I wildcraft them.

CAUTIONS

Too high a dose of the seeds can cause nervous-system damage, so do not exceed traditional dosages.

The seeds are abortive (Farnsworth et al. 1975: 535–98) because they inhibit implantation of the embryo (Prakash 1984) and thus should be *strictly avoided during pregnancy*. They should also probably be avoided during lactation.

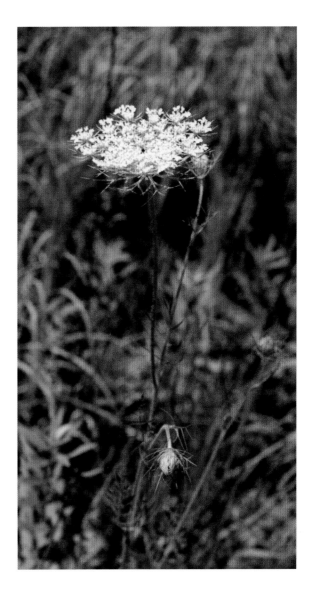

Contact with the leaves may cause dermatitis in sensitive individuals.

Wild carrot's leaf and flower pattern allows this plant to be easily confused with toxic relatives such as water hemlock (*Cicuta* spp.), fool's parsley (*Aethusa cynapium*), and poison hemlock (*Conium maculatum*). (Only the first-named species, however, generally occurs in the Midwest.) *Be absolutely certain of identification* before attempting to use any plant you think to be Queen Anne's lace, as a mistake could be deadly—review the important identifiers in the text and in other plant manuals. ↞

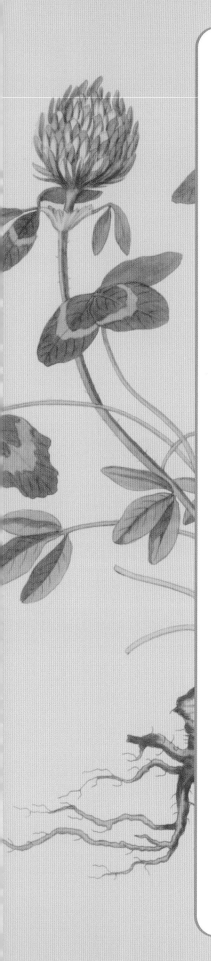

Red Clover

TREFOIL

Trifolium pratense

DESCRIPTION

This familiar perennial grows 6–18 inches tall and has a hairy, branching stem.

The alternate leaves are pinnately compound, possessed of three leaflets that are dark green in color and oval in shape. (The genus name, *Trifolium*, is named after this three-lobed structure.) The leaflets usually have a pale V shape, or chevron mark, in their center portions.

Many rosy-red or magenta flowers appear clustered into a round, compact flower head. These tiny individual flowers lack any sort of stalk.

RANGE AND HABITAT

Red clover is ubiquitous throughout North America. It flourishes in old fields, waste places, roadsides, trailsides, and lawns.

MAJOR CONSTITUENTS

Over 125 chemicals! Some chief constituents of red clover include coumarins (medicagol, coumestrol, and coumarin); isoflavones (1–2.5 percent, including genistein, daidzein, formononetin, biochanin A); flavones (including pectolinarin); salicylic acid; trifoliin (a phenolic glycoside); trifolianol (a saponin); pratol; phytosterols; an essential oil (inclusive of methyl salicylate and furfural); clovamide (trans- and cisclovamide conjugated with L-dopa); and carbohydrates (xylose, arabinose, rhamnose, and glucose). Nutrients include substantial amounts of calcium, chromium, copper, magnesium, potassium, and phosphorus. Vitamins such as C and several of the Bs (niacin, thiamine, riboflavin) also occur in high amounts.

FOOD

Fresh flower heads make a nice trail nibble. (However, see Cautions.) Not only do they taste good, but they are extremely high in water, and this is compounded to the nth degree by morning dew or after a good rain, since the design of the flower head is such that it can retain a lot of H2O.

HEALTH/MEDICINE

Red clover blossoms have traditionally been used as a salve to heal **sores**, **ulcers**, and **burns**. The famed seventeenth-century herbalist Nicholas Culpeper also noted: "Boiled in lard and made into an ointment, the herb is good to apply to the bites of venomous beasts" (Potterton 1983: 194). Nowadays, however, the *vulnerary* ointment or paste is usually made from a solid extract, available commercially from several sources.

A reliable *alterative*, red clover—and from here on, I mean the part of the plant traditionally used in herbal medicine, the blossoms—is helpful in many **skin problems** (especially **psoriasis** and **eczema**, concerning which herbalist David Hoffmann points out that the plant has an especial affinity toward children: Hoffmann 1986: 221) because of *depurative* effects. The plant's ability in this regard includes a strong *lymphatic* component. Consequently, an ointment has been a standard for softening **hard milk glands** (Lust 1974: 395) and **lymphatic swellings** characterized as "firm and hard" (Ody 1993:

105; Tilgner 1999: 99). As the plant has an affinity to the area of the body running from the bronchioles to the head, it is also often of value in **tonsillitis** as well (Winston 1999: 50).

Red clover may also possess *antifungal* properties. An infusion has been used as a folk treatment for **vaginal irritation** and **anal irritation** (Hutchens 1991: 234; Ody 1993: 105), and a poultice of the fresh plant has been a traditional remedy for **athlete's foot** (Lust 1974: 395).

The Cherokee have utilized red clover for **Bright's disease**, **fever**, and **leukorrhea** (Hamel and Chiltoskey 1975: 29). Interestingly, in England, Culpeper likewise used it for leukorrhea (Potterton 1983: 194).

The Midwest's Ojibwe have imbibed red clover tea for **persistent coughs** (Naegele 1980: 117). Most famously, it has traditionally been used as a strong infusion—dosed at ½ ounce at a time—for **whooping cough** (Wren 1972: 255; Millspaugh 1974: 188; Black 1980: 188; Bolyard 1981: 73), for which it is tailor made due to its *sedative, expectorant,* and *antispasmodic* effects (Wren 1972: 255; Bradley et al. 1992: 183). (The drug company Parke-Davis even marketed it as a sedative in the 1890s: Parke, Davis and Co. 1890: 149.) It is regarded as a specific for **bronchitis**, for which it should be taken in the form of a hot infusion (Willard 1993: 253).

Iroquois women have drunk a cold infusion of red clover when experiencing the "change of life" (Herrick 1995). It has also long been a favorite of both British and American herbalists for reducing hot flashes in menopausal women (Rogers 1995). Several clinical trials have confirmed this implementation (Coon et al. 2007). In studies by scientists from the University of California San Diego and the University of Illinois's College of Pharmacy, red clover was discovered to possess a high level of *estrogenic* activity (Liu et al. 2001; Oerter Klein et al. 2003; Overk et al. 2005). Despite this, it appears to be safe for those at risk for breast cancer (Pitkin 2004) and has even historically been used to fight reproductive cancers in both sexes.

Indeed, one of red clover's most famous applications has been for **cancer**. The Shinnecock found that a tea of this herb was helpful for that dreaded disease (Carr and Westey 1945), while an infusion has been used specifically for stomach cancer by the Thompson (Turner et al. 1990). Thomsonianism, the branch of herbal medicine founded by Samuel Thomson in early America, utilized it thusly but in the form of a salve. Writing in 1841, Morris Mattson described this application as follows: "The blossoms boiled in water ... and the liquid simmered over a slow fire until it becomes about the consistency of tar, forms the cancer plaster of Dr. Thomson, which has gained so much reputation in the cure of cancers" (Mattson 1841: 282–83). The flower heads were marketed in the late 1800s and early 1900s as the major ingredient in Merrell's Trifolium Compound, a skin salve suggested for various dermatological problems, including skin cancers.

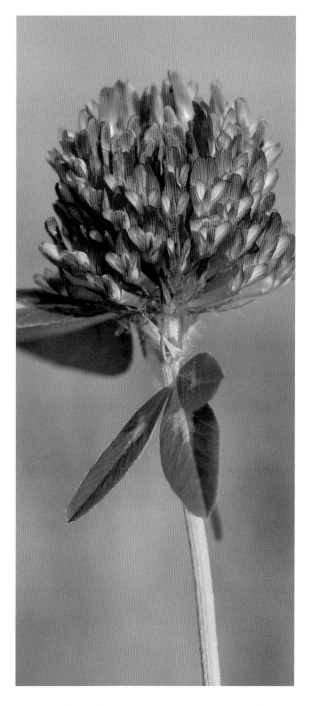

The Eclectic physician Harvey Wickes Felter observed that red clover "unquestionably has a retarding effect upon malignant neoplasms" (Felter 1922). In American folk herbalism, this herb has been viewed as the most important botanical for cancer, especially for gastric cancer, reproductive cancers (ovaries, breast, and prostate), colorectal cancer, and melanoma. The American folk herbalist Jethro Kloss extolled its use exceedingly, calling it "one of God's greatest blessings to man" in his million-seller health guide entitled *Back to Eden*, which was one of the chief texts among

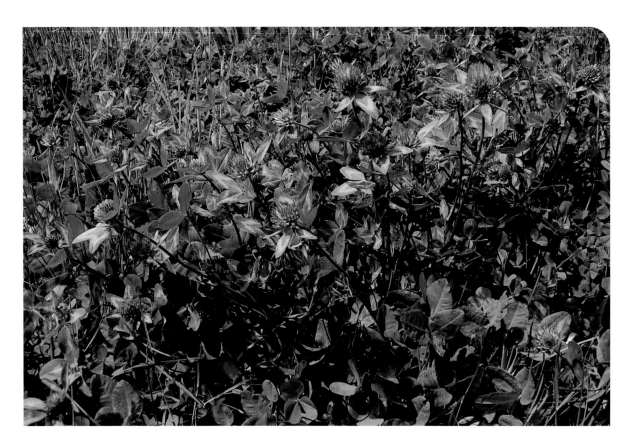

hippie herbal enthusiasts of the 1970s. He found it especially valuable as a simple in gastric cancer and as a gargle in throat cancer. He advised, however, that the tea, besides being drunk, should also be injected into the vagina for uterine cancer and likewise into the rectum for colorectal cancer (Kloss 1975: 301).

Not surprisingly, red clover's traditional uses as outlined above now have scientific support. In the late 1980s, an in vitro experiment isolated a carcinogenic-protective effect in the plant (Cassady et al. 1988). Red clover's isoflavones biochanin A and formononetin have both been shown to transactivate the aryl hydrocarbon receptor (AhR) that can drive cancer cells to apoptosis (Medjakovic and Jungbauer 2008), while biochanin A has been demonstrated to inhibit the activity of aromatase, the enzyme that converts testosterone into estrogen and is a target for pharmaceuticals that have been developed for patients with estrogen-sensitive cancers of the breast or endometrium (Wang et al. 2008). Research of late has focused more on the demonstrated anticancer effects of formononetin, however, which has been shown to inhibit the growth and proliferation of tumors. Its antiproliferative effect has proven especially powerful against estrogen-receptor-positive breast cancer cells (much less so against estrogen-receptor-negative cells), cervical cancer cells, ovarian cancer cells, non–small cell lung cancer cells, bladder cancer cells, colorectal cancer cells, glioma cells, osteosarcoma, and the major cell lines (PC-3, DU-145, and LNCaP)

of prostate cancer (Jiang et al. 2019). As to the latter, in a clinical trial of Asian men with low- to moderate-grade prostate cancer, red clover's four chief isoflavones induced apoptosis in cancer cells to a greater extent than had occurred in tissue controls obtained from radical prostatectomies (Jarred et al. 2002).

Red clover also contains coumarin, which has been shown to optimize macrophage activity, induce changes in lymphocyte-mitogen responsiveness in cancer sufferers, and inhibit any androgen-induced increase in prostate size in lab animals (Omarbasha et al. 1989).

Red clover was official in US drug literature until the late 1940s.

PERSONAL AND PROFESSIONAL USE

Clinically, I most often recommend red clover for persons suffering from cancer of the breast, prostate, stomach, colon, or ovaries. Overall, I would say that it is the most important herb for use with these various cancers; I specifically call to mind several cases where it proved to be the protocol item that turned a poor prognosis into a favorable outcome.

CAUTIONS

Because of hormonal effects, *this herb is contraindicated in pregnancy.*

The plant should *never be used* when *only wilted.* ⤺

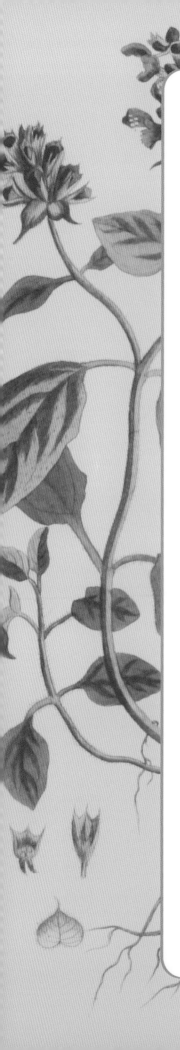

Self-Heal

HEAL-ALL; WOUNDWORT; CARPETWEED; CARPENTER-WEED

Prunella vulgaris

DESCRIPTION

Here we have a perennial mint of varying height—all the way from 3 inches to occasionally 3 feet, though usually 6–12 inches. Erect or sometimes matted in appearance, several square stems arise from a single base.

As is characteristic of the mint family to which this herb belongs, the leaves grow in pairs (i.e., opposite each other on the stem). They are lance shaped to egg shaped, 1–4 inches long, and less than 1 inch wide. The edges may be either smooth or a bit indented (wavy).

Flowers are small, numerous, short stalked, and snapdragon-like in appearance, with an arched upper lip and a three-part lower lip. They vary in color from violet (most common) to blue to pink to white (rarely) and are borne in a dense, spike-like cluster at the tip of the main stem, with smaller flowers usually appearing at the tips of any stem branches. Five greenish sepals surround the blossoms.

RANGE AND HABITAT

Self-heal prefers moist places, such as trailsides in damp woods and on streambanks. But it can also be found in drier areas, such as meadows, pastures, and wasteland. It is found throughout most of the United States and Canada. In the Midwest, it can be found everywhere except for the southwestern part of the region.

MAJOR CONSTITUENTS

In the past, not much work has been done in analysis, but currently this is changing. Self-heal is known to contain flavonoids (rutin, hyperoside, and others); rosmarinic, ursolic, caffeic, oleanolic, betulinic, and galactonic acid; prunellin; essential oil (containing cineol, pinene, camphor, and other chemicals); a resin; and tannins (up to 50 percent!). Nutrients include pro-vitamin A and vitamins B, C, and K as well as calcium, copper, iron, magnesium, manganese, potassium, sodium, and zinc.

FOOD

Raw leaves from the plant may be sprinkled onto a salad or eaten sparingly as a trail nibble. (As with any mint, use for food should not be overdone.) The plant may also be boiled as a potherb—a popular Appalachian repast. James Duke reports feasting on the herb prepared in this way at a West Virginia home, where the plant was called by a corrupted form: "eel-oil" (Duke 1992: 158).

HEALTH/MEDICINE

Self-heal has a fascinating history of medicinal applications among European, Chinese, and Native American cultures, having been used so widely and with such good results that it derived the name of "heal all [maladies]."

Various Native tribes have utilized it to treat a whole host of afflictions (Moerman 1986: 1:370). The Quinault have rubbed its juice onto **boils** (Gunther 1973: 45), while the Blackfoot have used it to wash a **burst boil** and **sores on the neck** (Hellson and Gadd 1974: 78). The Bella Coola have used a weak decoction of the root and of the aerial

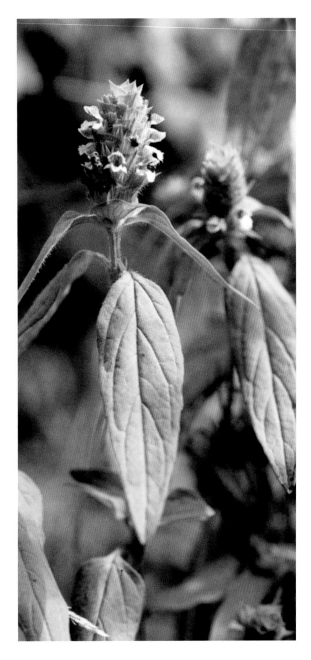

to treat a raging contagion—a type of **quinsy** that spread throughout the imperial armies in 1547 and again in 1566. The feverish affliction was called *die Braüne* ("the browns") because it was characterized by a brown-coated tongue. Our herb derived its genus name, *Prunella*, from the German word for "brunellen," a designation given to the herb because of its ability to cure this contagion (Germans, in fact, still call self-heal *Gemeine Brunelle*) (Dobelis et al 1986: 207; Keville and Szolkowski 1991: 154). Several ingredients in the plant may have come to the fore for this affliction, including prunellin, which has been found to be an active *antiviral* compound. Interestingly, a standard infusion of self-heal has been shown to be the most effective method of preparation to obtain the antiviral effects (Yamasaki et al. 1996), and such is what was primarily used during this contagion.

Modern Western herbalists have been little inclined to use self-heal for the spectrum of afflictions as delineated above. Because of its blatant *astringent* properties, however, they have recommended it for **sores**, **wounds** (hence its alternative common name, woundwort), and **leukorrhea** and as an ingredient in an ointment for **hemorrhoids**. Internally, it has been employed by way of infusion (tea) as a gargle for **sore throat** and for **diarrhea** and as a *styptic*. In the latter regard, **internal bleeding** has been treated by steeping 1 ounce of the herb in 1 pint of water and drinking 2 fluid ounces at a time. Regarding its amazing overall *vulnerary* properties, the famed European horticulturist John Gerard had summarized it thusly: "The decoction of Prunell made with wine or water doth joine together and make whole and sound all wounds, both inward and outward" (Gerard 1975: 507–8).

Scientific research from the 1990s to the 2010s is uncovering some astounding things about self-heal relative to its effects on the immune system, something of great interest to clinical herbalists like me. For one thing, it is now known that the plant is one of the very richest sources of rosmarinic acid, a phenylpropanoid that has powerful *antioxidant* and antiviral activities (the latter especially against **herpes simplex**; one study even found an ophthalmic form of self-heal to cure, or significantly improve, herpes simplex Type 1 keratitis in sufferers: Zheng 1990). Other studies have demonstrated *antiherpetic* effects also (Chiu et al. 2004; Zhang et al. 2007).

Interestingly, a number of Chinese studies have demonstrated *immunomodulating* effects from self-heal (Marková et al. 1997; Fang et al. 2005a; Fang et al. 2005b; Sun, N. X. et al. 2005; Harput et al. 2006), including antiallergic activity (Ryu et al. 2000; Shin et al. 2001; Kim et al. 2007). Research in the 1980s even found its prunellin content to display activity against HIV (Tabba et al. 1989). Then, in an important study published in 1992, a crude extract of the whole plant was found to significantly inhibit HIV-1 replication (Yao et al. 1992). When the active factor was purified, it was observed to block cell-to-cell transmission of the virus,

portions to support a **weak heart** (Smith 1929: 63). The Cree found it invaluable as a chew or as a gargle for a **sore throat** (Holmes 1884: 303), while the Midwest's Ojibwe have implemented the root in a compound decoction as a "female remedy" (Smith 1932: 372). The Iroquois have found many uses for self-heal: as a wash for **piles**, as an astringent for **diarrhea**, as a digestive aid for **stomachache**, and as a treatment for **venereal disease** (Herrick 1977: 423–25). Self-heal has also been an esteemed *febrifuge* in the materia medica of both the Iroquois and the Lenape (Delaware) (Tantaquidgeon 1972: 37; Herrick 1977: 424).

The herb rose in popularity among Europeans in the sixteenth century when German military physicians used it

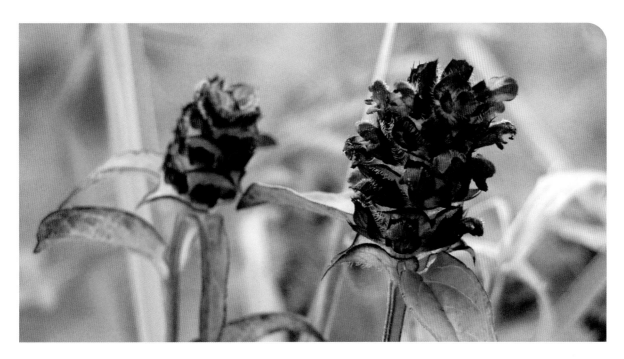

which it accomplished by preventing it from attaching to CD4 receptors (Yao et al. 1992). A 1993 study revealed further that a simple hot-water (as opposed to cold-water) extract was the preferred method for maximizing the inhibiting effects against HIV replication (Yamasaki et al. 1993). A study published one year later found the hot-water extract to provide protection against HIV-induced cell damage (cytotoxicity) and to enhance protection when used in conjunction with the standard HIV drugs zidovudine and didanosine (John 1994). Later research verified and enhanced our knowledge of how self-heal thwarts HIV (Yamasaki et al. 1998; Xu et al. 1999; Kageyama et al. 2000).

Self-heal's antiviral effects do not stop with HIV, however. A joint Chinese-American study published in 2017 found our herb to inhibit the entry of Ebola virus into host cells (Yang et al. 2017). Given the fact that no effective prophylactic medicines have been developed for this deadly, fearsome virus, this research is most exciting. Self-heal has also demonstrated effects against urinary tract infections caused by *Escherichia coli* (*E. coli*), the most common bacterium infecting urinary structures (Komal et al. 2018).

A 1988 study demonstrated that self-heal possesses powerful *antimutagenic* activity (Lee and Lin 1988). It contains, for one thing, ursolic acid, a triterpenoid saponin that manifests *antitumor* activity (Lee et al. 1988; Harborne and Baxter 1993: 687). Then, too, a Korean study published in 2014 isolated powerful antiestrogenic effects for self-heal, attributed to its content of both ursolic acid and betulinic acid, and concluded that it shows potential for use against estrogen-dependent tumors (Kim et al. 2014). Interestingly, the Chinese have traditionally used the blossom for **cancer**, beginning long before this information was known (Lee et al.

1988). Indeed, Traditional Chinese Medicine (TCM) finds self-heal flowers (but not leaves) to be a staple in its repertory. Feeling that it has an affinity for the liver and for the gallbladder and understanding it to be a cooling herb, TCM practitioners utilize it to treat **jaundice** (Reid 1992: 94) and various other "liver-heat" conditions manifested by **dizziness**, **irritability**, **headache**, **eyeball pain**, and **ringing in the ears** (Reid 1992: 94; Holmes 1997–98: 1:541). Health conditions popularly treated by TCM with *Prunella vulgaris* include **hypertension**, **gout**, **edema**, and **swollen lymph nodes** (Reid 1992: 94; Tierra 1992: 182; Holmes 1997–98: 1:541).

Chinese scientific research has also revealed *antidementia* activity for self-heal. In a rat study, it attenuated scopolamine-induced memory impairment by powerfully reducing acetylcholinesterase—the enzyme that breaks down the main neurotransmitter for cognition and memory, acetylcholine—and increased the important antioxidant enzymes glutathione peroxidase (GPx) and superoxide dismutase (SOD) (Qu et al. 2017). In another rat study, an aqueous extract attenuated diabetic renal injury by reducing inflammation and fibrosis of the kidneys, leading the study authors to conclude that self-heal has potential to thwart **diabetic nephropathy** (Namgung et al. 2017).

All in all, this is certainly an herb that deserves to be better known and used!

PERSONAL AND PROFESSIONAL USE

I have witnessed self-heal's benefits for my clients afflicted with hypertension manifested by painful pressure in the eyes and/or ringing in the ears; sore mouth or throat; allergies; hyperthyroidism (in conjunction with other herbs); and HIV infection (used only as an infusion). ⋘

self-heal

202 ❦ 203

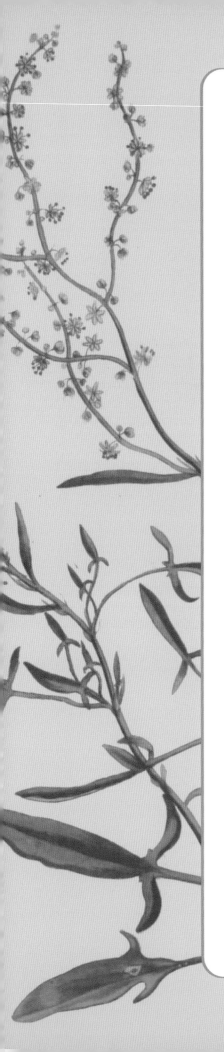

Sheep Sorrel

Rumex acetosella

DESCRIPTION

Sheep sorrel is a common perennial herb that is usually encountered growing in colonies. It possesses a slender, erect, four-angled stem and tops off at 4–15 inches.

The plant starts as a basal rosette with sessile and halberd-shaped leaves—it has two outward-pointing basal lobes that present the appearance of a sheep's head, thus the herb's common name. When summer arrives, the plant shoots up, bearing leaves that are alternate, lanceolate, and squared off at the point of attachment.

Many small blossoms can be found in slender racemes at the apex of the upper leaves, with male and female flowers appearing on separate plants (the former being greenish and the latter being more reddish orange).

RANGE AND HABITAT

This is a very common weed, occurring in the eastern five-sixths of the Midwest. It is an inhabitant of old fields, pastures, meadows, abandoned gardens, and untamed lawns. It requires some acidity in the soil and prefers partial to full sunshine.

SEASONAL AVAILABILITY

Look for this plant in practically every month of the year except for those experiencing heavy snow. It can be found, for instance, in the late fall, although died back to its basal leaves, in which form it hugs the ground, sheltered by grass. When the snow abates in the spring, it can be found in such a low-lying form once again.

MAJOR CONSTITUENTS

Sheep sorrel contains organic acids (malic, tannic, tartaric, citric, oxalic); auxin; calcium oxalate; potassium oxalate; catechin; flavonoids; and considerable amounts of chlorophyll. Anthraquinones occur in both the aerial portions (physcion) and the root (emodin and chrysophanic acid). The root also contains tannins. Nutrients include a broad spectrum of vitamins (B-complex, D, E, K, and very high amounts of C and pro-vitamin A [8–12 percent]) and minerals (including high amounts of iron).

FOOD

This plant makes a superb, lemony-tasting trail nibble. (However, see Cautions.)

Alternatively, the leaves can be simmered (or steeped) and then chilled for a delicious "sorrel-ade," tasting as good as the very best of lemonades! One can also add the leaves to soups and stews as a thickener or to fish and potatoes as a seasoning.

Sheep sorrel can be made into a soup as well. However, due to the oxalate content, this can be dangerous if prepared too strong, eaten in excess, or eaten too frequently. (Again, see under Cautions.)

This herb can also be frozen for future use. It needs only to be blanched in boiling water for one minute, then drained, cooled, and stored in a freezer bag.

HEALTH/MEDICINE

The revered horticulturist John Gerard discussed sheep sorrel in his famous herbal of the late sixteenth century, noting that it had *drying* and *cooling* properties (Gerard 1975: 318–21). In harmony with such drying properties, the plant has proven its worth throughout history as an *astringent*, having been utilized in the full variety of ways in which plants with such a property have been employed: First, sheep sorrel has been put to use for **diarrhea.** Secondly, the Cherokee have poulticed the leaves and blossoms onto **old sores** that refuse to heal (Hamel and Chiltoskey 1975: 56). Thirdly, the Russians have long used a compress of sheep-sorrel tea for **bleeding wounds** and even a decoction of the root given orally for **internal bleeding** (Hutchens 1991: 256). A decoction for this latter purpose has been used by other cultures as well, and it has been especially thought to be helpful for **stomach hemorrhage** (Callegari and Durand 1977: 37). Fourthly, a decoction of the root has held a valued place in the folk medicine of various cultures for **menorrhagia** (Callegari and Durand 1977: 37).

Gerard, as noted above, also mentioned the plant's cooling properties. Here, the *refrigerant* nature of the herb, combined with some possible *diaphoretic* ability (Grieve 1971: 2:754), has proven useful in **fevers**, as Gerard went on to observe (Gerard 1975: 318–21; cf. Potterton 1983: 178; Foster and Duke 1990: 214).

This delightful and versatile plant has experienced a variety of additional applications throughout history, many of which have related to either the gastrointestinal tract or the urinary tract—two body systems for which sheep sorrel seems to display an especial affinity (Potterton 1983: 194). As to the former, the Oklahoma Lenape (Delaware) have chewed fresh leaves of sheep sorrel as a *stomachic* (Tantaquidgeon 1972: 75, 132–33). Then, too, the Iroquois have given a decoction of the root to settle **upset stomach** (Herrick 1977: 311). Finally, a tea of the flowers has been reverenced by all sorts of people as an excellent treatment for **ulcers** in the GI tract (Callegari and Durand 1977: 37).

As to uses relative to the urinary tract, sheep sorrel has proven its merit as a *diuretic* (Mockle 1955: 38; Wren 1972: 278), finding application by various cultures for **kidney** and **bladder stones** (Hutchens 1991: 255) and sundry other **urinary conditions** (Wren 1972: 278). Some authorities would not recommend it for kidney stones—at least for those of the oxalate variety—because of the plant's own high oxalate content. See further under Cautions.

Our herb would also appear to have *vermifuge* properties (Hutchens 1991: 255). The raw leaves have even been eaten by the Squaxin in Washington State to inveigh against **tuberculosis** (Gunther 1973: 29).

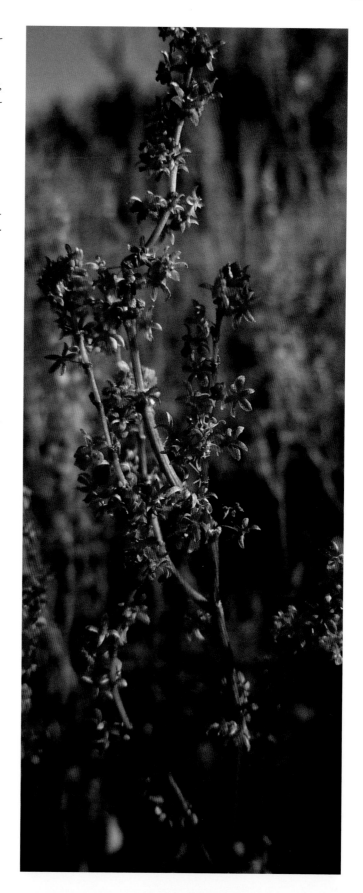

Sheep sorrel's best-known application, however, has been for **cancer.** Here, the roasted leaves have been poulticed onto **skin cancers** (Foster and Duke 1990: 214). The juice expressed on bread has been used by Native Americans as a plaster on same (Erichsen-Brown 1989: 420), which application, along with others, was catalogued by National Cancer Institute scientist Jonathan Hartwell in his series of articles on "Plants Used against Cancer" as published in the scientific journal *Lloydia* in the 1960s and 1970s and republished in book form in 1982 (Hartwell 1982).

Then there is the incredible story of Essiac, an herbal brew containing sheep sorrel and several other herbs (burdock, slippery elm, and Turkey rhubarb), which merits some detail to do it justice. (The history that follows is a synthesis from Thomas 1993; Walters 1993: 105–19; Olsen 1996; and Moss 1998: 103–15.) It begins in the 1890s, when an Ojibwe medicine man used an herbal tea containing sheep sorrel to help heal a woman with breast cancer. It seems that the woman recovered fully and, thirty years later, during an unrelated hospital stay in Ontario, met a nurse named Rene Caisse to whom she told her story. Caisse was intrigued and sought to secure the formula in the event that she herself might someday wind up with cancer. Her efforts were successful.

Several years later, in 1924, when Caisse's own aunt was diagnosed with advanced stomach cancer, Rene asked the attending physician, R. O. Fisher of Toronto, whether he would approve her attempting a trial with it. When he agreed, she dug out the formula, prepared it, and used it. After two months of drinking the concoction, the aunt got well and even went on to live another twenty-six years! Fisher was so impressed that he agreed to partner with Caisse in treating other cancer patients with the brew. At the same time, the two humanitarians worked nights and weekends experimenting with the formula on mice that had been inoculated with human cancer, modified it slightly to achieve optimum results, and eventually named it Essiac (Caisse spelled backward).

As word of their many successes with the brew began to spread, opinions for and against the tea began to crystallize. As to the former, nine physicians who came to be acquainted with its successes petitioned the Canadian federal health department to allow Caisse to test the herbal remedy on a wide scale. Rather than receiving a dignified response, two hatchet men were dispatched by Ottawa's Department of Health and Welfare to arrest Caisse or at least to restrain her from continuing with the treatment. When they realized that she was seeing only terminal cases and not charging for her services, they balked at arresting her.

Caisse next went on to treat her own mother, who at seventy-two years of age had developed inoperable liver cancer and was given a mere two days to live by a highly rated physician in Ontario. After ten days of daily injections with Essiac, Mrs. Caisse began to convalesce, finally being restored to full health and going on to live another eighteen years.

Eventually, fifty-five thousand people petitioned Ontario's parliament to allow Caisse to treat cancer patients freely and without fear of medical reprisals. The bill was presented in 1938 and failed to pass by a paltry three votes. Caisse began growing disillusioned by her opposition and decided to close her clinic in 1942, although she continued to treat patients privately out of her home. In 1959, however, Essiac saw new life: it was then that Caisse was invited by a famous New England physician, Charles Brusch, to test her formula at his prestigious medical center in Massachusetts, both on cancer patients and in lab mice. Brusch (who was knighted by Pope Paul VI and who was at the time the personal physician for John F. Kennedy) and his medical director, Charles McClure, found that the brew reduced pain and tumor size in human patients and reduced the mass of tumors in the mice as well as changed their cell formation. Some time later, Brusch himself would develop cancer, for which he would make the decision to use Essiac as his sole treatment. On April 6, 1990, he provided a statement to be notarized that declared: "I endorse this therapy even today for I have in fact cured my own cancer, the original site of which was the lower bowel, through Essiac alone."

Although, as we have earlier seen, burdock (see page 60) has shown documented activity against cancer, some of the key researchers involved with Essiac offered the opinion that the synergy between the various herbs is the best reason for the alleged efficacy of the brew, although some of these have also opined that sheep sorrel is the most powerful single antineoplastic herb in the mix. Thus, it was this herb that Caisse submitted to the Sloan Kettering Institute for Cancer Research for testing in 1973. That institute, after doing some testing, acknowledged to Caisse (by means of a letter from Chester Stock, its vice president for academic affairs) that sheep sorrel had indeed produced regression of sarcoma 180 in mice but also claimed that the results were not sufficient to warrant further study. Caisse responded that the institute had been freezing the herb and not boiling it as she had directed.

In 1977, Caisse, tired and frustrated and on her deathbed, sold the formula to a Canadian corporation that eventually began marketing it. Another source began to market a slightly different version of the formula in the late 1980s, claiming to have secured this version from Brusch. This product, called Flor-Essence, included red clover (see page 198), watercress (page 254), kelp, and blessed thistle (*Cnicus benedictus*). Countless other versions have appeared since. As there is no consensus among unbiased herbal researchers as to the precise measurements of the herbs used in the genuine formula developed by Caisse, I will not offer any here.

Although Caisse's formula has often been castigated by oncologists, more recent studies have lent some weight to a possible efficacy against cancer. For example, in the late

1990s, researchers from the University of Texas–Center for Alternative Medicine (UT–CAM) sent out a survey requesting feedback from 1,211 cancer patients who had used Flor-Essence. The tally revealed that the tonic was reported to have produced very good to excellent benefits in 71 percent of these people, including a retardation of cancer growth in 40.6 percent and a purported cure in 16.2 percent. Moreover, 53 percent felt better with the tonic, 31.5 percent had more energy, and 22.3 percent found that it improved the symptoms of their cancer (Richardson et al. 2000). Then, in a scientific study published in 2006, Essiac was shown to exert potent *antioxidant* and *DNA-protective* ability (Leonard et al. 2006). In yet another study, both it and Flor-Essence demonstrated *antiproliferative* activity in vitro at high concentrations (Tai et al. 2004).

As to preparations of sheep sorrel by itself, an infusion is made from 28 grams (1 ounce) leaves to 1 pint (568 milliliters) of boiling water and is usually administered in doses of 2 fluid ounces (56 milliliters) (Potterton 1983: 178).

PERSONAL AND PROFESSIONAL USE

I enjoy nibbling on fresh sheep sorrel from the field—especially on hot days, when it serves as a cooling and refreshing trail snack.

I will sometimes add sheep sorrel to protocols for passive gastric hemorrhage, gastric cancer, and various other afflictions of the stomach.

CAUTIONS

Due to the potential toxicity of the plant's oxalates in quantity, caution must be used in any ingestion of sheep sorrel for food. Keep fresh leaves to a minimum and as a trail nibble only. Prepared as a potherb, sheep sorrel should always be cooked in more than one water, to reduce toxicity, and quantity of intake should be kept down, for as little as 500 grams of garden sorrel prepared as a soup evidently proved to fatal to one man (Farré 1989). Medicinal doses of the plant are generally regarded as safe as long as traditional dosages are strictly observed.

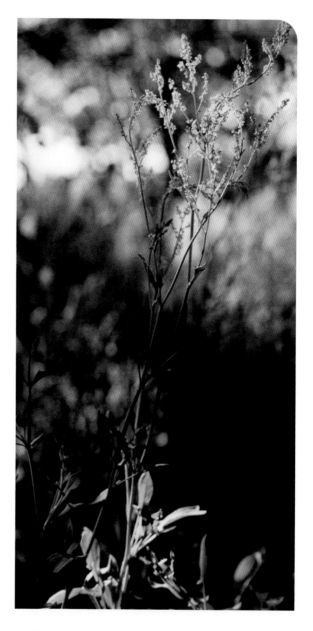

Those with a history of oxalate kidney stones should probably not be ingesting sheep sorrel (as food or as medicine), at least at any frequency more than occasionally. ⋘

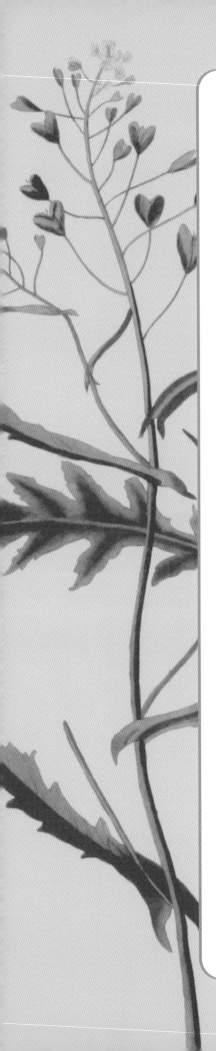

Shepherd's Purse

Capsella bursa-pastoris

DESCRIPTION

This is an annual weed growing 4–20 inches tall with an erect and branching stem. It starts life under the sun as a basal rosette of long-stalked, dandelion-like leaves, 2–5 inches long. Eventually, the stem starts to form and, with it, a number of alternate, sessile, arrowhead-shaped leaves that tightly clasp the stalk.

Shortly after the stem starts to sprout, the flowers begin to appear. These are small and white, with six stamens and four petals arranged as a cross. They are borne as elongate racemes at the end of the stem's branches. The lower ones open first, leaving green buds at the top of the raceme.

Triangular, two-parted seedpods (i.e., fruits) transition from the blossoms at the bottom of the raceme and then also from other flowers as the process moves upward at a rapid pace. Measuring 5–8 millimeters long, these fruits are flattened, notched, or indented at their tips and attached at their apex. The plant's common name, shepherd's purse, derives from the fact that these pods resemble the purses that medieval shepherds used to wear.

RANGE AND HABITAT

Shepherd's purse is a cosmopolitan weed, thriving in dry, open places such as old homesteads, old fields, gardens, ill-kept lawns, and wasteland.

MAJOR CONSTITUENTS

Shepherd's purse contains flavonoids (including rutin, quercetin, and diosmetin); choline; acetylcholine; tyramine; histamine; polypeptides; bursi[ni]c, fumaric, thiocyanic, malic, and pyruvic acid; bursine (an alkaloid) and other unidentified crystalline alkaloids; hyssopin; sinigrin (a mustard-oil glycoside); beta-sitosterol; saponins; and tannins. Nutrients include goodly amounts of protein (shepherd's purse is one of the best-known sources among greens!), pro-vitamin A and vitamin C, iron, thiamine, riboflavin, and potassium. It may or may not contain vitamin K as well; sources vary.

FOOD

Leaves may be consumed raw—sparingly as a trail nibble or in salads with other greens. They are best when consumed before the plant flowers and taste peppery like those of the related peppergrass, *Lepidium* spp. (see page 173).

The heart-shaped seedpods are also edible and instantly recognizable by taste as something that, when dried and ground, would make a marvelous pepper substitute. Fresh from the plant, they impart pizzazz to other greens when mixed in a salad. Fresh or dried, they make a superb seasoning when added to a camp stew at the tail end of its simmer.

Native Americans used to dry the pods and then crush them to free the seeds. They would then winnow and parch them and finally grind them into flour or cook them into mush. That's a lot of work for today's less enterprising soul!

Food can be procured from the roots of shepherd's purse, too, which can be dried and ground for use in soups, in stews, or even as a ginger substitute.

HEALTH/MEDICINE

Shepherd's purse is a unique and powerful plant that has played a major role in the history of herbal therapeutics but is tragically underused nowadays.

Best known is the plant's celebrated role as a hemostat. Here it is shepherd's purse's amines that yield powerful *vasoconstrictive* and *hemostatic* effects (Stuart 1982: 38). In the late 1960s, an animal experiment evinced shepherd's purse's *hypotensive* and hemostatic effects in rats (Kuroda and Kaku 1969: 151). A study in the early 1990s expanded on this research, providing further clarification as to the active agents (Vermathen and Glasl 1993). Historically, shepherd's purse has been utilized for **bleeding wounds** (it was used as such by soldiers on the battlefield during World War I), **nosebleeds** (wadded cotton soaked in the plant's juice was inserted into the nostrils), **fibroid tumors**, and **hematuria**. Its most famous use, however, has been for **uterine bleeding**, including **menorrhagia** (especially with heavy bleeding on the first few days, if the discharge is constant and colored bright red or is colorless, as opposed to being brownish) and **metrorrhagia**.

Aside from stemming blood flow, however, shepherd's purse has also been implemented to offset the **tendency to hemorrhage**. The German physician and phytotherapist Rudolf Fritz Weiss cited research demonstrating a stronger effect in this regard than could be derived from decoctions of either plantain (see page 180) or yarrow (page 282)—two other classic hemostatic herbs (Weiss 1988: 311). In a clinical review published in the medical journal *The Lancet* in 1940, details were presented on how this botanical had been successfully used as a hemostat before and after suprapubic and transurethral prostatectomy, specifically in 728 cases (patients age forty-seven to ninety-six) over a span of ten years, with only four cases of hemorrhage occurring, none of which were fatal (Greenberger and Greenberger 1940).

The plant's *astringent* effects have played a role in its utilization for **diarrhea**, the tannin content undoubtedly playing a large role here; in addition, other chemicals in the plant have been shown to exert a smooth-muscle-contracting effect on the small intestine (Kuroda and Takagi 1969a; Iurisson 1971). Its astringency has also led to its use for **atonic, catarrhal conditions** (Millspaugh 1974: 95, 96; Ellingwood 1983: 354; EthnobDB).

This herb seems to have an especial affinity for the genitourinary system, on which it most directly acts, supporting the tone of the tissues. Here it has been successfully used by herbalists for **children's bedwetting**, often in conjunction with even more astringent herbs, such as agrimony (*Agrimonia eupatoria*) (Clymer 1973; Carse 1989: 60; Hutchens 1991: 248). G. F. Parks, an Eclectic physician practicing in the early twentieth century, found it especially indicated when people were passing profuse urine loaded with thick material that was slimy or dusty in nature. He found that it worked best in women of a "high-strung, ambitious nature," but that it was also applicable to men who had acute gonorrhea "where they just slobber" (Parks 1909). It has also traditionally been used in China for **dysuria** (EthnobDB).

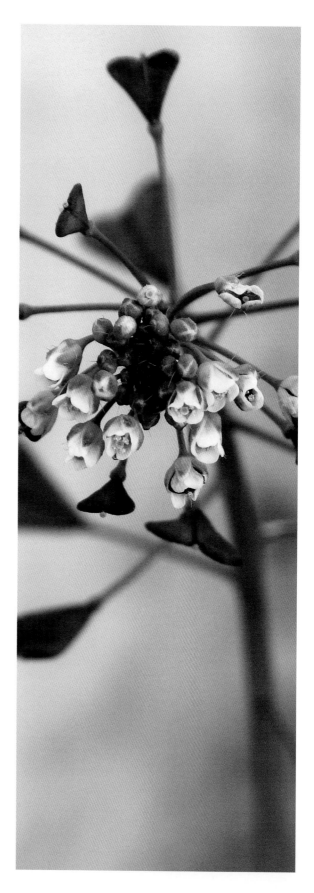

Another important study demonstrated that uterine tone is improved by the plant's polypeptides, which were shown to possess *uterine-contractile activity* similar to that of oxytocin (Kuroda and Tagaki 1968: 707). This was confirmed, and further elucidated, in a Bulgarian study published in 1981 (Shipochliev 1981). It's not surprising, then, that shepherd's purse has historically been used as a *parturient* to assist the birthing process. (Here its hemostatic properties can also help to manage any unusual bleeding, or even **postpartum hemorrhaging**, that may occur. However, herbalist Susun Weed cautions that it should only really be used to deal with an existing problem in this regard, not as a mere hemorrhagic preventive, citing several instances when two dropsersful of the tincture given by midwives during labor as a preventive resulted in huge blood clots that were painfully hard to excrete and made it difficult for the uterus to clamp down during the birthing process: Weed 1986: 72.)

A lab study published in the late 1960s showed that our herb is possessed of *anti-ulcer* effects (Kuroda and Tagaki 1969b). This investigation revealed that shepherd's purse, while not directly affecting the secretions of the stomach, yet speeded the recovery of **stress-induced ulcers**. This is interesting in that the Mohegan have used an infusion of the plant's seedpods as a *stomachic* (Tantaquidgeon 1928: 265), while the Midwest's Ojibwe have similarly employed shepherd's purse for **cramps** in the gastrointestinal tract (Densmore 1974: 344). Over half a century prior to the lab study, too, the Eclectic physician Finley Ellingwood had noted: "Dr. Heinen of Toledo treats non-malignant abdominal tumors in women with better results by adding five drops of capsella three times a day to the other indicated treatment" (Ellingwood 1983: 354).

In the same 1960s lab study referred to above, it was also demonstrated that shepherd's purse is possessed of both *anti-inflammatory* and *diuretic* effects (Kuroda and Tagaki 1969b). The former has been avidly appreciated by the Menomini, who have used an infusion of the herb as a wash for **poison ivy** (Smith 1923: 33). As to the plant's diuretic capabilities, which were appreciated by the Eclectics (Ellingwood 1983: 33), the previously cited study showed that such an effect results from a palpable increase in the glomerular filtration apparatus of the kidneys. This combination of anti-inflammatory and diuretic effects explains why the plant also has a cherished reputation for offsetting **gout**. Both Ellingwood and Charles Millspaugh observed, as well, that the bruised plant has been most gratefully applied to **rheumatic joints** (Millspaugh 1974: 461; Ellingwood 1983: 354).

Various Native American tribes have insisted that the seedpod serves as a reliable *anthelmintic*, with said ability being attributed to its pungency (Speck 1917: 319). *Antimicrobial* activity against certain gram-positive organisms has also been documented (Kuroda 1977; Moskalenko 1986). This may be due, in part, to the isothiocyanates. It is

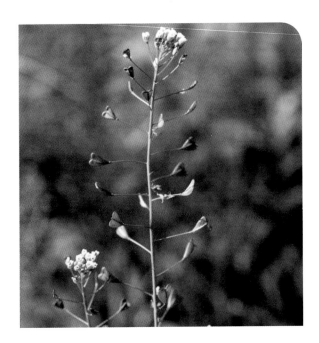

of interest here that the herb has traditionally been implemented as a urinary *antiseptic* (Wren 1988: 250).

Finally, shepherd's purse has been used for ages in Poland in the treatment of cancer (EthnobDB). Again, modern science has shed some light on this use: laboratory studies conducted in the mid-1970s found *antineoplastic* effects against Ehrlich solid tumors, which were originally attributed to the herb's content of fumaric acid (Kuroda et al. 1976). However, this acid occurs in many plants, very few of which have been shown to exert antineoplastic activity. Current research, therefore, has focused more on the plant's content of bursine and bursinic acid.

PERSONAL AND PROFESSIONAL USE

I enjoy adding shepherd's purse to wild salads or, more often, just eating it straight from the fields as a solitary menu item.

Shepherd's purse is one of my favorite herbs to help offset menorrhagia. Here I often use it half and half with yarrow (see page 282) in the form of a tincture and start it a few days before the anticipated menstrual flow, usually continuing it throughout the menses.

I'll often add shepherd's purse to a formula for hypertension, too, especially if the cause is unknown.

CAUTIONS

Because shepherd's purse is a member of the mustard family, skin contact with the seeds or the leaves for any length of time could cause blistering.

As this plant has uterine-stimulant properties, *do not use in pregnancy* except at end of term as an aid to parturition or earlier in term as an emergency hemostat during an episode of hemorrhaging. (Any such use, however, should be done under a qualified practitioner's care.) ⥸

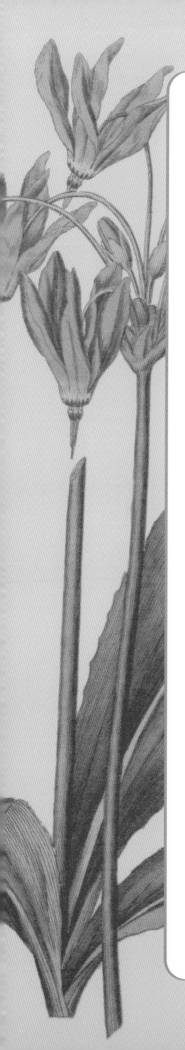

Shooting Star

AMERICAN COWSLIP; PRAIRIE POINTERS

Dodecatheon spp.

DESCRIPTION

Shooting star is an extremely beautiful native perennial that grows 10–20 inches high and bears a single, smooth stalk.

The leaves are entirely basal, spatula shaped, and smooth edged, and they grow to 6 inches long. The inch-long flowers are nodding and possessed of five long, backswept petals as well as five protruding yellow stamens growing to a common point. These flowers, which can be likened to badminton shuttlecocks in appearance, occur long stalked in clusters at the tip of the stem.

Two species occur in the Midwest:

Dodecatheon meadia has 6–30 flowers (rose, purple, or white in color) per umbel and leaf bases that are red.

D. amethystinum, also known as *D. radicatum* (amethyst shooting star), has two to eleven rose-purple (or occasionally white) flowers per umbel and green leaf bases.

RANGE AND HABITAT

The lovely shooting star thrives in medium to dry open woods, meadows, and prairies. In the Midwest, it flourishes from southeastern Minnesota eastward into southwestern Wisconsin.

FOOD

Fresh leaves can be added to salads (Willard 1992a: 171). The texture is tender, and the taste is pleasant.

The leaves and roots can also be prepared as a potherb, either by roasting them or by boiling them (Kirk 1975: 195). The Yuki have enjoyed both of these plant parts, roasting them in campfire ashes (Chestnut 1902: 378).

HEALTH/MEDICINE

When Blackfoot children develop **canker sores**, their parents may make an infusion of the western species *Dodecatheon pulchellum* ssp. *pulchellum* and have them gargle it to help heal the painful ulcers (Hellson and Gadd 1974: 76). The Blackfoot have also utilized a lukewarm infusion of the leaves as drops for **sore eyes** (Hellson and Gadd 1974: 81). For the same discomfort, the Okanogan-Colville have preferred an infusion of the roots (Turner et al. 1980: 117).

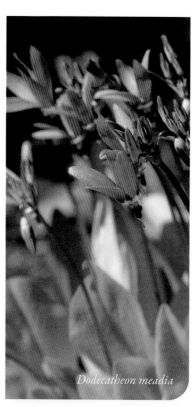

Dodecatheon meadia

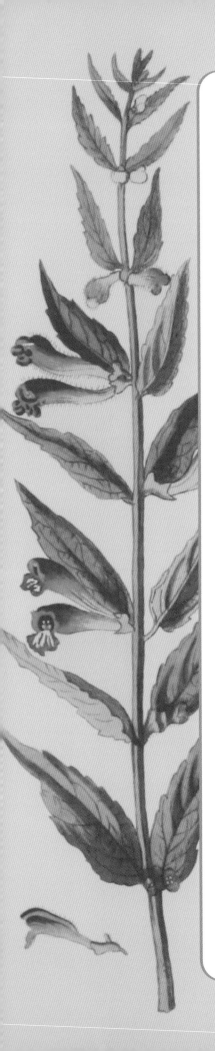

Skullcap

DESCRIPTION

Skullcap is a perennial member of the mint family, possessing that family's characteristically square stem and paired leaves.

The two-lipped blue flowers are bell shaped to horn shaped, with a "hump" on top of the calyx surrounding the base that looks somewhat like the skullcap worn by the Romans (hence the plant's common name). This hump is an important feature distinguishing skullcap from lookalikes.

Two major species inhabit the Midwest:

Scutellaria epilobiifolia, also known as *S. galericulata* (common skullcap, marsh skullcap, hooded skullcap), has a slender stem and grows 6–23 inches tall. Its short-stalked or sessile leaves are lanceolate to ovate. The lower lip on its inch-long flowers is flat and three-lobed. These blossoms are sessile (or nearly so) and appear singly in axils of the upper leaves.

S. lateriflora (mad-dog skullcap, blue skullcap, bushy skullcap) has pointed oval leaves that are barely stalked. Its flowers are smaller than those of the above species (only ½ inch long) and appear clustered on one-sided racemes that spring from the leaf axils.

RANGE AND HABITAT

Skullcap flourishes throughout the Midwest in moist places such as marshes, swamps, bogs, shores, wet woods, and thickets.

MAJOR CONSTITUENTS

Skullcap contains flavonoid glycosides (including scutellarin, scutellarein, apigenin, baicalin, dihydrobaicalin, lateriflorin, and luteolin); iridoid glycosides (including catalpol); flavonoid aglycones (lateriflorein, wogonin, oroxylin A, and baicalein); an essential oil (consisting of cadinene, calamenene, beta-elemene, alpha-cubenene, alpha-humulene, and alpha-bergamotene); phenylpropanoids (ferulic, caffeic, *p*-coumaric, and cinnamic acid); clerodane triterpenoids (ajugapitin, scutelarin A, B, and C, and scutecyprol A); and tannins. Nutrients include significant amounts of potassium, magnesium, phosphorus, and calcium.

HEALTH/MEDICINE

Here is an herb that, although widely marketed (though only *S. lateriflora*, unfortunately) in both North America and Europe, is incredibly understudied and underutilized as to its full potential. In clarifying its plethora of applications, I would like first to discuss its value as an *emmenagogue*, and to do so by pointing out that both the Cherokee and the Cree have used it for improving the quality of menstruation (e.g., blood flow, emotional stability, etc.) (Hamel and Chiltoskey 1975: 55; Goodchild 1984: 145). While it is perhaps a bit inferior in strength to a few other herbs discussed elsewhere in the present work—plants such as motherwort (see page 156), blue cohosh (page 33), and horsemint (page 132)—it is nonetheless of great value, especially when applied appropriately. It is definitely an herb of choice where the **amenorrhea** is accompanied by nervousness, **anxiety**, and **worry** (McIntyre 1995: 273) and *the* herb of choice when exhaustion enters the picture as well.

In fact, skullcap is the remedy par excellence for **nervousness, restlessness, anxiety, worry, PMS tension**, and **neurasthenia (nervous exhaustion)**. It was official as a *tranquilizer* in the *United States Pharmacopeia* from 1863 to 1916 and thereafter in the *National Formulary* until 1947. It is still official in most European pharmacopeias for epilepsy, hysteria, and nervous tension. All of this underscores the strangeness that only two clinical trials have ever been conducted with this herb. The first, published in 2003, demonstrated *anxiolytic* effects, verifying the herb's time-honored reputation for anxiety (Wolfson and Hoffmann 2003). (A rat study published the same year found the same effects, which were attributed to the plant's flavonoids: Awad et al. 2003.) The second clinical trial, published in 2014, involved forty-three physically and mentally healthy volunteers who were only mildly anxious or less and who used 350 milligrams of skullcap three times daily or a placebo over a period of two weeks. The result was that the herb significantly enhanced the study group's global mood, and that without reducing their energy, over the placebo group (Brock et al. 2014).

Skullcap is often quite helpful, too, in **irritable bowel syndrome** (Mills and Bone 2000: 175, 180) due to its nervine effects and to some carminative properties owing to its essential oil. People with **nervous heart disorders** may also benefit from this herb (Moore 1994b: 5.4; Smith 1999: 51; Tilgner 1999: 107). In fact, *S. epilobiifolia* has been used by the Midwest's Ojibwe in this very regard (Smith 1932: 372). Then, too, skullcap has proven itself to be a real gem for helping people to break addictions to recreational drugs. In this regard, one of America's Eclectic physicians observed: "In treating heavy drinkers who wish to give up the habit, I know of nothing better than Scutellaria. It steadies and sobers the patient and brings on sleep and appetite" (Felter and Lloyd 1898). Indeed, in view of its unique combination of minerals, essential oil, and glycosides, skullcap can be said to possess—as herbalist Peter Holmes points out—a *trophorestorative* effect on the nervous system (Holmes 1997–98: 2:535).

Herbalists find skullcap also to be indicated, as did America's Eclectic physicians, for any "nervous disorder characterized by irregular muscular action, twitching, tremors and restlessness, with or without incoordination" (Ellingwood 1983: 124). The herb has thus been classically used for **cerebral palsy**, **chorea**, **delirium tremens**, **stress-caused muscular spasms**, **Parkinson's disease**, **tension headaches**, and **epilepsy** (especially to offset petit mal seizures, but also grand mal ones to some extent) (Bradley et al. 1992: 197). In a letter to the *British Medical Journal*, William Bramwell of Liverpool noted of skullcap: "In many cases a simple infusion or extract in correspondingly suitable doses will lessen the severity of the [epileptic] fits and reduce their number equally with bromides and without any

of the disadvantages of the latter.... The medicinal qualities of this simple remedy are even more marked in chorea than in epilepsy" (Bramwell 1915). In harmony with these traditional uses, scientific studies have demonstrated *antispasmodic* and *anticonvulsant* effects for our herb (Claus 1961: 219–20; Peredery and Persinger 2004; Zhang et al. 2009).

S. lateriflora was also formerly used for **rabies**, which manifests symptoms like those we have been discussing (muscular tension and spasms). According to the Natura physician R. Swinburne Clymer, the classic application here was to use it as a poultice immediately after a rabid bite and also to take it internally as a tea of the fresh plant four times a day for seven days, along with a tea of purple coneflower (*Echinacea* spp.), or by way of a tincture of 2–15 drops combined with an *Echinacea* tincture of 15–30 drops, as frequently as indicated (Clymer 1973: 110).

Modern scientists have assumed that this application could not possibly possess any efficacy, and so skullcap has never actually been tested for action against rabies. While any actual curative action might seem improbable, it is interesting to note that it was a physician, Lawrence Van Derveer, practicing in New Jersey during the 1770s, who is credited

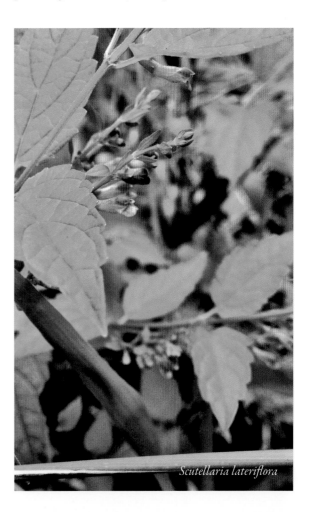

Scutellaria lateriflora

by historians as having pioneered just such a rabies-healing campaign with this herb. Van Derveer, who, according to the historical records, is said to have healed both rabid humans and animals, understandably created quite a stir in his area at the time. Unfortunately, one of his patients, a Mr. Daniel Lewis, who was so impressed with apparently having been healed of hydrophobia by the doctor, endeavored to capitalize on the cure, styling himself "Mad Dog Lewis" and shamelessly attempting to market the skullcap medicine surreptitiously in his own state of New York as "Lewis' Secret Cure." As botanical historian Virgil Vogel noted, the skullcap treatment thus "fell into disrepute when it was adopted by quacks who promoted it by advertising" (Vogel 1970: 367).

However, shortly after Van Derveer's death, L. Spalding, in 1819, collected case histories from the good doctor's work and calculated that of the 850 rabid patients whom this physician had treated with skullcap (some of whom were animals), only three had died! (Spalding 1819) Renowned botanist Constantine Rafinesque, writing in 1830, summarized this matter as follows: "[*Scutellaria lateriflora*] is lately become famous as a cure and prophylactic against hydrophobia. This property was discovered by Dr. Vandesveer [*sic*], towards 1772, who has used it with the utmost success, and is said to have till 1815, prevented 400 persons and 1,000 cattle from becoming hydrophobus, after being bitten by mad dogs. ... Many empirics and some enlightened physicians have employed it also successfully" (Rafinesque 1828–30: 2:82–83).

That is an enthusiastic endorsement and from the pen of a respected botanical scholar. What prompted such assuredness on Rafinesque's part? Charles Millspaugh informs us that Rafinesque was greatly impressed by the testimony of a Dr. White, who had assured him that he himself had been cured of rabies with skullcap after having been bitten by a mad dog, while others likewise bitten by the same animal had died without the treatment (Millspaugh 1974: 470). Yet there is more. The Eclectic pharmacist John Uri Lloyd investigated this chapter in medical history in still greater depth and uncovered some additional details that would likewise seem difficult to ignore: for instance, he highlighted a particular case of Van Derveer's in which "a man, two hogs, and two cattle, were bitten by a mad dog. Scutellaria was given the man and one hog. Both recovered. The other animals died of hydrophobia" (Lloyd 1929).

Might, then, skullcap actually possess some activity against rabies after all? Lloyd would spend the rest of his life trying to get the scientific community to set up controlled studies to answer that very question, but to no avail. Until such a time as those studies are undertaken, this question cannot be positively answered. Still, the evidence we have from historical records is surely most intriguing.

Having sung its praises, however, I would be remiss not to point out that skullcap should almost always be used as a fresh-plant extract rather than as a tea or an encapsulation of the dried herb. Eclectic physician John Scudder elaborated well in this regard: "Here we have another remedy that loses its medicinal properties by drying, until by age they are entirely dissipated. I have seen specimens furnished physicians by the drug trade that were wholly worthless—no wonder they were disappointed in its action. ... I value the remedy highly, but only recommend it when prepared [as a tincture] from the fresh [flowering] plant" (Scudder 1870: 213). I might add that this difference seems to be especially pronounced with reference to the plant's antispasmodic properties.

On a final note, our American skullcap species are markedly different in chemical structure from the Chinese baikal skullcap (*Scutellaria baicalensis*). The latter plant's variety of applications also differ greatly from those of our own skullcap species. What is more, the Chinese skullcap has the advantage of having had numerous scientific studies performed on its behalf, something that is conspicuously lacking for our American species. Indeed, the situation has changed little since Rafinesque's days of the early nineteenth century when he lamented concerning our American species: "We lack ... a series of scientific and conclusive experiments made by well informed men" (Rafinesque 1828–30: 2:83). Hopefully, however, this great deficit in plant research will someday be remedied, especially with reference to its historical uses for both rabies and epilepsy.

PERSONAL AND PROFESSIONAL USE

This remarkable plant has been a mainstay in my own herbal practice for many years. I have probably used it most for its nervine properties, with the observation that it supplies great strength to the nervous system. Here I have found that 1 teaspoon of the tincture used every hour and combined with 1 or 2 teaspoons of oat (*Avena sativa*) milky-seed tincture can often pull the most terribly addicted person through withdrawal. As for its renowned neuromuscular-relaxing effects, although it is weaker in this regard than a powerhouse such as kava (*Piper methysticum*)—which, in my experience, seems to possess the strength of diazepam to relax the neuromuscular system—it is safer for long-term use. While I thus often prefer to use kava as an initial treatment for anxiety and tight muscles, and almost always for acute episodes of either, I much prefer skullcap for sustained use. I value it highly for its antispasmodic properties and find that it combines well, in this regard, with another spasmolytic herb, blue vervain, *Verbena hastata* (see page 41), especially relative to problems experienced during the menstrual period.

CAUTIONS

Skullcap is contraindicated in pregnancy due to its emmenagogue and antiplacental action. ⋘

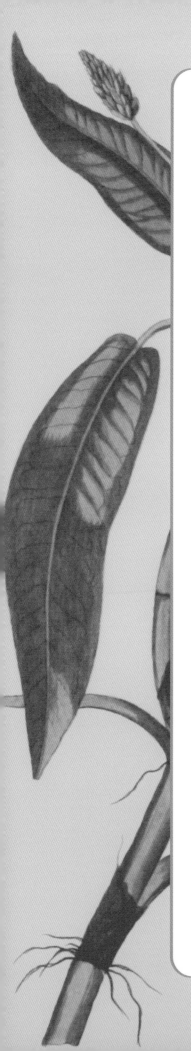

Smartweed

Polygonum spp.

DESCRIPTION

The smartweeds are a group of annual and perennial species of the *Polygonum* genus possessing branched stems with sheathed joints, flowers arranged in terminal spikes, an acrid juice, and a preference for damp ground. A number of species exist in the Midwest, including the following:

Polygonum amphibium (water smartweed) dwells either in water-soaked ground or on the surface of a body of water (where its stem can reach a length of 8 feet!). It has pink flowers arranged in clusters that are one to four times longer than they are wide.

P. coccineum (swamp smartweed) is a perennial that reaches a height of 1–3 feet. It possesses hairy, alternate leaves and pink, rosy, or white flowers.

P. hydropiper (common smartweed, water pepper) grows 8–24 inches high and has wavy-edged, lanceolate leaves with a reddish tinge. Its flowers are green, and their spiked arrangement is very slender, reaching 1–3 inches in length and sagging at the tip.

P. lapathifolium (dock-leaved smartweed, pale smartweed) is an annual species growing 3–4 feet tall with smooth and branched stems. Its leaves are elongate and pointed at both ends. The flowers are white to rosy in color, and the spike on which they are clustered nods quite blatantly at its tip.

P. pennsylvanicum (pinkweed, Pennsylvania smartweed) is an annual that may take on either an erect or a sprawling nature, reaching 1–5 feet. It has a branching stem and lanceolate leaves. The flowers are rose, pink, or white, and they do not nod but maintain an upright posture.

P. persicaria (lady's thumb): See the separate profile for lady's thumb (page 143).

RANGE AND HABITAT

One or another species grows throughout the Midwest in wet, open places—the shores of ponds, streams, and lakes and in marshes, swamps, roadside ditches, and wet fields.

MAJOR CONSTITUENTS

Smartweeds contain tannin (21 percent in the roots of some species, and 18 percent in their stems!), gallic acid, ellagic acid, acetic acid, malic acid, polygonic acid, valerianic acid, flavonoids (including high amounts of rutin), beta-sitosterol, sesquiterpenes, polygonolide (an isocoumarin), and an essential oil (inclusive of borneol, camphor, carvone, fenchone, p-Cymol, terpineol, and other chemicals).

FOOD

The peppery leaves can be added, in small quantities, to camp stews, but the noted wild-foods authorities Merritt Lyndon Fernald and Alfred Kinsey remarked that even so cooked and diluted, they tend to cause tearing of the eyes owing to their pungency and should therefore be used with caution (Fernald and Kinsey 1958: 173).

HEALTH/MEDICINE

The twenty-first edition of the *United States Dispensatory* (1926) noted that *P. hydropiper* possesses "medicinal properties" and that it is "esteemed diuretic, and ... used with asserted success in ... uterine disorders." It then notes its use by physicians in the treatment of **uterine hemorrhages** (Wood et al. 1926: 1228–29). Concordantly, the Menomini of our own area have used *P. pennsylvanicum* for **oral hemorrhage**, implementing a tea of the dried leaf (Smith 1923: 47). The *hemostatic* effects, acknowledged of late in the *PDR for Herbal Medicines* (Fleming 1998: 1059), perhaps partly occur due to the plant's rutin content, which strengthens capillary walls (Foster and Duke 1990: 214), but undoubtedly mainly because of an *astringency* owing to smartweed's high tannin content. Indeed, the twenty-sixth edition of the *US Dispensatory* cites the research of physician B. Woodward to the effect that dried *P. punctatum*, also known as *P. acre* (water smartweed), contains an unusually high amount of tannin for an herbaceous plant (18 percent), which content and consequent astringency allowed him to implement a tincture of that species to most successfully treat **diarrhea** and **dysentery**.

Smartweed's astringency has lent its use to the Midwest's Meskwaki (Fox), enabling them to utilize *P. pennsylvanicum* for **piles** (Smith 1928: 236). It has also allowed *P. coccineum* (common swamp smartweed or bigweed lady's thumb) to be implemented in Canadian folk medicine—the stems and leaves soaked in cold water for **diarrhea** and the root tea as a mouthwash for **canker sores** (Angier 1978: 160). Early American botanical writer Manasseh Cutler even informs us that William Withering, credited with the discovery of digitalis, was adamant that smartweed *relinquishes* these sores (Cutler 1785). Not incongruously, herbal journalist Will Messenger relates how a gargle of smartweed tea healed, almost overnight, a bad gash in his cheek that had been

brought about by an overbite (Messenger 1992: 3). Then, too, children's **flux** has been treated by the Cherokee with an infusion of *P. hydropiper*'s roots (Hamel and Chiltoskey 1975: 55). Traditional Chinese Medicine also uses *P. hydropiper* for diarrhea and even for **bacterial dysentery**, for which it is regarded as a specific (Anonymous 1977: 927).

The twenty-first edition of the *US Dispensatory* also noted that *P. hydropiper* has proven itself of value in the treatment of **amenorrhea.** This *emmenagogue* effect, in fact, was a favorite use of the plant by nineteenth-century and early twentieth-century physicians (Clapp 1852: 854; Johnson 1884: 237; Ellingwood 1983: 482–83). The Eclectic physician John Scudder wrote, in the 1870s, that it was "one of the best emmenagogues, especially when the arrest is from cold" (Scudder 1870: 181). John Gunn, in his popular household medical guide of the nineteenth century, recommended a strong tincture for this complaint, dosed at 1 or 2 teaspoonfuls, taken three times a day (Gunn 1859–61: 858). Alma Hutchens adds that internal use can be accompanied by a fomentation of the hot tea on the lower back where the menstrual pain is particularly emphatic (Hutchens 1991: 294). The use for amenorrhea remains smartweed's most popular application in the United Kingdom today (Wren 1988: 252–53).

Alabama herbalist Tommie Bass used smartweed for **kidney problems** (Crellin and Philpott 1990b: 171, 176). The Cherokee found that it stymied **painful** or **bloody urination** and that it also helped to dislodge **urinary gravel** (Hamel and Chiltoskey 1975: 55), an application that Gunn also endorsed (Gunn 1859–61: 858). Indeed, Charles Millspaugh remarked that it was a most "powerful diuretic when fresh" (Millspaugh 1974: 567). This *diuretic* effect was

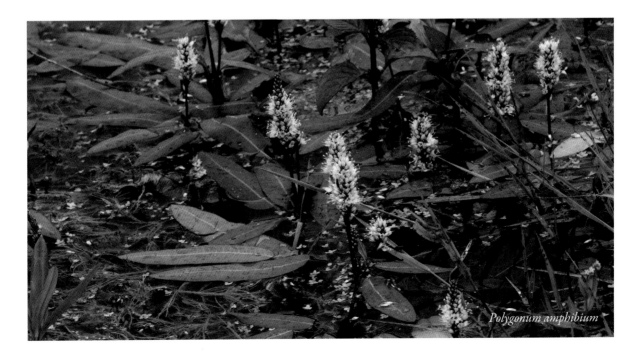

Polygonum amphibium

also undoubtedly partly responsible for the plant's many successes with **dropsy**, as the Malecite and Micmac discovered (Mechling 1959: 244); with **gout;** and with **rheumatism** (Fleming 1998: 1059), as implemented by the Mexicans, who bathed rheumatic limbs in a bath into which an infusion of smartweed had been poured (Millspaugh 1974: 567). Still, direct *anti-inflammatory* activity is no doubt contributory as well, since the Cherokee have poulticed **swollen** or **inflamed body parts** with this plant (Hamel and Chiltoskey 1975: 55). The Houma have implemented the boiled roots of *P. punctatum* for **pain** and **swelling** in the **legs** and **joints** (Speck 1941: 58). Will Messenger even tells of an eighty-two-year-old acquaintance who swears that smartweed soaked in vodka makes the best rubbing liniment around for **sore muscles**, **bruises**, and **sprains** (Messenger 1992: 3). Not surprisingly, then, an in vitro study demonstrated that *P. hydropiper* exerted powerful anti-inflammatory activity by suppressing the release of nitric oxide, tumor necrosis factor alpha, and prostaglandin E2 (Yang et al. 2012).

In both Western and Eastern herbalism, smartweed is thought to possess *heating* and *drying* energies (Grieve 1971: 2:743; Gerard 1975: 360–62; Anonymous 1977: 478). As such, it has traditionally been used for **respiratory problems** of a cold, damp nature, such as by the Potawatomi, who found it especially helpful for a **cold**—specifically one accompanied by a **fever** (Smith 1933: 72). Although it is a warming herb, smartweed's classic use for fever has undoubtedly been popular because the herb is, as John Scudder explained, "one of our most certain stimulant diaphoretics" (Scudder 1870: 181; cf. Grieve 1971: 2:743; Johnson 1884: 237). In other words, as the Iroquois explained, it is the presence of "fever when you are continually cold and cannot sweat" that calls for the use of this herb (Herrick 1995: 144).

The tops of *P. pennsylvanicum* have been used as a tea by certain Native American tribes to help deal with **epilepsy** (Foster and Duke 1990: 160). South Carolinian folk healers have wet this species' leaves with vinegar and then wrapped them around the head to relieve a **headache** (Morton 1974: 115). Various smartweed species have enjoyed a long tradition of folk-medicinal use for **cancer** (Hartwell 1970: 373).

As to form and dosage best used (see Cautions), David Potterton says to infuse 1 ounce of leaves in 1 pint of water (Potterton 1983: 281). Alma Hutchens writes of cutting up the herb into small pieces and then infusing 1 teaspoonful in 1 cup of warm (not hot) water, imbibing it thereafter in wineglassful amounts (Hutchens 1991: 294). Southwest American herbalist Michael Moore says to make a standard infusion, utilizing 2–4 ounces per dose, as needed (Moore 1994a: 18). M. Grieve and Gunn both note that any tincture must be made from the fresh plant and that a cold-water infusion is the best form for **gravel**, **gout**, **colds**, and **coughs** (Gunn 1859–61: 858; Grieve 1971: 2:743).

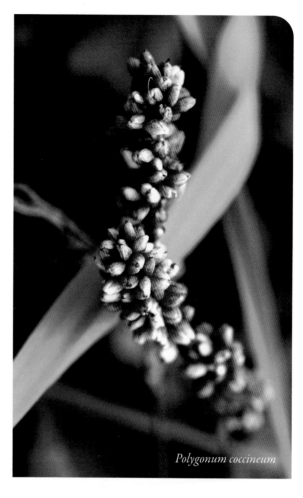

Polygonum coccineum

PERSONAL AND PROFESSIONAL USE

This valuable genus is not typically available on the herb market, but several species grow plentifully in the Midwest, so I am able to wildcraft them.

I can confirm that a tincture of *P. punctatum* does indeed make an excellent rubbing liniment, especially for chronic muscle aches and pains. I've also found it helpful for amenorrhea from cold, for infectious diarrhea, and as a swish or compress for sores or soreness in the oral cavity.

CAUTIONS

This plant produces very painful and rubefacient effects when the fresh plant or undiluted juice comes in contact with mucous membranes. Because of the severe acridity of this plant and the consequent dangers in handling it, it is best used only by way of a professional preparation and under professional guidance. In other words, this is *not* a plant for the layperson to wildcraft! Identify it if you will, see where it grows, admire its beauty, but *leave it alone*. (The exception here would be if such a layperson could accompany someone experienced in its identification, collection, and preparation.) Due to its emmenagogue effects, smartweed *should not be used during pregnancy*. ⤜

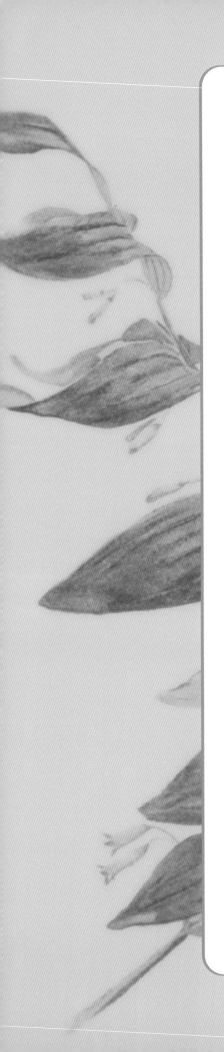

Solomon's Seal

Polygonatum biflorum, P. pubescens

DESCRIPTION

Solomon's seal is a lovely perennial herb that grows anywhere from 1 to 6 feet (usually 3–4 feet). Its elongate and unbranched stem is strongly arched so that the plant grows practically horizontally.

Its leaves are oval to elliptical, smooth and waxy, and parallel veined, and they lack any serration. They are about 4 inches long and about 2 inches wide and are arranged alternately along the stem. Smooth veins occur on the undersides of *Polygonatum biflorum*, whereas pubescence (hairiness) marks those of *P. pubescens*, as its Latin name suggests.

Flowers of *P. biflorum* are greenish white and ½–1 inch long. Those of *P. pubescens* are a bit smaller and more yellowish green. *Polygonatum* flowers may dangle from the leaf axils singly, as is the case with *P. officinale* (a European species) and sometimes with *P. pubescens*; in pairs, as with *P. biflorum* and sometimes *P. pubescens*; or in clusters, as with *P. multiflorum* (an Asian species) and sometimes *P. biflorum*. Six short, green-spotted lobes hang from the bottom of each flower, so that the blossom has an overall "bell-like" look.

In late summer, the flowers are replaced by berries. At first colored green, they finally—after quite a long time—turn blue or blue-black. They remind one of blueberries but are larger, being three-celled and carrying one or two seeds in each chamber.

The rootstock is a creamy-white, fleshy rhizome on which can be found one or more rounded scars—the "seals" in the name Solomon's seal, as they resemble wax seal impressions. One can tell the age of the plant by counting the number of "seals," for the rhizome has one for each year of life.

RANGE AND HABITAT

Solomon's seal thrives in moist woods and on riverbanks. It can be found in the eastern and midwestern parts of both the United States and Canada. In the Midwest, *P. pubescens* thrives in the eastern half, while *P. biflorum* can be found throughout, except for the far northeast.

MAJOR CONSTITUENTS

The rhizome contains polysaccharides (including mucilage, pectin, and gum); convallarin (a cardioactive glycoside); alkaloids; saponoside A and B (steroidal saponins); triterpenoid saponins; polyphenols; flavonoids (including homoisoflavanones); lectins; and a variety of vitamins. The berries contain anthraquinone glycosides (with saponins in the seeds).

FOOD

The rhizomes of Solomon's seal can be eaten after being boiled or baked. One should be prepared for a strong, unpleasant odor, however. In marked contrast to that bad smell is the taste, which is highly agreeable to many.

The rhizome is a useful survival food to know because, like many roots and tubers, it provides long-burning fuel in contrast to the quick and short-lived energy provided by leaves and berries. The wild-foods writer Oliver Medsger, in fact, refers to Francis Parkman's comment that this plant helped stave off starvation for French colonists in America (Medsger 1972: 163). Very young shoots can also be prepared as a potherb by cooking them in water for ten minutes.

HEALTH/MEDICINE

This lovely woodland plant shows significant *anti-inflammatory* properties (Fleming 1998). Thus, a poultice made from the rhizome has been used in many different cultures to treat inflammatory conditions such as **poison ivy**, **arthritis**, **gout**, and **rheumatism** (Naegele 1980: 206). The juice from the rhizome has been implemented to soothe **sunburn** as well as droppered into ears to treat **earache.**

Probably the plant's best-known use is as a treatment for **bruises.** Often cited here is sixteenth-century herbalist John Gerard's statement about it proving able to heal—in a mere day or two—bruises occurring from domestic abuse (Gerard 1975: 906). Gerard had noted that the fresh rhizome was, in these cases, mashed and applied topically in conjunction with cream or milk. Writing a century and a half later, botanical scholar J. Hill would call Solomon's seal "a vulnerary of the first rank" but go on to elucidate, most interestingly, that "our country uses it *internally* in cases of bruises from blows" (Hill 1751: 654). A number of Native American tribes have also used it for bruises, but chiefly by way of topical application. The Rappahannock, for example, have used two methods to make a salve: (1) boiling down the roots and (2) stewing the berries and mixing them with elder bark and hog grease (Speck 1942: 30). The Cherokee have bruised and heated the rhizome and applied it topically (Youngken 1924: 407).

Both mildly *astringent* and highly *demulcent* in its effects, Solomon's seal has an *affinity to mucous membranes* and thus has been used to treat various problems involving these, as well as the skin in general. Thus, in 1884, Laurence Johnson observed: "In decoction, [Solomon's seal] is employed as a domestic remedy to allay irritation of mucous surface, and in rhus [poison ivy/sumac] poisoning" (Johnson 1884: 276). The Iroquois have put a smashed rhizome in a glass of water, soaked a cloth in this solution, and squeezed the fluid into **sore eyes** (Herrick 1995: 244). The Russians have long used a decoction of the dried rhizome to treat internal **ulcers** (Hutchens 1991: 254–55).

Benefits would not seem to be limited to the upper gastrointestinal tract, however: Constantine Rafinesque, the brilliant nineteenth-century botanist who wrote a tome on the medicinal uses of American plants, made the observation that the powerful mucilaginous effects of powdered *Polygonatum* roots "appear to be equivalent to *Ulmus fulva* [slippery elm] and may perhaps be used in bowel complaints" (Rafinesque 1828–30: 2:85). The gastrointestinal applications would become well established in American practice, so much so that the popular nineteenth-century household guide by John Gunn could succinctly note that the rhizome is "good in ... irritable conditions of the stomach and bowels" (Gunn 1859–61: 860). In fact, the most revered application proved to be for **piles.** M. Grieve elucidated the classic method used: "4 ozs. Solomon's seal, 2 pints water, 1 pint molasses. Simmer down to 1 pint, strain, evaporate to the consistency of a thick fluid extract, and mix with it from

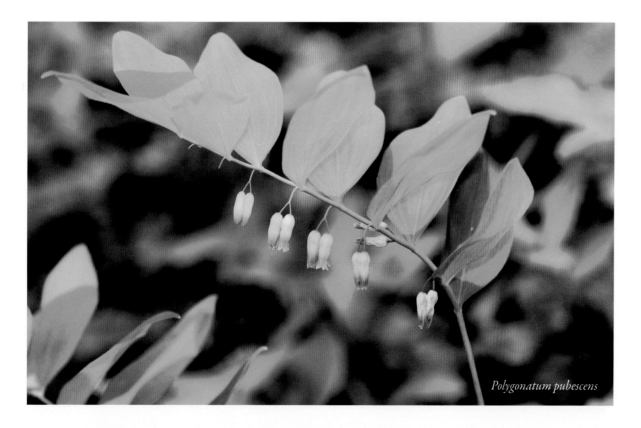

Polygonatum pubescens

½ to 1 oz. of powdered resin. Dosage: 1 teaspoonful several times daily" (Grieve 1971: 2:751).

Rafinesque observed that "coughs and pains in the breast" yielded to the magic of Solomon's seal (Rafinesque 1828–30: 2:85). Our own area's Ojibwe have appreciated its demulcent effects for **respiratory soreness** (Smith 1932: 363).

Solomon's seal has also been judicially employed for a wide variety of "**female problems.**" Gunn noted: "Very useful in female weakness and disease, as in leucorrhea or whites, and excessive and painful menstruation" (Gunn 1859–61: 860). This was in accord with the applications of this plant made by the Cherokee (Hamel and Chiltoskey 1975: 56). Another fascinating use of Solomon's seal was implemented by both the Fox and the Menomini: a smudge of the rhizome, often heated on a coal, was utilized to revive an **unconscious** person (Smith 1923: 41; Smith 1928: 230).

There appears to be a valuable *tonic* effect from the plant as well. Gunn noted that Solomon's seal was "good ... in general debility," while modern herbalists Michael Tierra and Peter Holmes find it invaluable as a nutritive tonic for what Traditional Chinese Medicine calls **qi deficiency**, which manifests as debility (Gunn 1859–61: 860; Tierra 1988: 322–23; Holmes 1997–98: 2:453–54). Interestingly, modern science has verified a powerful *antifatigue* effect from one species of Solomon's seal, native to Taiwan, attributed to the content of polysaccharides (Horng et al. 2014). The antidebility effect seen by herbalists may also relate to the genus's demonstrated ability to regulate blood sugar, with *Polygonatum officinale* significantly decreasing the blood glucose of diabetic mice (Miura and Kato 1995) and *P. odoratum* demonstrating an *antihyperglycemic* effect by way

of optimizing peripheral insulin sensitivity but without affecting the secretion of insulin (Choi and Park 2002).

Other effects demonstrated in scientific studies for at least the Chinese species include *antiosteoporotic, hypolipidemic, antioxidant, neuroprotective, immunosupportive, antibacterial*, and *antineoplastic* (Cui et al. 2018; Zhao et al. 2018).

PERSONAL AND PROFESSIONAL USE

I cooked and ate my first rhizome of Solomon's seal in 1972 and can still remember how much it stunk up the house! The taste, however, was oh so good. Since then, I've eaten quite a number of the rhizomes and have relished every single bite.

In my clinical herbal practice, I commonly implement Solomon's seal in formulas designed to support joint and spinal-disk integrity, healthy ligaments, a comfortable menopause, and an optimal utilization of glucose by the body's cells to make energy. I have found it to be very reliable in all of these respects.

CAUTIONS

The berries have a long tradition of being inedible or even toxic—sometimes provoking diarrhea and/or vomiting. Research has uncovered the presence of anthraquinone glycosides in them, which exert powerful cathartic effects (North 1967: 144; Lewis and Elvin-Lewis 1977; Woodward 1985: 38). There is also a particularly high concentration of irritating saponins in the seeds (Cooper and Johnson 1988: 60).

Solomon's seal should not be used during pregnancy. ⌇⌇

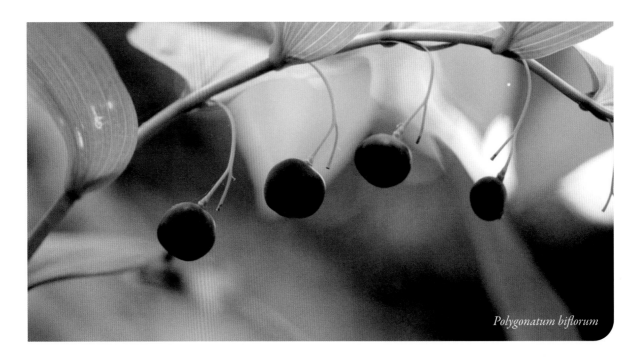

Polygonatum biflorum

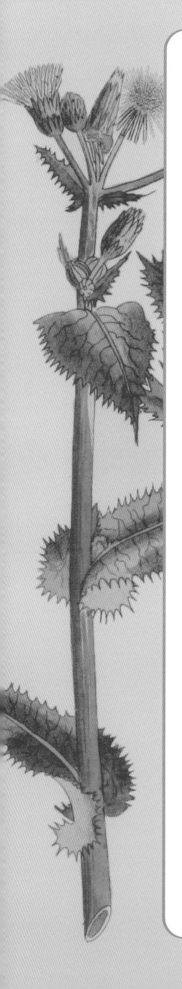

Sow Thistle

Sonchus spp.

DESCRIPTION

This is an annual or perennial herb growing to 3 feet high. The upright stem is smooth, hollow, and possessed of a milky sap in its walls.

The leaves are alternate, 4–14 inches long, 1½–5½ inches wide, and spiny toothed. Their bases clasp the stem.

The flowering heads are produced in loosely branched, elongated, erect, terminal clusters. Each head is 1–2 inches across, with lance-shaped bracts on the outside and many small yellow ray flowers within.

Several species abound in the Midwest as well as throughout North America.

Sonchus asper (spiny-leaved sow thistle) is an annual with a smooth, angled stem. It has very spiny leaves marked by rounded and curled lobes similar to those displayed by some of the true thistles. Viewed from the side, the base of each leaf looks like a human ear.

S. arvensis (field sow thistle) is a perennial with weak spines and hairy bracts and stalks. It has a horizontal rootstock and sharp leaf lobes. Its flower heads are larger than those of the above species. Many gland-tipped hairs appear on the bracts.

S. oleraceus (common sow thistle) is a hairless annual bearing leaves that have sharp-pointed basal lobes, the terminal one of which looks like a large triangle.

RANGE AND HABITAT

Sow thistle is a common weed growing throughout much of North America. It can be found throughout the Midwest in fields, roadsides, and waste places.

MAJOR CONSTITUENTS

Sow thistle contains flavonol glycosides, sesquiterpene lactones (at least four of them in *S. asper*), carbohydrates, flavonoids, tannins, saponins, and unsaturated sterols. Nutrients include fatty acids, carotenoids, a goodly amount of vitamin C, and a variety of minerals.

FOOD

Sow thistle was a popular food among the Romans, something that was mentioned by contemporary herbal writers such as Dioscorides and Pliny the Elder. The North American palate, however, has yet to get with the program.

Practically every portion of the plant is edible. First, young (spring-gathered) sow-thistle leaves can be collected, carefully trimmed of their thorny spines, and added to salads. When boiled in salted water for three to five minutes and then transferred into another pot and boiled for an additional five minutes, they also make a fair potherb. Alternatively, the young leaves can be added to casseroles or to soups. Autumn-gathered plants, especially their uppermost leaves, are likewise not too bad when cooked, *but only after a frost has touched them*. (Warm-weather sow thistle is far too bitter to be palatable, even after having been boiled in several waters.)

The peeled stalks of young *S. oleraceus* plants—harvested after the plant has reached a height of 1 foot and before it flowers—can also be boiled for a few minutes and then doused with butter and devoured. Sow-thistle roots are also edible and can be chopped and added to stews.

HEALTH/MEDICINE

The Kayenta Navajo (Diné) found *S. asper* to be helpful with **heart palpitations** (Wyman and Harris 1951: 50), as did European herbalist Juliette de Bairacli Levy (de Bairacli Levy 1974: 137). Success here may be due to *nervine* properties in the herb, since the Cherokee have also used *S. arvensis* to arrest **nervousness** (Hamel and Chiltoskey 1975: 59). (In my practice as an herbalist, I have noted that heart palpitations are often caused by overworked adrenal glands in their interweaving with the autonomic nervous system.) Many herbalists have discovered that the whitish sap is so potent in this regard that it can even be used to break **addictions!** The Chinese also value sow thistle for its calming ability, which is thought to accrue most effectively from the herb's yellow flowers (Silverman 1990: 15).

Much scientific research has been done on sow thistle of late, substantiating a number of its traditional applications. *S. oleraceus* has demonstrated *anxiolytic* effects in mice (Cardoso Vilela et al. 2009), *antidepressant* activity in mice comparable to the pharmaceutical amitriptyline (Vilela et al. 2010a), *antinociceptive* effects in mice (Vilela et al. 2009), *antidiabetic* effects in rats (Teugwa et al. 2013; Chen et al. 2019), and *antioxidant* activity comparable to that demonstrated for blueberries (McDowell et al. 2011; Ou et al. 2013). Both this species and *S. arvensis* have also shown antibacterial effects against *Streptococcus mutans*, *Staphylococcus aureus*, *Escherichia coli*, and *Salmonella enterica* (Xia et al. 2010; Xia et al. 2011). *S. asper* has been demonstrated to be *nephroprotective* and *hepatoprotective* (Khan et al. 2010; Khan et al. 2011; Khan et al. 2012c), to display *antidiabetic* and *hypolipidemic* effects (Khan 2017), and to manifest *antioxidant* activity (Khan 2012; Khan et al. 2012a, Khan et al. 2012b).

The noted European horticulturist John Gerard believed sow thistle to be possessed of powerful *refrigerant* properties and thus useful for "inflammations or hot swellings" and "gnawing of the stomach" (Gerard 1975: 232). Confirmatory in this regard are 2010 and 2019 scientific studies evincing *anti-inflammatory* effects for *S. oleraceus* (Vilela et al. 2010b; Chen et al. 2019) and a 2018 study showing a powerful *anti–ulcerative colitis* activity for this same species (Alothman et al. 2018).

PERSONAL AND PROFESSIONAL USE

I've found that a tincture of the flowering tops is useful as a cardiac nervine. I usually add it to formulas inclusive of herbs such as hawthorn (*Crataegus* spp.) flowers, motherwort (see page 156), and skullcap (see page 212). However, because

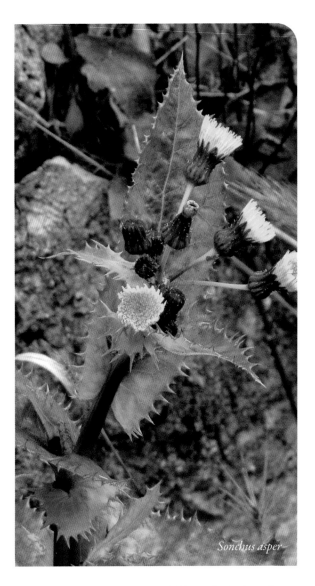

Sonchus asper

sow thistle is not commonly available on the herb market in the United States (although it can usually be purchased from some commercial sources of Chinese herbs), I tend to wildcraft it locally.

CAUTIONS

Be sure that you have trimmed off all the thorns from the leaves of this plant before consuming any of them.

While no plant for human consumption should ever be picked from a roadside owing to issues of heavy-metal contamination, this is especially true of *Sonchus* species, which tend to absorb heavy metals like a magnet!

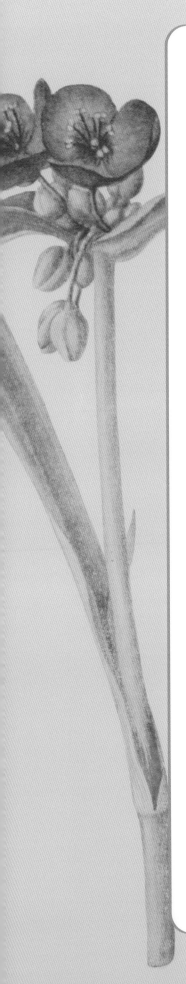

Spiderwort

DESCRIPTION

Spiderwort is a pretty summer perennial growing from 8 inches to 2½ feet tall, with several succulent stems that are usually erect but are sometimes bent.

Leaves are lanceolate—long and narrow, being onion-like to iris-like in their appearance. Large sheathes can be found at their bases. The tendency of both these and the stems to bend gives the appearance of a spider on the hunt, which may be the origin of the herb's name. Others say that the name arose because the herbage, when pulled apart, reveals a sticky, juice-like substance that appears in strands quite similar to a spider's web.

Largely responsible for the plant's legendary beauty is the three-petaled, purplish-blue flower, about 1¼ inches long and possessed of six blue stamens with prominent yellow anthers. These flowers, situated singly at the tips of the plant stems, open only in the morning, while in the afternoon a real sight to see transpires: the flower head closes up, and, in its place, the plant exudes a sticky, gel-like mass. This is due to enzymatic action within the herb and has given spiderwort its alternative common name, widow's tears.

RANGE AND HABITAT

This lovely plant is found in fields, meadows, prairies, open woods, thickets, and roadsides. Various species blanket the entire United States, except for the uppermost northeastern states: *Tradescantia virginiana* (with slightly hairy sepals and stamens) and *T. ohiensis* (with a whitish bloom on the leaves and the stem) preside in the east, and the latter in the very southeastern tip of Minnesota. *T. occidentalis* is dominant in the West and Midwest. Yet another species, *T. bracteata*, is ubiquitous in the southern two-thirds of Minnesota.

MAJOR CONSTITUENTS

To my knowledge, no known chemical work has ever been done on this species, although astringent chemicals are suspected.

FOOD

This plant's succulent leaves, stem, and flowers are quite edible and, in the opinion of many, very tasty. Not surprisingly, then, spiderwort makes an excellent trail snack—especially on a hot summer day, in that it is conveniently high in moisture and quickly chews into a mucilaginous mass. A fine potherb as well, spiderwort can be added to stews or eaten by itself after being boiled in salted water for about five to ten minutes.

It is said that George Washington Carver, the famed food scientist, raved about the flavor of this succulent herb (Fernald and Kinsey 1958: 124). Carver was right—it's downright delicious!

HEALTH/MEDICINE

A tea made from spiderwort has been used by the Cherokee to ease **stomachaches** (especially from overeating), as a *laxative*, and as part of a compound formula for **kidney trouble** as well as for **disorders of the female reproductive system** (Bank 1953: 12–13; Hamel and Chiltoskey 1975: 56, 57). The Cherokee have also poulticed leaves onto **skin**

cancers and rubbed them onto **insect bites** to obtain relief (Hamel and Chiltoskey 1975: 56, 57).

The Meskwaki (Fox) and Kayenta Navajo (Diné) also found medicinal uses for this lovely prairie plant: The former have utilized it as a *urinary* aid (Smith 1928: 209), while the latter have prepared a decoction of the root to treat **internal injuries** (Vestal 1952: 20). The Kayenta Navajo (Diné) also implemented a cold infusion of the root to treat what they called "deer infection" in humans, drinking it and applying it topically in a lotion (Vestal 1952: 20). I sometimes catch myself wondering: Might this have been what we now know as Lyme disease?

UTILITARIAN USES

Spiderwort has been implemented as a pollution indicator, in that its stamen filaments will transform from blue to pink in a period of one and a half to two and a half weeks in the presence of significant levels of pollution or radiation. It has been used extensively by the Environmental Protection Agency.

This herb is also often the plant of choice for cell studies conducted in cytology classrooms because its chromosomes are unusually large, enabling the nucleus and flowing cytoplasm to be viewed with relative ease.

PERSONAL AND PROFESSIONAL USE

I enjoy the taste and texture of this plant very much and eat it extensively while it is available, supplementing my water rations with it (ditto thistles and a few other such fluid-valuable plants), so that sometimes I don't even need to carry a water canteen. Indeed, it is a plant that makes me ache for summer!

I've used spiderwort topically on insect bites and on other skin afflictions, with noticeably good results. My strong suspicion, however, is that this plant possesses nervine properties not as yet elaborated, in that plants with blue-violet or blue-pink flowers—such as skullcap (page 212), blue vervain (page 41), lobelia, chicory (page 78), and pasque flower—tend to be nervines, just as plants with red flowers, fruit, or bark (such as hawthorn, pomegranate, cinnamon, rose, and cayenne) tend to be helpful to the heart and blood and plants with yellow-orange flowers (such as dandelion, page 99) tend to aid the hepatobiliary system. In fact, an association of plant use with colors seems to have been one way that the ancients learned how to implement herbs for healing, being one aspect of what has been called the "doctrine of signatures." ⫷

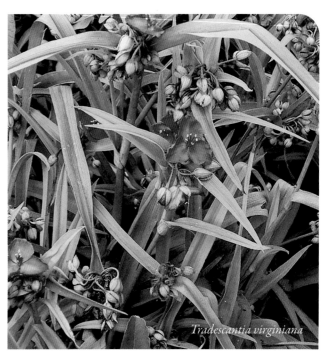

Tradescantia virginiana

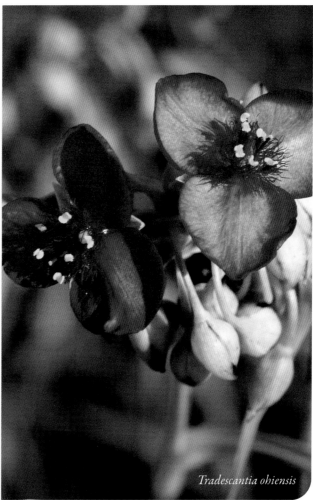

Tradescantia ohiensis

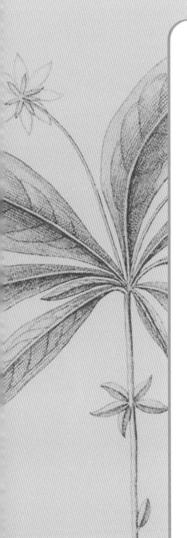

Starflower

STAR ANEMONE; CHICKWEED WINTERGREEN

Trientalis borealis

DESCRIPTION

Starflower is a lovely woodland plant that grows 2–8 inches tall. Its slender, upright stem arises from a horizontal underground rhizome.

This plant is appropriately named: the strikingly star-like flowers have pointed, white petals—usually seven of them, but they can number anywhere from five to nine. The showy stamens project well above the blossoms on hair-like stalks and are tipped with golden anthers.

Shiny, distinctly veined leaves are whorled from the stem. They number anywhere from five to nine (but, again, tend to be usually seven) and are lanceolate, pointed, and of uneven size. Their arrangement and pointed tips add to the overall star-like appearance of this delicate herb.

A small-scale leaf is also present below the whorl and near the middle of the stem.

RANGE AND HABITAT

This plant likes to grow in rich woods and at the edges of bogs—especially in shaded areas. In the Midwest, starflower grows from the east-central region of Minnesota to the west-central area of Wisconsin, and then northward in both states.

HEALTH/MEDICINE

The Montagnais of the Quebec region have steeped an infusion of this species to allay **general sickness** and to help manage the dreaded **tuberculosis** (Speck 1917: 314; Vogel 1970: 271). In the early 1800s, Native American tribes of the Arkansas Territory (including Oklahoma, Missouri, and parts of Kansas) also utilized starflower medicinally, but the details are not known (Vogel 1970: 107).

The Cowlitz of the northwestern United States squeezed the juice from the western species, *Trientalis latifolia*, into water and used it as an eyewash—whether for **infected eyes** or just **sore eyes** is not known (Gunther 1973: 44).

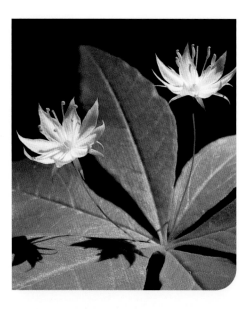

Herbalist Michael Tierra has found the root of our species, *T. borealis*, to be a *qi tonic* (in the model of Traditional Chinese Medicine) and a *stimulant*. He thus uses it for **fatigue, weakness**, and **exhaustion**. He says that it affects the heart, spleen, and lung meridians. Energetically, Tierra finds starflower to be acrid, sweet, and warm (Tierra 1988: 297–98).

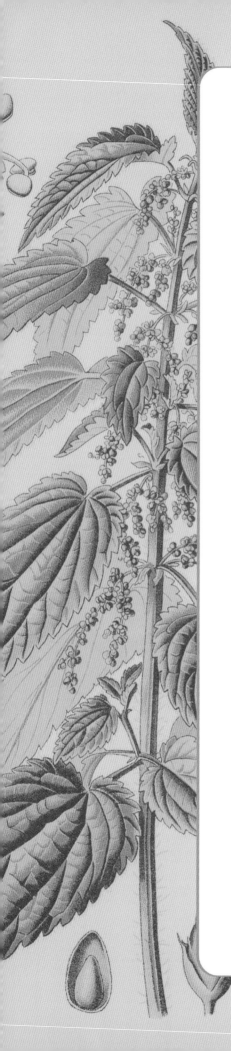

Stinging Nettle

Urtica dioica

DESCRIPTION

Undoubtedly, most persons are familiar with this plant, remembering it well from painful encounters in childhood, during which they suffered a painful, whitish rash from brushing against its stinging hairs! (The rash usually lasts about seven minutes, from which the nickname "seven-minute itch" has arisen for this plant.) But for the few who may not know it, the *Urtica* genus is a tall perennial (2–6 feet, averaging 3¼ feet) with creeping roots and a square stem that doesn't branch.

Its leaves are opposite, ovate to lanceolate, pointed at the tip, and deeply serrated, and they grow to 6 inches long. Dark green in color and prominently veined, they—like the stems on plants of this genus—are covered all over with tiny stinging hairs. Note that two similar-looking plants with which nettle is often confused lack the stinging hairs. These are false nettle, *Boehmeria cylindrica*, and clearweed, *Pilea pumila* (see page 84).

Tiny cream-colored flowers, lacking petals, droop in loose clusters from the leaf axils, the male (with stamens only) and female (with pistils only) often appearing on different plants (though occasionally both on the same). Contrariwise, flowers of the similar-looking false nettle are dark green, while those of clearweed are medium green.

Wood nettle, *Laportea canadensis* (see page 277), also a perennial, has a more succulent look, with wider—and alternate—leaves that are more broadly and conspicuously toothed. However, like its cousin, stinging nettle, it also bears flowers in the leaf axils (although it always has both sexes on the same plant) and stinging hairs on leaf and stem.

RANGE AND HABITAT

Stinging nettle can be found growing on disturbed ground—waste places, vacant lots, garbage dumps, woodland edges, streamsides, roadsides, and trailsides. It is ubiquitous in the Midwest in such environs.

MAJOR CONSTITUENTS

Aboveground portions contain glucoquinones; caffeic, *p*-coumaric, chlorogenic, and carbonic acid; organic acids (acetic, citric, butyric, malic, oxalic, fumaric); sterols (beta-sitosterol); essential oil; carotenoids (lycopene, violaxanthin); flavonoids (quercetin, kaempferol, isorhamnetin, rutin); betaine; lecithin; mucilage; and the enzyme secretin. The seeds contain fatty acids (linoleic, linolenic, oleic, and palmitic). The roots contain saponins, a coumarin (scopoletin), phenolic acids, phenylpropanoid aldehydes, polysaccharides, monoterpenes, triterpenes, and tannins. The stinging hairs contain acetylcholine, histamine, 5-hydroxytryptamine, and possibly formic acid. Nettle's vitamins include pro-vitamin A (in a very high amount), B_1, B_2, B_5, C, D, E, K_1, choline, and folic acid. (The presence of vitamin D is quite notable.) A smorgasbord of minerals includes iron, phosphorus, potassium, sulfur, manganese, calcium, sodium, and silica. It has an extremely high protein content (41 percent by dry weight and 7 percent fresh) and one of the highest contents of both chlorophyll and crude fiber in edible North American plants.

FOOD

Nettle's stinging hairs often discourage both man and beast from having anything to do with this plant. Still, with proper cautions, one need not be balked. Gloves and scissors can reap one a bountiful harvest that can be put to good use!

First, the entire plant can be harvested if under 8 inches tall. If over that height, only the tender young leaves at the top should be taken. This is because mature nettles become tough and develop a grittiness to them due to the formation of tiny, hard calcium crystals called cystoliths, which can irritate the kidneys. To harvest nettles (and many other plants, for that matter), I like to use a large plastic ice-cream pail, through which I have bored two holes and strung some twine in order to loop the bucket around my neck, which leaves my hands free for probing, bending, and clipping the desired plants.

Of course, even when taking reasonable care in harvesting nettles, there are no guarantees that one will not be stung. For example, although I myself have developed collecting techniques whereby I have not been stung by nettles in many years, once while lying over what I thought was simply a bed of dead, bent-over grass stalks in order to photograph some newly emerged nettles for the present work, I arose with the characteristic feel of nettle stings all over my elbows and forearms! I thereby discovered that the grass stalks lay across, and thus hid, an extension of the newly emerging nettle colony that I hadn't figured on and that the pressure of my arms had brought me into direct contact with some of the obscured plants. Needless to say, my entire arms were quickly covered with characteristic nettle welts!

What to do in such a situation? Foragers have traditionally looked for the leaves of dock, jewelweed (see page 136), or plantain (page 180), with which the sting can, it has long been claimed, often be successfully "rubbed out." In my own case, as summarized above, these plants were not readily to be found, so I implemented another age-old remedy—nettle *juice*! Whether it was the high amount of lecithin contained in the juice or some other factor, the traditional cure really did work, to my great delight!

I know of at least one foraging manual that urges the reader to remove nettle leaves from their stems and to rub them with gloved hands to rupture the stinging hairs, thereafter using them in a spring salad. The author of another foraging manual says that he has masticated raw leaves and that the stinging stopped by the time the nettles proceeded down his throat. *I consider these statements to be rash and unmerited in a foraging manual, possibly inviting dangerous experimentation.* While some persons might emerge unscathed from such an experience, others might suffer severe reactions. My background in physiology has alerted me to the fact that everyone's body chemistry is different and that one person's food could be another person's poison. Moreover, this principle is certainly compounded when dealing with the known toxins contained in raw nettle leaves. The possibility of some active stinging

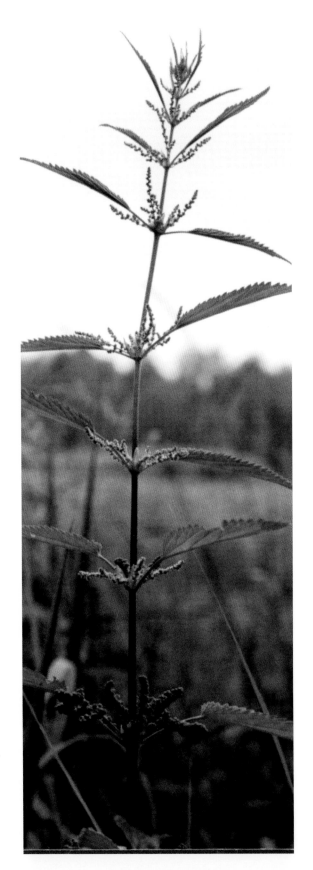

hairs making it through even a thorough glove rubbing or a mastication is quite real, in that they are small, numerous, and quite dexterous. Please, then, do *not* experiment with raw nettles—the results could be truly disastrous. Always remember the forager's rule: safety first!

Nettle's sole culinary use, then, should be as a cooked plant. The leaves can be boiled or steamed, which kills the stinging element; a few minutes is all that is required. They can then be eaten as is (they taste like spinach, but better!) or combined with cream of mushroom soup or other food(s). To avoid a bronze color forming in the leaves, leave the top off the kettle or use more water. This unappealing color change, experienced with bewilderment by foragers when cooking nettles in times past, is now known to be triggered by the high amount of chlorophyll in nettle reacting with natural acids present in the leaves and the cooking water, which then further react with carotenoids in the leaves (Rinzler 1991: 114).

A tea made from dried nettle leaves is quite good, and the reconstituted pieces in the brew can be chewed and eaten while the tea is being drunk. In fact, dried nettles (at least *U. dioica*) reconstitute readily, freshly, and nearly fully in water.

The fleshy pink section between the stem and the rootstock is an especially favored part of the plant for wild-foods foragers.

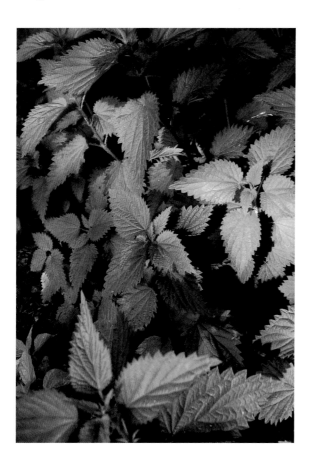

Nettle broth can be made from the roots. A better use of them, however, is to transplant the autumn-dug ones to a cellar or basement in a container of sand, secreting them away in a very dark place and watering them every few days. This procedure, called forcing, fools the plants into putting up shoots through the winter, all of which can be clipped for food or for tea, and this usually two or three times throughout the cold months.

Of course, what greens you have collected in the wild can be frozen, too. Blanch them for two minutes, then cool, pat dry, and freeze.

Nettles are incredibly healthful, containing many vitamins and minerals (see the list under Major Constituents). Two of the more interesting are vitamin D and phosphorus: Vitamin D is available from mushrooms but from very few green plants and is important for the absorption of calcium from the gastrointestinal tract into the blood and for immune function. The phosphorus content accounts, perhaps in part, for the herb's traditional good effect upon teeth and gums.

Interestingly, too, Euell Gibbons found nettle to contain more protein per unit of measurement than any other edible leafy green plant! (Gibbons 1971: 165) The precise numbers are 6.9 percent fresh (Gibbons 1971: 165) and 42 percent by dry weight (Tull 1987: 150). No wonder that inmates of notorious Nazi concentration camps like Malchow and Gross-Rosen found this weed to be so nourishing and helpful: although it often had to be gathered surreptitiously, it no doubt provided more nourishment than all the slop the Nazis tossed their way.

HEALTH/MEDICINE

The truly amazing nettle has a wide variety of therapeutic uses, often related to problems of a **burning** or **stinging** nature—similar to the feeling produced by its own stinging hairs! (Smith 1999: 47)

First, this despised weed serves as an excellent *styptic/hemostat*, both for external **wounds** and for **internal bleeding.** Regarding the former, the Eclectic scholars Harvey Wickes Felter and John Uri Lloyd said concerning topical use of the leaves: "Applied to bleeding surfaces, they are an excellent styptic" (Felter and Lloyd 1898). The Physiomedicalist physician William Cook observed of the latter: "As a local arrester of bleeding, it has few equals; and its infusion or tincture is of much power, used inwardly, for bleeding from the nose, lungs, or stomach, and may also be used for excellent advantage in bleeding from the bowels" (Cook 1985). In fact, both the tea and the fresh juice are useful for internal bleeding, with naturopath Donald Lepore having recommended a teaspoon of the juice every hour (Lepore 1988: 183), a dosage that might be committed to memory for any serious internal injuries that might occur in the wilderness when medical help is too far away. A scientific article published in 1990 reported that lectins isolated from this plant were observed to display hemagglutination activity (Willer and Wagner 1990), thus providing some scientific testimony for the plant's traditional use as a styptic/hemostat.

Then, too, this herb is considered the supreme *blood tonic* of Western herbalism. Chemical analysis has shown that it holds a high amount of iron and vitamin C (the latter necessary for the absorption of the former from plant sources) as well as an unusually high amount of chlorophyll, which chemical's structure resembles that of hemoglobin. Not surprising, then, are the results of an interesting study published in 2003, in which rats received subcutaneous injections for forty-five days of a chemical to lower their hematological values, and then fifteen of these received an intraperitoneal injection of 2 milliliters per kilogram of nettle-root "oils" for forty-five additional days, while fifteen others received a saline solution over the same time frame. The nettle-root-treated group displayed improved red blood cells, white blood cells, packed cell volume (PCV), and hemoglobin levels over the control group (Meral and Kanter 2003).

Then, too, nettle in the form of a tea has been advised for **itchy crotch** (Manning et al. 1972: 79). In fact, it is often recommended by herbalists to treat **skin conditions** in general, owing to a perceived *depurative* effect (Kresanek and Krejca 1989: 196). The *British Herbal Pharmacopoeia* says the herb is specifically indicated for **psychogenic eczema** as well as for **infantile eczema** (Hyde et al. 1976–79: 1:217). Further as to youngsters, Celsus, a medical-wise scholar of the late first century, found (as reported in his *De Medicina* 4.24) that mashed nettle seeds in water served as a *vermifuge* for **threadworms** in children.

This herb has also long been acknowledged as a valuable *diuretic* (Fyfe 1903; Weiss 1988: 255; Kresanek and Krejca 1989: 196; Bradley et al. 1992: 166), which action has been confirmed in a clinical trial (Kirchoff 1983). Another scientific experiment confirmed that the juice produced a diuretic effect in sufferers of both chronic venous deficiency and myocardial deficiency (Leung and Foster 1996: 384), supporting nettle leaf's use by Western herbalists for edema arising from congestive heart failure or from chronic venous insufficiency (Weiss 1988: 261). This diuretic effect has also allowed herbalists to recommend it for a condition much more common than the either of the above: **premenstrual bloating** (McQuade-Crawford 1996). Then, too, the Eclectics lauded the use of this common weed for **chronic cystitis**, especially when manifesting as a mucoid discharge (Fyfe 1909; Felter 1922). It is also one of the more frequently used herbs for **interstitial cystitis** (Tilgner 2000).

Nettle's most famous and traditional application has been in the treatment of **hay fever (allergic rhinitis).** Interesting here is that a randomized, double-blind study of a freeze-dried preparation of the plant found it to be about as effective in the human test group as hay fever medications of the standard over-the-counter and prescription variety (Mittman 1990; cf. Fisher 1997). The freeze-dried form preserves the histamine content, which many feel is vital to halting the allergic process—either by interfering with the body's release of histamine or by stimulating the body to make its own antihistamines. Interesting as this theory is, the clinical experience of numerous herbalists throughout history reveals that nettles do not need to be freeze-dried to produce relief for allergy sufferers. I, myself, have been privileged to have helped scores of hay fever sufferers with just plain ol' nettle tea, tincture, or capsules! I can't help but wonder whether this is due, at least partly, to the plant's renowned strengthening effect upon the adrenal glands, so important in the body's immune balance. As the famed endocrinologist John Tintera was so fond of communicating to his readers, a lack of potency in these glands allows allergic reactions to proceed unchecked (Tintera 1959).

From time immemorial, the nettle plant has been used by sufferers of **arthritis**, **rheumatism**, and **gout** as a counterirritant, with claimed results of fair to excellent. The Quinault have used the related species *Urtica lyallii* in the same fashion (Gunther 1973: 28). Celsus even urged the use of nettle whips to resolve or ameliorate **paralysis** owing to "stimulating the skin of the torpid limb" (Celsus 1938: 3.27). Orthodox medicine has summarily dismissed this practice as ignorant and useless. But herbal writer Donald Law cannot agree, pointing out: "In that mysterious acid of the sting lie some curative properties which both the Romans and the Aztecs have recorded quite independently of one another, and as a young man I experienced myself" (Law 1976: 32). Interestingly, the results proceeding from a late-1990s exploratory study suggested some clear benefits from this self-flagellation: eighteen persons undergoing a trial of nettle-sting therapy for joint pain were interviewed by researchers, with the result that all but one of those interviewed expressed praise for the therapy, and several even considered it a cure! The authors concluded the study with the stated impression that the therapy was safe, useful, and inexpensive and that it should be investigated in more detail (Randall et al. 1999).

Some have suggested that nettle, applied as a poultice to rheumatic joints, draws uric acid out of the body (Lepore 1988: 183; Ody 1993: 108). In a British study published in 2000, a poultice of nettle leaves on osteoarthritic joints of the thumb and fingers of twenty-seven people greatly reduced their pain in such spots after merely a week of treatment! (Randall et al. 2000) A goodly number of Native American tribes utilized a tea of the herb for rheumatic pains (Moerman 1986: 1:498). It is even endorsed for this use by the *Commission E Monographs*, prepared by a panel of German scientists (Blumenthal 1998). Moreover, some good scientific evidence exists for *anti-inflammatory* activity: the coumarin scopoletin and several of the plant acids in nettle have shown anti-inflammatory effects in scientific studies. Two clinical trials have even shown that ingestion of nettle leaf reduced the amount of anti-inflammatory drugs needed to moderate arthritic pain (Ramm and Hansen 1995; Chrubasik et al. 1997). A more recent study demonstrated that an extract from nettle leaf inhibited the proinflammatory transcription factor NF-κB (Riehemann et al. 1999).

Scientific research way back in the 1920s demonstrated a *cardiotonic* action for nettle (Hermann and Remy 1922). A tea of this herb has been a traditional treatment for hypertension in Morocco and in some other lands. Several modern scientific studies have elucidated stinging nettle's positive effects on the cardiovascular system: in a study published in 2002, both the aqueous and the alcoholic extracts of the root elicited a negative-inotropic effect in spontaneously beating atria of guinea pigs, a vasodilatory action in aortic-ring preparations with intact endothelial layers, and a significant and transient hypotensive effect in anesthetized rats. The conclusion of the researchers was that the root induced a *vasorelaxant* effect, mediated by three factors: a negative inotropic action, a release of endothelial nitric oxide, and an opening of potassium channels (Testai et al. 2002; cf. Legssyer et al. 2002). In another study involving male Wistar rats, an intravenous perfusion of the herbage created a reduction of blood pressure accompanied by a correlative increase of diuresis and of natriuresis. It was concluded that the herbage produced an acute *hypotensive* action with direct action on the cardiovascular and the renal systems (Tahri et al. 2000). Research published in 2016 has further clarified nettle's hypotensive activity (Qayyum et al. 2016).

Nettle leaf is also a time-honored *galactagogue*—stimulating the production of breast milk in lactating women (Ellingwood 1983: 355; Ody 1993: 108).

A good number of scientific studies have found the root of nettle to be of great help in offsetting urinary retention associated with **benign prostatic hypertrophy**, a condition affecting many elderly men (Belaiche and Leivoux 1991; Krzeski et al. 1993; Schneider et al. 1995; Lichius and Muth 1997; Sökeland and Albrecht 1997; Safarinejad 2005). The same has been demonstrated when this botanical was taken along with either saw palmetto (*Serenoa repens*) (Schneider et al. 1995; Sökeland and Albrecht 1997; Engelmann et al. 2006) or pygeum (*Pygeum africanum*) (Melo 2002; Safarinejad 2005). It has also shown equivalent effects to finasteride and to other prescription medications for BPH but without the undesirable sexual side effects often associated with the pharmaceuticals (Bartsch et al. 1998). Nettle root has been shown to act via at least two different pathways: (1) interrupting binding of sex hormone–binding globulin (SHBG) to its receptor site on the prostate, thus decreasing the amplification of the androgen signal by estrogen, and (2) inhibiting prostate Na+/K+-ATPase enzyme, preventing

prostate cells from multiplying (Belaiche and Leivoux 1991; Hirano et al. 1994; Wagner et al. 1994; Gansser and Spiteller 1995b; Hryb et al. 1995; Schöttner et al. 1997; Lichius et al. 1999). In one study, a combination of stinging-nettle root and pygeum bark inhibited metabolism of testosterone into both dihydrotestosterone (DHT) and estradiol (Hartmann et al. 1996).

Nettle root's effects on the prostate have suggested to some that it might be helpful in prostate cancer, and, indeed, a lab study published in 2000 demonstrated that it exerted an *antiproliferative* effect on human prostate cancer cells (Konrad et al. 2000). In a later study, even an aqueous extract of the leaf inhibited adenosine deaminase activity in prostate tissue derived from patients afflicted with prostate cancer (Durak et al. 2004).

Furthermore, the evidence demonstrating that nettle root is a DHT blocker might explain another traditional use of this herb: as a warrior in the battle against male-pattern baldness (in both men and women), since an excessive amount of DHT has been shown to damage hair follicles. Not only that, but the leaf's high content of quality protein, not to mention its silica, would undoubtedly contribute to the normal growth and health of hair, as well as to its strength.

Scientific research is also finding nettle root to exert *cytotoxic* and *antiproliferative* effects in **colorectal cancer** (Ghasemi et al. 2016; Mohammadi et al. 2016).

Lastly, the benefits of the seed must be mentioned: it has been found to reduce serum creatinine levels in those suffering from various forms of renal disease (Treasure 2003). Much of the modern-day clinical research on its benefits in this regard has been pioneered by an American herbalist named David Winston.

PERSONAL AND PROFESSIONAL USE

I could probably write for days on the ways that I have utilized stinging nettle but will try to condense that information into a few paragraphs here.

Firstly, I have enjoyed cooking and eating nettles since I was a teen. There are few tastes to match that of a properly cooked mess of nettle greens topped with a dollop of organic butter! (Just writing about it here now has gotten my appetite going something fierce.)

I also drink a strong infusion of nettle leaves from time to time—not only for its rich taste but also for its blood-building and adrenal-supportive effects. I often recommend the infusion to clients for its blood-building effects, too, especially to those undergoing chemotherapy to the point where their red blood cells and hemoglobin have been knocked down too low.

Because of nettle leaf's abundance of minerals, I also advise the use of the capsules to those who manifest mineral deficiencies or who test low in minerals via laboratory hair analysis.

Probably my most frequent recommendation for the leaf, however, has been for hay fever, for which it almost always makes a significant impact. Other complaints for which I have used it to good benefit have included psychogenic eczema, gout (as a formula ingredient), and interstitial cystitis (as a formula ingredient).

I use the root a lot for benign prostatic hypertrophy (BPH), prostate cancer, polycystic ovary syndrome (PCOS) marked preeminently by male-pattern baldness, and low libido in which laboratory analysis of the blood shows an elevated level of sex hormone–binding globulin (SHBG). For all of these conditions, it typically provides marked relief.

Finally, for the past decade or so, I have advised the use of nettle seed for kidney concerns manifested by an elevated serum creatinine level. (This marker should never exceed 1.2 milligrams per deciliter; when it does, each tenth of a point represents a significant loss of kidney function.) On all of those occasions, about two dozen by now, it has served ably to reduce the serum creatinine. (Coincidentally, just as I am writing this, one of my clients with a history of elevated creatinine has called for a refill of his nettle-seed tincture. His creatinine was at 3.4, but with the use of nettle seed it has been reduced to 1.9! He and I have no doubts that his level will continue to go down with sustained use.)

CAUTIONS

Do not eat fresh, raw nettle plant parts. Do not eat whole plants after the height of 8 inches is reached (see under Food) or even individual leaves from plants over that height except uppermost newly emerging leaves, which can be snipped off and boiled throughout most of the growing season.

Use gloves to collect so as to avoid being stung. If stung, rub leaves from dock (see page 104) or plantain (page 180) on the sting to allay. Nettle juice itself can be used instead, if it can be procured without further stinging. The hairs that transmit the sting are actually small capillary tubes, composed of silica at the upper end and calcium at the lower end. As to the exact mechanism of the sting, even the technological wonders of today's phytochemists have not explicated its mysteries in full, despite tedious work. Many herbals allege that the chemical agent responsible for the sting is formic

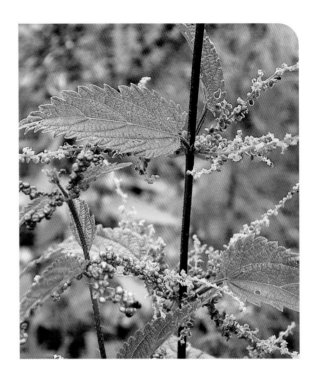

acid (the toxin found in red ants), which, depending on the analysis one consults, may or may not occur in the plant. However, a growing body of evidence since World War II has suggested that the sting is due to several compounds not inclusive of formic acid, with the consensus being histamine, acetylcholine, 5-hydroxytryptamine (5-HT), and at least one other unidentified substance—perhaps a histamine liberator (Emmelin and Feldberg 1947; Collier and Chesher 1956). Work by Saxena et al. in the mid-1960s buttressed the hypothesis of a histamine liberator (Saxena et al. 1965), arguing for an endogenous release of histamine to account for the persistent itching. Some European researchers have opted for a substance with the potential for secondary release of other mediators or even a nerve toxin because they also agree that histamine, acetylcholine, and 5-HT could not be responsible for the persistence of the sting but only for the initial phase of it (Oliver et al. 1991; cf. Kulze and Greaves 1988). ᘓᘓᘓ

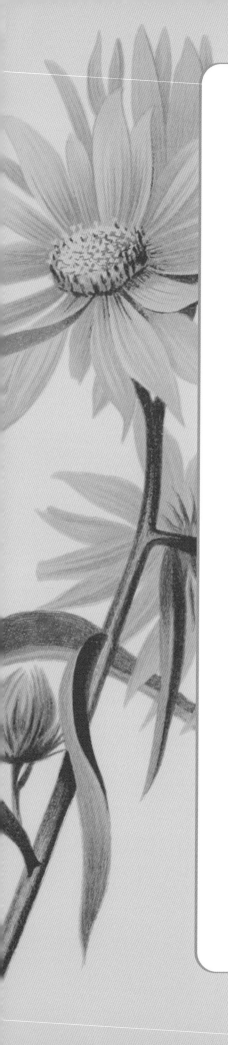

Sunflower

Helianthus spp.

DESCRIPTION

Sunflowers are tall annual or perennial plants with firm and upright stems, composite flowers consisting of a disk flower with ten to twenty-five yellow ray flowers, and dark-green leaves that are serrated.

A large variety of species exists throughout the United States and Canada, with a dozen or more thriving in the Midwest, including the following:

Helianthus annuus (common sunflower) is an annual growing 3–9 feet tall that is possessed of a brownish disk flower 3–9 inches wide and alternate, oval, or heart-shaped leaves that reach 3–7 inches.

H. giganteus (giant, great, or tall sunflower) grows to 11 feet tall and sports a rough reddish (or purplish) stem, sessile or short-stalked leaves that are lanceolate and mostly alternate (but occasionally opposite), and numerous light-yellow flower heads (1½–3 inches wide) having ten to twenty ray flowers, long-pointed bracts, and hairs on the flower stems just below the blossoms.

H. grosseserratus (saw-toothed sunflower) grows 4–10 feet tall and is possessed of hairless stems. Its leaves are lanceolate and coarsely toothed—like saw blades, thus its common name. Their undersides are covered with a whitish down.

H. × *laetiflorus* (stiff, showy, perennial, or cheerful sunflower) grows 2–8 feet tall. Its stem is covered with stiff hairs. Leaves are alternate. Its disk flower is yellow or even purple.

H. hirsutus (hairy sunflower) grows up to 7 feet tall. Its leaves and stems are covered with stiff hairs. The disk flower is yellow.

H. maximiliani (Maximilian's sunflower) is a prairie perennial 3–9 feet tall sporting a yellow disk flower on a head that is 2–3 inches wide. It has alternate, narrow, downy, and tapering leaves that grow 4–6 inches long and are often folded lengthwise and reflexed downward at the tips.

H. strumosus (pale-leaved wood sunflower) reaches 3–7 feet and has a smooth and branching stem that is often covered with a whitish bloom. It displays a yellow disk flower that is surrounded by nine to fifteen ray flowers. Its leaves are mostly opposite and grow 3–8 inches long on winged stalks, while its basal leaves reveal downy undersides.

Yet other species in the Midwest include *H. petiolaris*, *H. occidentalis*, and *H. rigidus*. Jerusalem artichoke (*H. tuberosus*) is also a sunflower but is discussed under a separate profile (see page 134).

RANGE AND HABITAT

Sunflowers can be found throughout most of the United States and Canada. Their preferred habitat is dry fields, prairies, waste places, and dry plains. One or another species is pretty much ubiquitous throughout the Midwest.

MAJOR CONSTITUENTS

The plant contains quercimetrin (a flavonoid), tannins, potassium carbonate, and potassium nitrate. The seeds contain lecithin, betaine (trimethylglycine), and albumin and are rich in vitamin E (75 milligrams per 100 grams), fatty acids (oleic and linoleic), and free-form amino acids (they are especially high in phenylalanine and S-Adenosyl methionine [SAMe] and are perhaps the highest known source of arginine).

FOOD

Sunflower seeds (available generally from *H. annuus* and *H. maximiliani* only) have been a favorite food of many Native American tribes. After knocking the sunflower head with a stick to loosen the seeds into a collecting implement, they would parch them over a fire. Next, they would pound them to loosen the hulls and then winnow these in the breeze. Finally, the kernels would be eaten as is or else powdered into meal and then prepared as a mush or gruel or made into cakes and cooked. The explorers Lewis and Clark described eating one of these repasts in their journal, under the date of July 17, 1805: "The Indians of the Missouri ... first parch and pound [the sunflower seed] between two stones, until it is reduced to a fine meal. ... They add a sufficient portion of marrow-grease to reduce it to the consistency of common dough, and eat it in that manner. This ... composition we ... thought ... at that time a very palatable dish."

Native tribes also found that the seedhead, or fruit, can be crushed and boiled to release sunflower oil, which can then be skimmed off the surface of the water and used as a salad oil or mixed with other foods as advisable.

Although nearly everyone knows about the edibility of sunflower seeds and oil, few realize that the best investment from the plants in the way of total food volume and accessibility is the unopened flower buds, which can be prepared as a potherb. As such, however, these must be boiled in several changes of water in order to remove their bitter principles. I personally find these buds quite tasty when prepared as described but practically unpalatable otherwise.

Available occasionally from species such as *H. laetiflorus*, *H. maximiliani*, and *H. strumosus* are edible tubers, which can be dug, cleaned, and consumed raw on the spot or else prepared in various ways at home. Another tuberous sunflower is the well-known Jerusalem artichoke (see page 134). However, tubers of the first three species are easier to clean in the field and less likely to produce flatulence when eaten raw than are those of Jerusalem artichoke since they contain less of the indigestible carbohydrate inulin than do those of the latter. In fact, I have frequently enjoyed them as a trail nibble.

HEALTH/MEDICINE

The common sunflower, *H. annuus*, has been the species most used medicinally. Most of its applications would seem to suggest that it has an affinity to the region of the chest and neck. For example, **pulmonary troubles** have been

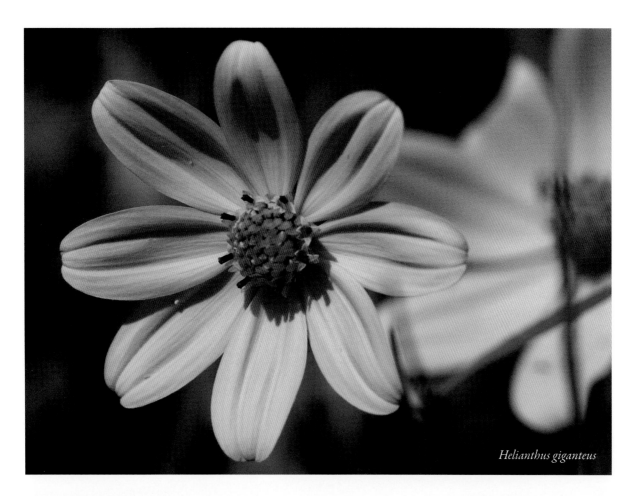

Helianthus giganteus

addressed by the Teton Dakota with this plant by boiling the flower heads (minus bracts) and drinking the resultant decoction (Gilmore 1991: 78). The Houma discovered that sunflower stalks could be made into a tea that was particularly useful for **whooping cough** (Speck 1941: 60). White herbalists have also used an infusion or syrup of the plant for the same, as well as for related respiratory complaints such as **bronchitis**, **coughs**, **sore throat**, and the early stages of **tuberculosis** (Wren 1972: 297; Hutchens 1991: 269). Sunflower seeds have also long been regarded as being *expectorant* (Wren 1972: 296), with an infusion of them having been used as such by America's Eclectic physicians of the late nineteenth and early twentieth centuries (Millspaugh 1974: 330).

As noted in the centennial edition of the *United States Dispensatory* and in other sources, this plant has a long tradition of use—and some scientific support—for treating **malaria** (Millspaugh 1974: 330; Carse 1989: 162). Interestingly here, sunflower contains bitter sesquiterpene lactones, the same chemicals found in boneset (*Eupatorium perfoliatum*), another plant traditionally and effectively used for malaria (see page 44). American healers have typically preferred an infusion of the stems for dealing with malaria (Millspaugh 1974: 33), while the British have tended to use an infusion of the leaves (Wren 1972: 297) and the Russians a decoction of the seeds, flowers, and leaves (Hutchens 1991: 271). Soft, pulpy parts of the stems have also been implemented by Russian healers for **fever** in general (Hutchens 1991: 271).

Sunflower has been much appreciated by Native Americans as a *vulnerary*. The Ojibwe have pounded the roots in order to poultice them onto **bruises** and **contusions** (Hoffman 1891: 199). The Thompson found that mixing the dried and powdered leaves of the common sunflower with some animal grease makes a healing ointment for both **sores** and **swellings** (Turner et al. 1990: 46). The Zuni have poulticed the chewed roots of this plant, along with those of three other plants, onto snakebites (Youngken 1925: 17). Various tribes have used a sunflower infusion as a wash for both **rheumatism** and **gout** (Hutchens 1991: 268). None of the abovementioned uses are surprising in view of a 1976 study that showed an extract from this plant was *anti-inflammatory* in the carrageenan-induced, rat-paw edema lab test (Benoit et al. 1976: 164). Perhaps sunflower's phenylalanine content is a factor in reducing pain.

The seeds manifest *diuretic* activity (Wren 1972: 297), and hence the Russians have used a decoction of them for **heart problems** as well as for **kidney** and **bladder ailments** (Hutchens 1991: 271). Likewise, the Physiomedicalist physician William Cook observed: "A decoction of the bruised acheniae [seeds and husks], made by boiling an ounce in a quart of water to a pint, acts quite efficiently upon the kidneys—promoting the flow of urine, and soothing inflamed and irritable conditions both of the kidneys and bladder. They are suited for acute cases, and deserve more attention than what they have received. It also acts well on irritable coughs" (Cook 1985).

PERSONAL AND PROFESSIONAL USE

Cooked sunflower buds (prepared in several waters, as outlined under Food) are one of my favorite potherbs. I have also often enjoyed eating raw tubers from the three sunflower species that are known to produce them. ✍

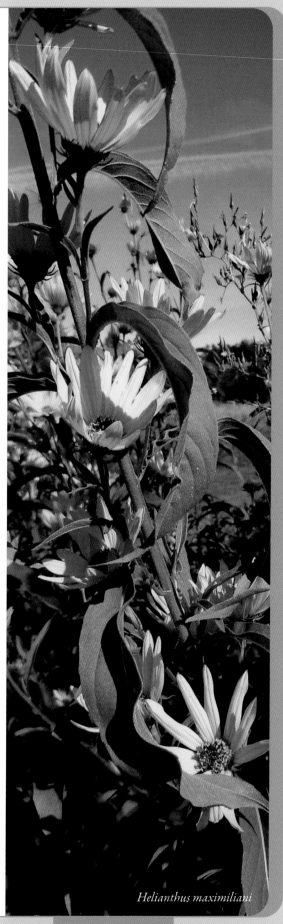

Helianthus maximiliani

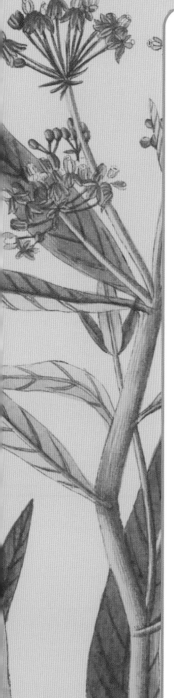

Swamp Milkweed

MARSH MILKWEED; ROSE MILKWEED; SWAMP SILKPLANT

Asclepias incarnata

DESCRIPTION

Swamp milkweed is a lovely native perennial growing 1–4 feet high and bearing a smooth, erect stem. Inside the stem flows a milky-white juice possessed of a strong odor.

The top part of this plant is branched and quite leafy. The oblong to lanceolate leaves are stalked, opposite, hairy (especially below), cordate, and lacking teeth, although they are sharp edged. They grow 4–7 inches long and 1–2 inches wide.

The gorgeous flowers, blooming from May to August, are pink to pink-red and clustered into several small umbels. In the fall, these are replaced by smooth, erect pods that are 3 inches long and that ultimately burst asunder, releasing many seeds that are tufted with silky hairs.

The plant's rhizome is oblong, 4–6 inches long, yellowish brown, knotty and hard, and covered with a thin, strong bark through which many tiny rootlets emerge.

RANGE AND HABITAT

Swamp milkweed thrives in sunny, wet areas, such as bogs, marshes, moist meadows, swamps, and the borders of streams and ponds. It is found throughout the Midwest.

MAJOR CONSTITUENTS

Swamp milkweed contains cardioactive glycosides (cardenolides), including asclepiadin, as well as resin, essential oil, albumin, and pectin.

HEALTH/MEDICINE

This plant's rhizome was listed in the *United States Pharmacopeia* from 1820 to 1863 and from 1873 to 1882. It was a favorite medicine of the Eclectic physicians who practiced in America in the late 1800s through the early 1900s. Finley Ellingwood, as a representative of such, found it to be *emetic, anthelmintic, stomachic,* and *diuretic.* He especially valued this species for the latter property, diuresis, finding it to be "speedy and certain" in that regard (Ellingwood 1983: 451). The Iroquois have likewise appreciated this aspect of swamp milkweed, holding that the plant's rhizome was helpful either where there was too much urine or where there was too little of it! (Herrick 1977: 418) Even the dreaded **dropsy** yielded to swamp milkweed, Ellingwood found—not simply because of the plant's diuretic properties but because it "affects the heart and arteries … strengthens the heart" (Ellingwood 1983: 451). (This is due to the presence of cardioactive glycosides and perhaps to additional factors.) Then, too, both the Iroquois and the Meskwaki (Fox) discovered that a wash or bath made from swamp milkweed rhizome was "strengthening" to the human system, perhaps referring here to some sort of *cardiotonic* (as per above) or otherwise stimulating assist (Densmore 1974: 364–65; Herrick 1977: 418).

As with many milkweeds (see page 151), this species has also been deemed anthelmintic, with Ellingwood advising ten to twenty grains of the root for vanquishing **worms** (Ellingwood 1983: 451), while other Eclectics found that 2–4 fluid ounces of the tea, taken three times a day, did the trick (Felter and Lloyd 1898). There is an ethnobotanical study that weighs in on this, too: Huron Smith, in his study of the Meskwaki (Fox), related that a healer working with this tribe—a Potawatomi medicine man named

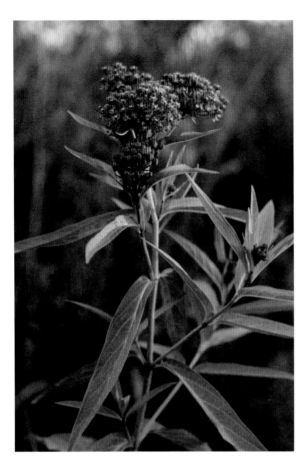

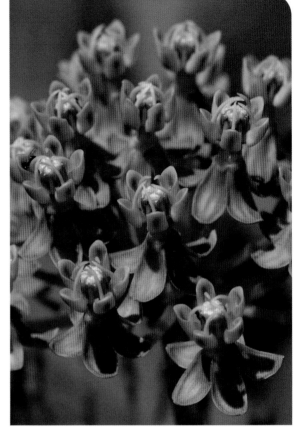

John McIntosh—had "recovered four long tape worms from a woman by its use. The root is said to drive the worms from a person in one hour's time" (Smith 1928: 205). If there is no exaggeration involved here, this would indeed mark swamp milkweed as a *taenifuge* of the first rank! (Smith relates further that McIntosh had also achieved fame by stabilizing a case of dropsy with swamp milkweed when regular physicians had failed. As we noted above, this would not be out of line with what Ellingwood and other Eclectic physicians found to be possible for this species of *Asclepias*.)

The dreaded **erysipelas** was likewise treated by the Eclectics with swamp milkweed, using it both internally and externally on the eruptions (Ellingwood 1983: 451). The Eclectics also used swamp milkweed for many **respiratory afflictions**, especially relative to **catarrhal inflammation** in the respiratory structures (Ellingwood 1983: 451). The botanical scholar Constantine Rafinesque noted that western Native American tribes had used the roots for **asthma** (Rafinesque 1828–30: 1:76). In the east, the Iroquois appreciated swamp milkweed for its beneficial effects upon **urinary stricture** (Herrick 1995: 198).

As it was held to improve digestion, *Asclepias incarnata* was often prescribed by the Eclectics when **chronic gastric catarrh** and/or **diarrhea** was present (Ellingwood 1983: 451). Earlier, too, Rafinesque noted that western tribes had used it

for **dysentery** (Rafinesque 1828–30: 1:76). Although swamp milkweed is seldom used by modern herbalists, the *PDR for Herbal Medicines* notes that the usage for **digestive disorders** has persisted in some areas up until the present day (Fleming 1998).

PERSONAL AND PROFESSIONAL USE

This is the only milkweed species growing in the Midwest with which I have no experience, other than admiring its beautiful flowers and watching the monarch butterflies alighting on them! For other milkweeds in the Midwest, see pages 66 and 151 for butterfly-weed and milkweed, respectively.

CAUTIONS

Owing to its content of both resin and cardioactive glycosides, this plant can prove to be strongly *emetic*. In view of this, and because of the very presence of cardioactive glycosides that can powerfully affect the heart, swamp milkweed *should not be used by the layperson*. Dosage can be crucial with plants containing glycosides such as these, and erring on the side of too much could prove to be disastrous. Use *only* under professional guidance, preferably somebody well practiced and skilled in its use. ⤺

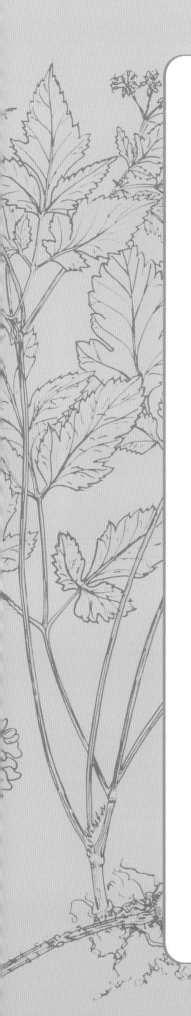

Sweet Cicely

WILD ANISE

Osmorhiza spp.

DESCRIPTION

The American sweet cicely—not to be confused with the European sweet cicely, *Myrrhis odorata*, sometimes to be found in the spice section of the supermarket—is a perennial plant growing 1–4 feet tall. It springs from a fleshy, carrot-like root that can grow to 6 inches in length.

The alternate leaves, spreading out from long leafstalks, are compound and fern-like. There are three leaflets, which are bluntly and irregularly toothed. All in all, the leaves have an appearance similar to that of carrots.

The long-stalked flowers are tiny, white, five-petaled, and arranged in flat-topped, long-stalked clusters. Each umbel is divided into three to eight rays.

Fruits are linear, oblong, and curved, resembling string beans. They are about an inch long and possessed of an anise scent and flavor. In the fall, they become more tapered, turn black, and develop stiff, clinging hairs. At this stage, they can easily wind up clinging to clothes and to fur.

Several species occur in the Midwest, including the following:

Osmorhiza longistylis (anise root) has very fleshy roots that are strongly scented and flower styles that are long, slender, and plainly visible while the plant is flowering.

O. claytonii (scent root), has a root that is less fleshy and less scented than the above species. Its flower styles are barely visible at first. The fruits end in two points.

Two other species—*O. chilensis* and *O. obtusa*—occur only in the extreme northeastern tip of Minnesota. The latter is pubescent, and its fruit styles are bent sharply outward.

RANGE AND HABITAT

Sweet cicely can be found in moist woods throughout the Midwest.

MAJOR CONSTITUENTS

Sweet cicely contains an essential oil consisting chiefly of anethole.

FOOD

I enjoy nibbling on this plant's fruit pods and young stems and being rewarded with their rich, anise-like flavor. (These parts can also be steeped to make a pleasant-tasting tea.) The roots are also edible and can be dug into late fall or early winter—that is, if the ground is not frozen. They can be either eaten raw or grated and cooked. The Midwest's Menomini have relished these roots (Black 1973: 163). They've looked upon them as being a marvelous fattener for skinny people; however, they've felt that they must be consumed slowly—only one section at a time (Smith 1923: 72).

Both the seeds and the roots can be used as seasoning for baked goods and for other dishes. Here the roots are dried and stored, then scraped or powdered when ready to use. (Such a methodology best preserves the potency of the essential oils and thereby the full, rich taste.)

Before you use what you think to be sweet cicely, be absolutely certain that you have the right herb, because it closely resembles a most toxic plant (see under Cautions).

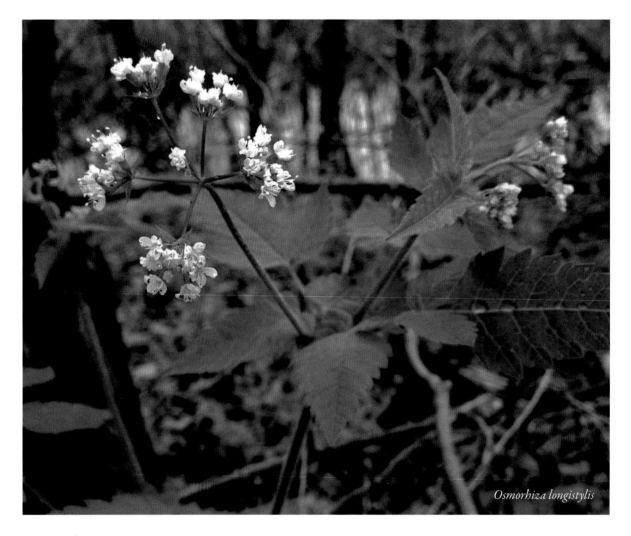

Osmorhiza longistylis

HEALTH/MEDICINE

Herbalist David Winston regards this herb as a valuable *adaptogen* (Winston 1992: 98). It seems to have been used by several Native American tribes for this very purpose—the Pawnee, for instance, regarding it as a staple for **debility** and for **general weakness** (Gilmore 1991: 55) and the Iroquois treasuring the autumn-harvested roots as a **tonic** (Herrick 1995: 196).

Sweet cicely has also been used as a wash for **sore eyes** by several Native tribes (Smith 1928: 249; Smith 1933: 86). Our own area's Ojibwe have esteemed the plant as a topical treatment for **ulcers** and for **running sores** (Densmore 1974: 354) and used the root for a gargle for **sore throat** (Smith 1932: 391). For **colds**, the Thompson and Okanogan have chewed the root of the western species, *O. occidentalis* (Turner et al. 1980: 158; Turner et al. 1990: 45). The Bella Coola of British Columbia found the root of this species to be invaluable for treating **pneumonia** (Smith 1928: 61). The Iroquois have regarded *O. claytonii* as an important **fever** medicine, boiling two medium-sized roots in 3 quarts of water until 1 quart remained—or, for children, steeping a lone root in 1½ quarts of water until it turned blue and then giving the youngsters a little bit at a time (Herrick 1995: 196).

Winston feels that sweet cicely strengthens what Traditional Chinese Medicine refers to as *wei qi*, defined as the body's defensive energy that can help offset pernicious influences, such as colds (Winston 1992: 98).

Sweet cicely would appear to support the gastrointestinal system most ably. The Potawatomi have treasured an infusion of the root as a *stomachic* (Smith 1933: 86). The Iroquois have appreciated it as a treatment for **diarrhea** (Herrick 1995: 196), as have tribes of the Nevada region (but utilizing a related species) (Train et al. 1988: 73). Here the typical preparation and dosage for a child is to steep two pieces, each about 2 inches long, for five minutes in a cup of water, then to give a teaspoonful (Herrick 1995: 196). Yet sweet cicely has been most especially esteemed by the Native tribes as a carminative for **flatulence** and for **colicky pains** (Train et al. 1988: 73). The Physiomedicalists shared this appreciation, with William Cook of their number observing: "It is gently warming to the stomach, and may be used in mild dyspepsia and in flatulent colic." He added that it is best used as a tincture "treated with thirty percent alcohol," as opposed to "treating it with hot water" (i.e., as an infusion), which would "render it worthless" (Cook 1985).

The Omaha have mashed the roots of sweet cicely as a poultice for **boils** (Gilmore 1991: 55), whereas the Winnebago (Ho-Chunk) have done the same for **wounds** (Gilmore 1991: 55).

The Ojibwe have utilized a tea made from the roots as a *parturient* (Smith 1932: 391). The Blackfoot have used *O. occidentalis* for the latter purpose as well (Hellson and Gadd 1974: 61).

The Kawaiisu discovered that an infusion of a related species, *O. brachypoda*, killed **fleas** when used as a hair wash (Zigmond 1981: 47).

Some herbalists (including Terry Willard, one of my early herbalism teachers) have found sweet cicely to be helpful as one plant in a compound tea (inclusive also of licorice and sassafras) to control **sugar-metabolism problems** (Willard 1992a).

PERSONAL AND PROFESSIONAL USE

There are few trail nibbles that are more pleasant to my palate than the seeds of sweet cicely! In the summer of 2011, I found a huge stand of the plant, to which I returned day after day for ten days straight to relish the incredible anise taste of the seeds.

Medicinally, I have observed that at least the root seems to exert a trophorestorative effect upon the adrenals and upon how they regulate blood sugar—in other words, it exhibits a true adaptogenic effect. It is a shame that it is not regularly available on the herb market, although I am glad that it is available in my area via wildcrafting.

CAUTIONS

Do not confuse this plant with the deadly water hemlock (*Cicuta* spp.), which also grows in the Midwest and has similar-looking leaves and umbelliferous flowers. (See page 197 for more information on this plant and another lookalike.) The flowering stage of baneberry (*Actaea* spp.), another plant with some toxicity, looks quite similar to sweet cicely as well.

In short, do not ingest what you think may be sweet cicely unless the plant exudes a strong anise-like or licorice-like scent. Even then, *be absolutely sure of identification* before using any such plant. ⋙

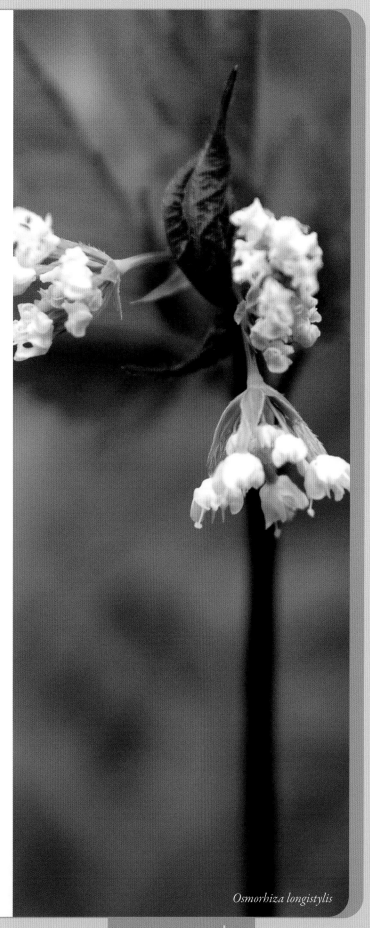

Osmorhiza longistylis

sweet cicely

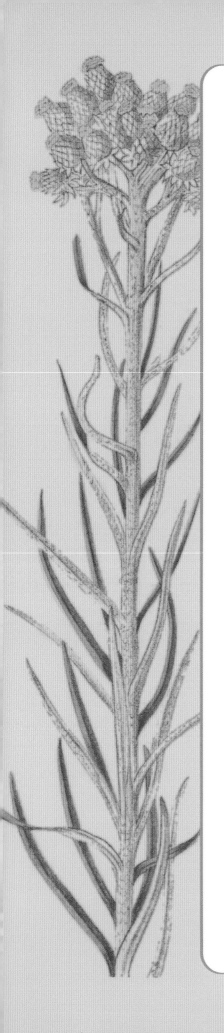

Sweet Everlasting

LIFE EVERLASTING; CUDWEED; RABBIT TOBACCO; OLD FIELD
BALSAM; CATFOOT; INDIAN POSY; POVERTY-WEED; SWEET BALSAM

Pseudognaphalium obtusifolium [formerly *Gnaphalium obtusifolium*]

DESCRIPTION

Sweet everlasting is an annual or a biennial plant 12–36 inches tall with a balsam-like fragrance. It has a woolly white stem that is erect, slender, and many-branched (especially near the top).

The plant is possessed of spatula-like basal leaves arranged in a rosette and numerous, alternate stem leaves that are sessile, smooth edged, linear to lanceolate, 1–4 inches long, less than ½ inch wide, and whitish underneath due to being covered with dense, woolly hairs.

The tips of this herb's many branches bear spreading clusters of numerous globular heads of yellowish-white disk flowers surrounded by papery brown bracts.

RANGE AND HABITAT

Sweet everlasting can be found in open, sunny places—dry fields, disturbed ground, sandy prairies, open woodlands, and roadsides.

SEASONAL AVAILABILITY

The plant is available in August, while flowering.

MAJOR CONSTITUENTS

Sweet everlasting contains monomethylgnaphaliin, an essential oil, gnaphaliin, and tannins.

HEALTH/MEDICINE

Sweet everlasting is primarily known for its *astringent* properties, especially with reference to its ability to increase the tone of the body's mucous membranes. "In cold preparations, its action is mainly expended upon mucous membranes," said the Physiomedicalist physician William Cook in 1869, adding, "It soothes and strengthens these tissues" (Cook 1985). Charles Millspaugh, writing a few decades after Cook, noted that it was commonly implemented in his time as a cold infusion for **diarrhea**, **leukorrhea**, and **bowel hemorrhage** (Millspaugh 1974: 351–52), the first two of which Cook had also said were benefited by the use of sweet everlasting (Cook 1985).

In addition to its astringent qualities, sweet everlasting is held to be *anti-inflammatory* and consequently useful for conditions such as **laryngitis**, **tonsillitis**, or **quinsy** (Hoffmann 1986: 189). The Cherokee have even used sweet everlasting topically for **diphtheria** (by gently blowing the warmed liquid into the clogged throat through a stem), chewed the plant for **sore mouth**, and even smoked it for **asthma** (Hamel and Chiltoskey 1975: 52). For the latter condition, famed Alabama herbalist Tommie Bass recommended putting a large clump of the herb in the sink, running hot water over it, and then inhaling the steam. He was also fond of explaining that this sort of treatment could likewise relieve **plugged sinuses**, **migraines**, and many other kinds of **headache** (Crellin and Philpott 1990a: 365).

Bass's biographer, John Crellin, noted that sweet everlasting has an excellent reputation as a *pectoral* (Crellin and Philpott 1990b: 140). Millspaugh had likewise drawn attention to its application in this regard, noting that the dried flowers were used in the pillows of **tuberculosis** victims in order to allow them a good night's sleep (Millspaugh 1974: 352), as, earlier, had the medical doctor Asahel Clapp (Clapp 1852: 802). British herbalist David Hoffmann writes that the related species *Gnaphalium uliginosum* is especially indicated as an *expectorant* for **upper respiratory catarrh** (Hoffmann 1986: 189; cf. Ody 1993: 191), with an infusion of the dried herb generally being used for this purpose. Our own species has been used similarly, and in both species the essential oil may be the active agent (Crellin and Philpott 1990a: 365–66). Not surprisingly, in view of the above, this herb—under the common name of rabbit tobacco—has been the most popular folk remedy among whites in the Carolinas for **colds** (Morton 1974: 66), as well as having been used by the Cherokee for this purpose (Hamel and Chiltoskey 1975: 51). Millspaugh also listed the hot decoction as *sudorific* and thus helpful in the early stages of a fever (Millspaugh 1974: 351–52). To this day, various species in this and in the related *Gnaphalium* genus (the latter to which our species used to belong) are a popular *febrifuge* in the southeastern United States, especially having been used there during the flu epidemic of 1941 (Morton 1974: 66).

Because several *Gnaphalium* species have been used for the above-listed complaints in Mexican traditional medicine, Mexican scientists decided to test two species (*G. oxyphyllum* and *G. americanum*) against six common respiratory and other pathogens (*Staphylococcus aureus*, *Enterococcus faecalis*, *Streptococcus pneumoniae*, *Streptococcus pyogenes*, *Escherichia coli*, and *Candida albicans*) and found the herbs to exert powerful antimicrobial activity against every one of them (Rojas et al. 2001).

Millspaugh further remarked that sweet everlasting has *anodyne* qualities (Millspaugh 1974: 351–52). In this regard, it is probably not without coincidence that the Cherokee have used the plant for **muscular cramps**, **rheumatism**, and **local pains** (Hamel and Chiltoskey 1975: 51). Millspaugh added that a hot fomentation has also been used for **sprains**, **bruises**, **tumors**, and **skin ulcers** (Millspaugh 1974: 351–52).

Undoubtedly, the plant's astringent, anti-inflammatory, and anodyne properties have been prime factors in offsetting another classic discomfort historically treated by it, **stomachache**—although here the plant's bitter qualities may be an even more significant factor (Kindscher 1992: 250). Another of the herb's alternative common names, cudweed, even supposedly arose because farmers discovered that feeding the herb to their cows allayed the sort of stomach inflammation that was capable of causing them to lose their cud.

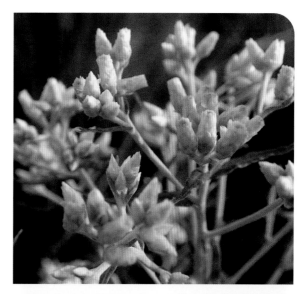

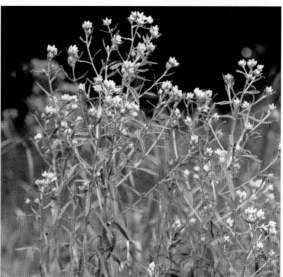

Finally, the Midwest's Meskwaki (Fox) used to steam the plant to revive a person from **unconsciousness** (Smith 1928: 214). I would guess that the pleasant scent may have had something to do with any successes in that regard!

PERSONAL AND PROFESSIONAL USE

I implement sweet everlasting most often for its astringent effects and for its stomachic abilities. For my clients, I have found that its anticatarrhal effect is quite pronounced and most welcomed by them. In fact, I remember directing one of my very first clients to use sweet everlasting for a chronically plugged nasal cavity and sinuses; he found it to be not only successful but also most pleasantly scented.

CAUTIONS

Internal use of this plant is *contraindicated in pregnancy*. ⁂

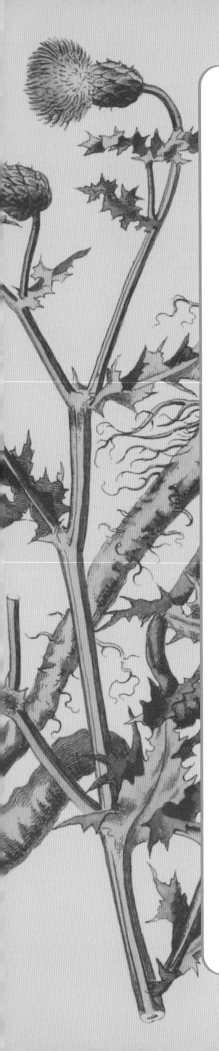

Thistle

Cirsium spp.

DESCRIPTION

The thistle is a well-known prickly biennial or annual, with most species possessed of a stout taproot and basal leaves arranged in a rosette. Flowers are composite and pink, pink-red, purple, or white.

A number of species flourish in the Midwest, including the following:

Cirsium arvense (Canada thistle) is a perennial that is often found in patches. It reaches a height of 1–4 feet, bears a smooth stem, and has slender, creeping white roots. The alternate leaves are oblong to lanceolate, 5–8 inches in length, and green on their surface but gray on their underside. They are deeply cut (lobed) and wavy edged (perhaps best described as crinkled), with their teeth extending into prickly spines. Sessile, they often clasp the stem. The numerous flower heads are ½–¾ inch across and pink to violet (or occasionally white) in color. This species is dioecious, i.e., male and female flowers are to be found on separate plants. Hugging the flower heads are involucral bracts that lack spines, in distinction from most other thistle species.

C. discolor (field thistle, pasture thistle) is a native perennial topping off at 3–6 feet. Its alternate, prickly leaves are elongate, grow 6–12 inches long, and are nearly flat. Their undersides are densely woolly and white. Five to twenty pale purple flower heads occur on the plant, with bracts bearing long spines that stick out at an angle.

C. vulgare (bull thistle, hog thistle, spear thistle) is a biennial forming a large rosette of basal leaves in the first year and then in the second year shooting forth a powerful, upright, branching stem that is winged and armed with spines. It eventually reaches a height of 2–6 feet (3–4 feet being average). Its alternate leaves are 3–9 inches long and quite narrow—only 1–1½ inches wide. They are coarsely lobed along their margins and possessed of stiff hairs on their surface. The undersides of the leaves display brownish hairs and a fat, swollen midrib. Each leaf lobe ends in a sharp spine. Blossoms (several per plant, but usually one per branch) occur as vivid reddish-purple flower heads, 2 inches high and 1–2 inches in diameter. These are surrounded by very spiny bracts with yellow tips on the spines.

C. altissimum (tall thistle) is a native biennial that grows 3–10 feet tall. Its leaves are toothed but not lobed (except that occasionally the lowermost leaves are lobed), and their undersides are covered with white hairs.

C. muticum (swamp thistle) is a biennial 3–8 feet tall possessing mature, hairless leaves and bracts that lack spines.

RANGE AND HABITAT

Most species occur throughout the Midwest in pastures, roadsides, fields, wasteland, vacant lots, and ill-kept lawns. They thrive in complete or partial sun. Bull thistle prefers to grow near water.

MAJOR CONSTITUENTS

Most thistles contain phenolic acids, flavonoids, sterols, tannins, and triterpenes. Contents of specific thistles are as follows. *C. arvense*: Alkanes, taraxasterol, stigmasterol, glucuronides of apigenin and acacetin, linarin, cnicin (a glycoside), coumarins, and an unidentified alkaloid can be found in the leaves; flavonoids (kaempferol, luteolin, apigenin) occur in the flowers; and a phototoxic compound occurs in the root.

C. vulgare: Flavonoids (including luteolin, apigenin, kaempferol, and the rare genkwanin-4'-O-glucoside); *p*-coumaric acid, caffeic acid, ferulic acid, vanillic acid, *p*-hydroxybenzoic acid, gallic acid, protocatechuic acid, triterpenes, and sterols in the leaves and stems; the flowers contain fourteen different flavonoids.

FOOD

Carefully trimmed leaves of *C. arvense* can be eaten raw (see Cautions). They are absolutely delicious and chock-full of water to help sustain the thirsty forager! I look forward to partaking of them on nearly every foraging trek, carrying a pair of round-tipped children's scissors with me to trim them so that I can consume them on the spot. Leaves of most other species are, unfortunately, too hairy or prickly to trim and eat as a trail nibble.

Young stems of most any thistle species in the Midwest can, before having gone to flower or even budding, be trimmed of their leaves, peeled, cut crosswise into pieces, and then boiled for five to ten minutes in salted water. The taste is reminiscent of cooked artichokes or celery, depending on the species and other factors. These can also be eaten raw and often make a great addition to a tuna salad. Older stems are too fibrous and tough to prepare as a main menu item. Still, depending on the species, they may possess edible pith, which can be separated from the stalk and then consumed—raw or cooked. Often, however, these older stalks are infested with vermin, not to mention the fact that the labor of removing the pith can be quite time consuming.

The flowers of *C. arvense* make a delicious chewing gum, and one that will not promote tooth decay either. I enjoy the flavor very much and always pick a few when I am out foraging. These flower heads, especially those of *C. vulgare*, can even serve, like rennet, to curdle milk! To do this, simply gather a number of them and mash them until a chestnut-like liquid is released. Only a tiny amount of this fluid is necessary to curdle a rather large amount of milk.

Did you know that artichokes are really the flower bracts of a cultivated species of thistle? 'Tis true, and as with artichokes, the bracts that surround the Midwest's thistle burs can be trimmed, cooked, and eaten—never eat them raw, in view of the thorns!—as can the base of the flower head, corresponding to the artichoke "heart."

The roots of all species, before or after flowering, can be peeled and eaten raw or cooked. Simply cut the peeled roots into disks as if slicing carrots, then boil them in two waters for twenty minutes total. Alternatively, they can be boiled for several hours until soft and mushy and then dried and ground into flour.

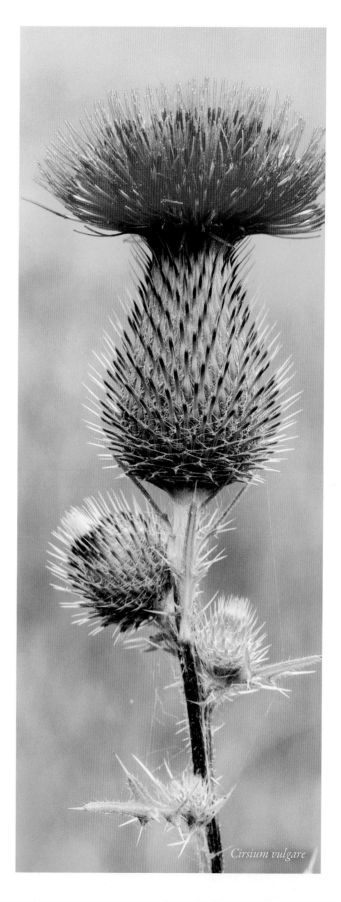

Cirsium vulgare

All in all, thistles are one of the most usable of wild foods and certainly one of the most nutritious, as a thrilling incident in human survival has well evinced. In 1870, during an expedition to Yellowstone, a man named Truman Everts was separated from his companions, thrown from his horse, and badly injured. Unable to walk but courageously fending off panic, he survived on thistle roots for more than a month until he was rescued (Medsger 1972: 201; Coffey 1993: 254–55). Yet this life-saving plant is castigated, cursed, and assaulted as a noxious weed by our local governments! Surely our officials could do better than to bad-mouth the Midwest's thistles and to spray them with what is truly noxious—herbicides! Why not educate the populace on the edible and medicinal benefits of thistles so that they could be put to good use instead?

HEALTH/MEDICINE

Thistles have predominantly been used by herbalists as *alteratives* (Lewis and Elvin-Lewis 1977: 277). North Carolinian folk use has also recognized and culled *tonic*, *diuretic*, and *hepatic* effects from the plant (Jacobs and Burlage 1958). The *United States Dispensatory* for 1926 said that scientist Herman Pierce's research finding Canada thistle to be *diaphoretic*, *emetic*, and *tonic* "merited attention" (Wood et al. 1926: 1506). Such toning, detoxifying, and normalizing activities tend to elucidate why thistles have been an important tool in the materia medica of herbalists for healing sufferers of toxic conditions.

Foremost among such healers were Native Americans. For example, *C. discolor* (field thistle) has been used by the Iroquois to heal **boils.** The procedure is to combine seven thistle roots with one root of burdock and 1 quart of water and then boil this mixture down to 1 pint, after which one-half wineglassful is taken every hour, followed by salts (Herrick 1995: 231).

The aerial portions of Canada thistle have been appreciated by Oklahoma Lenape (Delaware) as a *pectoral* (Tantaquidgeon 1972: 71). Several tribes, including the Mohegan, have even employed it as part of a regimen for **tuberculosis** (Speck 1917: 314; Tantaquidgeon 1928: 269). Our own area's Ojibwe have utilized this species as a *bowel tonic* (Smith 1932: 364). The Abenaki have given a decoction of the roots to children infested with **intestinal worms** (Rousseau 1947: 173). The Oklahoma Lenape (Delaware) made an infusion of the leaves to wash out the mouths of infants, probably because they were afflicted with **thrush** (Tantaquidgeon 1972: 71). East Indian research has revealed that an extract of Canada thistle is both *spasmolytic* and *hypotensive* (Asolkar et al. 1992: 205).

Another species common to the Midwest, *C. vulgare* (bull thistle), has been utilized for **stomach cramps** by the Ojibwe and as a steam treatment for **rheumatism** by the Oklahoma Lenape (Delaware) (Tantaquidgeon 1942;

Shemluck 1982: 328). This same species has been put into service by the Iroquois for both **bleeding piles** and **cancer** (Herrick 1995: 231). The Cherokee have used an infusion of its leaves for **neuralgia** (Hamel and Chiltoskey 1975: 58).

According to field research conducted by ethnobotanist Scott Camazine, the Zuni drank an infusion of the thistle species *C. ochrocentrum* and then ran as heartily as possible for 1 mile, thereafter bundling themselves with blankets—all in order to raise their body temperature to a point necessary to destroy **syphilis.** Camazine cites research showing that the infectious spirochetes that cause this disease die in a sustained temperature of 105.6 degrees Fahrenheit, and that jogging 3 miles on a hot day could produce a rectal temperature of 106 degrees. One wonders whether the thistle infusion might somehow have accelerated all of this.

Then, too, as **Lyme disease** is also caused by a spirochete and has even been called "deer syphilis," might there be a possible application of this herb to that debilitating condition? As it causes what has been called "floating arthritis," it is of interest that North Carolinian folk medicine has traditionally viewed thistle root and leaves as being *anti-inflammatory* (Jacobs and Burlage 1958), something that can be considered scientifically validated by a 1976 lab study that found Canada thistle was powerfully anti-inflammatory in the carrageenan-induced, rat-paw edema test (Benoit et al. 1976: 164).

A bevy of other applications for various species of thistle has been appreciated by Native American tribes. A tea of thistle leaves has had wide and varied use in external application for **skin eruptions** and **skin ulcers** (Foster and Duke 1990: 166). A strong decoction of the root of various species of thistle, too, has served many persons as a disinfectant and healing wash for **poison ivy rash** and for other **skin infections** (Brown 1985: 202). An unidentified species of thistle was used by the Midwest's Ojibwe for women who had "pains in the back" as well as for "male weakness" (Densmore 1974: 356). The Lumni have given a saltwater decoction of the roots and tips of a *Cirsium* species to women at childbirth (Gunther 1973: 49). The Costanoan have used the roots of an unidentified species of thistle for **stomach pain** (chewed raw) or for **asthma** (given as a decoction) in addition to soothing **sores** on the face or dried **infected sores** with a poultice made from the pounded stems (Bocek 1984: 254).

PERSONAL AND PROFESSIONAL USE

I relish eating the trimmed leaves of Canada thistle, which is something that I do quite a bit! To me, the taste is exquisite; moreover, they tend to yield a rich amount of water, a side benefit that is always good for me because I tend to sweat so heavily. I also find it fun to chew on the flowers to elicit their bubble gum–like taste!

Since 2006, I have utilized a tincture of the fresh first-year leaves of bull thistle to support the tendon-ligament-joint

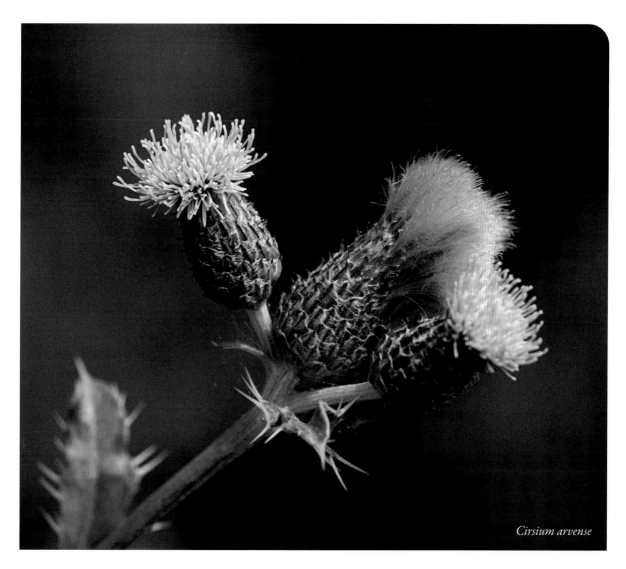

Cirsium arvense

health of persons suffering from a painful group of diseases grouped under the umbrella name of spondyloarthropathies, which includes psoriatic arthritis, juvenile spondyloarthropathy, ankylosing spondylitis, and the arthritis sometimes experienced by people afflicted with inflammatory bowel disease (enteropathic arthritis). In that a microbial origin has long been suspected by the scientific community for these conditions, I wonder whether the bull thistle might be nullifying whichever organism is responsible as well as exerting anti-inflammatory action. Such effects would not be out of line with either the chemical constituents or the historical applications of thistles as reviewed in the preceding section. In fact, several studies have demonstrated antibiotic activity on the part of this thistle species for a variety of infectious organisms and especially against *Pseudomonas aeruginosa*, for which it proved more effective than gentamicin! (Nazaruk et al. 2008; Borawska et al. 2010; Sabudak et al. 2017)

CAUTIONS

Be *absolutely sure* you have trimmed off *all* thorns from thistles before consuming them. When I feel I am done trimming the leaves of *C. arvense*, I always flip them over to view them from both sides before popping them in my mouth. (Invariably, upon doing this, I find a remaining thorn or two!)

Be wary of sun exposure when consuming thistle roots, as some of them contain a phototoxic compound that could conceivably cause severe sunburn. ⋙

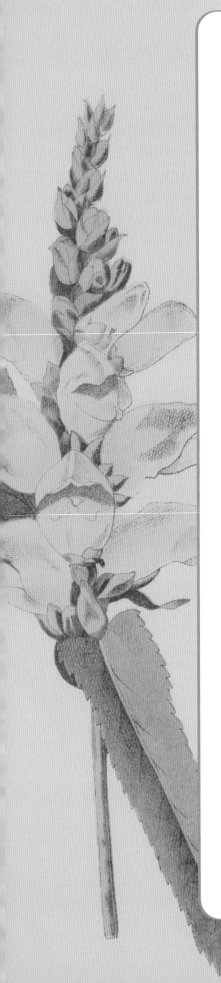

Turtlehead

BALMONY

Chelone glabra

DESCRIPTION

Turtlehead is a lovely perennial possessed of a slender, upright, almost square stem that sometimes branches. It grows 1–3 feet tall.

The strap-like leaves are opposite, sharply toothed, and possessed of prominent veins. Sessile, or nearly so, they grow 3–6 inches long and ½–1 inch wide.

Inflorescence is in the form of a number of large, two-lipped tubular flowers arranged in a tight, spike-like cluster at the tip of the stem. These blossoms are creamy white to purple in color.

Altogether, this plant presents the appearance of a turtle's head, hence its common name. The older herbalists preferred to call it balmony, however.

RANGE AND HABITAT

Turtlehead thrives in wet areas—streamsides, lakeshores, ditches, swamps, and wet meadows. It can be found throughout the Midwest, except for the western one-third of both Minnesota and Iowa.

MAJOR CONSTITUENTS

Little chemical work has been done on this plant, but it is known to contain iridoid glycosides, bitter principles, and a resin.

HEALTH/MEDICINE

Turtlehead's leaves, stem, and flower (aerial parts) have long been appreciated by herbalists as being a bitter *tonic* and thus a gentle *laxative*, working to improve the secretions of the salivary glands, the stomach, and the hepatobiliary system, and such is how it has been implemented by various Native American tribes, including the Cherokee (Hamel and Chiltoskey 1975: 59). Likewise, the Physiomedicalist physician William Cook, writing in 1869, noted that the leaves "are fairly laxative. ... Few tonics are equal to balmony in cases of enfeebled stomach, with accompanying indigestion, biliousness, costiveness, and general languor. ... It arouses the gastric and salivary secretions, and decidedly improves digestion; also favors the biliary and fecal discharges, and leaves the whole assimilative organism toned" (Cook 1985). The Eclectics described it in like manner, with Harvey Wickes Felter adjudging it to be "a useful remedy for gastrointestinal debility with hepatic torpor or jaundice" (Felter 1983).

The early-nineteenth-century American naturalist and botanist Constantine Rafinesque noted that turtlehead "is useful in ... jaundice, hepatitis, eruptions of the skin & c," adding, "In small doses it is laxative, but in full doses it purges the bile and cleans the system of the morbid or superfluous bile, removing the yellowness of the skin in jaundice and liver diseases. The dose is a drachm of the powdered leaves 3 times daily. ... Few plants promise to become more useful in skillful hands" (Rafinesque 1828–30: 2:118).

As to the abovementioned application for jaundice, the noted Natura physician R. Swinburne Clymer, who practiced from the early 1900s until the middle of the twentieth century, considered balmony to be one of the finest treatments for this condition when it was chronic, finding this herb to serve as a stimulating *cholagogue* (Clymer 1973: 115).

The Cherokee have found turtlehead useful as an *appetite stimulant* (Hamel and Chiltoskey 1975: 59). Implementation among white herbal healers of the mid-nineteenth century pretty much echoed the Native uses here, as *Gunn's Domestic Physician*, a common home-remedy guide of the time, informs us: "This herb ... is employed in costiveness, dyspepsia, loss of appetite, and general languor, or debility. Given to children afflicted with worms, it will generally afford relief. ... An even teaspoonful [of the tea] is a dose" (Gunn 1859–61: 740).

Anthelmintic properties have been culled from this plant by the Cherokee (Hamel and Chiltoskey 1975: 59). Some modern herbalists even revere turtlehead as one of the best expellers of parasites around. Such ones often advise a dose of 1 ounce of the leaves to 1 pint of boiling water taken in a wineglassful dose in the evening before retiring and in the morning on an empty stomach, with a purge to be expected—or, if not consequently accomplished, to be induced at the end of the day after fasting (Clymer 1973: 115; Carse 1989: 167; Hutchens 1991: 22).

The Indigenous peoples of the Maritimes have used turtlehead in an undisclosed way as a *contraceptive* (Mechling 1959). Native peoples, in fact, have used so many, many plants to prevent conception that this is an area that is assuredly overripe for detailed investigation, given our overflowing population at present (see the index to physiological functions in the rear of this volume, under "contraceptive").

PERSONAL AND PROFESSIONAL USE

Unfortunately, turtlehead is not readily available on the market, necessitating that I wildcraft it. It is difficult to find in abundance in my area, so I have had little experience in using it clinically. The few exceptions have been for skin problems, where it seems to have done at least some good. ⤺

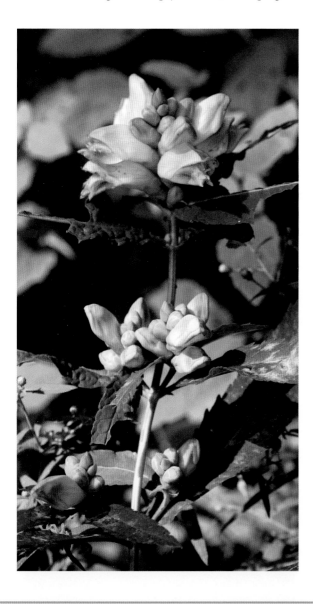

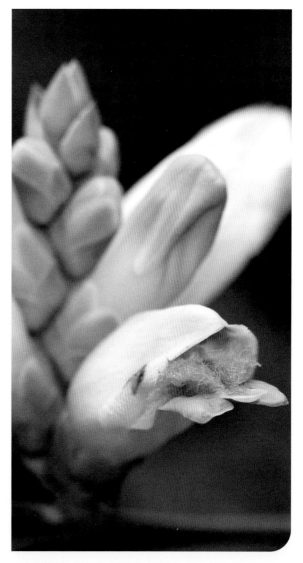

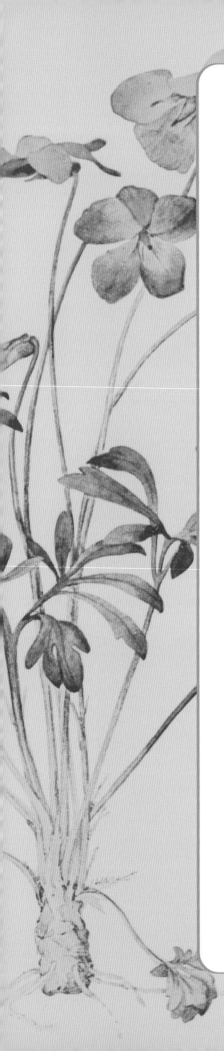

Violet

Viola spp.

DESCRIPTION

There are over seventy species of this delicate perennial herb growing in the United States and over twenty in the Midwest alone! Although the various species differ a bit in detail, they all share some common features, including the fact that their blossoms bear some distinctive earmarks: five sepals, five stamens, and five petals, with the lower petal terminally positioned and usually larger than the rest, as well as possessing noticeable veins (usually purple in color) and displaying a backward-projecting spur. The blossoms of most species are situated on a separate stalk from the leaves, which on most species are basal.

In the Midwest, the most common violet species is *Viola sororia*, known as the common blue violet, the woolly blue violet, or the sister violet, which grows 3–6 inches high. It possesses heart-shaped basal leaves about as wide as they are long, with scalloped margins (i.e., rounded teeth). The long-stalked, blue-violet blossom bears bilaterally symmetrical petals, with the lateral petals being "bearded." The whole plant is finely pubescent, especially the stem and the underside of the leaves.

A second blue violet growing in the Midwest is the marsh violet, *V. cucullata*, which resembles the former except that its blossoms grow taller than its leaves, the center of its blossom is a darker shade of blue than are the exterior portions, and the lower petal is shorter than the others, rather than being longer as in other species.

Another blue-flowered species in the Midwest is the dog violet, *V. conspersa*, which sports its blossoms and leaves on the same stalk. Still another is *V. pedata*, called the bird's-foot violet because its leaves are deeply dissected and thus somewhat resemble the foot of a bird. Its petals have no beards, and the upper ones curve backward.

A yellow-flowered species common to our area is *V. pubescens*, the common yellow violet, which reaches a height of 4–14 inches. It has leaves and blossoms on the same stalk and occasionally features a basal leaf besides. Its heart-shaped, scalloped leaves are 2–5 inches wide, while the lateral petals on its flowers are bearded. The whole plant is pubescent, but it is especially so along the stem and the leaf veins. A variant yellow-blossomed species, *V. pensylvanica*, the smooth yellow violet, possesses smooth stems and one or more basal leaves.

A white-blossomed species in the Midwest is *V. canadensis*, the Canada violet or tall white violet, which grows larger than our other species: 8–16 inches. It features both basal leaves (2–4 inches long, 2–4 inches wide, and pointed) and stem leaves. Its flower has a yellow center, while the backs of its petals are tinged with violet. Its stems are purplish and hairy. This species may have a light wintergreen-like odor.

Violets bear self-pollinating flowers situated close to where the stalk emerges from the root. Called *cleistogamous* by botanists, these flowers, which produce numerous seeds, do not open until they release those seeds and thus are difficult to spot by the untrained eye. While windblown seeds initiate new violet colonies, the existing colonies spread largely by means of subterranean rhizomes.

RANGE AND HABITAT

One or another species of violet occurs, often in large colonies, throughout the Midwest and indeed throughout most of the United States and Canada. The preferred habitat is open woods, trailsides, pastures, moist meadows, swamps—in short, wherever the combination of shade and moist soil can be found.

SEASONAL AVAILABILITY

Violets should be gathered in the spring, while in flower, for fear of mistaking them for inedible or mildly toxic plants having leaves resembling theirs.

MAJOR CONSTITUENTS

Violets contain saponins, eugenol, salicylic acid, flavonoids (including both rutin and anthocyanins in goodly quantities in blue-flowered species), mucilage, and a bitter, purgative principle in the root. Methyl salicylate occurs in *V. canadensis*, giving rise to its faint wintergreen odor and/or taste. Nutrients include incredibly high amounts of pro-vitamin A (15,000–20,000 imperial units per 100 grams—much more carotene than in spinach, which has one of the highest contents of any marketed vegetable) and C (150–250 milligrams per 100 grams—in other words, in ½ cup of violet leaves, there is more vitamin C than in four oranges!).

FOOD

The raw leaves are often excellent as a trail nibble or mixed into salads, although at certain stages of their growth they can be too bitter. The blossoms are also edible in moderation (in not so moderate doses they can be laxative) but are usually not as tasty as the leaves.

The leaves can also be eaten as a potherb by boiling them in a small amount of water for ten to fifteen minutes. Then, too, a tea made from the leaves has a pleasant, mild taste. Chilled, it makes an excellent iced tea. Euell Gibbons raved over the taste of violet jam and jelly (Gibbons 1970: 64–68).

HEALTH/MEDICINE

The most acclaimed use of violet has been the application of its flowers along respiratory lines—to help ease **colds**, **bronchitis**, **sore throat**, and **chronic cough.** Here the blossoms are prepared by soaking for three minutes in cold water and then brought to a boil for ten minutes, after which the tea is cooled to a drinkable temperature. Combined with a tincture of blue vervain (see page 41), violet blossoms have also been used to treat **whooping cough** (Potterton 1983: 196).

Violet's mucilage is helpful in these conditions as a soothing, protective agent for the mucous membranes—thus the tea is gargled for sore throat, as done by the Ojibwe (Hoffman 1891: 201)—while the saponins in the herb serve as an expectorant because of irritating the respiratory system by means of reflex action from the stomach. In other words, violet is a *moistening expectorant*. Not surprisingly, too, persons with **asthma** have been known to benefit from this herb. The Blackfoot, for instance, have given an infusion

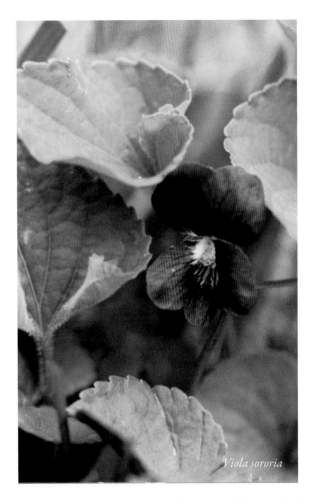

Viola sororia

of the leaves (as well as a very small portion of the roots) of *V. adunca*—another species scattered throughout the northern part of the Midwest—to asthmatic children (Hellson and Gadd 1974: 74).

Violet blossoms are also renowned in folk medicine as a safe and effective *laxative* for children. For this purpose, British herbalist Mary Carse recommends pouring 1 cup of boiled water over 1 cup of fresh violet flowers, steeping this for twelve hours, then straining, sweetening with 1 pound of honey, and giving ½–1 teaspoon of the syrup to constipated youngsters at bedtime so as to induce a morning bowel movement (Carse 1989: 170).

A much-appreciated *refrigerant*, violet tea has proven useful as an oral swish for **inflamed gums** and in compress form for reducing **fever**, the latter commonly used by French physicians in the early 1900s. A Pakistani study found violet leaf extracts comparable to aspirin in reducing pyrexia in animals (Khattak et al. 1985). The compress remedy has also been used for **headache**, especially where the head feels "hot." It is especially effective for hangover headaches, as the Roman naturalist Pliny the Elder acknowledged, pointing out that a garland of violets around the forehead would banish headaches and dizziness from too much drinking! Centuries later, and undoubtedly unaware of Pliny's remarks, the Cherokee likewise poulticed violet leaves onto aching heads (Hamel and Chiltoskey 1975: 60). Certainly here, the salicylic acid and the eugenol are factors in relieving headache pain and may also help elucidate why violet (especially its blossoms) has traditionally been valued for *anodyne* activity in general.

In accord with this pain-dulling property, the Midwest's Ojibwe have employed a decoction of Canada violet *(V. canadensis)* for **bladder pain** (Hoffman 1891: 201). This species also contains methyl salicylate, as noted under Major Constituents, which is the analgesic chemical well known from wintergreen. Then, too, a poultice of the leaves of various violet species has traditionally been used to ease the pain of **rheumatism** (the Blackfoot have used a compress of a root and leaf infusion to the painful area: Hellson and Gadd 1974: 79) and of **gout** (Pliny related that a liniment made from violet roots and vinegar had proven helpful here). Especially significant in this regard is that violet tea is a mild *diuretic* (confirmed in animal studies: Dobelis et al. 1986: 316) and *blood purifier*, thus enabling it to drive excess uric acid from the body. These physiological activities also lend violet for use with **swollen lymph nodes**, **boils**, and **pimples** (de Bairacli Levy 1974: 148). The Iroquois have used it for the latter affliction, taking a decoction internally and also using it as a facial wash (Herrick 1977: 387). The Cherokee have appreciated the use for boils, applying a poultice of the crushed roots of one or another species to them (Hamel and Chiltoskey 1975: 60). The effect on the lymphatic system can be quite pronounced: this is the herb of choice in stagnant lymph conditions and in chronic lymphatic swelling when, as present-day herbalist David Winston points out, such is accompanied by constipation (Winston 1999: 54).

Some of violet's other topical uses have been as a chewed-leaf poultice for **cracked nipples** and for **sore eyes.** Manasseh Cutler, an early American botanical author, also noted that Native Americans commonly bruised the leaves of a yellow-blossomed species as a topical application to **boils** and other **painful swellings** in order to ease the pain and to cause these to suppurate (Cutler 1785: 485). Then, there is a vivid personal account from an American missionary working among Native Americans in the early 1800s, which reveals that its author "once suffered the most excruciating pain from a felon or whitlow on one of my fingers, which deprived me entirely of sleep. I had recourse to an old Indian woman who in less than half an hour relieved me entirely by the simple application of a poultice made of the root of the common blue violet" (Heckewelder 1820: 229). It should be noted that when suppuration is not the goal, mashed violet blossoms should not be left on painful body areas for longer than two or three hours, in order to prevent blistering.

Violets have traditionally been used topically to soften almost any kind of hard lump in the body, especially **swollen**, **lumpy breasts** and even including **tumors**. A poultice of the fresh or dried leaves has long been used as an application to **skin cancers.** Jonathan Hartwell, an American scientist with the National Cancer Institute, collected voluminous accounts of the many uses of violets in anticancer regimens from around the world (Hartwell 1971; Hartwell 1982). In fact, in the five-year period from 1901 to 1906, five different articles even appeared in British medical journals on violet treatments for cancer! (Mockle 1955: 50) While naysayers may claim that the salicylic acid in violet simply acts as a dissolvent to rid the physical structure of these cancerous growths—as, indeed, a violet ointment has been a favorite treatment for removing **warts** and **corns**—the incredible range and variety of cultural uses strongly suggests that there is more to it than merely that. Such a conclusion is reinforced by a 1960s lab study wherein a violet extract (from *V. striata*) brought about genuine damage to cancer in mice (Farnsworth 1968: 237–48).

Because of violet's above-noted anodyne properties, the herb has been used to help ease the **pain** of cancer as well, especially when it is in the throat. For this purpose, a strong tea is sought. A recipe popular in India and Pakistan consists of 2 ounces of leaves infused in 1 pint of boiled water, which is left to stand twelve hours and then is strained and taken in doses of 2 fluid ounces every two to three hours (Potterton 1983: 196; Hutchens 1991: 288). Then, too, *sedative* abilities (especially where there is **restlessness**: de Bairacli Levy 1974: 148) have also been ascribed to our little plant, and thus a violet footbath has been a favored treatment for **insomnia.** The plant is especially indicated for restlessness in children.

Violet flowers contain a large amount of the bioflavonoid rutin, which has been recognized by medical science for over half a century now as providing support to the walls of blood vessels. Former US Department of Agriculture scientist James Duke, in calculating the content of this bioflavonoid in violet, says that a few tablespoons of the plant could provide biologically significant amounts for rectifying **atonic blood vessels** (e.g., **varicose veins**) (Duke 1997: 446).

Another circulatory affliction traditionally benefited by violet has been **heart problems.** The Potawatomi have used the root of our *V. pubescens* as a cardiac medicine (Smith 1933: 87–88), while the Flambeau have preferred the entire aerial portions of dog violet, *V. conspersa* (Smith 1932: 392). *V. tricolor*, the garden pansy or Johnny-jump-up, has even been known by the common name of "heart's ease" owing to its traditionally understood cardiotonic effects. This species was at one time official in the *United States Pharmacopeia* (1883 edition), as have been our *V. pedata* (1820–70) and Europe's *V. odorata* (the Midwest's *V. cucullata* being the American equivalent to this latter species).

UTILITARIAN USES

Juice from crushed violet blossoms can be used as a natural litmus paper—to test whether a substance is primarily acidic

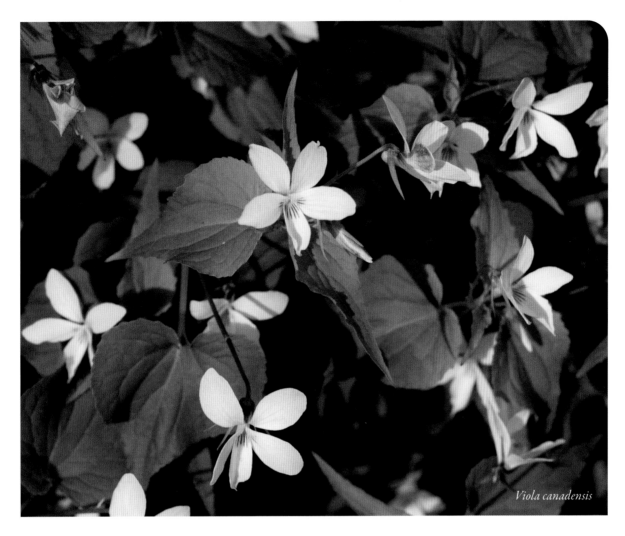

Viola canadensis

or alkaline. The juice turns red when contact with an acid is made, but green when touched by a base (alkaline substance).

PERSONAL AND PROFESSIONAL USE

I very much look forward to the appearance of violets in the spring, as I so relish the taste of their flowers and leaves!

For purposes of healing, I've used the crushed fresh plant topically for acute, painful swellings in the fingers, hands, wrists, feet, toes, or ankles, as per traditional use.

In my clinical practice, I use violet in formulas to be taken by mouth for lymphatic congestion as well as for cancers of the breast, lymph, throat, and esophagus. My experience has convinced me that this plant is most helpful in these disorders.

CAUTIONS

Yellow violets have been known to cause stomach upset or diarrhea in some persons. Proceed with caution in attempting to use any non-blue/non-purple-flowered violets.

Violet roots of any species should never be eaten, as they are all purgative to one degree or another.

Collect violets only when blooming so as to avoid confusing these species with toxic or inedible plants whose leaf structures resemble those of violets.

Bear in mind that the common houseplant known as African violet is not related to wild violets and is strictly inedible. Do *not* eat African violets! ⚞

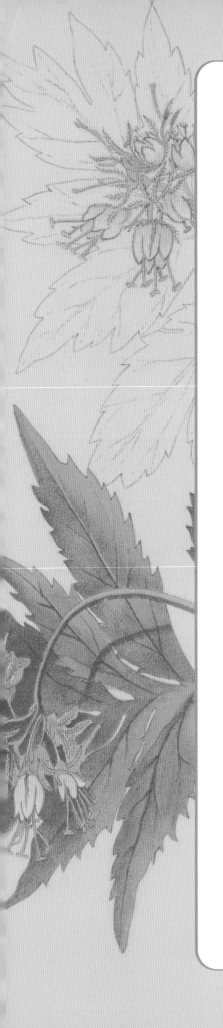

Virginia Waterleaf

INDIAN SALAD; JOHN'S CABBAGE

Hydrophyllum virginianum

DESCRIPTION

This is a perennial herb that grows 1–2½ feet tall. It is possessed of an erect—though weak—stem.

Its leaves are irregularly serrated and pinnate, and they display five to seven ovate or lanceolate leaflets (lobes) per leafstalk. Each leaflet is 2–5 inches long.

In early spring, the leaves appear to be mottled with striking blotches of gray-green, giving the impression that they have been stained with water droplets. These pseudowatermarks are one excellent identifier of the waterleaf plant.

As summer progresses, these "water spots" sometimes fade. But visual resplendence is not lost, for this herb then puts forth its dazzling purple to purplish-white flowers, which are in the shape of bells, bearing five petals, and characterized by stamens with long filaments that protrude beyond the rim of the body of the flower. The blossoms grow in dense clusters on long stalks in the leaf axils, arising noticeably above the leaves.

RANGE AND HABITAT

Virginia waterleaf grows in rich, moist woods and often in colonies, as it spreads via rootstocks. It flourishes in southern Canada (Quebec to Manitoba) and throughout much of the northern two-thirds of the United States east of the Mississippi. A variety of related species grow in the same vicinity, as well as in sandier soils in the west. The plant grows throughout the eastern two-thirds of the Midwest, except in the northernmost strip.

SEASONAL AVAILABILITY

The leaves are available from spring to early summer, while the root is typically harvested in the spring or in the autumn.

MAJOR CONSTITUENTS

It would appear that this plant has been largely ignored by phytochemists—at least, I am not aware of any chemical profile that has been done. It is certain, however, that it contains tannins. Known nutrients include pro-vitamin A and vitamins C and E.

FOOD

Both this species and a near relative, *Hydrophyllum appendiculatum*, make good salad ingredients when the leaves and/or shoots are collected before flowering. In fact, in my vicinity, this is one of my most awaited spring greens, and I have several guarded patches to which I return year after year!

The leaves also make a fine potherb when boiled or steamed for five to ten minutes. Wild-plant cook Adrienne Crowhurst recommends cooking the plant initially for three minutes, afterward throwing off the water, submerging the plant in a second pot of boiling water (this time salted), and cooking it for five more minutes (Crowhurst 1972: 47). According to Merritt Lyndon Fernald and Alfred Kinsey, the renowned ethnobotanist Huron Smith asserted that it was very important to throw off the first water (Fernald and Kinsey 1958: 327). Some excellent recipes for this plant can be found in the foraging manual *The Wild Plant Companion* by Kathryn and Andrew March (March and March 1986: 121, 143).

After Virginia waterleaf flowers, the leaves are usually too bitter to eat raw. At this stage, they are not too appealing as a trail nibble anyway, for whenever I have passed this herb during its flowering stage I have noted that it seems particularly attractive to flies, which are continually landing upon it.

In the autumn, various Native American tribes would dig, cook, and eat the thick roots.

As mentioned, very little research seems to have been done on this herb, although it is known that it contains pro-vitamin A and vitamins C and E. My personal suspicion is that a complete chemical profile would yield some impressive data. All in all, waterleaf is a plant not given nearly enough attention in the foraging manuals.

HEALTH/MEDICINE

This plant has been sadly ignored not only by chemists but by herbalists, which is unfortunate, in that it is a first-rate *astringent*. This is especially the case with the roots but also appears to be true of the leaves to a certain extent. Thus, a decoction of the root or simply the chewed root has been used by the Iroquois for **mouth sores** and for **cracked lips** (Herrick 1977: 420; Herrick 1995: 203). The Menomini from the Midwest have implemented the root for **flux** (Smith 1923: 37), as have our area's Ojibwe (Smith 1932: 371). As such, it has been utilized and deemed safe for adults and children (Smith 1932: 371).

An analgesic element may be present in the root, since the Menomini have also used a root decoction as part of a compound formula for **chest pain** (Densmore 1932: 130). The Ojibwe have done likewise, finding it helpful for **back pain** (Hoffman 1891: 201).

A tea is the most common method of treatment, as noted above, but a tincture can also be used (the procedure for making such being outlined by Charles Millspaugh in his tome *American Medicinal Plants*: Millspaugh 1974: 478).

PERSONAL AND PROFESSIONAL USE

For decades now, I've enjoyed munching on Virginia waterleaf's leaves during spring, looking forward to each year's crop with great anticipation!

Then, too, when I need a good astringent for oral sores in clients, Virginia waterleaf is always at the top of my list.

I suspect that it would make an excellent antidiarrheal—and perhaps antifungal as well—owing to its tannin content. ⚘

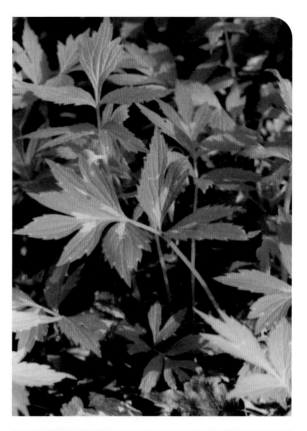

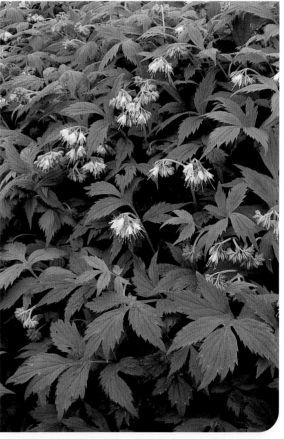

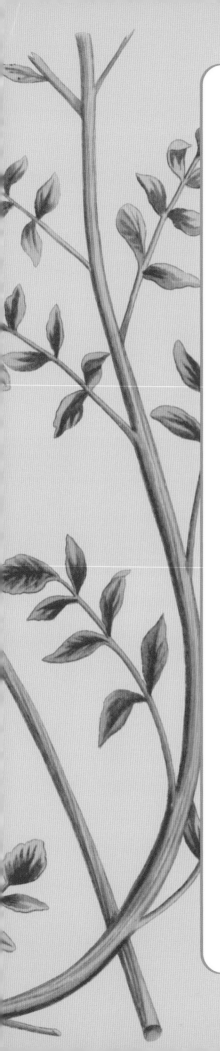

Watercress

Nasturtium officinale

DESCRIPTION

Watercress is a creeping or floating perennial herb, averaging 4–10 inches long and possessed of a pungent odor when bruised. The hollow stems are succulent and have white rootlings at their nodes.

The alternate leaves are pinnately compound, with three to nine leaflets. As with mustard-family relatives such as wintercress (*Barbarea vulgaris*) the end leaflet is the biggest one.

Also characteristic of its mustard-family membership is the fact that watercress's tiny white flowers have four petals and six stamens. These blossoms display themselves in clusters but usually only toward the last half of the growing season.

RANGE AND HABITAT

Watercress grows in colonies in running—although quiet—waters, such as can be found in brooks and streams. It flourishes throughout the Midwest.

MAJOR CONSTITUENTS

Watercress contains gluconasturtin (a glycosidal isothiocyanate precursor); isothiocyanates; flavonoids (quercetin, apigenin, and kaempferol); lutein; and an essential oil consisting chiefly of myristicin (at 57.6 percent!). Nutrients include protein, free-form amino acids, pro-vitamin A (4,900 imperial units per 100 grams), thiamine, riboflavin, niacin, pantothenic acid, folic acid, biotin, vitamin C (104 milligrams per 100 grams), vitamin E, calcium (151 milligrams per 100 grams), manganese, copper, iodine, iron, zinc, phosphorus (54 milligrams per 100 grams), and sulfur.

FOOD

This plant is one of the most nutritious of all vegetables, as can be ascertained from its nutritional profile as provided here. I have savored it since I was a teen, and I doubt that I will ever lose my taste for its wonderful tang!

Watercress can be lightly steamed for a few minutes or chopped and added to stir-fried dishes. Ideally, however, it should be eaten raw, as this form best preserves its nutrients. I think that it tastes much better this way, but because it is a member of the mustard family, most will find that eating it by itself is much too pungent to the palate. This is why it is usually added to a salad of blander greens or layered onto a sandwich—to somewhat disguise its pungency.

It is important to be aware, however, that this plant can accumulate harmful parasites if taken from infected waters (see Cautions), which can easily be transferred to humans. Thus, in wildcrafting it, one runs some risks. In view of this, it may be best to secure it from commercial sources, where it is grown in protected beds.

Watercress can also be blanched for two minutes, drained, patted dry, put in labeled freezer bags, and frozen for future use.

HEALTH/MEDICINE

This plant is a nutritional powerhouse, and many of its therapeutic benefits are related to its vast array of nutrients. First, due to its goodly amount of iron, it has long served as a revered treatment for **anemia** (de Bairacli Levy 1974: 150). Second, the high vitamin C content explains the traditional use of this plant as an *antiscorbutic* (Dobelis et al. 1986: 327). The vitamin may also explain why watercress has a tonic effect on the gums when chewed (Mabey et al. 1988: 53).

The plant's flavonoids and its sulfur may also play a role in its traditional aid for the gums. Watercress strengthens the lungs and acts as an *expectorant* (Winston 1999: 54), to which fact Hippocrates alluded, several centuries before the birth of the common era. Thus, macerated in honey, this water-loving plant has been used as a **cough** remedy (Krochmal and Krochmal 1973: 156) and to rid **fluid** from the **lungs** (Tierra 1988: 225). There was even some use of the herb by various communities (including the Chinese laborers working on the railroads in nineteenth-century America) to help ease the ravages of **tuberculosis** (Grieve 1971: 2:845; Krochmal and Krochmal 1973: 156; Duke 1997: 218).

Spanish-speaking communities in New Mexico have long used our herb for **heart trouble** (Krochmal and Krochmal 1973: 156). Its aid in this respect may be due to its high content of vitamin E, which increases the body's utilization of oxygen and is helpful for the heart in other respects as well (Hutchens 1991: 293).

Watercress's pungency stimulates digestive function (Johnson 1884: 94), so that it is often helpful for **indigestion** (Tierra 1988: 225) or even for a **lack of appetite** (Grieve 1971: 2:845; de Bairacli Levy 1974: 150). The plant is also a *cholagogue* and has thus been used for "biliousness" (digestive discomfort from poor fat metabolism). Traditional Chinese Medicine hails it as a remedy for **liver congestion** (Winston 1999: 54).

Watercress is real food for the kidneys (Landis 1997: 188) and has long been appreciated by Spanish-speaking communities of New Mexico for **kidney troubles** (Krochmal and Krochmal 1973: 156). It is a reliable *diuretic* (Johnson 1884: 95; Stuart 1982: 100; Tierra 1988: 225), although it can be too irritating for some (see Cautions). It has historically been used for **edema** (Tierra 1988: 225). Its diuretic activity may at least partly explain its historic utilization for both **rheumatism** and **gout** (de Bairacli Levy 1974: 150; Lust 1974: 390; Foster and Duke 1990: 34). Direct anti-inflammatory activity may also, or instead, be involved, in that an Iranian study from 2014 demonstrated potent *anti-inflammatory* activity from a hydroalcoholic extract, both systemically and topically (Sadeghi et al. 2014).

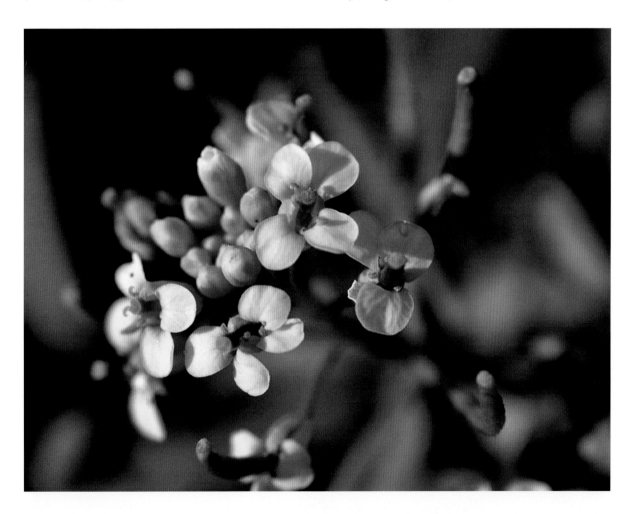

The fresh plant is somewhat *laxative* (Krochmal and Krochmal 1973: 156), probably due to its content of mustard oil. This oil is also *antibacterial* (Winston 1999: 54).

Watercress is also mildly *antipyretic* (Stuart 1982: 100). It has also been used in some lands, such as in Africa, as an *aphrodisiac* (Krochmal and Krochmal 1973: 156). The ancient Romans found it of value in this regard as well, calling it *impudica*, meaning "shameless." (It is interesting, in this regard, that another member of the mustard family, peppergrass [*Lepidium* spp.], has been used by the Lumbee as an aphrodisiac—see page 173.) Could watercress's purported ability in this regard be due, at least partly, to its long-recognized *stimulant* effects? Then, too, what role—if any—does its high content of vitamin E play in this regard?

Much research of late has focused on the abundance of anticancer chemicals that can be found in watercress, especially its isothiocyanates. At least two studies have shown that this herb helps protect the lungs from changes that can lead to lung cancer, even in smokers (Hecht et al. 1995; Hecht 1996). There have even been a few laboratory studies that have demonstrated that watercress causes human breast cancer cells, cervical cancer cells, and liver cancer cells to undergo apoptosis (suicide) (Park et al. 2007; Pledgie-Tracy et al. 2007). New research, however, has shown that cooking watercress reduces its anticancer potential (Aksornthong et al. 2019).

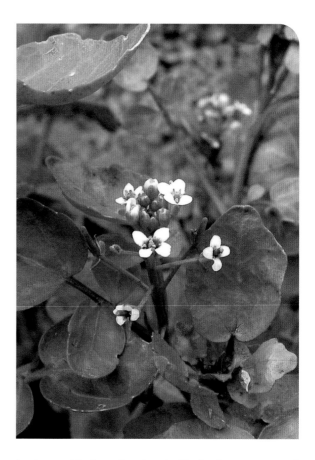

PERSONAL AND PROFESSIONAL USE

I recommend watercress to clients most often for one of two reasons: to stimulate libido or to expectorate fluid that has accumulated in the chest. I am also fond of recommending that it be regularly incorporated into the diet of those at risk for cancer or for its reoccurrence because of its anticancer chemicals. Then, too, owing to the research cited here, I also now use it in formulas for clients with cancer of the breast, cervix, or lungs.

CAUTIONS

Wildcrafting watercress presents some danger in areas where cattle or sheep graze, as it can harbor liver flukes in the waters where it grows due to the excrement of contaminated livestock. If gathered from these areas, then, it should always be thoroughly cleaned and cooked before being consumed. Logically, however, it would be wisest to secure it from commercial sources, where it is grown in protected beds.

Caution in pregnancy: It is thought that this plant could possibly cause miscarriage if used in quantity during pregnancy (Krochmal and Krochmal 1973: 156). Some Native American women have even eaten it during labor to hasten delivery (Scully 1970: 285).

Excessive use may cause bladder irritation. This is because, as botanist and physician Laurence Johnson so well put it: "The [plant's] acrid principles ... appear, clinically, to be eliminated by the kidneys, and hence, incidentally they produce a decided diuretic effect. The urine is not only increased in quantity, but partakes also of the acrid character of the plant" (Johnson 1884: 95). ⤺

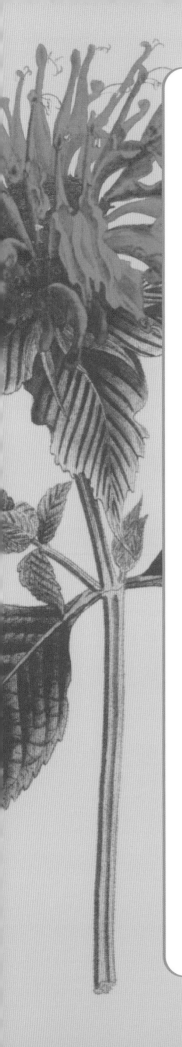

Wild Bergamot

Monarda fistulosa

DESCRIPTION

Wild bergamot is a perennial mint that reaches a height of 1–4 feet. It has a square stem that is hairy at the nodes. The leaves are opposite, lanceolate in shape, and coarsely toothed. They grow to 3 inches long and spring from short stalks.

Many tubular, inch-long lavender flowers appear clustered into dense, rounded heads at the ends of the stems. These flowers are two-lipped—the upper lip being hairy, erect, toothed, and two-lobed and the lower lip three-lobed and sagging.

The entire plant is permeated with a powerful, perfume-like scent.

RANGE AND HABITAT

Wild bergamot thrives in dry, open places—prairies, meadows, thickets, fields, or open or upland woods. It flourishes throughout the Midwest except for the central portion of South Dakota and the southern quarter of North Dakota.

MAJOR CONSTITUENTS

Wild bergamot contains rosmarinic acid and an essential oil that includes alpha-pinene, geraniol, alpha-terpinene, alpha-terpineol, beta-pinene, camphene, carvacrol, formaldehyde, limonene, linalool, myrcene, p-cymene, pulegone, sabinene, thymol, and nerol.

HEALTH/MEDICINE

This interesting plant has long been appreciated for the *carminative* and *diaphoretic* effects that all mints exert to some extent. Like its cousin horsemint, *Monarda punctata* (see page 132), it is also a *stimulant*.

Wild bergamot's carminative effect was greatly appreciated in colonial America, where its essential oil was extracted and two drops of it were added to a sweetened glass of water to alleviate **gas pains** (Rafinesque 1828–30: 2:37–38). The South Ojibwe have valued a decoction of the root for **gastrointestinal pain** (Hoffman 1891: 201). The Teton Dakota have implemented a decoction of the leaves and the flowers for same (Gilmore 1991: 59). The Meskwaki (Fox) have used a lone plant in a compound formula for **stomach cramps** (Smith 1928: 225).

The Ojibwe have also utilized an infusion of the flowers as a *febrifuge* (Densmore 1974: 270), while the Lakota have appreciated wild bergamot for both **fever** and **colds** (Rogers 1980: 50; Munson 1981: 236). The Koasatis have even bathed a feverish patient having **chills** with a decoction of this herb's leaves (Folsom-Dickerson 1965: 64). Nineteenth-century medical botanist Constantine Rafinesque likewise alluded to its use for fevers, especially those that were intermittent, noting the work of Johann David Schoepf in just such a regard (Rafinesque 1828–30: 2:37–38). The Cherokee have even used a bergamot infusion to "bring out measles" (Hamel and Chiltoskey 1975: 39). The Navajo (Diné) found that a cold tea served as a healing wash for **headaches** (Elmore 1944: 73).

Undoubtedly the plant's noted *diaphoretic* property lent a hand to reducing fevers in these instances. Yet there seems to be another factor at work here, too—more along an energetic line. As herbalist Matthew Wood explains, in his wonderful *Book of Herbal Wisdom*, Native American tribes have always viewed bergamot as a plant that can "draw

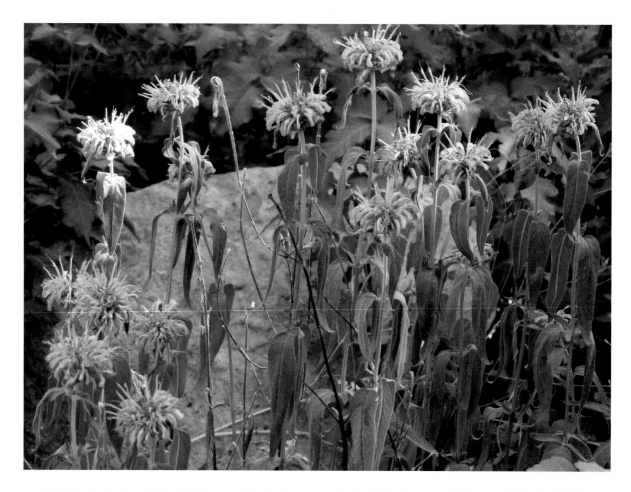

out fire." They've believed, Wood informs us, that the heat of an affliction will go into a "hot" plant like bergamot. And hot it is, for if applied directly to the skin, there is a strong *rubefacient* effect. (Among the American colonists, the extracted oil was dissolved in alcohol and used as a rubefacient liniment for **periodic headache** as well as for **chronic rheumatism**, **deafness**, **paralysis**, and **typhus**: Rafinesque 1828–30: 2:158.) Native healers feel that bergamot is especially indicated for interior heat and where the body surface is cold, so it is specific for a fever accompanied by chills or a cool, clammy skin. Some tribes have even used it for **burns**, probably where a cold sweat accompanies such. Our own area's Ojibwe seem to have applied a poultice of the plant's flowers and leaves to such a burn, finding it especially effective for **scalds** (Densmore 1974: 354).

Other "hot" conditions have been treated similarly with bergamot: The Lakota have wrapped bergamot leaves in a soft cloth and positioned such over **sore eyes** to bring relief (Rogers 1980: 50; Munson 1981: 236). Then, too, the Crow discovered how to take the sting out of **insect stings** and **bites**: they simply crumpled bergamot leaves, mixed the powder with spittle, and applied the mixture directly to the painful areas (Vestal and Schultes 1939: 49). The Blackfoot have poulticed bergamot flower heads over a **burst boil** until

it healed, thus drawing the fire out of this "hot" affliction, while the plant's thymol and other chemicals no doubt serve to quell any new infection.

As for the plant's stimulant potential, the Iroquois have treasured just such an effect for **general lassitude** (Herrick 1995: 208). The Lakota have even implemented our herb as a nasal stimulant for tribe members who have **fainted** (Rogers 1980: 50; Munson 1981: 236). Such a property has also been of value in treating **congestion** due to a **cold**, for which various tribes have used the plant, including the Meskwaki (Fox) and the Teton Sioux (Oceti Sakowin) (Densmore 1918: 270). The Flambeau Ojibwe have inhaled vapor from the boiled plant to resolve **catarrh** and for **bronchial affections** (Smith 1932: 372; Smith 1933: 61). The Menomini have used the leaves and the flowers for **catarrh** (Smith 1923: 39). The Blackfoot have treated **coughs** with an infusion of the plant (Hellson and Gadd 1974: 67). The Crow have used the same infusion for various **respiratory problems** (Hart 1976: 70). Bergamot's high content of essential oil is no doubt largely responsible for its benefits for respiratory afflictions.

The Iroquois have steeped a handful of roots in 1 quart of water and instructed children with both **headache** and **constipation** to drink ½ cup three times a day (Herrick 1995: 208).

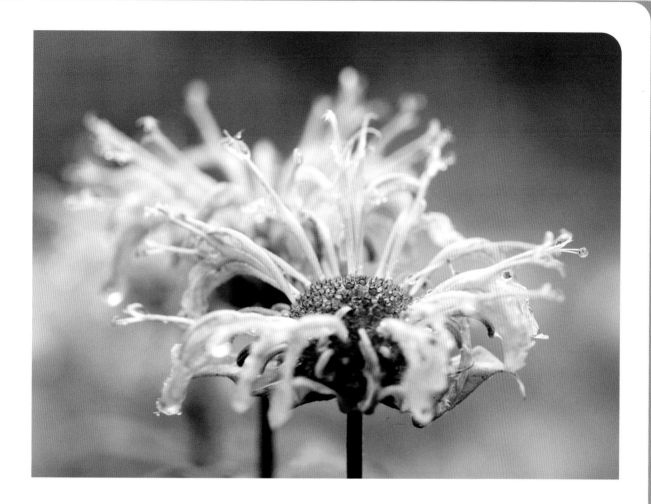

The Blackfoot have imbibed bergamot tea for **aching kidneys** (Hellson and Gadd 1974: 67). Interesting in this regard is the *United States Dispensatory*'s observation that our herb is "an active diuretic" (Wood et al. 1926: 1386). Thymol is also a *urinary antiseptic*, as we saw with horsemint, earlier (see page 132). Undoubtedly, too, bergamot's energetics are involved in the Blackfoot's use for painful kidneys, with the herb "drawing" out the heat from what Traditional Chinese Medicine might call a *kidney fire* situation.

The Winnebago (Ho-Chunk) have splashed a decoction of the leaves onto **pimples** and other **skin eruptions** (Gilmore 1991: 59). Scientific studies suggest that bergamot seems to counter **herpes-family infections** (Keville and Szolkowski 1991: 132). (Probably this is owing to its content of rosmarinic acid, as another plant containing that in abundance, self-heal—see page 201—also inhibits this virus.) The Blackfoot have chewed bergamot roots when experiencing **swollen lymph nodes** (Hellson and Gadd 1974: 67, 72, 77, 84). Then, too, the chemical geraniol, found in goodly amounts in this plant, is a decay-preventive compound. Coupled with the high content of the antibacterial thymol, this suggests—says former US Department of Agriculture

scientist James Duke—that wild bergamot might serve as a good oral rinse (Duke 1997: 431).

Like its cousin horsemint, wild bergamot is also a *vermifuge*. Because of this, the Midwest's Ojibwe have utilized a decoction of the flowers and of the roots to expel **worms** from the intestinal tract (Densmore 1974: 346).

PERSONAL AND PROFESSIONAL USE

There is a certain meadow within driving distance from my home that I hold special in my heart and to which I will travel, in midsummer, to sit and behold its mammoth colony of wild bergamot in all its glory, while taking in its wonderful perfume-like scent as it powerfully fills the air!

In the clinic, I use wild bergamot—either as a simple or as a formula ingredient—for nasal stuffiness, for flatulence, for oral thrush, for *Candida* proliferation in the gastrointestinal or genitourinary tract, and for herpes-family viral infections.

CAUTIONS

Because of wild bergamot's high content of both thymol and carvacrol and its classic use as an emmenagogue, it should be *excluded from use during pregnancy*.

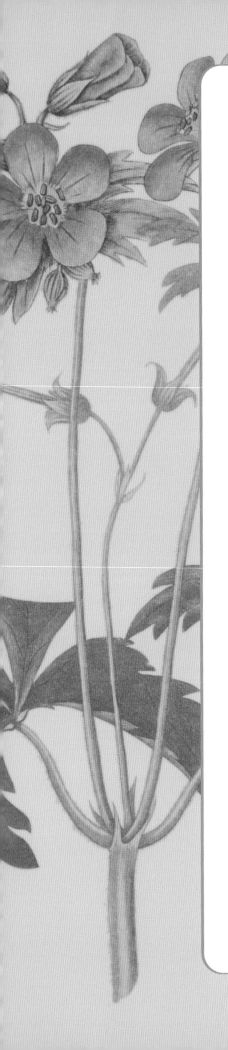

Wild Geranium

AMERICAN CRANESBILL; ALUM ROOT

Geranium maculatum

DESCRIPTION

Here we have an attractive native perennial topping off at 1–2 feet and possessed of a hairy and a branched stem.

The plant contains both basal leaves and stem leaves. The latter are short stalked and in pairs, while the former are long stalked and palmately divided into five to seven coarsely toothed segments that are etched with deep veins—the length of each leaf being 4–5 inches. At first light green with pale spots, the leaves eventually become, as woodsman Bradford Angier once so well phrased it, "an unforgettable red before dying" (Angier 1978: 285).

Two to ten rose- to violet-colored flowers appear in a loose corymb at the tips of the stems, just above the uppermost set of paired leaves. Like the leaves, these blossoms are heavily veined. They are 1–2 inches across and possessed of five petals, ten stamens, and a long pistil that develops into a slender, beaked, five-chambered seedpod. As the pod dries, its outer surface contracts, gradually building up tension until its segments dramatically curl upward, explosively releasing the precious seminal cargo.

RANGE AND HABITAT

Wild geranium can be found in dry, shaded areas, such as open woods and thickets. It thrives throughout the Midwest in such locales, although it is less common in our western third and around the Great Lakes.

MAJOR CONSTITUENTS

Wild geranium contains tannin (up to 30 percent!), gallic acid (upon drying, via decomposition of the tannin), pectin, calcium oxalate, gum, and resin.

HEALTH/MEDICINE

This gorgeous woodland plant is possessed of *cooling* and *drying* energies (Holmes 1989–90: 1:406), and its root has a cherished place in herbal medicine as an *astringent*, used by way of a strong decoction to the tune of 1–4 ounces, as needed, or as a 1:5 tincture of the dried plant with 50 percent alcohol and 10 percent glycerin, dosed at ½–1 teaspoon, also as needed (Moore 1993: 298). Wild geranium was even an official astringent in American drug literature for over a century, having been listed in the *United States Pharmacopeia* from 1820 to 1916 and subsequently in the *National Formulary* from 1916 to 1936. The *United States Dispensatory* for 1926 even praised our cranesbill heartily, noting: "Geranium is one of our best indigenous astringents, and may be employed for all the purposes to which these medicines are applicable" (Wood et al. 1926: 519).

This, however, was no news to Native Americans, who had all along been utilizing the plant or its root for the variety of purposes for which an astringent is typically used. For example, various tribes have utilized it for **diarrhea** (Smith 1928: 222; Smith 1932: 370–71; Gilmore 1933: 134). The Meskwaki (Fox) found that a poultice of the pounded root bound to a **hemorrhoid** caused it to recede (Smith 1928: 222). Some tribes have employed a douche of the decoction for **leukorrhea** (Winder 1846; cf. Moore 1994b: 13.8). The Cherokee found that a swish of wild geranium tea was a good medicine for **canker sores** (Hamel and Chiltoskey 1975: 35), while Pillager Ojibwe used it for **sore mouth** (Smith 1932: 370–71). The Iroquois found it helpful for sore mouth as well, even **trench mouth**, implementing the decoction from two pieces of roots about 3 inches long that have been boiled in 1 pint of water for just a bit or from boiling a small handful of roots in 2 quarts of water for a longer time (Herrick 1995: 190). The Meskwaki (Fox) discovered that a freshly sliced root portion could be poulticed directly onto an **aching** or **infected tooth** or onto **infected gums**, with fine results (Smith 1928: 222; cf. Moore 1979: 69).

The Eclectic physicians and later British and American herbalists built upon the astringent applications pioneered by Native tribes. With reference to its use for diarrhea, for instance, the Eclectics came to appreciate that it worked best with *chronic* diarrhea, especially when there were semiformed feces and frequent evacuations and when the inflammatory stage has passed and the mucous membranes have relaxed. Here the recommended dose was 10 drops of the tincture every two hours (Felter and Lloyd 1898; Ellingwood 1983: 347). Laurence Johnson, both a physician and a botanist who wrote in the latter part of the nineteenth century, commented glowingly on wild geranium (although he was generally critical of other botanicals in use by the Eclectics), pointing out regarding its application as an astringent:

"Although active and efficient, it is still mild and unirritating and devoid of all unpleasant or offensive properties. It is therefore particularly suited to the later stages of diarrhea and dysentery, especially in children. In such cases a decoction in milk has been found very serviceable" (Johnson 1884: 113). With reference to the common application of an injection or a douche for leukorrhea and for other genital discharges, he also made the pointed observation that "the decoction is much more serviceable than a simple injection of tannin, doubtless from the fact that there is present [in cranesbill] mucilaginous material which exerts a soothing influence" (Johnson 1884: 113).

Natura physician R. Swinburne Clymer came to appreciate that wild geranium root was especially helpful for the pain and distress characterizing **gastric ulcers** (Clymer 1973: 78). Southwest American herbalist Michael Moore likewise found wild geranium root helpful for gastric ulcers, especially when they were accompanied by vomiting (Moore 1994b: 10.24). However, a 2000 scholarly work by two of today's top herbalists opined that the plant might even be more useful for **duodenal ulcers** than gastric ulcers, perhaps even being too aggravating for the latter (Mills and Bone 2000: 176). Of interest here is that wild geranium has long been an important ingredient in the famed "Roberts formula," an herbal formula developed some time ago by noted

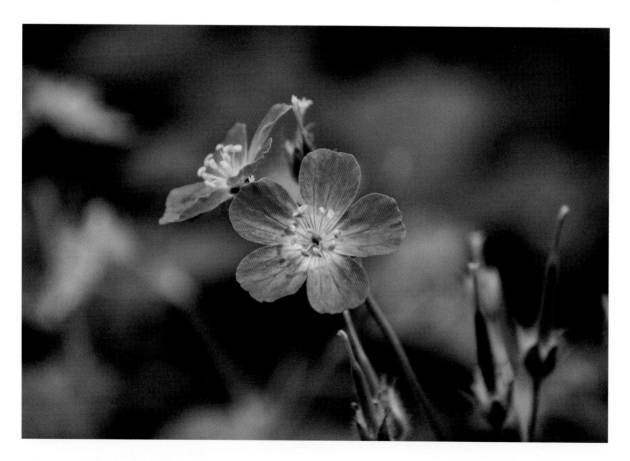

British herbalist Frank H. Roberts, which herbalists then and since have traditionally used for sores practically anywhere in the digestive tract but especially in the intestines.

In that wild geranium possesses *styptic* properties in view of its great astringency, many Native tribes and herbalists of various other cultures have found it helpful, as well, for **bleeding wounds**. In this regard, William Winder of Montreal remarked concerning the Native peoples of Great Manitoulin Island in Lake Huron that it was, for them, "a favorite external styptic, the dried root being powdered and placed on the mouth of the bleeding vessel" (Winder 1846: 11). In similar fashion, the Iroquois have used a chew of the root as a poultice for a **severed umbilical cord** (Herrick 1995: 190). Treatment of **menorrhagia** with wild geranium has also been traditional among herbalists of numerous cultures (Wren 1988: 95; Chevallier 1996: 214). Clymer found that it was "the remedy" for **lung hemorrhages**, dosed at 40–50 drops of the tincture—and, after success was obtained, repeated in doses of 10–15 drops and taken up to three times a day (Clymer 1973: 78). As if this plethora of treatments by widely differing cultures were not enough to demonstrate cranesbill's styptic abilities, a lab experiment conducted in 1938 found that it markedly increased clotting time in the blood of rabbits (Spoerke 1990: 65).

Wild geranium's very high amount of tannin allows it to serve as a useful *antimicrobial* agent, too. Here it is effective against *Candida* species and thus has been widely used for **oral thrush**, including by the Cherokee, who have used it in combination with chicken grape (*Vitis cordifolia*) for washing out the mouths of infants suffering from this condition (Hamel and Chiltoskey 1975: 35; cf. Moore 1979: 69). A 1954 study even revealed that it somewhat inhibited a virulent human strain of tuberculosis (Fitzpatrick 1954: 530). An even earlier antibiotic test revealed that it inhibited gram-positive bacteria (Suter 1951). Canadian research in the 1970s, followed by Bulgarian research since then with the European species *Geranium sanguineum*, has revealed that wild geranium also possesses powerful *antiviral* activity, especially against **herpes simplex infections** and **influenza** (Konowalchuk and Speirs 1976; Serkedzhieva et al. 1986; Serkedzhieva et al. 1987; Serkedzhieva et al. 1988). (The latter is interesting in view of early American use for **ague:** Vogel 1970: 390.) The Choctaw have considered it to be the most powerful natural agent against *venereal diseases* (Campbell and Roberts 1951: 287), and early American botanist-physician Benjamin Barton recommended it for *gonorrhea* (Barton 1810: 1:7, 2:1, appendix:45).

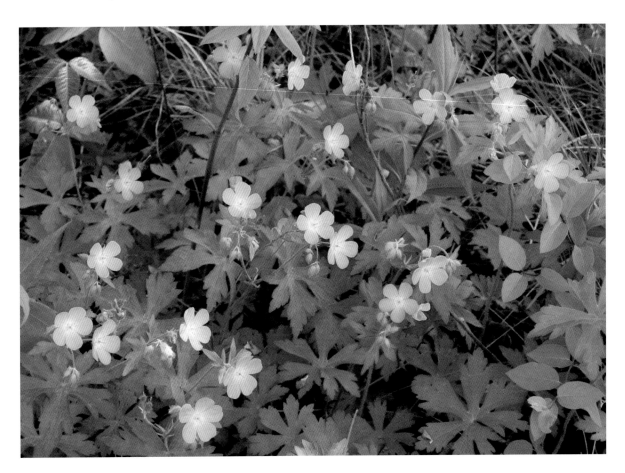

Applications for our gorgeous wild geranium seem almost endless. Michael Moore used to recommend it for both **tonsillitis** and **diverticulitis** (Moore 1979: 69). Yet others find it helpful in **irritable bowel syndrome** (Chevallier 1996: 21). Certain Native American tribes have applied a poultice of the mashed roots to breasts afflicted with **mastitis** in order to help relieve the pain.

Wild geranium has shown experimental *hypoglycemic* activity (Lewis and Elvin-Lewis 1977: 219). Canadian herbalist Terry Willard has even found that it can leach mercury from the body, should poisoning from that toxic element be suspected (Willard 1993: 266).

I predict that herbal birth control will be a wave of the twenty-first century, and wild geranium is certainly a plant to look at in this regard: the Nevada used to give the tea to a woman one month after childbirth to keep her from conceiving until the child was at least one year old (Scully 1970: 121). Virginia Scully, author of a popular book on Native ethnobotany, felt that the use of wild geranium tea was probably the most widely used method of *birth control* among tribes (Scully 1970: 178).

Finally, in view of this plant's cooling and drying properties, herbalist Peter Holmes recommends it for conditions of the urinary system viewed by Traditional Chinese Medicine as involving "kidney fire," such as **anuria** and **acute nephritis** (Holmes 1989–90: 2:821). Interestingly, these applications are in accord with speculation among early American physicians that wild geranium would be helpful "perhaps in nephritis" (Barton 1810: 1:7, 2:1, appendix:45). A bit later down the stream of time, the Eclectics put it to the test for "hot" urinary-tract afflictions and were most satisfied (Felter and Lloyd 1898). One of their number, Finley Ellingwood, once remarked in this regard that he "treated a case of hematuria for nearly two years with absolutely no permanent impression upon this condition. … All of the usual remedies were used. Finally fifteen drops of geranium were given every two hours, and in two weeks the blood was absent and had not returned at the end of three years, except mildly when the patient persistently overworked" (Ellingwood 1983: 347).

PERSONAL AND PROFESSIONAL USE

Just as the Meskwaki (Fox) have poulticed wild geranium root onto an aching or infected tooth, as mentioned above, I found occasion to use the same remedy, to my great relief, in the 1980s when I was bothered by a sore tooth and unable to get to a dentist. I was so happy with the results that I vowed never to allow the roots to be lacking in my cupboards!

Also in the 1980s, the Roberts formula successfully knocked out a duodenal protoulcer that I had developed, after lengthy trials of both cimetidine and ranitidine had failed miserably even to touch it.

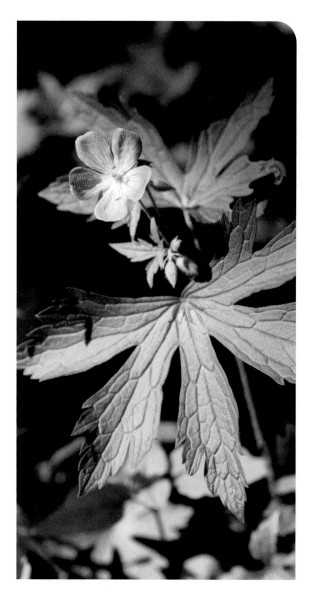

In my clinical practice, I've used wild geranium as a swish for both oral thrush (even once in an AIDS patient, for whom it worked marvelously after prescribed drugs hadn't improved the situation at all) and trench mouth, as well as via the Roberts formula for duodenal ulcers and ulcerative colitis. Although I also use other agents for these intestinal conditions, the Roberts formula always proves to be indispensable.

CAUTIONS

Wild geranium's extremely high content of tannin contraindicates its use for any length of time, as this substance may be harmful to the liver and in other ways if used injudiciously.

Because of its traditional use among Native Americans as a contraceptive, wild geranium *should not be taken internally during pregnancy.* ⋘

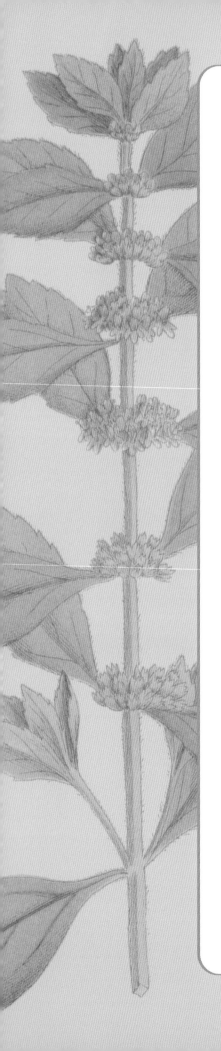

Wild Mint

CORN MINT; FIELD MINT; CANADA MINT;
BROOK MINT; NATIVE MINT

Mentha canadensis [alternatively, *M. arvensis var. canadensis*]

DESCRIPTION

Wild mint is a perennial herb that grows 6–24 inches tall and is possessed of a square stem that is usually not branched. That stem may be either hairy or smooth, and it often appears to be reclining at the base.

The plant has opposite, stalked, freely toothed leaves with a strong, characteristic minty odor, especially when disturbed (such as when stepped on!). They are lanceolate to ovate in shape, about 2 inches long, and tapered at their tips. Peculiar dotted glands adorn their surface.

This herb possesses tiny bell-shaped flowers that may be white, pale pink, or pale blue. These blossoms cluster in balls around the stem at the leaf nodes.

This is the Midwest's only native *Mentha*. Other *Mentha* species in our area (including peppermint) have either been introduced or are garden escapees.

RANGE AND HABITAT

Wild mint can be found predominantly in wet places or in damp soil such as occurs in moist woods, streambanks, ditches, wet fields, and on the perimeters of bodies of water. In the Midwest, the plant is ubiquitous in such terrain.

MAJOR CONSTITUENTS

Wild mint contains essential oil, consisting largely of menthol (65–80 percent, the highest source known—up to 26,000 parts per million), menthone (5–30 percent), piperitone, cineole, limonene, camphene, pulegone, carvone, eugenol, and menthol acetate). Also present are rosmarinic acid, flavonoids (luteolin, hesperidin), resin, oligosaccharides, and tannin. Nutrients include pro-vitamin A and vitamins C and K as well as calcium, iron, magnesium, zinc, and potassium.

FOOD

One can use this mint in all recipes for which the domesticated mints are prized—in a mint julep, as a garnish, and more.

HEALTH/MEDICINE

Native American tribes have widely used and cherished this highly scented herb, which ably proves its worth for infectious illnesses: the Mohawk, Potawatomi, Cherokee, Tête-de-Boule, and Pillager Ojibwe have implemented it as an *antipyretic* (Smith 1932: 371–72; Smith 1933: 61; Raymond 1945: 129; Rousseau 1945a: 58; White 1945: 562; Hamel and Chiltoskey 1975: 45), while the Midwest's Menomini have combined it with catnip and peppermint to treat **pneumonia**, drinking the mixture as a tea and poulticing it onto the chest (Smith 1923: 39). The Potawatomi have also used it for **pleurisy** (Smith 1933: 61; Vogel 1970: 340), while the Woods Cree have found it to be most effective for **infected gums**, combining the ground flowers with those of yarrow (*Achillea millefolium* [see page 282]), in a moistened cloth to use as a topical rub (Leighton 1985: 45). With reference to the abovementioned widespread use of wild mint for infections, it is of interest that scientific studies published since the late 1960s have verified that the plant and its essential oil are powerful *bactericides* and *fungicides* (Sanyal and Varma 1969; Kishore et al. 1993; Duarte et al. 2005; Coutinho et al. 2008; Johnson et al. 2011: 196; Makkar et al. 2018).

As to other applications, the Cheyenne, Flambeau Ojibwe, and Blackfoot have used an infusion of wild mint as a remedy for **heart problems** (Smith 1932: 371; Grinnell 1972: 186; Hart 1981: 27). Such a cardiac assist may be due to *stimulant* properties widely thought capable of being elicited from this plant. Such activity may also explain wild mint's cherished reputation as a *libido restorer*, which effects have been treasured especially by the Cheyenne (Hart 1981: 27).

Further with regard to sexual function, several animal studies have indicated that wild mint is a *contraceptive*, decreasing sperm concentration, motility, and viability but without negatively affecting libido. Moreover, these effects were found to be nontoxic and reversible within thirty days of a treatment period lasting sixty days (Sharma and Jacob 2001; Sharma and Jacob 2002).

Like most other mints, *Mentha canadensis* is a powerful *stomachic* and *carminative*. Tribes of the Missouri region have thus appreciated it for **flatulence** (Gilmore 1991: 60), as have our own area's Ojibwe (Gilmore 1933: 140). Tribes of the Nevada region found it invaluable for **diarrhea** (Train et al. 1988: 69). The Cheyenne have appreciated it for its remarkable *antiemetic* effects (Grinnell 1905: 39; Hart 1981: 27).

As to additional applications: The Lakota and Gosiute have relieved **headache** with a strong tea made from its roots (Chamberlin 1911: 351; Buechel 1983: 461, 799). The Kayenta Navajo (Diné) have poulticed the leaves onto **swollen areas** of the body (Wyman and Harris 1951: 40), as have the Kawaiisu (Zigmond 1981: 40). Finally, the Woods Cree have poulticed ground wild mint onto **aching teeth** (Leighton 1985: 45).

A sports-medicine study reported at the International Symposium on Essential Oils in Berlin in 1993 found that a gel made from the oil of this plant surpassed the usual salicylate treatment for the care of acute and subacute **sports injuries** based upon the level of *analgesia* experienced—78 percent receiving the wild-mint therapy reported good results, as contrasted with only 34 percent in the salicylate group (Bergner 1994–95: 12). Undoubtedly, both the menthol and the eugenol content in wild mint are prime factors in such a powerful pain numbing ability.

Finally, exciting new research out of the National Chemical Laboratory in Pune, India, has demonstrated that wild-mint leaves can reduce the postprandial release of glucose in the blood and thereby offset **postprandial hyperglycemia** (now understood to be more serious than fasting hyperglycemia) (Agawane et al. 2019).

PERSONAL AND PROFESSIONAL USE
I much savor the taste of wild-mint tea and of wild-mint julep—both of which I am fond of making!

In my clinical practice, I've implemented wild mint in formulas for upper-body eczema, irritable bowel syndrome, and cardiac weakness. I also like to use it as a simple for flatulence or for nausea.

CAUTIONS
This plant has demonstrated *abortive* effects in animals and thus *should not be used during either pregnancy or lactation* due to its high content of both menthol and carvone (Kanjanapothi et al. 1981: 559).

Never apply wild mint topically to the head, neck, or chest of an infant, as the significant levels of menthol possessed by this plant could cause *instant respiratory collapse* (Leung 1980: 232). ᐊᐊᐊ

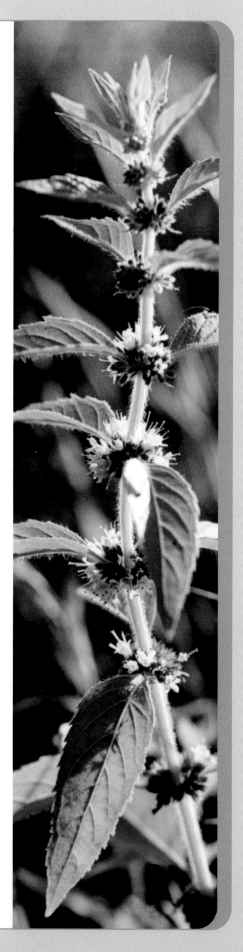

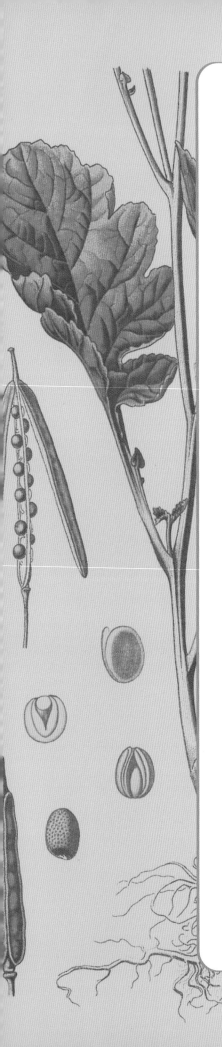

Wild Mustard

Brassica spp.

DESCRIPTION

Wild mustard is an annual weed with slender, erect, branching stems that are covered with stiff hairs.

The leaves are alternate and hairy. The lower ones are stalked and deeply divided, while the uppermost blades are sessile, coarsely toothed, and bristly.

The characteristic four-petaled yellow flowers, growing about ½ inch wide, are clustered atop the branched stems. As the petals fall, slender seedpods develop, containing minute, dark-colored, pungent seeds.

The Midwest's major species are as follows:

Brassica nigra (black mustard) is an annual that grows 2–6 feet tall and possesses a round stem. The lower leaves have four lateral lobes and a large terminal one. The upper leaves are lanceolate and serrated but lack lobes. The four-sided seedpods are about ¾ inch long and sharply angled upward, practically appressed against the stem. Most conspicuously, they are beaked at their tips. The seeds contained within the pods are brown in color.

B. alba (alternatively, *Sinapis alba*) (white mustard) is an annual reaching a height of 2–5 feet. Its leaves are smoother and its flowers larger than in other *Brassica* species. Unlike *B. nigra*, above, its seedpods are not beaked.

B. kaber (crunchweed, charlock) tops off at 8–30 inches and has green stems that are hairy near the base. The middle and upper leaves are toothed, while the lower leaves are deeply lobed. The fruits lack visible hairs or are very lightly pubescent.

Brassica species should be distinguished from the similar-looking wintercress (*Barbarea vulgaris*), which has hairless stems and rounded, glossy leaves—the lower of which are deeply lobed (the terminal lobe being especially prominent).

RANGE AND HABITAT

Brassica species thrive in fields, meadows, wasteland, and clearings throughout the Midwest.

MAJOR CONSTITUENTS

Black mustard contains sinapine (an alkaloid); myosin (an enzyme); sinigrin (a glycoside); irritant oil (allyl isothiocyanate, as a result of hydrolysis, which causes myosin to act on sinigrin, thereby producing the oil); fixed oils (up to 37 percent, including oleic, palmitic, erucic, arachic, and eicosenoic); alkanes; urease; arginase; lipase; and mucilage.

White mustard contains sinalbin, which winds up being enzymatically converted into the irritant oil isothiocyanate, exuding a less pungent odor than does black mustard's oil.

Mustard greens are rich in vitamins and minerals. A whopping 7,000 imperial units of pro-vitamin A occurs in a 100-gram portion, as well as 100 milligrams of vitamin C and goodly amounts of several vitamins B1 and B2. Minerals occurring in appreciable amounts include calcium (183 milligrams per 100 grams), potassium (32 milligrams per 100 grams), phosphorus (30 milligrams per 100 grams), and iron (3 milligrams per 100 grams).

FOOD

Very young leaves can be added to salads to give them more of a zing or else nibbled on sparingly in the field. Older leaves must be boiled in two waters for about twenty to thirty minutes total. Properly prepared like this, however, they are quite tasty and are especially relished by many people of Southeast Asian descent living in the Midwest.

Naturalist and herbalist Tom Brown Jr. relishes the taste of the unopened flower heads, which he cooks like broccoli. He says that they are best when steamed for five minutes; if accidentally cooked longer, they will lose their fine taste and become mushy. Later in the growing season, Brown enjoys the tender young seedpods added to salads or eaten as a trail nibble (Brown 1985: 151, 153).

HEALTH/MEDICINE

Undoubtedly, the most famous application of mustard for medicinal purposes is the ages-old mustard plaster, a treatment that has been used for **pneumonia**, **bronchitis**, **arthritic pains**, **rheumatic pains**, and general **joint stiffness** (de Bairacli Levy 1974: 102; Duke 1997: 386). Traditionally, 120 grams (4 ounces) of ground black-mustard seeds have been mixed with equal to thrice the amount of wheat flour and some water to make a paste that is sandwiched between two layers of muslin or flannel and then gently placed on the affected area, sometimes being covered by a towel to retain the heat. This is never applied to children under six years old, nor does the application for adults or older children ever exceed fifteen minutes, with five or ten minutes

being usually sufficient (Hoffmann 1986: 211; Jones 1991: 43; Willard 1992b: 131; Fetrow and Avila 1999: 447). After the plaster is removed and any mustard residue carefully wiped off, olive oil or egg white is applied to the area or it is sponged with cold water to minimize smarting of the skin. The Meskwaki (Fox) have even bound black-mustard leaves to an **aching tooth** or **head**, being ever mindful of its potential for burning the skin (Tantaquidgeon 1928: 265).

Yet how does a mustard plaster serve so ably to relieve the discomfort of the conditions delineated above? As a *rubefacient* (or counterirritant), the mustard oil induces the peripheral blood vessels to dilate, with the resultant rush of blood drawing the inflammatory chemicals away from the original, deeper site (Dobelis et al. 1986: 108). Laurence Johnson, a nineteenth-century physician and botanist often critical of herbal remedies of the day, nevertheless acknowledged of mustard that "as a rubefacient, its sphere of usefulness is practically unlimited" (Johnson 1884: 96).

The ancient Roman physician Celsus even urged that a mustard plaster be applied to **paralyzed limbs** in order to "stimulate the skin of the torpid limb," but he gave the customary caution that it be removed "as soon as the skin becomes red" (Celsus 1938: 3.27). Probably one of the most universally appreciated applications has been the addition of some mustard powder into a tub of water as a footbath

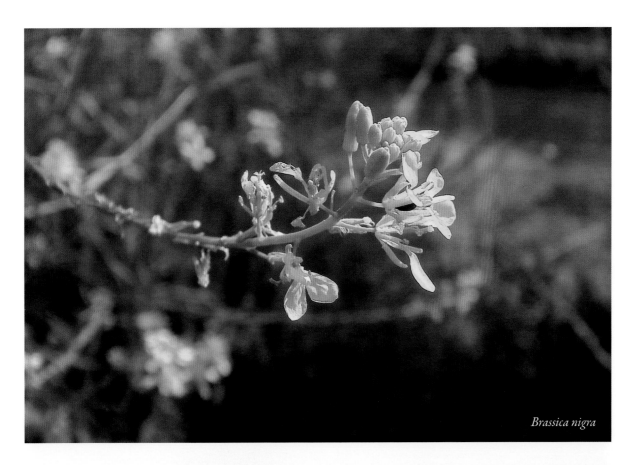

Brassica nigra

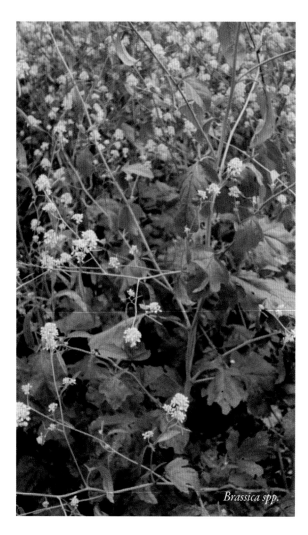
Brassica spp.

It is of interest in this regard that the seeds serve to improve digestion not only by marshaling the gastric juices but also by stimulating pancreatic secretions (Lewis and Elvin-Lewis 1977: 273, 278). Then, too, when there are infestations of microorganisms in the GI tract, the use of mustard in foods can lend a helping hand, since its irritant oil is powerfully *antimicrobial*, and that against many different kinds of bacteria and fungi (Fitzpatrick 1954: 531; Abdullin 1962: 75).

Going beyond the traditional culinary use, mustard can serve as a mild *laxative*—the usual dose here being ½ teaspoon of crushed seeds in a glass of warm water (Jones 1991: 43). A dose a bit stronger (1–3 drachms in 6–8 ounces of warm water, according to the Eclectics, or 1 tablespoon of mustard flour in a glass of tepid water, according to the herbal of Englishwoman M. Grieve: Felter and Lloyd 1898; Grieve 1971: 2:569) has long served as a "prompt and efficient emetic" for household poisonings (Johnson 1884: 96), although syrup of ipecac has replaced mustard as an emergency emetic in most modern American homes.

Mustard has long served as an important part of Dr. Coffin's Famous Formula for **dropsy**, which consists of ½ ounce of the crushed seeds and 1 ounce of fresh horseradish root, which mixture is covered with 1 pint of boiling water, steeped for four hours, strained, and then dosed at 3 tablespoons, repeated twice during the day (Hutchens 1991: 156; Willard 1993: 130).

PERSONAL AND PROFESSIONAL USE

I have long enjoyed adding a few wild-mustard leaves to a salad of wild greens when I am out foraging for wild foods.

CAUTIONS

Mustard is contraindicated as a medicine and as a food in quantity when there is hypothyroidism.

Those having venous disorders should not use mustard medicinally.

Do *not* use a mustard plaster on a *child under six years of age*. Do *not* leave a mustard plaster on an adult longer than fifteen minutes or on a child older than six longer than five minutes. In fact, in all cases, it should be removed as soon as a burning sensation is felt or the skin is observed to redden. Be sure to wash off any remaining mustard paste from the skin, even if not visible. The subsequent application of olive oil or egg whites to the area where it had been applied may dull any residual smarting, as may dabbing the region with cold water. ⪻

for **tired**, **aching feet**, **chilled feet**, or even a **chilled body** in general (Carse 1989: 136). Tom Brown Jr. experienced such a footbath as a lad and later enthused about it in his memoirs, although he was careful to note that he washed off all of the mustard water afterward to prevent his skin from being burned (Brown 1985: 151). The usual dose for a mustard bath is 1 tablespoon of bruised seeds to 1 quart of hot water.

Mustard flour can be of great assistance when gastrointestinal problems are occurring. It serves ably as a digestive *tonic* for **poor appetite**, **halitosis**, or **flatulence** (de Bairacli Levy 1974: 102; Brown 1985: 151). Such uses have a treasured pedigree in American domestic practice: writing in 1884, Laurence Johnson remarked that "as an aid to digestion, it [mustard] is used in every household" (Johnson 1884: 96).

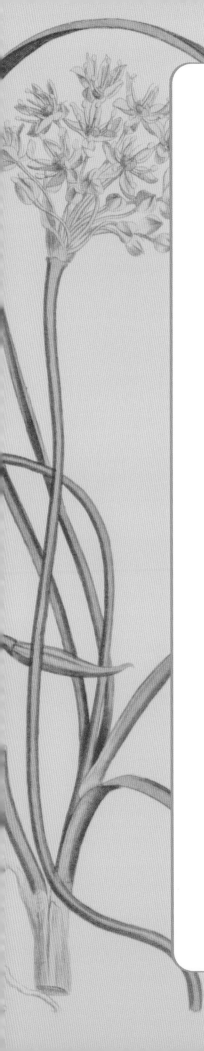

Wild Onion

Allium stellatum

DESCRIPTION

As might be expected, this is a strong-smelling herb, growing 1–2½ feet tall. It has a long, straight, tubular stem and usually two narrow, flat, grass-like basal leaves.

Individual flowers are star-like in shape, sporting three petals, three sepals, and six stamens. They are pink to purple in color.

The faded, autumn inflorescence is dotted with small, but showy, black seeds.

The related species *Allium cernuum* (nodding wild onion), thriving in a single county in Minnesota, has a drooping flower cluster because of a bend at the tip of the stem.

RANGE AND HABITAT

One species or another of wild onion occurs in every American state except Hawaii and in all of Canada except for the far north. *A. stellatum* thrives pretty much throughout the Midwest. Its preferred habitat consists of meadows, fields, prairies, plains, and open and rocky places.

SEASONAL AVAILABILITY

I have dug wild onions as late as the first week of December and found them to be crisp and delicious even at that time! Mostly, however, the bulbs start to decay in November.

MAJOR CONSTITUENTS

Wild onion contains flavonoids (especially quercetin), sterols, saponins, inulin, and sulfur compounds.

FOOD

Raw bulbs can be added to salads to give them a richer taste. They lend themselves to a variety of recipes, too; they can be boiled but need at least one change of water in order to reduce their otherwise overly strong flavor. A simpler and often more welcome method is just to roast them, something that is especially apropos in an outdoor setting. One can accomplish this by placing the unpeeled bulbs on a bed of medium-hot coals. When tender, the skin can be poked to allow the steam to be released. Then, the interior can be spooned out, flavored as desired, and added to hamburgers, sandwiches, or wild dishes.

A number of Native American tribes have appreciated the ability of the wild onion to add its pungent flavor to so many meals: the Cheyenne, Blackfoot, and others have often cooked meat with these onions in order to improve its flavor (as we do with domesticated onions).

Wild onions, like their domestic counterparts, also can be made into an excellent soup and can be added to stews during the last ten minutes of cooking.

HEALTH/MEDICINE

A. stellatum has been appreciated by the Midwest's Ojibwe for **respiratory complaints**, especially in children, to whom it is given by way of a sweetened decoction (Densmore 1974: 310–14).

The chewed aerial portions of the related *A. cernuum*—found in a few counties in the Midwest—have been placed on the chest of those suffering from **pleurisy** by the

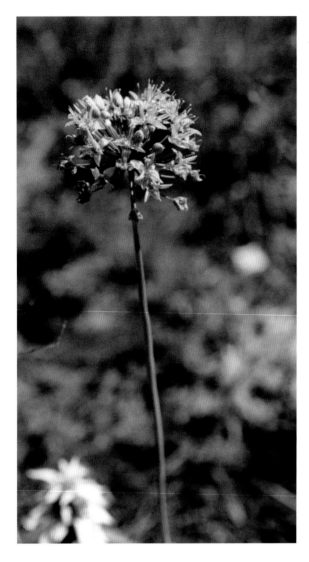

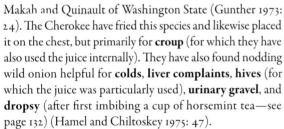

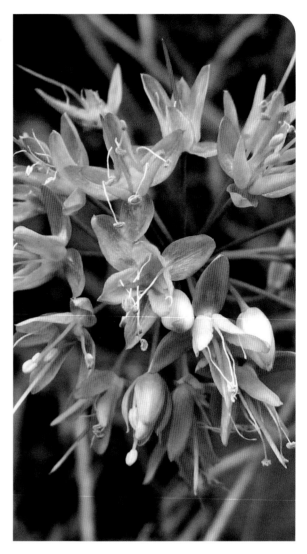

Makah and Quinault of Washington State (Gunther 1973: 24). The Cherokee have fried this species and likewise placed it on the chest, but primarily for **croup** (for which they have also used the juice internally). They have also found nodding wild onion helpful for **colds**, **liver complaints**, **hives** (for which the juice was particularly used), **urinary gravel**, and **dropsy** (after first imbibing a cup of horsemint tea—see page 132) (Hamel and Chiltoskey 1975: 47).

The bruised bulbs of various unspecified species of wild onion have been used by Native Americans—including our own area's Dakota and Winnebago (Ho-Chunk)—as a poultice for the **stings** of **wasps** and **bees**. A medical doctor named F. Andros, who observed this treatment for years, wrote that it "almost instantly relieves the pain" (Andros 1883: 117). Eclectic physician Finley Ellingwood offered similar observations: "The onion poultice stands in high favor with me for all swelling. ... Roasted[,] the cut surface [can be] applied hot to glandular inflammations and suppurating tumors" (Ellingwood 1983: 261).

PERSONAL AND PROFESSIONAL USE

I really enjoy digging and eating wild onions, which grow plentifully in my area in open, sunny, dry fields and meadows. In fact, as mentioned, I've dug and eaten them as late as early December!

CAUTIONS

Green portions of onions should probably not be eaten, as they readily absorb selenium from the soil and pollutants from the air. (Selenium in amounts above 600 micrograms per day can be toxic if ingested over an extended period of time.)

Persons sensitive to inulin may develop indigestion and/or flatulence from eating raw onions.

Do not collect any plants that may look like wild onions but *lack the characteristic odor*, as several inedible plants—including one very toxic one, death camas (*Zigadenus venenosus*)—resemble this herb, especially in the feature of its grass-like leaves. ⪻

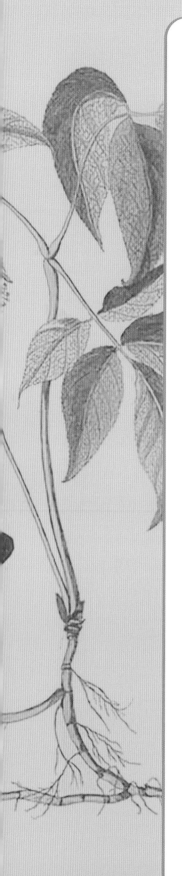

Wild Sarsaparilla

FALSE SARSAPARILLIA; AMERICAN SARSAPARILLA

Aralia nudicaulis

DESCRIPTION

Wild sarsaparilla is a pretty, leafy woodland plant that typically grows to about 1 foot high but can top off at 16 inches. The stems are thick, square, and lightly prickled.

The three branches of "leaves" are actually but one solitary leaf divided pinnately into three groups of five-toothed leaflets. Each leaflet tends to grow 2–4 inches long.

The leaf grows from a strongly aromatic underground rhizome, which also sends forth a leafless stem (shorter than the leaf stem) upon which the plant's globular flowers appear. As with the leaflets, the greenish-white flower umbels are in threes, with each cluster growing on a separate branch of the flower stem.

Round berries, dark blue to dark purple in color, replace the flowers in July.

RANGE AND HABITAT

This species can be found growing in moist to mesic woods in the northern half of the Midwest.

SEASONAL AVAILABILITY

The rhizome is collected in either the spring or the autumn.

MAJOR CONSTITUENTS

Little chemical work has been done, but research has revealed that the rhizome contains an essential oil, polyacetylenes (falcarinol and panaxydol), resin, pectin, and sugars. The berries contain a glycoside.

FOOD

The dried rhizomes make a very pleasant drink. One needs simply to powder three or four of them and to stir the results into a cup of boiling water. Afterward, the mixture is cooled, strained, and sweetened. Alternatively, one can decoct the roots until the water becomes a reddish color and then strain, sweeten, and serve as a hot beverage. The rhizomes are most famous, however, for the root beer that was made from them in colonial times. I might add that I can confirm the raw rhizome, contrary to many popular foraging manuals, is *not* edible but leaves a sting in the throat!

To humans, the plant's berries are toxic when eaten raw, as they contain a glycoside that also leaves a sting in the throat—as I can well attest. (This principle does not seem to bother animals such as foxes and bears, however, as these critters feast readily upon them.) Some say that the berries are edible when cooked because the heat breaks down the glycoside. I cannot say, as I have never tried doing that.

HEALTH/MEDICINE

This plant has a long history of use by both whites and Native peoples. As to use by the former, the renowned botanist Constantine Rafinesque, writing in the early 1800s, noted that the plant's then-current physiological affectations were as follows: *diaphoretic*, *stimulant*, *depurative*, *sudorific*, *pectoral*, *cordial*, and *vulnerary*. Regarding the latter, he wrote: "The fresh roots and leaves chewed and applied to wounds, heal them speedily;

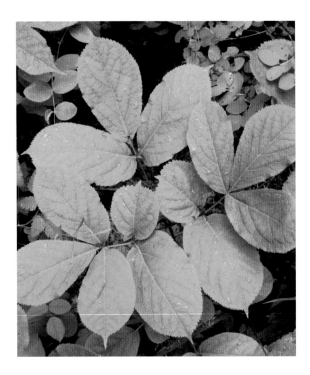

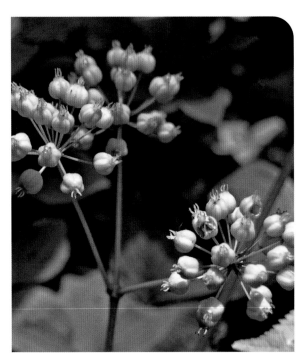

Dr. Sp. informed me that he was once cured by them alone of a desperate accidental wound by a broad axe" (Rafinesque 1828–30: 1:53–55). As to wild sarsaparilla's depurative abilities, John Gunn's famous *Household Guide* of the mid- to late 1800s explained that the plant is "useful in constitutional disease, such as scrofula, syphilis, skin diseases, and wherever an alterative and purifying medicine is needed" (Gunn 1859–61: 886). The rhizome of wild sarsaparilla wound up as official medicine in the *United States Pharmacopeia* for sixty-two years (from 1820 until 1882), where it was held to be diaphoretic and stimulant as well as *alterative*. Scientific research has also shown it to be *cytotoxic* to human leukemia and colon-cancer cells (Huang et al. 2006; Wang et al. 2006).

As for Native American uses of *Aralia nudicaulis*, there have been many. The Midwest's Ojibwe have utilized it to treat **nosebleeds**, for which the rhizome was dried, powdered, and used as a snuff; on some occasions, however, the fresh root was chewed and inserted into the bleeding nostril. They also found it helpful for **amenorrhea** and for various **blood disorders** (Reagan 1928: 231; Densmore 1974: 340–41, 350–51, 356–57, 366–67). **Fits** and **fainting** were yet other conditions for which they implemented it (Reagan 1928: 231).

Vulnerary applications were the most frequent kind of use by Native tribes, however. Thus, the Ojibwe have pounded the rhizome and applied it to **sores** (Densmore 1974: 350). The Meskwaki (Fox) have done the same (Smith 1928: 203), while the Potawatomi have poulticed it onto **swellings** and **infections** (Smith 1933: 40–41). The Ojibwe of the Flambeau region have poulticed the pounded, fresh root onto **boils** to bring them to a head and also to resolve **carbuncles** (Smith 1932: 356).

The Creek have found it helpful for **pleurisy** (Swanton 1928: 658), while the Penobscot and Kwakiutl have utilized the dried, powdered rhizome to make a **cough** syrup (Vogel 1970: 361). The Iroquois have added a decoction of the rhizome to parts of other plants to make medicine for the cough of **tuberculosis** (Herrick 1977: 393). Interestingly here, scientific research has found the rhizome's polyacetylenes to exert *antimycobacterial* activity (Li et al. 2012; Li et al. 2015). The Woods Cree have used the whole plant in decoction for **childhood pneumonia** (Leighton 1985: 29).

Numerous Native tribes have also made use of wild sarsaparilla's *nephritic* and *urinary* functions: the Creek have implemented wild sarsaparilla for **difficult urination**, **bloody urination**, and **pain in the back or lower abdomen** (Swanton 1928: 658). A number of tribes have valued the plant as a *tonic*, including the Thompson (Steedman 1928: 471), Okanogan (Perry 1952: 42), Mohegan (Tantaquidgeon 1972: 70), Montagnais (Speck 1917: 315), Blackfoot (EthnobDB), Meskwaki (Fox) (Smith 1928: 203), and Lenape (Delaware) (Tantaquidgeon 1942: 74).

PERSONAL AND PROFESSIONAL USE

Decocting wild-sarsaparilla tea on the stove is a pastime that I greatly enjoy, although drinking it afterward is even more fun because it tastes so very good!

CAUTIONS

Raw berries or rhizomes should not be consumed. ⤺

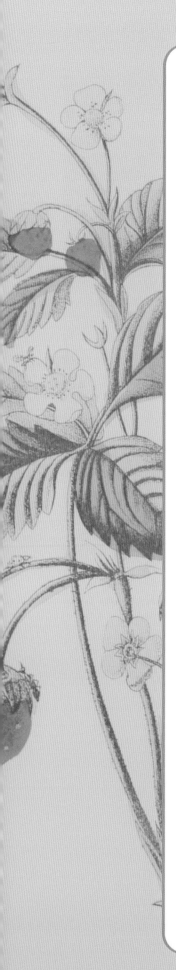

Wild Strawberry

Fragaria virginiana

DESCRIPTION

This is a low perennial herb (3–6 inches tall) possessed of roots that send out runners, so that it is often found in colonies.

The dark-green leaves are wholly basal and are divided into three coarsely toothed, broadly elliptical leaflets, each growing 1–1½ inches long. The leafstalks are quite hairy.

The pleasantly scented flowers—each possessing five rounded petals, five sepals, and five bracts—are in stalked clusters. The many yellow stamens create the illusion that the blossoms possess a yellow center disk.

The fruits consist of small, dark, hard achenes embedded in a fleshy-red receptacle shaped like a top—a berry. Each berry rests on a hull of ten small calyx lobes. The thin, filament-like stems on which the berries form can't help but droop under their weight, so that the ruby-red morsels often wind up being somewhat obscured by the leaves.

A related species, wood strawberry (*Fragaria vesca*), has more elongate berries, with achenes standing out a bit from the fleshy receptacles. Its sepals point backward.

RANGE AND HABITAT

This plant is found throughout the United States and southern Canada except in arid regions. The preferred habitat is roadsides, open woods, and old, grassy fields.

SEASONAL AVAILABILITY

Berries are available in the Midwest for only about three weeks, from mid-June to early July.

MAJOR CONSTITUENTS

The berries contain glycosides (arbutin), flavonoids (including anthocyanins), lutein, pectin, organic acids (citric, malic), salicylates, mucilage, and the amino acid arginine. Nutrients include vitamins (pro-vitamin A, B-complex, C, and E) and minerals such as calcium, potassium, magnesium, sulfur, and iron. The leaves contain ellagic acid and are extremely high in vitamin C. The roots contain ellagitannin.

FOOD

The berry of this lovely little wild plant is universally acknowledged to be tastier than its domestic counterpart. The famed English writer Izaak Walton (1593–1683), in quoting a certain Dr. Boteler, put it well: "Doubtless God could have made a better berry, but doubtless God never did!"

Excellent pies and jam can be made from the berries, but it is difficult to save enough of the gathered jewels to do the job, since one is tempted to eat five berries on the spot for every one saved! What berries one does manage to collect should have their hulls pinched off immediately upon picking, since this is difficult to accomplish later when the weight of so many berries in the collecting vessel has crushed those on the bottom.

Dried leaves can be steeped to make a tea that is pleasant and mild to the taste. See Cautions on wilted leaves.

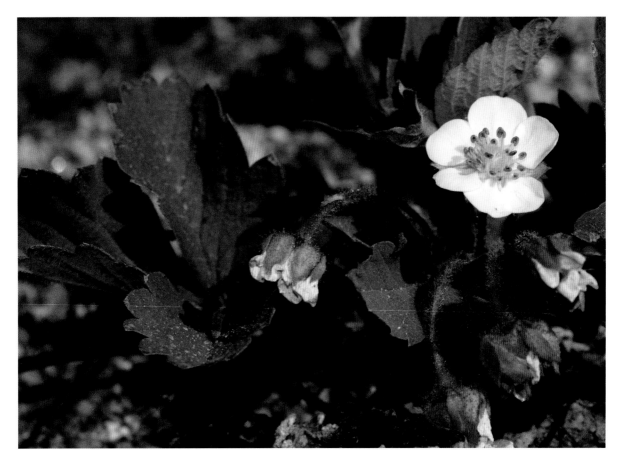

HEALTH/MEDICINE

The berry juice is a powerful *refrigerant*, useful internally for **fevers** and topically for **sunburn**. For the latter, M. Grieve's herbal recommends rubbing the juice well into the sun-burned area and leaving it there for half an hour, afterward washing it off with warm water into which a few drops of tincture of benzoin have been added (Grieve 1971: 2:777). The significant amount of iron in the berries also allows these little rubies to be used in the diet to help offset iron-deficient **anemia**, especially in that their high vitamin C content helps assure the iron's absorption. The overall high nutrient content, in fact, may at least partly explain the historic use of both the fruit and the leaves to treat **nervous debility** (de Bairacli Levy 1974: 140).

The Cherokee discovered that holding the fruit in the mouth helped to remove **tartar** from the teeth (Hamel and Chiltoskey 1975: 57). This seems to work quite well, especially if the fruits are rubbed on the teeth and the juice allowed to remain there for about five minutes, followed by a brushing of the teeth with baking soda (to neutralize the acidity of the strawberries so that they don't damage the teeth) and water (Schofield Eaton 1989: 183). Because of the high sulfur content of strawberries and because they possess a similar pH as the skin, Virginia Castleton, in her *Handbook of Natural Beauty*, advised mixing a cup of mashed strawberries with a cup of water and spreading this on the skin of the face, hands, arms, shoulders, and chest before bed to enhance beauty, rinsing it off in the morning (cited in Schofield Eaton 1989: 183). This technique has also been used to diminish **freckles**.

The leaves are so enormously high in vitamin C that when Euell Gibbons had a sample analyzed for its content of this vitamin at Penn State, the lab tech thought he had doctored the sample because the amount turned out to be so incredible to her. When she proceeded to retest with her own sample, she was shocked to find an even greater amount of vitamin C! (Gibbons 1971: 158) Not surprisingly, strawberry-leaf tea has been used in folk medicine to prevent **colds**. Fortunately, as Gibbons reminds us, strawberry leaves are evergreen and thus continue to thrive right underneath the snow during winter. If found at this time, they can be harvested and dried to provide a rich source of vitamin C during these cold months when other avenues have largely disappeared.

Strawberry-leaf tea seems to have an affinity for the genitourinary system, proving helpful for **bladder**, **kidney**, and **urethral problems** (especially **dysuria**), as various Native American tribes discovered (Scully 1970: 267; Hamel and Chiltoskey 1975: 57). The berry, for its part, contains arbutin, the same chemical occurring in the renowned urinary herb uva ursi (bearberry), *Arctostaphylos uva-ursi*, which hydrolyzes in the system into hydroquinone, a powerful disinfectant for the urinary tract. It is also somewhat *diuretic* (Wren 1988: 260). Then, too, **gonorrhea** and **irregular menstruation** have been treated with this herb by the Malecite (Mechling 1959: 258).

Wild strawberry has a cherished reputation for helping to alleviate both **rheumatism** and **gout**. It is possible that the salicylate content may be mildly helpful here (Phillips and Foy 1990: 65). Surely of greater importance, however, is the herb's diuretic effect, serving to leach out the excess uric acid characterizing these most painful conditions (Ody 1993: 60). Modern research would also highlight the importance of the anthocyanin content. Yet, whatever the exact combination of mechanisms involved, we know that it works; in fact, the famed Swedish botanist and physician Carolus Linnaeus assured us that he cured himself of gout simply by subsisting for a time on a diet of wild strawberries! (Scully 1970: 267)

This herb has also traditionally been used for **jaundice** (Hamel and Chiltoskey 1975; Ody 1993: 60). Probably this is due to the digestive stimulation that the plant supplies, which also explains why it has traditionally been used for both **poor appetite** and **dyspepsia** (Dobelis et al. 1986: 339). The digestive-stimulating effect is probably also at least partly responsible for wild strawberry's long-appreciated application to **eczema**, a condition that seems to have a connection with a sluggishness of stomach function, liver function, and/or pancreatic-enzyme production. The Natura physician R. Swinburne Clymer, in fact, considered it to be the remedy par excellence for this irksome condition. Interestingly, he found it to work best in combination with other digestion-stimulating plants, such as the roots of dandelion (see page 99), burdock (page 60), and rhubarb (Clymer 1973: 137).

The type and amount of tannins in the leaves and especially the root allows an infusion of either part to be implemented for a variety of purposes owing to their powerful *astringency*. Thus, **sore gums** can often be alleviated by swishing a tea of wild strawberry leaves or root in the mouth or even simply by pressing a raw root against the gums. The tea also makes an excellent gargle for **sore throat**. **Diarrhea** often yields to its power as well, an application that has been a favorite among the Blackfoot, Cherokee, Thompson, and Micmac (Hellson and Gadd 1974: 66; Hamel and Chiltoskey 1975: 57; Turner et al. 1990: 259; Lacey 1993: 116). British herbalist Mary Carse discusses an application of the leaf tea to infant diarrhea, noting that ½ cup of the carefully strained and unsweetened tea can be put into a baby bottle three or four times a day but that no food should be given for twelve hours (Carse 1989: 161). (That last part is easier said than done!)

The Micmac have also appreciated the tea for **stomach cramps**, using 6 teaspoons of fresh or dried leaves to a pint

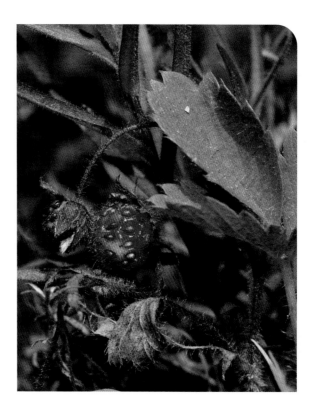

of boiled water and steeping such for fifteen minutes, then drinking 2–3 cups a day (Lacey 1993: 116). Several different Native tribes, in fact, have used the infusion for **stomachache** and even for **infant colic** (Smith 1932: 384; Turner et al. 1990: 259).

Externally, a powder made from the leaf has been dusted onto **sores** by the Okanogan-Colville (Turner et al. 1980: 125). The Quileute have chewed wild strawberry leaves and spit them onto **burns** (Gunther 1973: 36).

Finally, a Canadian study published in 2008 evinced potent *antifungal* activity from an aqueous extract of this plant. In fact, it was the only plant of fourteen analyzed to show activity against every one of the twenty-three different fungal isolates tested! (Webster et al. 2008)

PERSONAL AND PROFESSIONAL USE

It's hard to disagree with Walton, quoted earlier, about the exquisite taste of these little red jewels. In fact, I know of several patches in the wilds to which I return each and every June.

I've used wild-strawberry leaves in formulas for eczema and as a simple for diarrhea in both toddlers and adults and have not been disappointed by the results.

CAUTIONS

If you're allergic to cultivated strawberries, bear in mind that you will no doubt be allergic to the wild ones.

When drying the leaves for tea, be sure to dry them fully, as mere *wilted leaves can produce a dangerous mold*.

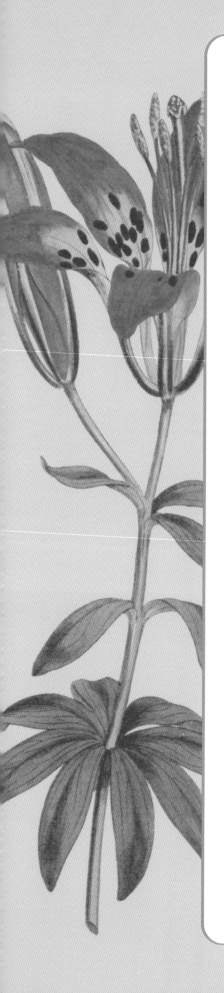

Wood Lily

PRAIRIE LILY; ORANGE-RED LILY; WILD LILY

Lilium philadelphicum

DESCRIPTION

This is a native perennial that grows 1½–2½ feet tall. The people of Saskatchewan, Canada, so appreciate its breathtaking beauty that they have made it their floral emblem.

The lanceolate leaves grow 1–4 inches long and are whorled in groups of three to eight (sometimes the lower leaves are not whorled, but merely scattered). The orange-red, bell-shaped corolla is erect, 2½ inches long, and 2–3 inches across. There are three petals and three sepals tapering to a stalked base, which is dotted inside with black or purplish brown. Six long stamens can be observed. The blossoms are single or in umbels of two to five.

RANGE AND HABITAT

Wood lily can be spotted in open and brushy places—meadows, prairies, thickets, clearings, and dry and open woods. It is most common in pine-forest country. It grows in scattered spots throughout the Midwest in such environs but is getting scarcer.

FOOD

The straight, bulbous roots have been gathered by the Meskwaki (Fox) and prepared and eaten like potatoes (Smith 1928: 262). The Woods Cree have consumed segments of the bulbs or sometimes dried them for a nibble when traveling; they have also relished the plant's seeds (Leighton 1985: 43). The Blackfoot have likewise feasted on the fresh bulbs, although sometimes they have saved them for stews (Hellson and Gadd 1974: 103).

HEALTH/MEDICINE

The Algonquin of Quebec found that wood-lily roots were good for helping to alleviate **stomach disorders** (Black 1980: 138). Various other tribes have implemented a tea of the roots to treat both **cough** and **fever** (Mechling 1959: 251; Chandler et al. 1979: 58), to expel **afterbirth** (Herrick 1977: 282), and to apply topically to **wounds**, **swellings bruises**, and **sores** (Densmore 1932: 132; Gilmore 1933: 125; Mechling 1959: 245; Chandler et al. 1979: 58).

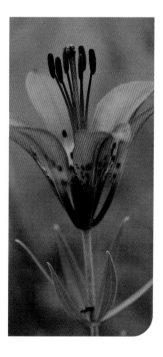

The Ojibwe of Michigan have used this plant topically, too—chiefly for **dog bites**, plastering it thereon with another (unidentified) plant species (Gilmore 1933: 125). The chewed or pulverized flowers of *Lilium umbellatum*, a thin-leaved subspecies of *L. philadelphicum* found in the southern tip of Minnesota and southward along the Missouri River region, have been poulticed onto the **poisonous bites** of a small brown spider by the Dakota, which quickly relieved the painful inflammation (Gilmore 1977: 19). ⤺⤺

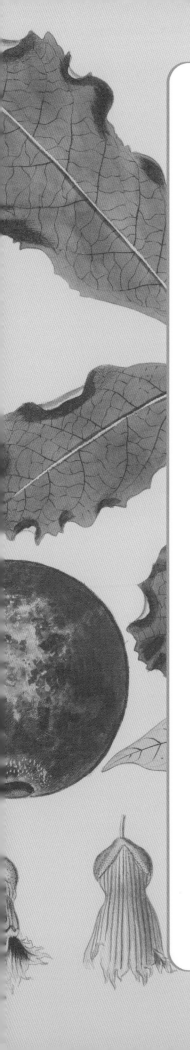

Wood Nettle

CANADA WOOD NETTLE

Laportea canadensis

DESCRIPTION

This is a large, conspicuous herb growing to 4 feet and possessed of a stem that is covered with stinging hairs.

The alternate, ovate leaves are noticeably long stalked and coarsely toothed. They grow 3–8 inches long.

The small greenish flowers occur in loose, branching clusters in the plant's axils: male blossoms (having five sepals and five stamens) in the lower axils and female ones (with four sepals and one pistil) in the upper axils. The flowers of both sexes lack petals.

RANGE AND HABITAT

Wood nettle can often be found growing in dense colonies on streambanks as well as on trailsides in wet woods. This species occurs throughout the Midwest in such environs.

FOOD

Wood nettle is edible when cooked and, indeed, quite scrumptious! For preparation and other particulars, the reader is referred to the profile on stinging nettle (page 226), since that information is entirely applicable here.

HEALTH/MEDICINE

Not nearly as widely used by either white or Native American herbal practitioners as stinging nettle (*Urtica dioica*), wood nettle has yet been appreciated by several Native American tribes as a *urinary* aid. Here the roots have been used by both the Pillager Ojibwe and the Meskwaki (Fox) as a *diuretic* (Smith 1928: 251; Smith 1932: 391). The latter found it to be serviceable for **urinary incontinence** as well (Smith 1928: 251). Interestingly, native peoples of the Caribbean region use a related species, *Laportea aestuans*, for **urinary obstruction** (Honeychurch 1980: 144). These three widely differing— even seemingly contradictory—uses relative to the urinary system merely give emphasis to what some of today's herbalists believe: namely, that this plant (as well as *Urtica* spp.) is actually a urinary *trophorestorative*, "fixing" the system regardless of the problem.

The Houma have taken a decoction of wood nettle to help relieve a **fever** (Speck 1941: 60). The Iroquois have revered wood nettle as a *parturient*. Again, it is the roots that are implemented: a handful of them are smashed and added to a teacupful of warm water. Afterward, the Iroquois advice is: "Drink immediately. Drink twice" (Herrick 1995: 132).

PERSONAL USE

I have a foraging friend who enjoys eating cooked wood nettle even more than he does its better-known relative, stinging nettle. I like it a lot, too, although I wouldn't say that it is markedly superior in taste to stinging nettle.

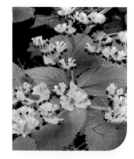

CAUTIONS

Do not eat fresh, raw nettle plant parts. Use gloves to collect so as to avoid getting stung. ⤶

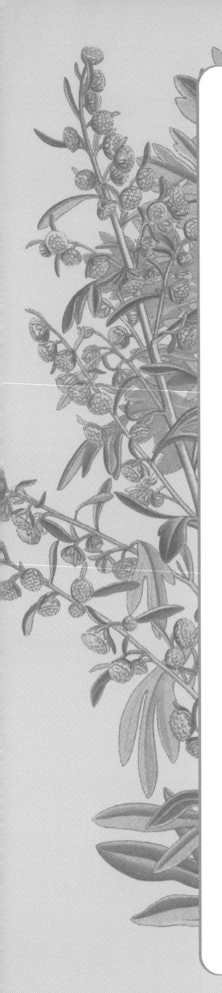

Wormwood

Artemisia spp.

DESCRIPTION

Wormwood is a pungently fragrant perennial, reflected by several species in our area, including *Artemisia absinthium* and *Artemisia ludoviciana*.

Artemisia absinthium is a species that spread to the Americas from the Old World and which grows 1½–3 feet tall. Its hoary stems are clumped and sometimes also a bit woody at their base.

This species' alternate leaves, growing 2–5 inches long, are divided once or twice and are whitish-gray on both sides, owing to the presence of soft, silky hairs. The leaflet segments are blunted at the tip.

Small, yellow-gray flower heads are situated in sagging, elongate, leafy panicles. The gray-to-tan fruits find form as smooth and flattened achenes, measuring ⅟₁₆ of an inch long.

A. ludoviciana (tall wormwood, Western mugwort, white sagebrush, Indian sage, prairie sage), our native species, grows taller than the former species—in some instances, as high as 3½ feet (2 feet being average).

This perennial possesses a woolly stem that branches toward its top and bears leaves that are linear and grow to 3 inches long—the top ones lacking teeth and the bottom ones pinnately lobed. Quite characteristic are the dense, white or silver hairs that cover the leaves and, in fact, the entire plant, giving it an overall silvery look.

Inflorescence consists of numerous, silvery-gray flower heads. Like *A. absinthium*, it exudes a pungent odor when crushed or otherwise damaged.

RANGE AND HABITAT

A. absinthium is a cosmopolitan weed, occurring throughout our region in old farmsteads, abandoned homesteads, pastures, dry fields, roadsides, waste places, and other open and dry areas.

A. ludoviciana flourishes in the western half of our region and can be found growing in loose colonies in fields, pastures, and prairies.

SEASONAL AVAILABILITY

In late summer, while flowering.

MAJOR CONSTITUENTS

A. absinthium: Essential oil (consisting of terpenes [thujone, pinene, sabinene, phellandrene, myrcene, cadinene, beta-carophyllene, azulenes] and sesquiterpene lactone-glycosides [santonin, absinthin, anabsinthin, artabsin, matricin]), polyacetylenes, phenolic acids (chlorogenic, *p*-coumaric, syringic, vanillic), lignans (diayangambin, epiyangambin), flavonoids, hydroxycoumarins, and tannins. Nutrients include pro-vitamin A and vitamin C and silica.

HEALTH/MEDICINE

A. ludoviciana has been used extensively by Native American tribes.

The Blackfoot applied a poultice of the plant to both **blisters** and **boils** and imbibed an infusion of the leaves when they felt **tightness** in the **chest** or in the **throat** (Hellson and Gadd 1974: 75).

The Cheyenne crushed the leaves and used this as a snuff for **sinus headaches** (Hart 1981: 18), while the Comanche applied the chewed leaves to the **bites** of both **insects** and **spiders** (Jones 1968: 7). The Poliklah poulticed them onto **sore eyes** (Merriam 1966: 173), while several different Native American tribes poulticed them or compressed them onto **sores** in general (Smith 1928: 211; Ray 1933: 217; Vestal and Schultes 1939: 56; Train et al. 1988: 40–42; Hart 1992: 44).

One of the more interesting topical applications was utilized by the Shoshone, who steeped the leaves and then used them as a poultice or a compress on the foreheads of babies with **fevers**, as well as implemented a decoction of the plant as a wash for **itchy rashes** and other kinds of **skin eruptions** (Train et al. 1988: 40–42). The Paiute soaked their **aching feet** in a foot bath made from a decoction of the plant, as well as implemented the steamed plant or bruised leaves as a poultice for **musculoskeletal aches** (Train et al. 1988: 40–42). (The Keres of the western United States utilized the latter application as well: Swank 1932: 28.) The Southern Carrier chewed the plant and poulticed the result onto sprains (Smith 1929: 65).

Both the Miwok and the Kiowa implemented an infusion of the herb for **stomach troubles** (including **indigestion**) (Vestal and Schultes 1939: 56; Merriam 1966: 353), while the latter tribe utilized the same to cut **respiratory phlegm** (Vestal and Schultes 1939: 56). The Flathead (Salish) appreciated the infusion for **colds** (Hart 1992: 44), as did the Lakota, who used it for both **sore throat** and **diarrhea** (Kraft 1990: 46). The Meskwaki (Fox) tended to use the infusion for sore throat also, as well as for **tonsillitis** (Smith 1928: 211). The Gros Ventre used it for **high fevers** (Hart 1992: 44), while the Shoshone preferred a decoction of the plant tops for **severe infections** and for **diarrhea** (Train et al. 1988: 40–42). The Paiute were able to implement the same for **venereal diseases** (Train et al. 1988).

Many of the above applications, it might be noted, suggest that this species possesses some *antimicrobial* activity, most likely owing to its essential oil and/or its sesquiterpene lactones. Such effects, in fact, have been verified in scientific studies, in which the plant has been shown to exert activity against *Campylobacter* spp. (Castillo et al. 2011), *Helicobacter pylori* (Castillo-Juárez et al. 2009), *Vibrio cholera* (Sánchez et al. 2010), *Entamoeba histolytica* and *Giardia lamblia* (Said-Fernández et al. 2005), *Mycobacterium tuberculosis* (Jimenez-Arellanes et al. 2003), *Plasmodium yoelii yoelii* (Malagón et al. 1997), and a variety of fungi (McCutcheon et al. 1994). It has been shown to offset diarrhea also by reducing small-intestine motility (Calzada et al. 2010).

A. ludoviciana was also used by several different tribes as a smudge to drive away **mosquitoes** (Smith 1928: 211; Turner et al. 1990). The Thompson, Lakota, Blackfoot, and Cheyenne smudged homes with it to drive away **evil spirits** (Kraft 1990: 46; Turner et al. 1990: 170; Hart 1992: 44),

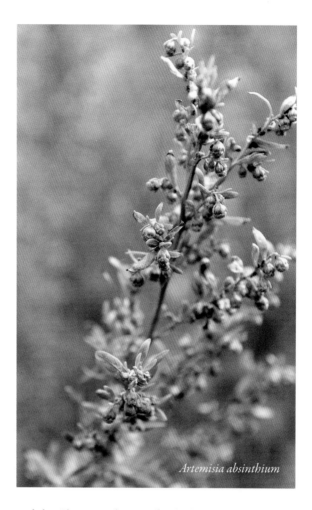

Artemisia absinthium

and the Cheyenne also to offset **bad** or **ominous dreams** (Grinnell 1972: 190); these practices seem to have spun off into modern Western society (at least here in the upper midwestern United States) in that so many people have called my herbal clinic to obtain "sage wands" to drive away demonic spirits from new or existing homes.

A. absinthium also has a rich history of use, even going back to Greco-Roman times: Dioscorides, a first-century herbalist who may have been a medical officer in the Roman emperor's employ, noted that this wormwood *(A. absinthium)* had a "warming, binding facultie." He observed that the vapor exuding from a decoction of the plant took the pain out of both a **toothache** and an **earache.** He further outlined its benefits for **bites**, including bites of "dragons of ye sea" (Dioscorides 1996: 3:26). Whichever venomous sea creature Dioscorides had in mind is difficult to say, but it is of interest that in Caribbean lands, a wormwood tincture is venerated as an emergency treatment for **jellyfish stings** (Honeychurch 1980). It has also been demonstrated to possess *anti-snake venom* activity in a mouse study (Nalbantsoy et al. 2013). Moreover, the late, great European herbalist Juliette de Bairacli Levy found it useful for easing the pain of stings and bites of just about *any* kind (de Bairacli Levy 1974: 159).

The thujone content may be partly responsible, since this chemical is analgesic owing to a narcotic property (Rice and Wilson 1976). Another major factor may be its content of azulenes, which are powerful anti-inflammatory agents. At any rate, the analgesic effects were also appreciated by our area's Ojibwe, who utilized a warm compress of the decoction of the plant for **sprains** that swelled (Densmore 1974: 362–63).

A powerful *stomachic,* wormwood was also highlighted by Dioscorides as an excellent herb for "taking away ye cholerick matter sticking to ye stomach, and ye belly" as well as for "pains of the belly & of ye stomach" (Dioscorides 1996: 3:26). It is most specifically a *tonic* relative to its stimulation of digestive juices (Johnson 1884: 183; Kresanek and Krejca 1989: 54). The German phytotherapist Rudolf Fritz Weiss praised it as one of the best herbs in this regard, noting its aid in **dyspepsia** and in **atony** of the **gastrointenstinal tract** (Weiss 1988: 80–81). The stomachic effects are, of course, due to the plant's poignant bitterness, which has been recognized since antiquity (even being referred to in the Bible on several occasions—"bitter as wormwood," Proverbs 5:4 and Revelation 8:11). However, just *how* bitter *is* wormwood? Russian research has revealed that a mere single part of wormwood in 10,000 parts of water still leaves a bitter taste! (Hutchens 1991: 311)

Pliny the Elder, a great naturalist who lived during the time of Dioscorides, outlined wormwood's usefulness for **colitis, bowel pain,** and **flatulent colic** (Pliny 1938: 27:28), while, centuries later, the Kashaya Pomo would implement it for **cramps** associated with diarrhea (Goodrich and Lawson 1980: 119). The Eclectics advised it for "obstinate diarrhea" (Felter and Lloyd 1898), as did the Okanogan and the Thompson (Perry 1952). All of these uses are understandable in light of the plant's *antispasmodic* activity (Millspaugh 1974: 349). Such an effect might also shed light on the traditional use of the infusion for **traveling sickness** (usually dosed at 5–30 drops, three to four times a day [Willard 1993: 214]), but here the plant's *disinfectant* effects are undoubtedly also an important factor (Kresanek and Krejca 1989: 54). Some herbalists regard wormwood as being helpful as well for intestinal permeability ("leaky gut"), because of its widespread antimicrobial effects (Fleming 1998). A recent, double-blind, placebo-controlled clinical trial showed that it exerted a marked *steroid-sparing effect* in sufferers of Crohn's disease, with complete remission of symptoms in 65 percent of test subjects after eight weeks of use as compared to no remission in the placebo group (Omer et al. 2007).

Wormwood's best-known use is probably as a *vermifuge* for **worms** in the intestinal tract. This application has been appreciated since ancient times. Celsus, a learned gentleman who lived during the time of Jesus and who may himself have been a physician, urged a wormwood decoction for **threadworms** in children (Celsus 1938: 4.24.2). Further down the stream of time, the Mohegan also employed the plant as a vermifuge (Tantaquidgeon 1972: 70, 128–29). So did the Cherokee, who poulticed it on the stomach to rid the gastrointestinal tract of worms (Hamel and Chiltoskey 1975: 62). This herb is most especially renowned for expelling **threadworms** (per Celsus) and **roundworms** (Felter and Lloyd 1898; Moore 1979: 162). Michael Moore, an herbalist who practiced in the American Southwest during the latter half of the twentieth century, noted that an effective regimen is to imbibe at least two cups of the infusion per day for one to two weeks (Moore 1979: 162). Alma Hutchens opts for a decoction used as an enema (Hutchens 1991: 312).

Wormwood's content of santonin and artemisin are thought to be the chief *anthelmintic* factors by most researchers, although the thujone content is highlighted by other authorities. Interestingly, the classic worm medicine known as "santonine" is derived from wormwood's cousin, *A. santonica.* Some feel that wormwood can also rid the body of both **fleas** and **lice** (de Bairacli Levy 1974: 159).

Rudolf Weiss further considered wormwood to be "a well-proven gallbladder remedy ... one of the best remedies for biliary dyskinesia or a gallbladder apt to cause trouble." He advised it especially for a gallbladder that was atonic, feeling that, for this condition, the tea should best be taken some time *after* meals because otherwise its energies might be more concentrated on stimulating the stomach instead (Weiss 1988: 80). Celsus regarded wormwood highly for **jaundice** (Celsus 1938: 3.24.2). Centuries later, so did the early-American medical botanist Constantine Rafinesque and also the Eclectic physicians (Rafinesque 1828–30: 2:184; Felter and Lloyd 1898). This application makes sense in view of the herb's demonstrated *cholagogue* ability (Baumann et al. 1975; Kresanek and Krejca 1989: 54; Willard 1993: 214; Fleming 1998)—although, as Weiss pointed out, the herb's quite minor abilities in this regard are not necessarily to be understood as the chief reason for its value as a biliary tonic (Weiss 1988: 80).

Herbalists have observed that wormwood's *hepatic* effects can sometimes help relieve a **frontal headache** when there is fatty indigestion; the herb even appears to halt lipid peroxidation, thus protecting the liver from the bad effects of rancid fats (Willard 1992a: 203). It also holds promise in treating **acetaminophen poisoning**, in that a 1995 study revealed that a crude extract ameliorated acetaminophen-induced liver toxicity in mice (Gilani and Janbaz 1995: 309). Wormwood, as Celsus observed, is also *diuretic* (Celsus 1938: 2.31), which may partly elucidate its time-honored benefits for **gout** (Millspaugh 1974: 349) and for **diabetes** (Jashemski 1999: 26).

In fact, one may not need acetaminophen at all for a fever if one has access to wormwood, as it is a powerful *febrifuge* in itself (confirmed via in vivo experiments with rabbits [Fleming 1998]), at least partly due to its azulenes, as well to its phellandrene content and perhaps to its thujone

(Moore 1979: 162; Potterton 1983: 203). In fact, chemicals in the plant directly fight **malaria** (Zafar et al. 1990), for which affliction the Eclectics sometimes used it, prior to the introduction of cinchona (Felter and Lloyd 1898). (However, wormwood's cousin, sweet annie [*A. annua*] is the superior *antimalarial*.)

The Cherokee found wormwood helpful for **dysmenorrhea** (Hamel and Chiltoksey 1975: 62). Michael Moore found it to be especially of aid for **amenorrhea** with **cramps**, particularly when occurring on the tail end of an illness or trauma (Moore 1979: 162).

It seems to be of aid in a general sense for almost any sort of **pelvic discomfort**, serving to stimulate blood flow in this region (Kresanek and Krejca 1989: 54).

Finally, two recent scientific studies on wormwood should be noted. One found it to cause apoptosis (self-destruction) of human breast-cancer cells in both an estrogen-sensitive cell line and a non-estrogen-sensitive cell line (Shafi et al. 2012). Another found it to exert powerful *neuroprotective* effects in **focal ischemia** and in **cerebral injury**, suggesting possible application in the treatment of **stroke** (Bora and Sharma 2010).

Wormwood was official in the *United States Pharmacopoeia* from 1831 to 1905 and in the *National Formulary* from 1916 to 1926.

PERSONAL AND PROFESSIONAL USE

In my herbal practice, I tend to use Old World wormwood (*A. absinthium*) in formulas for indigestion owing to poor biliary flow and/or to hypochlorhydria. I've also verified Weiss's observation, above, that it is the best thing out there for biliary dyskinesia, although I often combine it with artichoke *(Cynara scolymus)* for this to improve the taste, sometimes even adding a few drops of peppermint oil to the tincture combo for this purpose as well.

I also sometimes include this species in formulas I craft for colicky intestinal pains, such as occurs in irritable bowel syndrome (IBS) or inflammatory bowel disease (IBD). Of course, it is a staple in any formula meant to address intestinal parasites.

For bacterial or fungal infections in the gut, I prefer *Artemisia ludoviciana*, whereas if these infections are viral in nature, my herb of choice is fragrant giant hyssop (*Agastache* spp.) (see page 120), which is also effective for fungal infections.

CAUTIONS

Wormwood is absolutely contraindicated in both pregnancy and lactation. Those with kidney failure, or at risk for such, should also probably not use wormwood—especially the oil, since the latter has been implicated in renal failure.

The advice in the older herbal literature was to hold back from using wormwood on any long-term basis (longer than

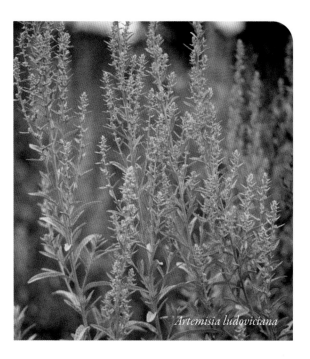

Artemisia ludoviciana

three to four weeks) because of possible negative neurological impact from its content of the chemical thujone (Weiss 1988: 81). In fact, in nineteenth-century France, a slick, green, alcoholic beverage known as *absinthe* that was largely derived from an extract of wormwood became the rage of the day, but sustained use was eventually connected with mental confusion, seizures, hallucinations, and other adverse neurological effects by a scientist named Valentin Magnan, who even demonstrated in the 1870s that an alcohol-soluble component of wormwood itself induced myoclonic jerks, tonic-clonic convulsions, and lapses of consciousness in laboratory animals. In fact, historians have generally speculated that Vincent van Gogh's slide into mental illness—climaxed when he severed his ear and mailed it to a lady friend—was as a result of his addiction to this drink. By the early 1900s, then, absinthe was banned in many European nations and finally in France (in 1915). (The United States banned it in 1912.)

Recently, however, a number of European nations have begun lifting the ban, arguing that the thujone content from absinthe samples tested in modern times is not as high as that which was reported from samples tested in the nineteenth- and early- twentieth centuries, that it falls within safe levels set by governmental authorities, and that hallucinogenic and convulsive effects that may have accrued from drinking absinthe in that earlier period resulted either from the alcohol content or from adulterants (including copper) that were popularly used at that time.

All of this may be true; but to my way of thinking, the course of wisdom would be to exercise caution with respect to either the imbibing of absinthe on any regular basis or the use of wormwood as a medicine on any regular, sustained basis. ◄◄

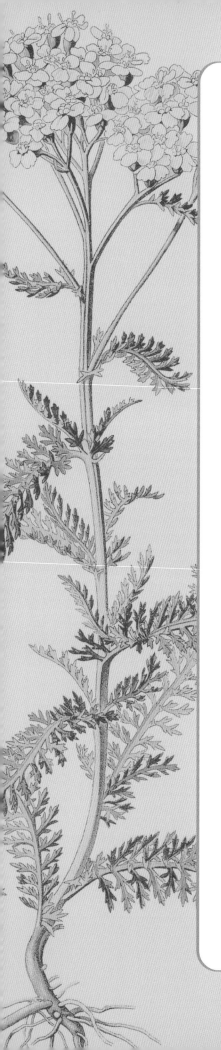

Yarrow

MILFOIL

Achillea millefolium

DESCRIPTION

Yarrow is a scented perennial herb growing 9–24 inches high that is entirely covered with soft hairs. Its square stem, characteristic of the mint family to which it belongs, is usually not branched but occasionally branches near the top.

The alternate leaves are finely divided (twice pinnate) into numerous narrow segments, looking almost like disheveled pipe cleaners. Strongly scented with a bitter, pungent odor (especially noticeable when handled), their divided form and scent are what distinguish this plant from lookalikes.

Yarrow's flowers form small heads that compact into a terminal, flat-topped cluster. They are almost always white in color but can occasionally be pink. With the aid of a magnifying glass, one can see that each individual flower is composite, made up of a yellow (female) disk flower and several white or pink (male) ray flowers.

RANGE AND HABITAT

Yarrow is one of those plants that are appropriately described as cosmopolitan, in that it can be found throughout North America. This herb likes to grow in loose colonies in fields, pastures, prairies, meadows, open woods, roadsides, and any exposed area that is sunny and well drained.

MAJOR CONSTITUENTS

Yarrow contains over 120 compounds, including alkaloids (achilleine, trigonelline, stachydrine); sesquiterpene lactones of the guaianolide and germacranolide types (achillicin, achillin, millefin); an essential oil (containing terpenes such as carophyllene, pinene, eugenol, linalool, borneol, camphor, limonene, menthol, cineole, sabinene, and a trace of thujone); saponins; polyacetylenes; alkanes (tricosane, pentacosane, heptadecane); furanocoumarins (including psoralcn); beta-sitosterol; flavonoids (rutin, isorhamnetin, apigenin, luteolin); salicylic acid; caffeic acid; isovalerianic acid; fatty acids (linoleic, oleic, palmitic); amino acids; sugars; and tannin. Nutrients include vitamins (pro-vitamin A, C, folic acid, choline) and minerals (especially potassium and silica but also some iron, magnesium, calcium, and phosphorus).

FOOD

Young leaves can be sparingly added to a salad to give it greater pungency. Their distinctive taste is also used to flavor several different alcoholic beverages.

HEALTH/MEDICINE

Yarrow abounds in my area and has, since my childhood, strongly held my attention due to its odd scent and appearance. My fascination with it ensured that it was one of the first herbs on which I concentrated when I initially found myself immersed in a concerted study of herbalism in the 1980s. (Here I was especially impressed when I learned that it had been used by over fifty-eight different Native American tribes!) It remains a fascination to the present day.

First and foremost, yarrow is a truly amazing *styptic*. According to Homer's account in the *Iliad*, the mighty Achilles used poultices of yarrow leaves on the **wounds** of fellow soldiers during the Trojan War (circa 1200 BCE). Subsequent peoples, then, appropriately called it soldier's woundwort, and here it has been observed that it especially excels for deep wounds, for which the tea is commonly used as a soak (Wood 1997: 65–67). Yet you don't have to be a warrior to benefit from yarrow, in that it has also long been used with success for **internal bleeding** in the **alimentary canal**, **nosebleeds**, **hemorrhages** (Millspaugh 1974: 336; Kresanek and Krejca 1989: 38), and especially **menorrhagia** (Felter and Lloyd 1898; de Bairacli Levy 1974: 160; Carse 1989: 176; Brooke 1992: 151), for which latter application it has been put to good use by the Cherokee (Hamel and Chiltoskey 1975: 62). Even that scholarly Roman naturalist of the first century, Pliny the Elder, drew attention to its use in this regard and noted that menorrhagia could be checked by taking a sitz bath in a decoction of yarrow (Pliny 1938: 7:377). Yarrow's styptic and hemostatic actions would seem to arise chiefly from its alkaloid achilleine, which has been shown to clot rabbit blood more quickly than usual and with such a hemostatic action persisting for up to forty-five minutes! (Miller and Chow 1954)

The plant's renowned *disinfectant* action—resulting from its essential oil, tannins, and other factors—keeps wounds and sores that have been poulticed with it from getting infected, as the first-century herbalist Dioscorides noted (Dioscorides 1996: 4:115). Yarrow is indeed a powerful *antimicrobial*, effective against a wide range of both gram-positive and gram-negative microorganisms (D'Amico 1950; Ibragimov and Kazanskaia 1981; Chandler et al. 1982; Goranov et al. 1983; Fleming 1998). An aqueous extract has been found to possess in vitro activity against *Staphylococcus aureus* (Mockle 1955: 85) as well as *Bacillus subtilis, Escherichia coli, Mycobacterium smegmatis, Shigella sonnei*, and *S. flexneri* (Moskalenko 1986). Its action against the *Shigella* organisms suggests that it would be specific for **shigellosis**—which it is, but it is most effective for that condition when, as herbalist Michael Moore noted, it is combined with echinacea (especially *Echinacea angustifolia*, I would think) in goodly amounts (Moore 1993: 274).

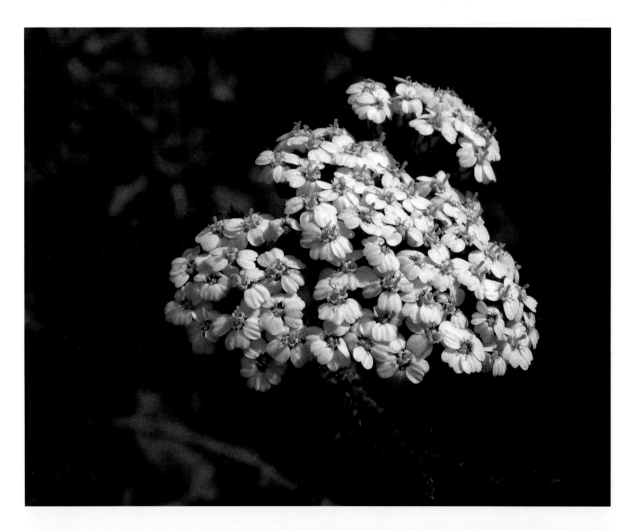

Another test-tube study revealed that yarrow had some minor inhibiting effect upon a virulent human strain of tuberculosis (Fitzpatrick 1954: 530), which could be due to its psoralen content, since this compound has been shown to be active against *Mycobacteria* (Harborne and Baxter 1993: 362). Yarrow also contains a natural peroxide that is a proven *antimalarial* (Rücker et al. 1991).

Interestingly, regardless of its styptic properties, a twirled leaf in the nose of a person with a **vasodilated migraine** or a **sinus headache** can *cause* a nosebleed and thus relieve the painful pressure (Jones 1991: 7), as the Woods Cree discovered (Leighton 1985: 23). Numerous writers have speculated that this is due to the plant's coumarins, which they hail as hemorrhagic. Normally, coumarin is not hemorrhagic when ingested or utilized in moderate amounts but only when acted upon in a complex combination of ways involving a wilting of the plant and the introduction of moisture, which then transforms it into dicoumarol (the compound upon which rat poison and medical anticoagulant has been patterned). It's difficult to fathom how this is likely to occur from simply plucking a leaf and twirling it in one's nose; yet, regardless of the mechanism or mechanisms involved, the procedure does often work.

A renowned *astringent*, yarrow has been greatly valued throughout history for **diarrhea**, **uterine fibroids** (Brooke 1992: 151; Harrar and O'Donnell 1999: 80; Mills and Bone 2000: 243), **cracked nipples** (Weed 1986: 91), **sore throat** (Hellson and Gadd 1974: 70), and **colitis** (Winston 1999: 55), proving helpful as well for the latter condition owing to *anti-inflammatory* activity (Goldberg and Mueller 1969; Verzan-Petri and Banh-Nhu 1977; Shipochliev and Fournadjiev 1984), possibly due to its essential oil (Mabey et al. 1988: 40; Pedersen 1998: 175), and/or to its protein-carbohydrate complexes (Goldberg and Mueller 1969) and/or to its flavonoids (Bruneton 1995: 290) and/or to its salicylic acid (Mabey et al. 1988: 40).

The anti-inflammatory benefits are legion. The Bella Coola have poulticed yarrow leaves onto **abscessed breasts** (Turner 1973: 201). The Micmac have poulticed pulped stems onto **swellings**, **bruises**, and **sprains** (Lacey 1993: 95). The Southern Carrier have chewed the leaves and applied them to same (Smith 1928: 65). The Malecite have boiled the plant down to a thick paste and used this as a liniment for these painful issues (Mechling 1959: 244), while the Blackfoot have preferred to use the chewed flowers as a poultice for them (Hellson and Gadd 1974: 74). The Winnebago (Ho-Chunk) have bathed swellings with an infusion of yarrow; members of this tribe have also wadded up leaves to stick into the ear canals of persons afflicted with an **earache** or sometimes simply poured a small bit of the infusion into the affected ear (Gilmore 1991: 82). Canada's Thompson tribe has implemented a decoction of the plant as a wash for **arthritic limbs** (Turner et al. 1990: 47). The Flambeau

Ojibwe have poulticed leaves onto **spider bites** (Smith 1932: 362). **Eczema** and various **rashes** have been treated topically by the Menomini with fresh yarrow tops (Smith 1923: 29).

As a topical painkiller, yarrow ranks most highly—perhaps even highest—among midwestern plants. (However, see Cautions.) The Thompson found that a poultice of the root brought relief to those afflicted with **sciatica** (Turner et al. 1990: 46). Throughout the ages, too, many persons have chewed yarrow leaves to relieve a **toothache** (de Bairacli Levy 1974: 160); the Osage and a few other Native tribes successively chewed a dozen or less leaves until a numbing sensation ensued (Kavasch 1977: 176). The Costanoan simply held the leaves in their mouths next to the painful tooth (Bocek 1984: 254), while Saskatchewan's Woods Cree preferred the root for the same purpose (Leighton 1985: 23). Yarrow is no doubt effective here because of the plant's content of eugenol, the famous drugstore remedy (formerly sold as "oil of cloves," but now marketed simply as the distinct chemical eugenol). The *analgesic* effect, which has been scientifically demonstrated (Gherase 2002), may also be partly due to the camphor content and perhaps, as well, to the plant's salicylic acid.

Yarrow flowers are *antiallergic* and thus useful for **hay fever**, probably chiefly because of the flavonoid content but perhaps as well due to proazulenes that occur in some subspecies—which, when the blossoms are prepared as an infusion, are converted by the steam into azulenes, which are powerful antiallergic substances (Ody 1993: 30; Bruneton 1995: 290; Fleming 1998).

Yarrow is a treasured *antipyretic* and thus has long been used for **fever**, for which it is also often recommended by present-day herbalists (Hyde et al. 1976–79: 1:145). It is generally agreed that this herb dilates the blood vessels in the outer surfaces of the body, causing a *diaphoretic* effect that flushes the skin of excess heat and wastes. Such an effect also makes yarrow useful for **pleurisy** (de Bairacli Levy 1974: 160). It is possible that the plant's alkaloids are partly responsible here (Pedersen 1998: 175). Most likely, however, the sesquiterpene lactones are largely responsible, as is probably the case with yarrow's cousin boneset, *Eupatorium perfoliatum* (see page 44), which has a similar diaphoretic effect. When one of these chemicals, achillin, was administered to rabbits, there was demonstrated a subsequent fall in rectal temperature (Falk et al. 1975).

Yarrow's application for fever has been appreciated and utilized by numerous Native American tribes, including the Woods Cree, who have used it by way of a compress on the head (Leighton 1985: 23). The Flambeau Ojibwe, on the other hand, have singed yarrow blossoms on hot coals and inhaled the steam to break a fever (Smith 1932: 362). The herb's fever-fighting power has also been utilized by the Micmac (Lacey 1993: 95), the Abenaki (Rousseau 1947: 154), the Menomini (Smith 1923: 28–29), the Cherokee (Hamel and Chiltoskey 1975: 62), and the Montagnais (Speck 1917:

315), all of whom have simply drunk an infusion of the herb to deal with the problem. For feverish infants, the Iroquois have steeped three or four leaves in ½ teacupful of cold water for one minute and given a little of it to the babes throughout the day (Herrick 1995: 227).

As for its indications in fever, herbalist Matthew Wood finds it most applicable with a red, flushed face and dry skin accompanied by a full and rapid pulse and a red, uncoated tongue that is drier in the center and wetter toward the edges (Wood 1997: 72–73). Somewhat similarly, the Eclectic physician Finley Ellingwood pointed to its use when there was "hot, dry burning skin, at the beginning of acute asthenic fevers, with suppressed secretion" (Ellingwood 1983: 355). However, because of its stimulant properties, the herb is felt by some other herbalists to be best applicable to a fever in which the skin is cold and the pulse is weak (Cook 1985; Willard 1993: 196). Personally, I haven't noticed that much difference in its effects with these different types of fever. My own experience over three decades of use is that it seems to work remarkably well for almost any kind of fever, simply because it is so extraordinarily diaphoretic. In fact, as I was writing the above, I remembered a summation that Ellingwood gave of the work of a Dr. Cole of Seattle, who "confirmed in a practical matter the action of achillea on the skin. ... When there is no abnormal temperature, he believes that it has little but a diuretic action. When there is a temperature of 100 or above, he *has never failed* to get profuse diaphoresis without depression. He considers it a *certain remedy*" (Ellingwood 1983: 356; emphasis added). I most heartily agree but also echo Ellingwood's admonition that "it acts best in strong infusion and its use must be persisted in" (Ellingwood 1983: 356).

Yarrow is a time-honored *bitter tonic* for **dyspepsia** and for **appetite loss** (Kresanek and Krejca 1989: 38). The Paiute have used it to treat **weak, disordered stomachs** (Palmer 1878: 651). The evidence for these effects is so good that the German *Commission E Monographs* give the seal of approval to yarrow for appetite loss, dyspepsia, and **mild, cramp-like pains in the abdomen** (Blumenthal 1998). The plant's antimicrobial action, along with its content of butyric acid, also lends it for possible use in helping to heal "**leaky gut" syndrome (intestinal permeability)**, much like its cousin wormwood, *Artemisia absinthium* (see page 278). It has also demonstrated healing effects on **gastric ulcers** that were experimentally

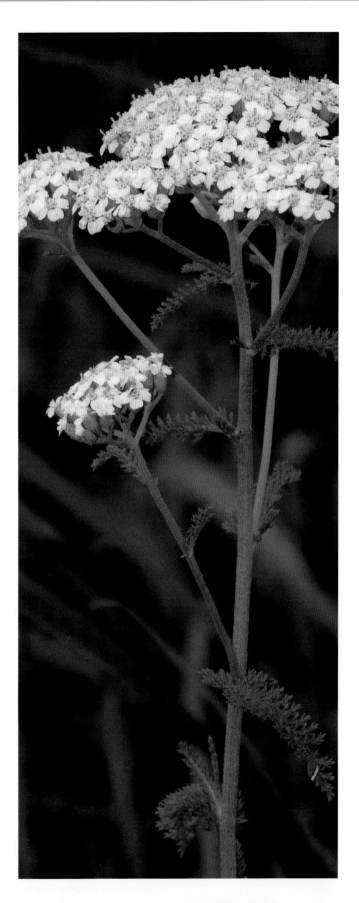

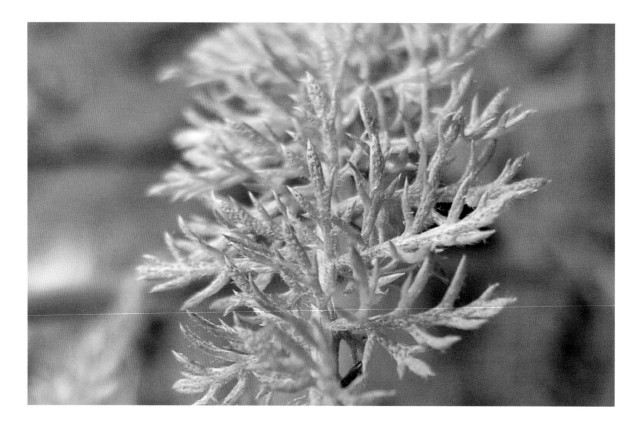

induced in rats (Cavalcanti et al. 2006). The Eclectics and the Physiomedicalists esteemed it for mild cases of **loose stools** (Ellingwood 1983; Cook 1985).

Yarrow is also *hepatic*. As such, it is first a *choleretic* (Bisset and Wichtl 1994; Benedek et al. 2006), which has allowed it to be used by the Gosiute for "biliousness" (Chamberlin 1911: 360). Secondly, scientific studies have demonstrated *hepatoprotective* activity (Yaeesh et al. 2006). Two clinical studies have even shown that the plant may help treat **hepatitis** or **cirrhosis** when used in a formula that also includes chicory (see page 78) (Harnyk 1999; Huseini et al. 2005). It should come as no surprise, then, that yarrow is sometimes considered an herb for the liver above all else (Holmes 1989–90: 1:282).

Yarrow has long been appreciated for **circulatory** disorders, especially for **Raynaud's disease** and for **thrombosis** (the herb's coumarins are *antithrombotic:* Pedersen 1998: 175), and it is the herb of choice for these conditions when **hypertension** is also involved (Hyde et al. 1976–79: 1:145), since yarrow has demonstrated *hypotensive* effects (Leung and Foster 1996: 327; Asgary et al. 2000; Khan and Gilani 2011: 577), mainly due to its alkaloids (Pedersen 1998: 175) and to its flavonoids (Mabey et al. 1988: 40). British herbalists find that it reduces hypertension most effectively, however, when combined with linden and/or hawthorn, two other classic antihypertensives (Hyde et al. 1976–79: 1:145; McQuade-Crawford 1996: 182). (As a point aside, linden is most specific when *emotional factors* are largely responsible for the hypertension, or at least are aggravating it in some way. I know more people than I could count who have had their blood pressure reduced by adding linden flowers to their otherwise failing regimen. Since it is a "cooling" herb, however, one should not fail to note that it works best in "hot"-bodied types. For "cold"-bodied types with hypertension aggravated by the emotions, valerian root, *Valeriana officinalis*, is the herb of choice.)

Further as to its circulatory assists, the plant has a special attraction to the venous system of the body (Felter and Lloyd 1898), so that it is much appreciated by those suffering from **hemorrhoids** or **varicose veins**, in which conditions it is employed internally and often as a wash as well (Moore 1979: 164; Carse 1989: 176; Kresanek and Krejca 1989: 38; Brooke 1992: 151; Fischer-Rizzi 1996: 303). Here, the Eclectics deemed yarrow specific for those hemorrhoids that manifested bloody or mucoid discharges (Felter and Lloyd 1898).

Yarrow also has a marked affinity for the pelvic region, a specificity widely acknowledged (Johnson 1884: 182; Millspaugh 1974: 336; Fleming 1998). A real gem for **pelvic discomfort** (Brooke 1992: 151; Fischer-Rizzi 1996: 303), it is approved by German Commission E in the form of a sitz bath for **painful cramps** in the lower quadrant of the pelvis (Blumenthal 1998). It is also an *emmenagogue* par excellence for **amenorrhea**, especially when of an atonic character (Scudder 1870: 60), and for **menstrual cramps**, especially when due to cold (Brooke 1992: 151; Harrar and O'Donnell 1999: 80) or when accompanied by spasms. It is also probably the single best herb to modulate the miseries of **endometriosis** (Bergner 1995–96). Yarrow is, further, one of several plants that modern herbalists find helpful in expelling a **retained placenta** (Harrar and O'Donnell 1999: 80), as the Blackfoot earlier discovered (Hellson and Gadd 1974: 60). Then, too, it often proves to be a real dandy for **leukorrhea** (Scudder 1870: 60; Carse 1989: 176), especially when this discharge is profuse and when it is accompanied by relaxed vaginal walls, in which case the Eclectics advised a douche propelled into the area (Felter and Lloyd 1898; Ellingwood 1983: 356).

A *diuretic* and a *urinary antiseptic* (Goldberg and Mueller 1969; Hellson and Gadd 1974: 69; Hyde et al. 1976–79: 1:145), yarrow can be helpful for **cystitis** (Brooke 1992: 151), for **urethral irritation** (Winston 1999: 55), for **hematuria** (Felter and Lloyd 1898), and as a cold infusion for **urinary incontinence** (Felter and Lloyd 1898). The Eclectics found that it especially fit the bill when there was "irritation of the kidneys and vesical and urethral irritation" (Scudder 1870: 60) and primarily when such symptoms were indicative of "chronic diseases of the urinary apparatus," as opposed to being acute (Felter and Lloyd 1898). Michael Moore agreed that it especially excels with both cystitis and urethritis when these have become low level and chronic, for which he says that 2 cups of tea a day for two weeks often proves to be therapeutic (Moore 1993: 275). Herbalist Peter Holmes finds yarrow of aid with urinary conditions when urination is *frequent*, *scanty*, and *dribbling* (Holmes 1989–90: 1:281). Not surprisingly, in view of its urinary properties as explicated previously, a Chinese species (*Achillea alpina*) proved marvelously effective in a clinical study with sixty-five cases of **urinary tract infection** (**UTI**) (Peng et al. 1983). Our herb is ideal for urinary problems because it strengthens the urinary organs without irritating them, unlike some other urinary herbs in popular use (Ellingwood 1983: 355; Fischer-Rizzi 1996: 303). It may also be appropriate for persons afflicted with **nephritis** (Ellingwood 1983: 355; Carse 1989: 176).

Yarrow flowers have an *antispasmodic* effect on smooth muscle due to their flavonoid content (Hoerhammer 1961; Weiss 1988: 92; Fleming 1998; Pedersen 1998: 175). The urinary system is lined with smooth muscle, so yarrow finds ideal application with **spasms** of the **bladder** and of the **urinary tract**. Smooth muscle also exists in the gastrointestinal tract and in the uterus, which facts undoubtedly at least partly account for yarrow's *stomachic* and *emmenagogue* effects as noted previously. The German phytotherapist-physician Rudolf Fritz Weiss drew attention to its application in "spastic conditions in the small pelvis, the parametrium, and neurovegetative disorders in that region" (Weiss 1988: 92). Its effect on muscular structures may also explain why it has classically been used for **trembling** (Felter and Lloyd 1898; de Bairacli Levy 1974: 160) and for **angina pectoris** (Kresanek and Krejca 1989: 38). The Iroquois even found our herb helpful for **convulsions** in babies; they would boil a whole plant in 1 pint of water until the fluid turned green and then feed 1 teaspoonful of the cooled decoction to the baby while rubbing the rest over its body (Herrick 1995: 227).

The plant's sesquiterpene lactones have shown an *antitumor* effect in lab studies with mice (Tozyo et al. 1994). We have observed in earlier profiles, such as boneset (see page 44) and burdock (page 60), that these chemicals, widely distributed in the Asteraceae family of plants, have been shown to be generally possessed of this ability. All in all, I would not be surprised should sesquiterpene lactones become the most widely investigated and publicized compounds in cancer phytotherapy research in the twenty-first century.

Yarrow flowers and leaves were official in the *United States Pharmacopeia* from 1836 to 1882 as tonic, stimulant, and emmenagogue. The herb is still official in the pharmacopeias of some European nations.

PERSONAL AND PROFESSIONAL USE
In my clinical herbal practice, I most often advise the use of yarrow for elevated diastolic blood pressure, pain in the pelvic region (including endometriosis), colitis, and menorrhagia. I also recommend topical use of the chewed or crushed leaves for tooth pain and bleeding cuts, a salve for hemorrhoids, and a sitz bath of the tea for perineal tears.

CAUTIONS
Yarrow is not to be used during pregnancy, as it can stimulate the uterus in larger doses. Even the trace amounts of thujone present may make yarrow a risk for miscarriage.

Touching bruised leaves can lead to contact dermatitis—some studies show up to half of the population is sensitive in this regard, a sensitivity that can be aggravated severely by sunlight.

Those on anticoagulants and antihypertensive drugs should use yarrow with caution and under supervision of a health-care professional. Persons with low blood pressure should also use this herb with caution, owing to its demonstrated hypotensive effect.

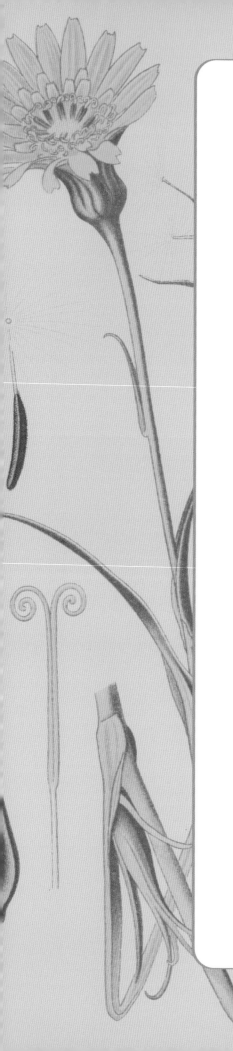

Yellow Goatsbeard

MEADOW SALSIFY; YELLOW SALSIFY; JACK-GO-TO-BED-AT-NOON

Tragopogon pratensis, T. dubius

DESCRIPTION

This is a common biennial or perennial herb 1–3½ feet tall with a smooth, branching stem. The first-year plant remains a rosette, but in the second year, the plant sends forth a long stem and herbage. At this point, the root has lost much mass and is finger-like.

Yellow goatsbeard has alternate, smooth-edged, narrow, and grass-like leaves that are parallel veined. Blue-green in color, they are 4–10 inches long and pointed at the tip, and they contain a milk-like juice. Each leaf wraps around the stem at its base.

A solitary flower head appears at the tip of the stem, situated on a long, slender, pointed bract. (There is a swelling on the stem just below the flower head in *Tragopogon dubius* that is lacking in *T. pratensis*.) It is 1–2½ inches wide and composed of many yellow ray flowers. Quite noticeably, the blossoms close up shop by early afternoon (banker's hours!), folding up into their bean-pod-shaped bracts. This feature was the impetus for one of its alternative common names: Jack-go-to-bed-at-noon.

One of the most noticeable features of yellow goatsbeard is its showy seedhead. When the plant is ready to seed, the flower heads transform into globular fuzzy balls similar to those put forth by dandelions, but much larger (approximately the size of tennis balls). The "dirty" white look of the seeds gives rise to the plant's most oft-used common name, goatsbeard. The seedhead's structure is loose, enabling the seeds to spread easily on breezy days, facilitated by the fact that each of them possesses a parachute-like structure, allowing for a thrill-packed ride along the air currents.

RANGE AND HABITAT

Tragopogon is found in sandy waste places, roadsides, railroad rights-of-way, vacant lots, and fields and meadows. It thrives in the eastern two-thirds of the United States and in Canada from Nova Scotia to Ontario.

MAJOR CONSTITUENTS

The plant's constituents have not been fully elucidated as yet, although the root is known to contain the following nutrients: vitamin C, potassium, and some smaller amounts of iron, phosphorus, calcium, and B vitamins. Inositol, mannitol, inulin, and sterols are also present.

FOOD

Young leaves are edible raw; if bitter in taste, a quick blanching in boiling water will take the "nip" out of them. The leaf crown, located at the bottom of the flower stalk, makes a fine potherb. Being tender, it needs to be simmered for only a few minutes in a little water. (Note that cooked crowns do not store well and should be used right away.)

Master forager and wild-plant author François Couplan enjoys the tender young flower buds, finding them to be most sweet. He notes that they can either be used as a trail nibble or lightly steamed to retain their crunchiness (personal communication June 2001).

The most renowned food use of the plant, however, involves the taproot of first-year specimens, which is quite tasty, either when boiled or when roasted. Roots from flowering plants can be used, too—contrary to popular belief. Tough and stringy, they look as if they wouldn't be very palatable, but experimenting with cooking times is all that is needed to render them appropriately tender. (Of course, one has to have access to a number of them to provide one with enough substance to make preparation worthwhile.)

HEALTH/MEDICINE

Largely abandoned by modern herbalists, *Tragopogon* yields several important physiological effects that persons of previous generations were evidently more humbly disposed to learn and to utilize. The celebrated seventeenth-century herbalist Nicholas Culpeper wrote of this plant: "A large double handful of the plant, roots, flowers, and all bruised and boiled, and then strained, with a little sweet oil, is an excellent clyster in the most desperate cases of **strangury** or **suppression of urine**, from whatever cause" (Potterton 1983: 86, emphasis added). Culpeper went on to add that yellow goatsbeard "expels sand and gravel, slime and small stones" (Potterton 1983: 86, emphasis added). Moreover, these were not isolated observations: famed botanical scholar Carolus Linnaeus also noted the plant's reputation for strangury, in his *Vegetable Materia Medica* of 1829 (Linnaeus 1829: 147). Naturopathic writer John Lust commented that the *diuretic* effects are particularly helpful relative to **urinary problems** or **water retention** (Lust 1974: 414). Probably largely responsible for alleviating the urethral stricture or swelling is the plant's experimentally verified *anti-inflammatory* effect, established in a 1976 study (Benoit et al. 1976: 165).

Culpeper observed further: "A decoction of the roots is good for **heartburn**, **loss of appetite**, and **liver** and **chest disorders**" (Potterton 1983: 86). The use for heartburn was adopted by Native Americans after the settlers shared with them the secrets of this European import (Dobelis et al. 1986: 196). Some such tribes would let the juice coagulate into a gum, which was then chewed to obtain the desired *anti-dyspepsic* effect. Notably, the *appetite-stimulant* and *hepatic* effects that Culpeper described above have been at least partially evidenced since his time (Stuart 1982: 146). It is thought that the herb serves to liquify thickened bile (Steinmetz 1957).

Culpeper added: "The roots cooked like parsnips, with butter ... strengthen the ... weak after a **long illness**" (Potterton 1983: 86). Today, we would call such use for debilitated persons a *tonic*; at least partly responsible for such effects must be the high vitamin C content (the plant has traditionally been implemented as an *antiscorbutic*). However, we know that it goes far beyond this: a 1990 Chinese study using mice discovered powerful *anti-fatigue* and *anoxia-tolerating* activities in *Tragopogon porrifolius* (Long and Tian 1990: 765). While the particular chemicals responsible have not yet been definitely isolated, further studies will undoubtedly shed additional light on these intriguing results. ⋘

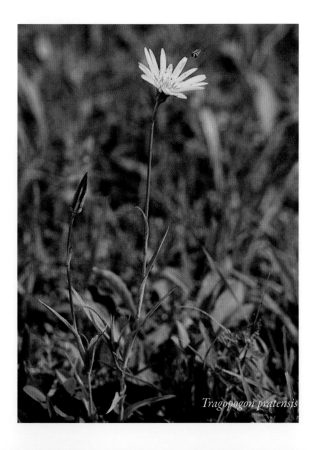

Tragopogon pratensis

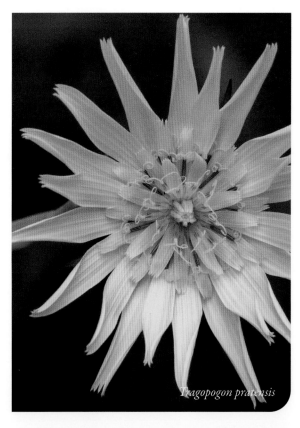

Tragopogon pratensis

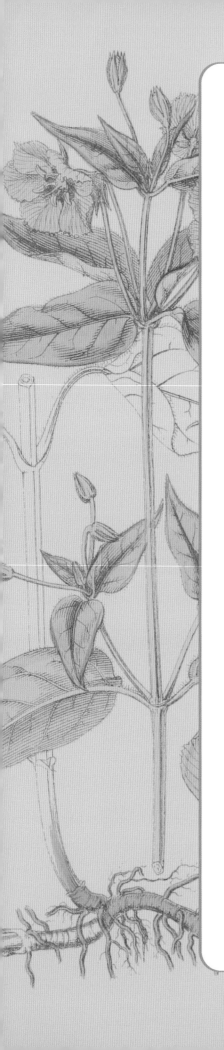

Yellow Loosestrife

Lysimachia spp.

DESCRIPTION

The plants of this genus sport yellow flowers with five (occasionally six) petals and stamens. The leaves are opposite (occasionally whorled) and sessile, while the blossoms almost always emerge from the plant's axils. *Lysimachia* is represented in the Midwest by several species, among which are the following:

L. ciliata (fringed loosestrife, tufted loosestrife) is a perennial that grows 1–3 feet tall and has a very weak stem. Its opposite, ovate, light-green leaves reach a length of 2–3 inches and are borne on long leafstalks that are fringed on the upper axils. The flowers, borne in groups of two or three, nod most conspicuously, and their petals are fringed.

L. quadriflora (prairie loosestrife) reaches a height of 1–2½ feet and possesses opposite, sessile, lanceolate leaves. These grow to 3 inches long, and their edges are smooth and slightly reflexed. The star-like flowers have reddish centers and grow singly on long, skinny stalks.

L. quadrifolia (whorled loosestrife) resembles the previous species, but its leaves are in whorls.

L. terrestris (yellow loosestrife, swamp candles) grows 6–20 inches tall and has opposite leaves and star-like blossoms with a circle of red spots. Unlike other species in this genus, its leaves are not borne from the leaf axils but are clustered into a terminal raceme.

L. thyrsiflora (tufted loosestrife) is a perennial that tops off at 6–30 inches and has opposite, lanceolate to elongate leaves that reach a length of 2–4 inches. It differs from the other species in that its flowers are arranged in ball-like clusters on short stalks.

RANGE AND HABITAT

L. terrestris and *L. thyrsiflora* thrive in swamps and marshes. *L. quadriflora* prefers moist prairies and shores. *L. ciliata* likes moist, shaded areas and can be found in woods and roadside ditches. One or another species can be found throughout the Midwest.

MAJOR CONSTITUENTS

Yellow loosestrife contains flavonoids, saponins, tannins, and a benzoquinone.

FOOD

During the period immediately preceding the Revolutionary War, the whorled loosestrife (*L. quadriflora*) was dried and steeped as a tea when the colonists refused to drink the heavily taxed British tea. As such, it was known (as were many other such alternatives) as "Liberty Tea." It is quite mild in taste, however, and often needs to be mixed with another herb or two to bring out its flavor.

HEALTH/MEDICINE

This genus has a long history of use as a medicinal plant. The first-century Greek herbalist Dioscorides wrote of the *astringent* applications of a European species, *L. vulgaris*, while seventeenth-century herbalist Nicholas Culpeper described such an activity in even more detail when he wrote that this plant was implemented widely for **nosebleeds**, **bloody diarrhea**, **menorrhagia**, **sore throat**, and **wounds** (for which it was said to "quickly close up the lips") (Potterton 1983: 115). Reflecting upon Culpeper's remarks, David Potterton notes that modern European herbalists use this species similarly, in the form of an infusion

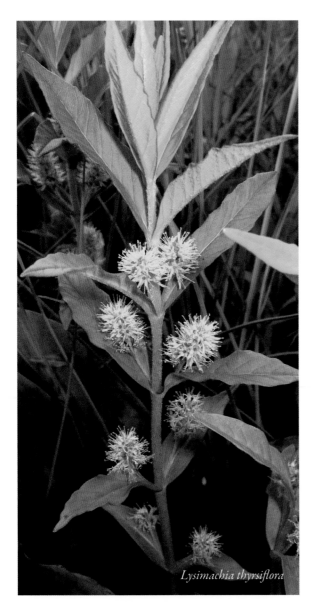

Lysimachia thyrsiflora

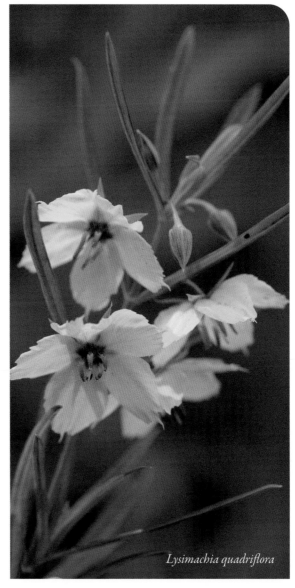

Lysimachia quadriflora

of the dried herb prepared from 1 ounce (28 grams) of herb to 1 pint (568 milliliters) of boiling water and dosed to the tune of 2 fluid ounces (56 milliliters) at a time (Potterton 1983: 115).

Traditional Chinese Medicine uses yet another species of yellow loosestrife, *L. christinae* (referred to in Chinese as *jin qian cao*), as a cooling herb to rid the body of pathogenic heat and dampness—factors thought to be connected with conditions such as **jaundice**, **edema**, **snakebite**, **abscesses**, **burns**, and **calculi** of the urinary tract and the gallbladder (Anonymous 1977: 719; Yanchi 1995: 108).

As for the midwestern species, *L. quadrifolia* has been held to be a powerful remedy for "female trouble" by the Cherokee, who have also used it for **bowel complaints** and for **kidney problems** (Hamel and Chiltoskey 1975: 43). For the latter, they have implemented an infusion of the roots (Taylor 1940: 50). The Iroquois have also occasionally employed an infusion of this plant's roots, but as an *emetic* when needed (Herrick 1977: 411). *L. terrestris*, another of our local species, has shown significant *anti-inflammatory* properties in the rat-paw edema lab test (Benoit et al. 1976: 167). *L. thyrsiflora*'s leaves have been applied by the Iroquois to the breasts to halt the flow of milk when such was desired (Herrick 1977: 411). ⤙⤙

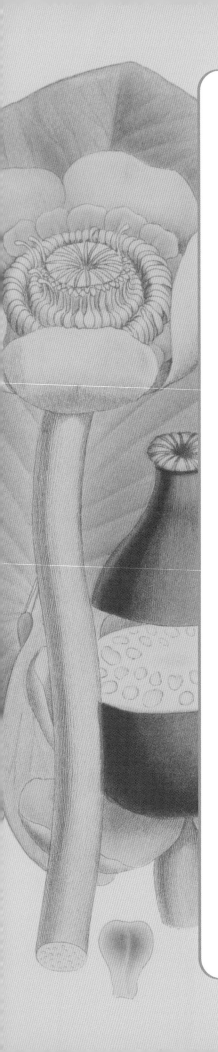

Yellow Pond-Lily

SPATTERDOCK; COW LILY

Nuphar variegata [alternatively, *N. lutea* ssp. *variegata*],
N. advena [alternatively, *N. lutea* ssp. *advena*]

DESCRIPTION

This is a common aquatic perennial with several large heart-shaped leaves (3–15 inches) possessing a conspicuous notch between their two basal lobes.

The leaves are situated at the tips of long, slimy leafstalks that arise from a huge rootstock or rhizome (some 1½–2½ feet long!) buried in the muck below. Many have described this rootstock as resembling a green pineapple.

The flowers, appearing individually on separate stalks and resembling the leafstalks, are yellow and cup-like, measuring 2 inches across and sporting five or six prominent sepals that resemble petals. (The real petals, however, are hidden inside and look more like stamens than they do petals.) Most noticeable is the disk-like stigma situated in the center of the flowers.

In autumn, sepals and petals fall away, and green fruits form that are filled with many seeds resembling corn kernels—which, however, are largely obscured from view.

RANGE AND HABITAT

Yellow pond-lily flourishes in the eastern four-fifths of the Midwest as well as in most of the midcentral and eastern states. It thrives in lakes, ponds, pools, and slow streams.

MAJOR CONSTITUENTS

Yellow pond-lily contains steroidal saponins, tannins, mucilage, and alkaloids (including nupharolutine) and pseudoalkaloids (nitrogenic sesquiterpenes, including nupharidine, desoxynupharidine, nuphacristine, nupharine, and thiobinupharidine).

FOOD

Foragers have long argued whether yellow pond-lily's large rhizomes make a passable food if prepared in a certain way or are just plain toxic regardless of how they are prepared. Of possible significance here is a mid-1980s experiment with rodents—reported in the *Journal of Ethnopharmacology*—that revealed that a mere boiling of *Nuphar luteum* poorly eliminated its toxins, while baking it in an oven at 180–200 degrees Celsius (212–232 degrees Fahrenheit) rendered it "well tolerated" by the rodents (Airaksinen et al. 1986).

One method for human consumption claimed successful by some begins with a boiling of the mass for about twenty minutes. Next, the water is changed, and the rhizome is peeled down to its core. Then, the core is either steamed for ten minutes or boiled in two waters. After this, it is baked in a slow oven. Another method, popular in a wilderness setting, involves leaving the whole, scrubbed rootstock wrapped in foil in hot campfire ashes for the day. By twilight, it is thought to be sufficiently cooked, enabling it to be peeled and eaten at that time.

There are enough variables, however (including the fact that the raw rhizome is indisputably toxic—see Cautions), that leave me hesitant to try to prepare yellow pond-lily rhizome as a food—even by baking it—and so I have never attempted to do so.

The elusive seeds, however, are not viewed as toxic and are frequently prepared by wild-foods foragers as "wild popcorn." To accomplish this successfully takes some skill and some practice. First, the mature seedpods need to be cut free from the plant; these fruits are frequently swarming with insects. Scatter them by placing fruits in a container, then beating the container with a stick and chanting, "Bugs, bugs, go away. Leave and live another day!" Before you know it, you'll feel like the Pied Piper of the pond-lilies. Next, the seedpods should be dried in the sun. Finally, these should be pounded to loosen the seeds. If still soft, however, the seeds can sometimes be rubbed free or removed by hand.

The fully dried seeds can be prepared like popcorn the old-fashioned way—that is, in a pan and not in a modernized popcorn popper! Here's how it is usually done: In a skillet, add vegetable oil and seeds to the tune of one or two layers. Place over high heat on the stovetop. Move (but do not shake) the pan as necessary in order to avoid burning the popping kernels. When finished, cool as necessary and eat the kernels, but not the shells. Although most would rate this snack a bit below popcorn in taste, you may still find yourself pleasantly surprised at the flavor. Famed wild-foods connoisseur Euell Gibbons often prepared and served this treat to youngsters, and he said that they always wanted more!

The seeds can also be parched, winnowed, and ground into flour. This flour can be added to soup as a thickener or made into a fair gruel.

HEALTH/MEDICINE

Yellow pond-lily manifests *astringent* activity (Tierra 1988: 341) and has been used by various peoples to treat **bleeding**, **diarrhea**, **dysentery**, **urethritis**, **gleet**, and **vaginal discharges**. It has also been appreciated as a topical *analgesic*. The Upper Tanana, for instance, have implemented a poultice of the sliced and warmed rhizome to control pain (Kari 1977: 17), while the Okanogan-Colville have applied the stem to an **aching tooth** to ease the agony of the sufferer

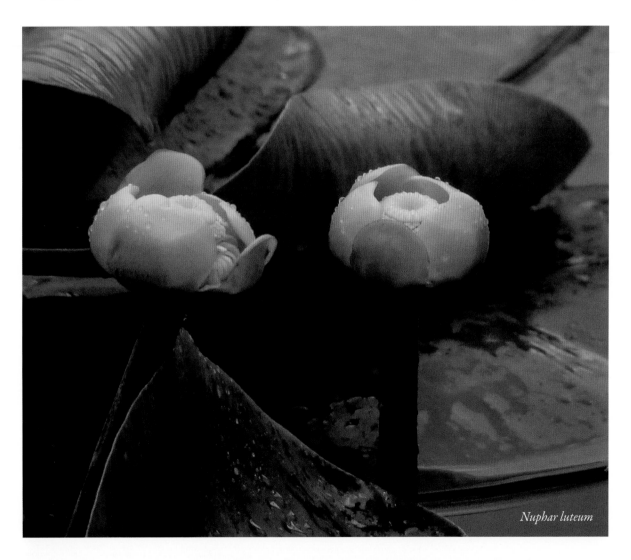

Nuphar luteum

(Turner et al. 1980: 110). The Bella Coola discovered that a decoction of the plant's rhizome soothed the **pain** of tuberculosis, heart disease, rheumatism, and gonorrhea, as well as that occurring in any part of the body! (Smith 1929: 56)

The *analgesic* effects may be due, in certain instances, either to an *antispasmodic* effect (Tierra 1988: 341) or to an *anti-inflammatory* activity possessed by this herb due to its content of steroidal saponins (Foster and Duke 1990: 88). Indeed, many inflammatory conditions have been treated with yellow pond-lily by a variety of peoples, and most especially an **inflamed uterus**. The Quinault and the Shuswap have employed a poultice of the heated rhizomes to ease the agony of **rheumatism** (Gunther 1973: 29; Palmer 1975: 64). The Kwakiutl have found the rhizomes helpful for **internal swellings** and for "sickness in the bones" (Turner and Bell 1973: 287). The Potawatomi have pounded the rhizome and used it, fresh or dried, for a variety of inflammatory diseases (Smith 1933: 65).

The most prominent use to which this plant has been put, however, is as a *vulnerary*. Numerous tribes have used it as such, in various ways: The Flathead (Salish) have applied a poultice of the baked rhizome to **sores** (Hart 1992: 33). The Micmac have pounded the rhizome into a mash and applied it to **swollen limbs** (Lacey 1993: 72). The Woods Cree have grated the rhizome, as well as that of both calamus (*Acorus calamus*) and cow-parsnip (*Heracleum lanatum*—see page 91), into a mixture with water or grease to use as a poultice for **headaches**, **sore joints**, **swellings**, **painful limbs**, and **worms in the flesh**. They have also poulticed a fresh or a rehydrated segment of the rhizome onto **infected skin lesions** to draw out the pus (Leighton 1985: 46, 47). The Algonquin in Quebec have also utilized a poultice of the boiled and mashed rhizomes for **infections** and for **swellings** (Black 1980: 163).

The application for infections is especially interesting since modern scientific research has substantiated that yellow pond-lily's alkaloids are strongly *antimicrobial*. For example, in a 1954 study of some three hundred plants tested to determine any activity against a virulent human strain of tuberculosis, yellow pond-lily was found to be among the very top botanicals that were active against this organism! (Fitzpatrick 1954: 529, 532) Interesting in this regard, too, is that the Bella Coola have long used yellow pond-lily

rhizome for **tuberculosis** (Smith 1929: 56). Then, too, the Nitinat discovered that placing large rhizomes of the plant in hot water and imbibing the resultant liquid acted as an impenetrable barrier against **epidemic diseases** (Turner et al. 1983: 114).

Yellow pond-lily evidently has powerful effects on the reproductive system as well: the Gitksan found that they could rely on either an infusion of the toasted rhizome or a decoction of the heart of the rhizome as a *contraceptive* (Smith 1929: 56). Some modern-day herbalists prefer to try it as an initial treatment for **menopausal symptoms**. The Abenaki have even implemented an infusion of the rhizome as an *anaphrodisiac*—especially for men, for whom it was said to curtail the sex drive for a full two months! (Rousseau 1947: 154, 167) One authority informs us that in some lands medical doctors still use this plant's rhizomes to curtail both **excessive sexual excitation** and **premature ejaculation** (Starý and Jirásek 1983: 140).

The Iroquois have used an infusion of the dried, grated plant for **heart problems** (Herrick 1977: 319). They have also combined an infusion of the rhizome with those of two other plants to improve the speed of blood circulation in adolescents (Rousseau 1945a: 43). These cardiovascular effects are no doubt due to the alkaloids, which are *cardioactive* as well as *vasoconstrictive* (Foster and Duke 1990: 88).

As to the form and the dosage usually used, the late Southwest American herbalist Michael Moore listed a 1:2 tincture of the fresh root to be taken at a dosage of 10–20 drops or a weak decoction of the rhizome to be used at a dose of 2–4 ounces, with either form to be taken up to three times a day (Moore 1994a: 17).

CAUTIONS

Due to the unpredictable content and nature of yellow pond-lily's alkaloids, the plant is potentially toxic. With the exception of the popcorn-like snack that can be prepared from the seeds as described, no other part of this plant should be prepared for food. As for herbal use in health conditions, only professionally prepared extracts of the roots should be used and with their intake best supervised by an herbal professional.

Yellow pond-lily should not be used as food or as medicine during either pregnancy or lactation. ᘓ

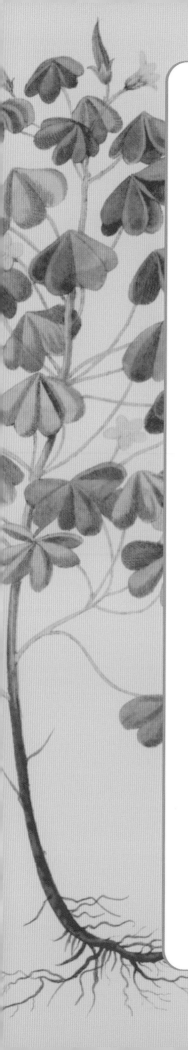

Yellow Wood-Sorrel

COMMON WOOD-SORREL; SOURGRASS; YELLOW OXALIS

Oxalis stricta, O. dillenii

DESCRIPTION

Yellow wood-sorrel is a delicate perennial herb with an upright, freely branching stem. It grows 4–14 inches high (average 5–8 inches). *Oxalis stricta* has blunt stem hairs, whereas the stem hairs on *O. dillenii* are pointed. Also, the former species spreads from underground stems, whereas the latter one lacks these.

The plant has alternate, light-green, smooth-edged leaves composed of three heart-shaped leaflets that are notched at their outer edges and sport a prominent midrib. All in all, the plant looks very much like common white clover. (In fact, some feel that the Irish shamrock was based on the *Oxalis* genus rather than on clovers as commonly believed.)

Two to five attractive yellow flowers grow on each plant. These display five petals, five sepals, and ten stamens.

The flowers are eventually replaced by pencil-shaped seedpods. These fruits are greenish tan and five-celled, with two or more seeds in each cell. In *O. stricta*, they are hairless (glabrous) or wide spreading, whereas in *O. dillenii*, they are pubescent with appressed hairs (occasionally with some spreading hairs). Also, the seedpods of the former species have straight stalks, whereas those of the latter species have bent stalks.

RANGE AND HABITAT

This is a cosmopolitan weed of the United States and southwestern Canada but is especially concentrated in the eastern two-thirds of the United States. In the Midwest, *O. stricta* is ubiquitous, whereas *O. dillenii* is scattered only around the southern half.

MAJOR CONSTITUENTS

Yellow wood-sorrel contains potassium oxalate, mucilage, and flavonoids (orientin, vitexin, and isovitexin). Nutrients include goodly amounts of vitamin C, phosphorus, and potassium.

FOOD

A wonderful trail nibble, this delicate little plant—full of a zestful, lemony flavor due to its oxalate content—has been appreciated as such by the Kiowa, Cherokee, Omaha, Pawnee, and other Native American tribes.

It is a popular salad ingredient among wild-foods foragers, especially the seedpods, which some liken to sour pickles. Then, too, *Oxalis* soup recipes abound in foraging manuals, although these should be treated with caution (see Cautions).

Outdoor enthusiasts appreciate yellow wood-sorrel as a stuffing for fish or made into a sauce as a condiment for such. The plant also makes an excellent stuffing for muskrat, porcupine, beaver, and other wild game. The Potawatomi have even made a tasty dessert out of it (Smith 1933: 106).

HEALTH/MEDICINE

Noted European herbalist John Gerard highlighted the main uses of this plant in reviewing the European species (*Oxalis acetosella*), which he recommended for

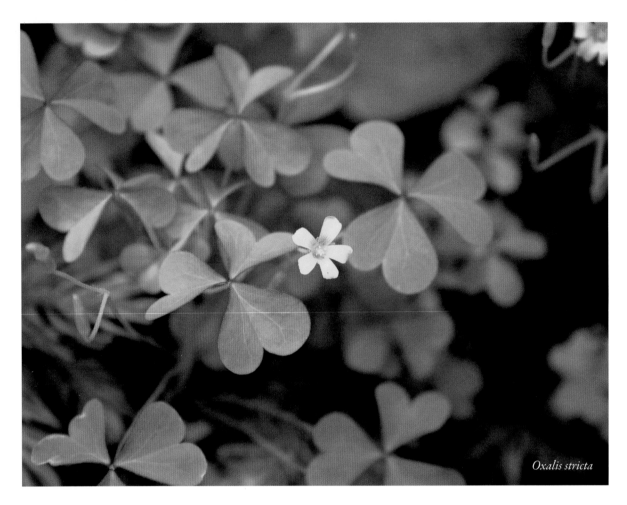

Oxalis stricta

"pestilential fevers," "sicke & feeble stomach," and "ulcers of the mouth" (Gerard 1975: 1031).

Looking at these recommendations in the light of study and experience since, we note the following: The plant, possessed of cooling energies—i.e., being a *refrigerant* (de Bairacli Levy 1974: 156; Wren 1988: 287)—is indeed a useful *antipyretic* (Stuart 1982: 104), especially for fevers producing a rash or pimples (de Bairacli Levy 1974: 156). It was much appreciated as a **fever** herb by early American healers (Crellin and Philpott 1990a: 459), as well as by the Iroquois (Herrick 1977: 365).

As to the second application enumerated by Gerard, yellow wood-sorrel is renowned as a *stomachic* (Grieve 1971: 2:752), appreciated in various herbal traditions to offset **heartburn**, **stomach cramps**, and various other **disorders of digestion** (Brown 1985: 215; Foster and Duke 1990; Crellin and Philpott 1990a: 459f). The Iroquois have found it useful for conditions such as **nausea**, **cramps**, and **diarrhea** (Herrick 1977: 365). Naturopathic physician Bill Mitchell pointed out that it contains an acid that research suggests may bolster gallbladder activity (Mitchell 2003).

As to Gerard's third recommendation, modern herbalists have indeed found an *Oxalis* mouthwash helpful for various problems in the oral cavity (Brown 1985: 215), especially for **cankers** (Grieve 1971: 2:752; Bolyard 1981: 102). The Iroquois have likewise appreciated the use of an infusion of this plant as a mouthwash (Herrick 1977: 366).

It is probable that an *anti-inflammatory* effect accounts, at least partly, for the applications to the alimentary canal. *Oxalis* juice has traditionally been used as a compress for **inflammation** (Grieve 1971: 2:752), which is a heat condition that would be offset by the plant's *refrigerant* powers. Other probable anti-inflammatory applications are as follows: Herbalist Tom Brown Jr. has found a strong tea to be useful as a wash for **skin afflictions** (Brown 1985: 215). A famed European herbalist recommended it as a poultice for **varicose veins**, to be held on by cabbage leaves and a cotton bandage over them and then left on overnight (de Bairacli Levy 1974: 156). Herbalists also use it for **hangover headaches** (Stuart 1982: 104).

There is evidently an *antimicrobial* aspect to this plant as well, which has also traditionally been used as an *antiseptic* (de Bairacli Levy 1974: 156). Lending support to this use, one study found that *O. stricta* strongly inhibited the tuberculosis bacterium in vitro (Fitzpatrick 1954: 530). Interestingly here, early American physicians applied the herb topically to "scrofulous ulcers" (Crellin and Philpott 1990a: 459). In the United Kingdom, it is used topically for **scabies** (Stuart 1982: 104).

Historically prominent has been its celebrated *diuretic* assist, an application that was much appreciated by early American physicians (Bolyard 1981: 102; Crellin and Philpott 1990a: 459). The Eclectics also found it useful in "urinary affections" (Felter and Lloyd 1898). More specifically, this powerful refrigerant has been used in folk medicine for **urethritis** or **cystitis** with **dysuria** and scanty flow and even for **acute nephritis** (de Bairacli Levy 1974: 156; Foster and Duke 1990: 88). Application for "urinary disorders" continues up until the present day in some circles (Wren 1988: 287). Thus, herbalist Peter Holmes notes that yellow wood-sorrel "promotes urination" and is especially helpful for what Traditional Chinese Medicine calls "kidney *qi* stagnation," marked also by fetid stool, a lackluster appetite, and dry skin. He also sees it as valuable in "kidney heat" conditions such as **acute nephritis** (Holmes 1997–98: 2:651).

Oxalis was also popular in early America as a topical treatment for **skin cancers** (Crellin and Philpott 1990a: 459), a tradition that has been perpetuated in Appalachian folk medicine. In this regard, naturalist and botanist Judith Bolyard interviewed Kentucky minister Alvin Boggs, a school superintendent, who relayed his family recipe in this regard: Boggs said that two bushels of the fresh plant's leaves and stems were boiled in water until a small black lump remained. This was to be applied daily to the skin cancer for two or three weeks until it disappeared (Bolyard 1981: 102). Dandelion leaves are typically added to decrease the pain of the wood-sorrel's destruction of the cancerous tissue (Bolyard 1981: 102). An almost identical application (including the use of dandelion to offset the pain) was elaborated in 1869 by the Physiomedicalist healer William Cook, who remarked that it "unquestionably has a decided power in causing the ejection of the cancerous deposits ('roots'), and promoting the healing of such degenerate sores" (Cook 1985). This treatment may have originally derived from the Native American tradition. In fact, a student of mine witnessed a Native American healer implement the herb in this manner for skin cancer, which she said resulted in success.

It is of possible interest here that other plants containing high amounts of oxalates have also been used for skin cancers. One of these, sheep sorrel (*Rumex acetosella*) (see page 204), is even a component of the famous Essiac herbal mix, which has proven popular as a natural treatment for cancer in lay circles.

Finally, being high in vitamin C, "the fresh plant, eaten raw, is useful in **scurvy**" (Wood et al. 1926: 1415).

PERSONAL AND PROFESSIONAL USE

For decades, I've appreciated yellow wood-sorrel as a trail nibble. Its lemony taste makes for an especially refreshing treat on a hot, humid day (as is often the case in my home state of Minnesota during the mid- to late summer).

In my clinical practice, I've used the herb as a refrigerant for acute gastric discomforts and for other acute inflammatory conditions.

CAUTIONS

In view of the high content of soluble oxalates, consumption of the fresh herb would best be restricted to light trail nibbling or sparing use as a salad ingredient. Nor should one use the extracts medicinally for an extended period of time. Also, yellow wood-sorrel should probably not be used in the presence of gout, rheumatism, or a tendency toward kidney stones of the oxalate variety. Finally, use of *this herb is best avoided during pregnancy*. ⋘

Physiological Actions of the Plants

Italicized plants are generally the superior ones in their respective categories

ADAPTOGEN
favorably modifies
stress response
Starflower?
Sweet cicely

ALTERATIVE
See Depurative

ANALGESIC/ANODYNE
reduces pain
Blue vervain
Bunchberry
Cattail
Mullein
Penstemon
Violet
Wild mint
Wild onion
Yarrow

ANAPHRODISIAC
inhibits sexual desire
Yellow pond-lily

ANTHELMINTIC
expels/destroys
parasites
Boneset
Horsemint
Pearly everlasting
Pineapple-weed
Purslane
Queen Anne's lace
Shepherd's purse
Stinging nettle
Swamp milkweed
Thistle
Turtlehead
Wormwood
Yarrow

ANTI-ANAEMIC
maintains
blood-iron levels
Chickweed
Dandelion
Dock
Jerusalem artichoke
Marsh marigold
Stinging nettle
Watercress
Wild strawberry
Yarrow

**ANTIBACTERIAL/
ANTIMICROBIAL**
inhibits/reduces
microbes
Bloodroot
Blue-eyed grass
Blue flag
Boneset
Bouncing bet
Burdock
Butter-and-eggs
Butterfly-weed
Catnip
Cattail
Chickweed
Chicory
Cleavers
Columbine
Creeping Charlie
Dandelion
Dock
False Solomon's seal
Fireweed
Hawkweed
Horsemint
Lamb's quarters
Milkweed
Mullein
Penstemon
Peppergrass
Plantain
Purple loosestrife
Purslane
Queen Anne's lace
Red clover
Self-heal
Shepherd's purse
Solomon's seal
Watercress
Wild geranium
Wild mint
Wild mustard
Wormwood
Yarrow
Yellow pond-lily
Yellow wood-sorrel

ANTICOAGULANT
reduces blood clotting
Cattail (raw pollen)
Motherwort

ANTICONVULSIVE
inhibits tendency to
convulse/seizure
Blue vervain
Burdock (seed)
Cow-parsnip
Marsh marigold
Skullcap

ANTIDIARRHEAL
See Astringent

ANTI-EMETIC
inhibits nausea/
tendency to vomit
Cow-parsnip
Fragrant giant hyssop
Horsemint
Mountain mint
Nutgrass
Wild bergamot
Wild mint

ANTIFUNGAL
inhibits/reduces fungi
Bloodroot
Burdock
Clearweed
Cow-parsnip
Dandelion
Fireweed
Fragrant giant hyssop
Goldenrod
Horsemint
Jewelweed
Milkweed
Plantain
Queen Anne's lace
Red clover
Wild bergamot
Wild mint
Yarrow

ANTIGALACTIC
reduces breast
milk production
Arrowhead

ANTIHISTAMINE
inhibits allergenic
release of histamine
from mast cells
Arrowhead
Burdock

Evening primrose
Plantain
Purple loosestrife
Self-heal
Stinging nettle
Wild onion
Yarrow

ANTI-INFLAMMATORY
reduces inflammation
Bloodroot
Blue cohosh
Blue vervain
Boneset
Bouncing bet?
Bugleweed
Bulrush
Bunchberry
Burdock
Butter-and-eggs
Chickweed
Chicory
Cinquefoil
Clearweed
Cleavers
Cow-parsnip
Creeping Charlie
Dandelion
Evening primrose
False Solomon's seal
Fireweed
Fleabane
Goldenrod
Gumweed
Hawkweed
Joe-pye weed
Knotweed
Lamb's quarters
Motherwort
Mullein
Penstemon
Plantain
Self-heal
Shepherd's purse
Smartweed
Solomon's seal
Stinging nettle
Sunflower
Sweet everlasting
Thistle
Violet
Wild mint
Wild onion
Wild strawberry

Yarrow
Yellow goatsbeard
Yellow loosestrife
Yellow pond-lily
Yellow wood-sorrel

ANTILITHIC
prevents or reduces/
eliminates calculi
(stones) in the biliary
or urinary system

Blue vervain
Cleavers
Goldenrod
Joe-pye weed
Knotweed
Wild strawberry
Yellow goatsbeard

ANTIMALARIAL
inhibits malarial
organisms or symptoms
of malarial infection

Boneset
Sunflower
Wormwood
Yarrow

ANTINEOPLASTIC
inhibits cancer cells

Bloodroot (skin)
Boneset
Burdock (breast, colon,
lymph)
Cleavers (breast, cervix,
lymph)
Dandelion (breast)
Fireweed (colon, lung,
prostate)
Goldenrod (breast, lung,
melanoma, prostate)
Gumweed (spleen,
stomach)
Knotweed
Plantain (breast)
Red clover
Sheep sorrel
Shepherd's purse
Spiderwort? (skin)
Stinging nettle (root)
(prostate)
Violet (breast, esophagus,
lymph, throat)

Watercress (colon, lung,
stomach)
Wild sarsaparilla (colon,
leukemia)
Yarrow?
Yellow pond-lily (testicles)
Yellow wood-sorrel (skin)

ANTIOXIDANT
enhances body's
scavenging of
free radicals

Chicory
Motherwort
Plantain
Self-heal
Sow thistle

ANTIPARALYTIC
reduces/inhibits
paralysis

Aster (facial)
Bunchberry?
Wild mustard?

ANTIPHLOGISTIC
See Anti-Inflammatory

ANTIPRURITIC
reduces/inhibits
itching

Chickweed
Dock
Knotweed
Nutgrass
Pennycress
Plantain
Turtlehead
Wild mint

ANTIPYRETIC
reduces fever

Arrowhead
Blue cohosh
Blue vervain
Boneset
Bunchberry
Butterfly-weed
Catnip
Chickweed
Cinquefoil
Cleavers
Fleabane
Goldenrod

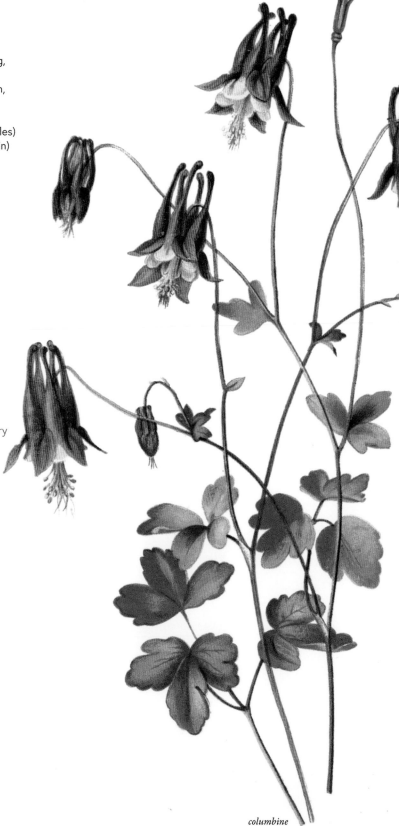

columbine

Horsemint
Lamb's quarters
Mountain mint
Pineapple-weed
Plantain
Self-heal
Sheep sorrel
Sunflower
Sweet everlasting
Violet
Watercress
Wild mint
Wild strawberry
Wormwood
Yarrow
Yellow wood-sorrel

ANTIRHEUMATIC
reduces rheumatic
inflammation
Arrowhead
Aster
Bloodroot
Boneset
Burdock
Butterfly-weed
Chickweed
Chicory
Cow-parsnip
Dandelion
False Solomon's seal
Fleabane
Goldenrod
Joe-pye weed
Lamb's quarters
Milkweed
Peppergrass
Plantain
Queen Anne's lace
Shepherd's purse
Smartweed
Solomon's seal
Stinging nettle
Sunflower
Wild sarsaparilla
Wild strawberry
Thistle
Yarrow
Yellow pond-lily

ANTISCORBUTIC
prevents vitamin-C
deficiency
Chickweed
Cleavers
Lamb's quarters
Peppergrass

Sheep sorrel
Watercress
Wild strawberry
Yellow goatsbeard
Yellow wood-sorrel

ANTISPASMODIC
inhibits/reduces spasms
Aster
Blue cohosh
Blue vervain
Butterfly-weed
Catnip
Cinquefoil
Cow-parsnip
Evening primrose
False Solomon's seal
Fireweed
Fleabane
Goldenrod
Gumweed
Marsh marigold
Skullcap
Sweet everlasting?
Wormwood
Yarrow

ANTITUSSIVE
inhibits/reduces
coughing
Blue vervain
Burdock
Red clover
Violet

ANTIVIRAL
inhibits/reduces
viral infections
Boneset
Burdock
Fireweed
Fragrant giant hyssop
Mullein (flowers)
Red clover
Self-heal
Wild geranium

APERIENT
See Laxative

APHRODISIAC
stimulates sexual desire
Cow-parsnip
Peppergrass
Watercress
Wild mint

APPETITE STIMULANT
stimulates hunger
Bunchberry
Chicory
Dandelion
Fleabane
Turtlehead
Yellow goatsbeard

ASTRINGENT
contracts/tightens
mucous membrane
or other tissue
Aster
Bugleweed
Bulrush
Butter-and-eggs
Catnip
Cattail
Cinquefoil
Cleavers
Creeping Charlie
Dock
Evening primrose
Fireweed
Fleabane
Goldenrod
Hawkweed
Knotweed
Lady's thumb
Lamb's quarters
Monkey-flower
Motherwort
Mullein
Pearly everlasting
Pigweed
Plantain
Prairie smoke
Puccoon
Purple loosestrife
Purslane
Self-heal
Sheep sorrel
Shepherd's purse
Smartweed
Sweet cicely
Sweet everlasting
Thistle
Virginia waterleaf
Wild geranium
Wild mint
Wild strawberry
Yarrow
Yellow loosestrife
Yellow pond-lily
Yellow wood-sorrel

CARDIOTONIC
enhances cardiac
tone/function
Bloodroot
Bluebead lily
Bugleweed
Chicory
False Solomon's seal
Fragrant giant hyssop
Gumweed
Milkweed
Motherwort
Solomon's seal
Sunflower
Violet
Watercress?
Wild mint
Yellow pond-lily

CARMINATIVE
inhibits/reduces the
spasms that cause
intestinal gas
Bunchberry
Catnip
Cow-parsnip
Creeping Charlie
Fragrant giant hyssop
Goldenrod
Gumweed
Horsemint
Motherwort
Mountain mint
Nutgrass
Pineapple-weed
Self-heal
Wild mint
Wild strawberry
Wild bergamot
Yarrow

CATHARTIC
See Laxative

CHOLAGOGUE
stimulates the
flow of bile
Blue flag
Burdock
Chicory
Dandelion
Watercress
Wormwood
Yarrow
Yellow goatsbeard

CHOLERETIC
stimulates the production/ excretion of bile
Culver's root
Dandelion
Yarrow

CONTRACEPTIVE
inhibits conception
False Solomon's seal
Puccoon
Wild geranium
Wild mint
Yellow pond-lily

DECONGESTANT
relieves or reduces congestion
Catnip
Creeping Charlie
Horsemint
Mountain mint
Sweet everlasting
Wild bergamot
Wild mint

DEMULCENT
locally soothes sore/ irritated mucous membranes
Evening primrose
Plantain
Solomon's seal

DEOBSTRUENT
removes obstruction
Butter-and-eggs
Peppergrass

DEODORANT
inhibits body odor
Cleavers
Wild mint

DEPURATIVE
cleanses the blood/lymph
Blue flag
Burdock
Chickweed
Cleavers
Dandelion
Dock
Evening primrose
Pigweed
Plantain

Red clover
Stinging nettle
Thistle
Violet
Wild sarsaparilla

DIAPHORETIC
stimulates sweating
Aster
Blue vervain
Boneset
Burdock
Butterfly-weed
Catnip
Columbine
Fleabane
Goldenrod
Horsemint
Joe-pye weed
Milkweed
Motherwort
Pineapple-weed
Sheep sorrel
Sweet everlasting
Wild bergamot
Wild sarsaparilla
Yarrow

DISCUTIENT
scatters tumor or coagulation
Bloodroot
Burdock
Cleavers
Dock
Red clover
Self-heal
Sheep sorrel
Shepherd's purse
Spiderwort?
Violet
Yellow wood-sorrel

DISINFECTANT
inhibits/reduces infection
Bloodroot
Burdock
Catnip
Cattail
Dock
False Solomon's seal
Fireweed
Fragrant giant hyssop
Goldenrod
Horsemint
Knotweed

Pigweed
Plantain
Shepherd's purse
Violet
Wild bergamot
Wild mint
Wild sarsaparilla
Wormwood
Yarrow
Yellow wood-sorrel

DIURETIC
stimulates reduction of water from body tissue by means of enhanced elimination through the kidneys
Arrowhead
Blue cohosh
Blue flag
Blue vervain
Bouncing bet
Burdock
Butter-and-eggs
Cattail
Chickweed
Chicory
Columbine
Creeping Charlie
Dandelion
Fleabane
Goldenrod
Hawkweed
Jerusalem artichoke
Joe-pye weed
Knotweed
Lady's thumb
Milkweed
Peppergrass
Plantain
Purslane
Queen Anne's lace
Self-heal
Sheep sorrel
Shepherd's purse
Smartweed
Swamp milkweed
Stinging nettle
Sunflower
Thistle
Watercress
Wild bergamot
Wild strawberry
Wood nettle
Wormwood
Yarrow
Yellow wood-sorrel

EMETIC
stimulates vomiting
Bloodroot
Blue cohosh
Blue flag
Blue vervain
Boneset
Butterfly-weed
Peppergrass
Solomon's seal
Swamp milkweed
Thistle

EMMENAGOGUE
stimulates menstruation
Bloodroot
Blue cohosh
Blue vervain
Catnip
Fleabane
Goldenrod
Horsemint
Joe-pye weed
Marsh marigold
Motherwort
Mountain mint
Pineapple-weed
Queen Anne's lace
Skullcap
Smartweed
Wild strawberry
Wormwood
Yarrow
Yellow wood-sorrel

ESCHAROTIC
locally dissolves tissue
Bloodroot

EXPECTORANT
stimulates coughing/ sneezing to eliminate excess mucus from the respiratory tract
Bloodroot
Blue vervain
Boneset
Butterfly-weed
Chickweed
False Solomon's seal
Gumweed
Marsh marigold
Milkweed
Mullein
Peppergrass
Plantain
Red clover

Sunflower
Violet
Watercress
Wild onion

FEBRIFUGE
  See Antipyretic

GALACTAGOGUE
  stimulates production/
  flow of breast milk
Blue vervain
Pineapple-weed
Stinging nettle

HEMOSTATIC/STYPTIC
  inhibits bleeding
Blue vervain
Bugleweed
Bulrush
Cattail (burnt pollen)
Cinquefoil
Cleavers
False Solomon's seal
Fleabane
Goldenrod
Knotweed
Pigweed
Plantain
Purple loosestrife
Self-heal
Sheep sorrel
Shepherd's purse
Smartweed
Stinging nettle
Yarrow
Yellow pond-lily

HEPATOPROTECTIVE
  protects the liver
  from toxins
Chicory
Nutgrass
Plantain
Queen Anne's lace
Wormwood

HERPATIC/HERPETIC
  inhibits/reduces
  lesions of the skin
Bloodroot
Bluebead lily
Burdock
Cattail
Chickweed
Cleavers
Dock

Evening primrose
Gumweed
Lamb's quarters
Peppergrass
Red clover
Stinging nettle
Thistle
Wild bergamot
Yellow wood-sorrel

HORMONAGOGUE
  affects hormone
  production, action,
  or levels
Bugleweed
Chickweed
Cinquefoil
Puccoon
Self-heal
Sweet cicely?

HYPOGLYCEMIC
  reduces levels of
  blood glucose
Bluebead lily?
Bugleweed
Burdock
Fleabane
Jerusalem artichoke
Joe-pye weed
Purple loosestrife
Solomon's seal
Sunflower
Wild geranium

HYPOTENSIVE
  reduces arterial
  blood pressure
Butterfly-weed
Cleavers
Joe-pye weed
Knotweed
Motherwort
Mullein
Purslane
Self-heal
Shepherd's purse
Stinging nettle
Sweet everlasting
Thistle
Wild onion
Yarrow (diastolic)

IMMUNOSTIMULANT
  stimulates or enhances
  immune-system function
Boneset

Bouncing bet
Burdock
Dock
Self-heal
Stinging nettle (root)

LAXATIVE
  stimulates defecation
  or maintains regular
  bowel movement
Arrowhead
Blue flag
Blue vervain
Boneset
Burdock
Chickweed
Chicory
Cleavers
Cow-parsnip
Culver's root
Dandelion (root)
Dock
False Solomon's seal (fruit)
Grindelia
Plantain (seed)
Purslane
Spiderwort
Turtlehead
Violet
Watercress
Wild mustard

LITHOTRIPTIC
  See Antilithic

LYMPHATIC
  stimulates or maintains
  healthy functioning of
  the lymphatic system
Blue flag
Burdock
Cleavers
Mullein
Red clover
Stinging nettle
Violet

MUSCLE RELAXANT
  relaxes tight/
  spastic muscles
Aster
Blue vervain
Nutgrass
Purslane
Self-heal
Skullcap

NEPHRITIC
  enhances kidney
  function
Bunchberry
Dandelion
Milkweed
Peppergrass
Shepherd's purse
Spiderwort
Stinging nettle
Thistle
Watercress
Wild strawberry
Yellow wood-sorrel

NERVINE
  soothes the nerves
Aster
Blue vervain
Bugleweed
Catnip
Chicory
Cinquefoil
Gumweed
Joe-pye weed
Motherwort
Pineapple-weed
Skullcap
Sow thistle
Wild strawberry

OPHTHALMIC
  enhances/preserves
  eye health
Hawkweed
Purple loosestrife
Self-heal

OXYTOCIC
  accelerates uterine
  contraction/childbirth
Blue cohosh

PARTURIENT
  aids childbirth
Bluebead lily
Blue cohosh
Motherwort
Shepherd's purse

PECTORAL
  relieves conditions in
  the region of the chest
Blue cohosh
Blue vervain
Butterfly-weed
Fragrant giant hyssop

Gumweed
Jerusalem artichoke
Marsh marigold
Mullein
Plantain
Red clover
Sunflower
Sweet everlasting
Thistle
Violet
Wild mint
Wild mustard
Wild onion
Wild sarsaparilla
Yarrow
Yellow pond-lily

REDUCENT
reduces body fat
and weight
Chickweed
Cleavers
Peppergrass
Queen Anne's lace

REFRIGERANT
cools the system
Dandelion
Lamb's quarters
Purslane
Sheep sorrel
Violet
Wild strawberry
Yellow wood-sorrel

REPELLANT
repels insects or vermin
Bluebead lily
Catnip
Mountain mint

RUBEFACIENT
irritates the skin by
enhancing the flow of
blood to the area
Horsemint
Wild bergamot
Wild mustard

SEDATIVE
tranquilizes the
nervous system
Blue vervain
Catnip (infants)
Chicory
Motherwort
Mullein

SIALAGOGUE
stimulates salivary
secretion
Blue flag
Cow-parsnip

STIMULANT
increases functional
activity, often of a
particular system,
e.g., circulatory
Boneset
Cow-parsnip
Gumweed
Horsemint
Mountain mint
Peppergrass
Queen Anne's lace
Watercress
Wild bergamot
Wild mint
Wild sarsaparilla
Yarrow

STOMACHIC
stimulates or improves
stomach function
Arrowhead
Blue vervain
Cow-parsnip
Creeping Charlie
Dandelion (leaf)
Evening primrose
Fireweed
Gumweed
Lamb's quarters
Nutgrass
Pineapple-weed
Plantain
Sheep sorrel
Shepherd's purse

Solomon's seal
Spiderwort
Swamp milkweed
Sweet everlasting
Wild mint
Wild strawberry
Wormwood
Yarrow
Yellow goatsbeard
Yellow wood-sorrel

SUDORIFIC
See Diaphoretic

TONIC
restores tone to a
particular body system;
especially used of the
gastrointestinal system
Arrowhead
Blue vervain
Boneset
Bunchberry (bladder)
Chicory
Creeping Charlie
Culver's root
Dandelion
Fireweed
Goldenrod
Gumweed
Jerusalem artichoke
Mullein (root) (bladder)
Plantain
Red clover
Solomon's seal
Starflower?
Stinging nettle
Thistle
Watercress
Wild mustard
Wild sarsaparilla
Wormwood
Yarrow
Yellow goatsbeard

VASOTONIC
improves the tone of
the vascular system
Dandelion
Purple loosestrife

Violet
Yarrow

VERMIFUGE
See Anthelmintic

VULNERARY
helps heal wounds
Bluebead lily
Blue flag
Butterfly-weed
Cattail
Chickweed
Cleavers
Cow-parsnip
Dock
Evening primrose
False Solomon's seal
Fireweed
Goldenrod
Gumweed
Joe-pye weed
Lady's thumb
Lamb's quarters
Monkey-flower
Mullein
Penstemon
Pineapple-weed
Plantain
Puccoon
Purple loosestrife
Purslane
Queen Anne's lace
Red clover
Self-heal
Shepherd's purse
Solomon's seal
Spiderwort
Stinging nettle
Sunflower
Wild bergamot
Wild onion
Wild sarsaparilla
Wormwood
Yarrow
Yellow pond-lily
Yellow wood-sorrel

How to Make Herbal Preparations at Home

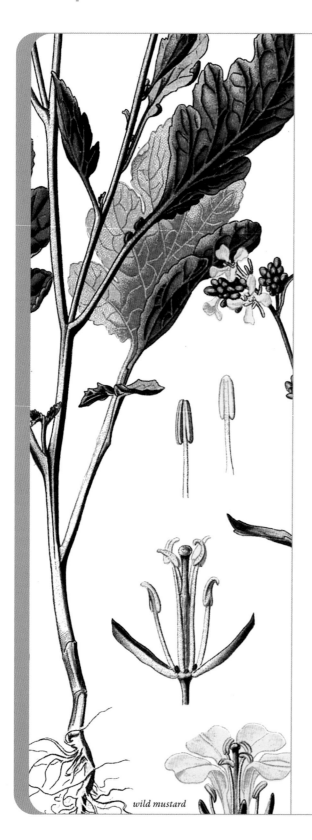

wild mustard

INFUSIONS

Infusions are aqueous extractions made by *steeping* the *soft* parts of an herb or herbs (i.e., leaves, flowers) in water that has been heated to the point of boiling but which is not actively boiling.

SUPPLIES
- Herb
- Mortar and pestle
- Pure water
- Tablespoon
- Teacup
- Creamer cup (teacup with a pour spout)
- Paper coffee filter or cheesecloth
- Stoneware or porcelain saucer plate
- Nonaluminum tea kettle

MEASUREMENT GUIDELINES
Usually, 1 tablespoon herb to 1 cup (8 ounces) water

STEPS
1. Lightly crush approximate amount of herb with mortar and pestle.
2. Measure required amount of herb and place in creamer.
3. Bring required amount of water just to boiling point.
4. Pour nearly boiling water into creamer until a bit below the rim.
5. Immediately cover cup with nonplastic, non-metallic saucer plate.
6. Steep herb 15 minutes to several hours, depending on herb and preparation needed.
7. Fit straining device (strainer, coffee filter, cheesecloth, etc.) over second cup and secure.
8. Carefully pour steeped fluid through filter into cup; remove filter.
9. Imbibe beverage per individual need or desire.

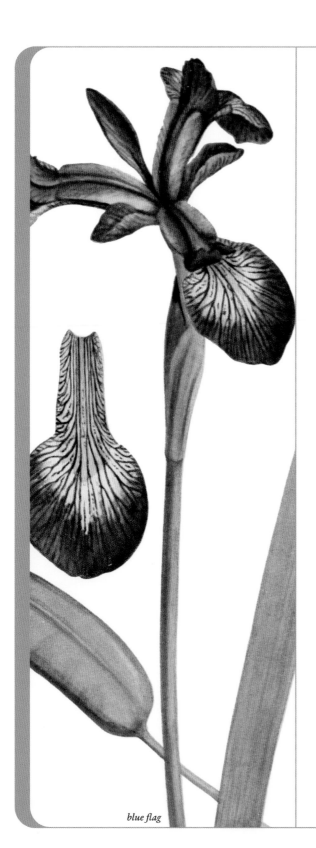

blue flag

DECOCTIONS

Decoctions are aqueous extractions of plants made by *actively boiling* their *hard, tough part*s (root, seeds, bark, fibrous stems) in water.

SUPPLIES

- Herb
- Mortar and pestle
- Kitchen scale
- Pure water
- Medium saucepan
- Tablespoon
- Creamer cup (teacup with a pour spout)
- Paper coffee filter or cheesecloth

MEASUREMENT GUIDELINES

Usually, 1 ounce (by weight) dried herb if using a pint (2 cups) water, or 2 ounces by weight fresh herb to the same amount of water; to make only a cup's worth, generally 1 rounded teaspoon dried plant parts to 1 cup water or 3 level teaspoons fresh plant part to the same amount of water.

STEPS

1. Break up plant part and crush with mortar and pestle.
2. Measure plant material and water and place in saucepan.
3. Heat to a boil, then lightly simmer for 15 minutes or more, or until mixture is reduced by one-third to three-quarters, depending on desired strength.
4. Fit straining device (strainer, coffee filter, cheesecloth, etc.) over creamer cup and secure.
5. Carefully pour fluid through filter into cup; remove filter.
6. Cool tea to desired temperature and then imbibe as needed or desired.

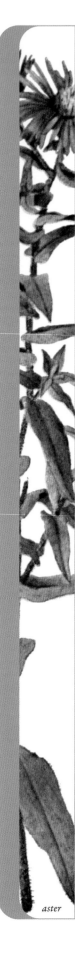
aster

TINCTURES

Tinctures are alcoholic extractions of plants, either fresh or dried.

SUPPLIES

- Herb
- Alcohol (100-proof vodka)
- Glass jar with lid
- Measuring cups
- Unbleached cheesecloth or tincture press
- Large beaker
- Small funnel
- Small amber glass bottles with glass droppers
- Stick-on label
- Felt-tip pen

MEASUREMENT GUIDELINES

Dried-Herb Tincture
(1:5 ratio = 1 part herb by weight to 5 parts vodka by volume)

This works out on a gram-to-milliliter basis as well as, correspondingly, on an ounce (by weight)-to-ounce (by volume) basis.

Examples (note how multiplying the grams by 5 equals the milliliters and how multiplying the weight in ounces by 5 equals the volume in ounces)
- 2 oz (60 g) herb to 300 ml (10 oz) vodka
- 4 oz (120 g) herb to 1 pint (600 ml = 20 oz) vodka
- 8 oz (240 g) herb to 1200 ml (40 oz) vodka

Fresh-Herb Tincture
(1:2 ratio = 1 part herb by weight to 2 parts vodka by volume)

This works out on a gram-to-milliliter basis as well as, correspondingly, on an ounce (by weight)-to-ounce (by volume) basis.

Examples (note how multiplying the grams by 2 equals the milliliters and also how multiplying the weight in ounces by 2 equals the volume in ounces)
- 2 oz (60 g) herb to 120 ml (4 oz) vodka
- 4 oz (120 g) herb to 1 cup (240 ml = 8 oz) vodka
- 8 oz (240 g) herb to 1 pint (480 ml = 16 oz) vodka

STEPS

1. For dried herb, place measured herb in bottom of glass jar; cover with appropriate amount of vodka. For fresh herbs, mix herb and vodka in blender and then place in jar. Seal jar tightly.
2. Use marking pen to write date on label; affix label to jar.
3. Store jar in a dark place. For dried-herb tinctures, shake 1–2 times daily for 2–4 weeks. For fresh-herb tinctures, let sit for 10–14 days. Top off with more vodka as liquid evaporates.
4. Strain steeped fluid through cheesecloth into beaker, squeezing excess fluid from filter into the beaker.
5. Use funnel to carefully pour strained liquid into tincture bottle and tighten dropper.
6. Indicate contents with marking pen on label; affix label to tincture bottle.
7. Store tincture in a dark place at room temperature and use when necessary. (Note: a dose of a tincture should always be diluted in a little water before being imbibed, so that the high alcohol content will not irritate the oral mucosa.)

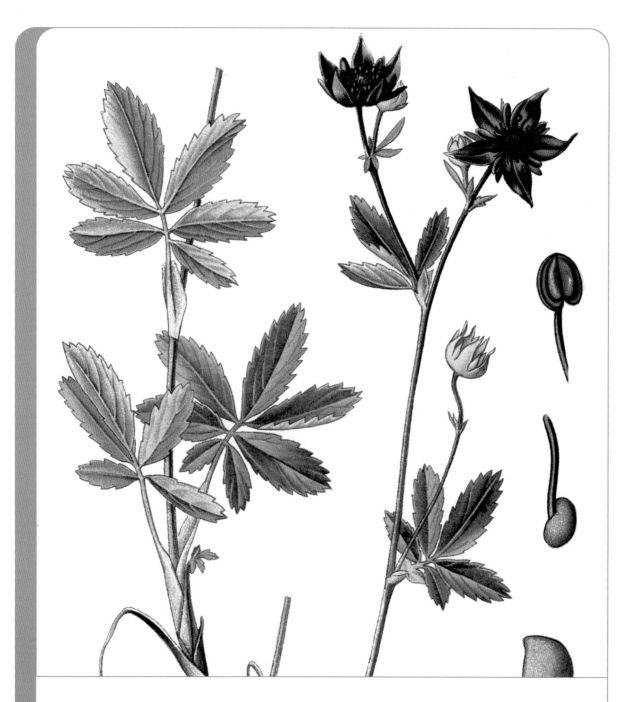

COMPRESSES

A compress is a porous wrapping (typically consisting of gauze, cloth, or cheesecloth) that is soaked in an herbal infusion or decoction, wrung out, and applied to a body part. (Plastic wrap is sometimes used as an overlay on the compress to keep it from drying out prematurely.)

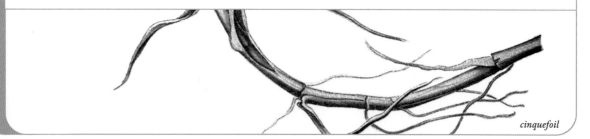

cinquefoil

Glossary

ABSCESS: a painful, swollen region of tissue where pus is forming

ACHENE: a small, hard, one-seeded fruit not splitting open at maturity

ADAPTOGEN: favorably modifying the stress response, or an agent for such

ALKALOID: a bitter, alkaline, nitrogenous, organic substance found in certain higher plants and often possessed of toxic and/or medicinal properties

ALLERGIC RHINITIS: allergic inflammation of the nasal passages; also called "hay fever"

ALTERATIVE: the "altering" of a body's condition so as to gradually restore health, or an agent for such

AMENORRHEA: where normal menstruation is absent or restricted

ANALGESIC: relieving pain, or an agent for such

ANAPHRODISIAC: inhibiting sexual desire, or an agent for such

ANNUAL: a plant that sprouts, lives, and dies all within one growing season

ANODYNE: reducing pain, or an agent for such

ANTHELMINTIC: serving to expel or destroy internally resident parasitical creatures, or an agent for such

ANTHER: club-like tip of a plant stamen and the site where the pollen is held

ANTHOCYANINS: pigments in plants responsible for the blue, violet, and red colors that occur in their flowers or other parts; sometimes grouped as a subdivision of *flavonoids*

ANTI-ANAEMIC: maintaining healthy blood-iron levels, or an agent for such

ANTICATARRHAL: reducing mucosal inflammation, or an agent for such

ANTICOAGULANT: reducing blood clotting, or an agent for such

ANTICONVULSIVE: inhibiting the tendency to convulse or seizure, or an agent for such

ANTI-EMETIC: inhibiting nausea or a tendency to vomit, or an agent for such

ANTIFUNGAL: inhibiting fungi, or an agent for such

ANTIGALACTIC: inhibiting the production or flow of breast milk, or an agent for such

ANTIHISTAMINE: inhibiting the allergenic release of histamine from the mast cells of the body, or an agent for such

ANTILITHIC: preventing, reducing, or eliminating calculi (stones) in the hepatobiliary or urinary systems, or an agent for such

ANTINEOPLASTIC: inhibiting cancer cells, or an agent for such

ANTIOXIDANT: enhancing the body's scavenging of free radicals, or an agent for such

ANTIPHLOGISTIC: reducing inflammation, or an agent for such

ANTIPRURITIC: reducing or inhibiting itching, or an agent for such

ANTIPYRETIC: tending to reduce fever, or an agent for such (see also under *febrifuge*)

ANTISPASMODIC: alleviating cramps or spasms, or an agent for such

ANTITUSSIVE: helping to settle or terminate a cough, or an agent for such

ANURIA: failure to urinate

APHRODISIAC: stimulating sexual desire, or an agent for such

ASTRINGENT: causing tissues to contract and tighten, or an agent for such

ATONY: lack of proper tone (of an organ, muscle, etc.)

AXIL: the upper angle of a leaf stalk and its stem

BASAL: referring to leaves emanating directly from the crown of a plant and thus at or near ground level

BERRY: a pulpy fruit evolving from a single ovary and having a thin skin and several or many small seeds that are often distributed throughout the pulp (The term is often misapplied to other kinds of fruits by modern herbalists and foragers who should know better. For example, fruits produced by hawthorn shrubs are not berries, although they are often designated by that term, but actually *pomes* and are properly referred to as "haws" or "hawthorn fruits"—*never* as "hawthorn berries.")

BIENNIAL: a plant that lives for only two seasons, growing only vegetatively in the first season and then flowering, seeding, and dying in the second season

BIPINNATE: twice pinnate (See *pinnate*)

BRACT: a reduced or imperfectly developed leaf growing directly beneath a flower

BULB: an underground food-storage structure consisting of leaves which are very tightly wrapped around the stem

CALYX: the green, outer, floral envelope consisting of sepals, the function of which seems to be to protect the flowers (especially when unopened)

CARDENOLIDE: a cardioactive glycoside

CARDIOACTIVE: any agent affecting the heart

CARDIOTONIC: enhancing cardiac tone/function, or an agent for such

CARMINATIVE: relieving or expelling intestinal gas, or an agent for such

CAROTENOID: a type of terpene (namely, a tetraterpene) found in plants and possessed of bioactive capabilities; beta-carotene, responsible for the orange-yellow coloring in some plants, is one example in that it is a precursor to vitamin A

CATARRH: inflammation characterized by a free discharge from mucous membranes (The term is derived from the Greek *katarrhein*, "to flow down.")

CATHARTIC: evacuating the intestines quickly and powerfully, or an agent for such

CHOLAGOGUE: improving the flow of bile in the digestive process, or an agent for such

CHOLECYSTITIS: inflammation of the gallbladder

CHOLERETIC: stimulating the production or excretion of bile, or an agent for such

CHOLESTASIS: sluggish or halted bile flow

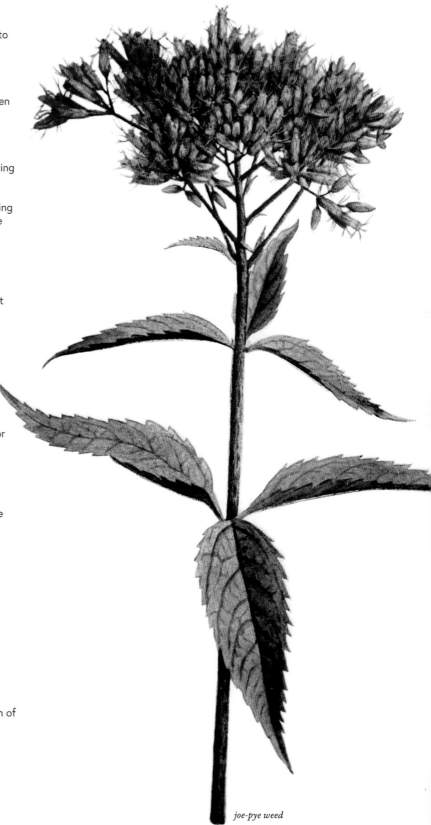

joe-pye weed

CHOREA: a nervous condition or disease marked by a sudden, severe, and involuntary twitching of the face or limbs

COMPOSITE FLOWER: a flower in the Asteraceae family consisting of a central disk with many ray flowers extending from it

COMPOUND LEAF: a leaf whose blade is divided into two or more parts called "leaflets"

COMPRESS: a cloth or bandage that has been soaked in a solution and applied externally to a body part to achieve relief of pain, infection, malady, or symptoms

CONTUSION: an injury to the skin where it does not break but simply bruises

CORM: an underground enlargement (especially vertically) of a plant's stem that resembles a *bulb* but lacks layers

COROLLA: the showy parts of a flower; the petals considered collectively

CORYMB: a flattened or convex flower cluster in which the outer flowers bloom before the central ones

CROUP: an acute infection that blocks the larynx, resulting in difficult breathing and a barking cough

CROWN: the base of a perennial plant from which the shoots grow upward and the roots downward

CYME: a flattened or convex flower cluster wherein the central flowers bloom before the outer ones

CYSTITIS: inflammation of the bladder

CYTOTOXIC: toxic to organs, tissues, or cells, or an agent for such (Cytotoxic agents are studied by scientists for any possible selective role they might possess; for example, in destroying cancer cells while leaving healthy cells intact.)

DEBILITY: a run-down state, with loss of vital strength, often due to stress, overexertion, or disease

DECIDUOUS: plants that grow through a cycle of growth and then shed parts and/or die back at the end of a growing season; in contrast to "evergreen"

DECOCTION: an herbal extract wherein a hard plant part (root, stem, seed, or bark) has been actively boiled in water

DECONGESTANT: breaking up excessive mucus in the respiratory tract that is making breathing difficult (especially in the nasal/sinus region), or an agent for such

DEMULCENT: locally soothing to sore mucous membranes, or an agent for such

DEOBSTRUENT: removing obstruction, or an agent for such

DEPURATIVE: cleansing impurities from the system (usually with reference to the blood/lymph), or an agent for such

DIAPHORETIC: promoting perspiration, or an agent for such

DIOECIOUS: possessing either male or female flowers only

DISCUTIENT: scattering tumors or coagulation, or an agent for such

DISK FLOWER: the central, rounded part of a *composite flower*

DIURETIC: increasing urination, or an agent for such

DROPSY: bygone term for an edematous state wherein fluids effuse into body tissues or cavities, typically caused by cardiac or renal failure

DRUPE: a fleshy fruit with a single seed encased in a hard, bony substance

DYSENTERY: diarrhea accompanied by painful inflammation of the colon, and thus often marked by the passing of mucus and blood

DYSKINESIA: failure to move or to exert activity

DYSMENNORHEA: painful menstruation

DYSPEPSIA: a bygone term for indigestion

DYSPNEA: difficult or labored breathing, arising from air hunger—whether from overexertion, respiratory malfunction, disease, or distress

DYSURIA: disordered, difficult, or painful urination

EDEMA: a condition of swelling resulting from retained fluids in the connective tissues of the body

EMETIC: inducing vomit, or an agent for such

EMMENAGOGUE: tending to normalize or stimulate menstruation, or an agent for such

EMOLLIENT: tending to soften (the skin, etc.), or an agent for such

ENTERITIS: inflammation of the mucous membrane of the small intestine

ERYSIPELAS: an acute infection caused by *Strep. pyrogenes* that results in a localized redness and inflammation of the skin and underlying tissue

ESCHAROTIC: locally dissolving tissue, or an agent for such

ESSENTIAL OIL: aromatic oil contained in many plants, e.g., the mint family

ETHNOBOTANIST: a person who studies the use of plants by Native peoples

EXPECTORANT: promoting the expulsion of mucus from the respiratory tract, or an agent for such

FEBRIFUGE: reducing fever, or an agent for such

FELON: also known as a "whitlow," an *abscess* occurring near a fingernail, usually caused by a bacterial infection

FIBROID, UTERINE: also known as a "leiomyoma," a bundle of fibers that forms within the uterus; typically manifested by an unusually heavy menses and clots

FILAMENT: in a plant's *stamen*, the hairy stalk on which rests the *anther*

FLAVONOIDS: pigments in plants, sometimes responsible for the yellow and white colors in their flowers or plant parts (They are all to some extent bioactive, often being anti-inflammatory, antiviral, *vasotonic,* or otherwise helpful to the organism.)

FOMENTATION: a warm dressing, ointment, or poultice

FURUNCULOSIS: an occurrence of many boils at once

GALACTAGOGUE: stimulating production of breast milk, or an agent for such

GALACTORRHEA: excessive or involuntary flow of breast milk

GALACTOSTASIS: sluggish or halted flow of breast milk

GLAUCOUS: covered with a fine, whitish film

GLEET: involuntary, non-seminal, non-urinous discharge from the urethra, usually pathogenic in nature, and typically used currently only of the mucopurulent discharge occurring in chronic gonorrhea

GLYCOSIDE: a plant compound decomposable into a sugar molecule and another molecule referred to as an "aglycone"

HALITOSIS: bad breath

HEMATURIA: urine tinted with blood

HEMOPTYSIS: an expectoration of blood from the respiratory system

HEMOSTATIC: checking or arresting the flow of blood, or an agent for such

HEPATIC: benefiting the liver, or an agent for such

HEPATOMEGALY: enlargement of the liver

HEPATOPROTECTIVE: protecting the liver from toxins, or an agent for such

HEPATOTOXICITY: toxicity of the liver

HERB: a tender, succulent plant having aboveground portions which are entirely nonwoody (thus dying back at the end of the growing season)

HERBALISM: the practice of using medicinal herbs to support health/healing

HERBOLOGY: the study or science of the use of plants to support health/healing

HERPATIC/HERPETIC: inhibiting/reducing lesions of the skin

HORMONAGOGUE: affecting hormone production, action, or levels

HYDROPHOBIA: fear of water, characterizing rabies infection

HYPOCHLORHYDRIA: low levels of hydrochloric acid in the stomach

HYPOGLYCEMIC: reducing levels of blood glucose, or an agent for such; also refers to a state wherein the blood-sugar level is suboptimal

HYPOKALEMIA: a low level of serum potassium

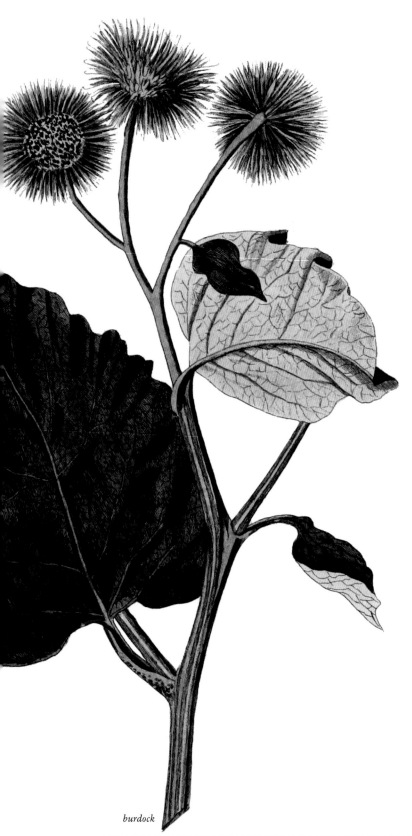

burdock

HYPOTENSIVE: lowering blood pressure, or an agent for such

IMPETIGO: a contagious, inflammatory skin condition, usually occurring around the nose, that is characterized by pustules that encrust and rupture

INCONTINENCE: reduced ability to hold urine in the bladder, with consequent involuntary leakage of urine from the urethra

INFLORESCENCE: the flowering portion(s) of a plant, applicable to either a simple blossom or a flower cluster; also, the particular arrangement of the flower cluster, whether as *cyme*, *panicle*, *raceme*, etc.

INFUSION: an extract made from steeping a soft plant part or parts in hot (but not actively boiling) water

INVOLUCRE: an arrangement of whorled *bracts* occurring in many plants, functioning as a shield for the plant's reproductive elements

LACTATION: the act of breastfeeding or the state wherein breast milk is readily available

LANCEOLATE: lance-shaped, i.e., leaves are longer than wide and taper to a point

LASSITUDE: weariness leading to lack of activity

LEAFLET: main subdivision of a compound leaf, looking like a small, entire leaf

LEUKORRHEA: a milky and viscous vaginal discharge, often resulting from mucosal inflammation (This can be a normal, physiological attendant to menses if occurring right before or after the flow.)

LITHOTRIPTIC/LITHONTRIPTIC: breaking up or dissolving calculi (stones) in the urinary or the hepatobiliary system, or any agent for such

LOBE: a rounded projection on a leaf formed by an indentation of its margin

LUMBAGO: a chronic ache in the lower back

LYMPHADENITIS: inflammation of a lymph node or nodes

LYMPHADENOPATHY: lymph-node enlargement

LYMPHANGITIS: inflammation in the lymphatic channels

LYMPHATIC: stimulating or maintaining healthy functioning of the lymphatic system

MACERATE: to soften or to separate a plant part by steeping it in water or other fluid in order to allow for extraction

MASTALGIA: pain in a breast (mammary gland) or breasts, such as can occur premenstrually in some women

MASTITIS: inflammation of a breast (mammary gland) or breasts, such as can occur from infection during lactation, etc.

MATERIA MEDICA: Latin for "medical material" and thus relating to the systematized corpus of healing agents in possession of a particular healer or group of healers

MENORRHAGIA: excessive menstrual flow

METRORRHAGIA: uterine blood flow occurring mid-cycle or at any time in the cycle when it would not normally be occurring

MUCILAGE: gelatinous substance occurring in certain plants (Mucilage has healing potential for irritated mucous membranes, which it can protect and soothe.)

MUCOLYTIC: dispersing mucus, or an agent for such

MUCUPURULENT: having mucus and pus

MYALGIA: pain in the muscles

NARCOTIC: depressing the central nervous system, or an agent for such

NEPHRITIC: enhancing function of the kidneys, or an agent for such

NERVINE: strengthening and/or soothing to the nervous system, or an agent for such

NEURALGIA: pain in the nerves

NODE: the marked joint of a plant stem where the branches or leaves attach

OPTHALMIC: enhancing or preserving eye health, or an agent for such

OXYTOCIC: accelerating uterine contraction for childbirth, or an agent for such

PALLIATIVE: providing relief but without effectively curing, or an agent for such

PALMATE: a leaf shaped like a human hand, with the blade having three or more fingerlike sections

PANICLE: a loosely branched flower cluster, often pyramidal in shape, and with each branch consisting of a *raceme*

PARBOIL: to boil briefly

PARTURIENT: aiding childbirth, or an agent for such

PECTORAL: relieving a condition in the region of the chest

PEDICEL: in a flower cluster, the stalk of a solitary flower

PEDUNCLE: the primary stalk of a flower cluster or of a solitary flower when it is the only one on the flowering stem

PERENNIAL: a plant that lives for several or more seasons, growing from the same root year after year

PERFOLIATE: when a plant has paired leaves lacking stalks so that it looks like they have been perforated by the stem

PERIANTH: where a plant's *calyx* and *corolla* are considered together, especially when they are visually similar

PETIOLE: a leaf's stalk

PHARYNGITIS: sore throat

PINNATE: a condition wherein a leaf is divided into leaflets resembling feathers arranged on a bird's wing

PISTIL: the central organ of a flower, consisting of the ovary, *stigma*, and *style*

POME: a fleshy fruit having a central core consisting of seeds enclosed in a hard, membranaceous capsule

POTHERB: an edible plant that is cooked before being consumed

POULTICE: a moistened mass of herb, or herbs, wrapped in a cloth and applied externally to a body part

PROPHYLACTIC: preventing or protecting against disease, injury, or other harm, or an agent for such

PRURITIS: inflammation of the skin marked by itching

PUBESCENT: hairy and soft

PULMONARY: pertaining to the lungs

PURGATIVE: forcefully emptying the colon, or an agent for such

RACEME: an inflorescence consisting of an elongate flower cluster of short-stalked flowers arising from a single axis

RAY FLOWER: in a *composite flower*, one of many petal-like flowers surrounding the central, disk-shaped flower

RECEPTACLE: the base of a flower, from which its parts extend (In some plants, the fruit wall is produced from this structure.)

REFRIGERANT: powerfully cooling, or an agent for such

RENAL: pertaining to the kidneys

RHEUMATISM: general term for inflammation of the joints, muscles, tendons, bursa, or suchlike structures

RHIZOME: a horizontal, and often elongated, underground stem of certain perennial plants. It is usually situated just below the surface of the soil and it possesses *nodes* (by which it is distinguished from a root)

ROOTSTOCK: an ill-defined term used by botanical writers which is sometimes used of the *crown* and root system of a perennial plant and at other times is used interchangeably—though perhaps arguably—for the plant's *rhizome*

ROSETTE: a circular cluster of *basal* leaves, often looking as if flattened against the ground

RUBEFACIENT: irritating the skin by enhancing the flow of blood to the area

SAPONIN: a *glycoside* chemical found in many plants which foams when shaken with water; many saponins are bioactive, often serving as *antiphlogistics*, *expectorants*, etc.

SCIATICA: pain in a leg along the path of the sciatic nerve (running from the back of the thigh to the inside of the leg)

SCROFULA: swollen cervical lymph nodes resulting from tuberculosis

SEPAL: a sort of floral "leaf," this is the outermost flower part, usually green in color and petal-like; it serves to protect the flower petals (especially when unopened) and is one of several like members of the *calyx*

SERRATE: when the edge or margin of a leaf is saw-toothed, as opposed to being round-toothed, lobed, or entire

SESSILE: lacking a stalk, i.e., where a leaf clasps the stem

SHOOTS: newly sprouted portions of a plant

SIALAGOGUE: stimulating salivary secretion, or an agent for such

STAMEN: the male (pollen-bearing) part of a plant, consisting of *anther* and *filament*

STIGMA: the pollen-receiving tip of a plant's *pistil*

STIMULANT: increasing functional activity, often of a particular system

STIPULE: a small appendage at the base of the leafstalk of certain plants

STOMACHIC: beneficially affecting the stomach, digestion, or appetite, or an agent for such

STYLE: in a plant's *pistil*, this is the middle portion connecting the *stigma* with the ovary

STYPTIC: serving to check blood flow by constricting the vessels, or an agent for such

SUDORIFIC: promoting perspiration, or an agent for such

TACHYCARDIA: chronically elevated heart rate, such as occurs in hyperthyroidism

TANNIN: an *astringent*, phenolic plant compound that possesses the ability to precipitate protein

TAPROOT: the stout, main, vertical root of a plant, which in turn gives rise to smaller roots

TENDRIL: a thin, coiling part of a vine that grasps onto other plants or structures for support

THROMBOSIS: formation or existence of a blood clot

TINCTURE: an alcoholic extract of a plant or plant part

TISANE: a bygone name for an herbal *infusion*

TONIC: strengthening and restoring tone, often with reference to the digestive or some other body system

TRIFOLIATE: a compound leaf possessed of three *leaflets*

TUBER: a subterranean swelling on a root or stem—a sort of modified branch, usually short and thick, with buds or "eyes" (It is used by the plant for storing food and may occur some distance from the aboveground portions.)

TUFTED: tightly clustered

UMBEL: a type of flower cluster wherein the individual flower stalks all rise from a common point, giving the appearance of an umbrella

URINARY: enhancing the tone or function of the urinary system

URTICARIA: outbreak of allergic, itching hives

VARIEGATED: leaves having the markings of a second color

VASOCONSTRICTIVE: constricting the blood vessels, or an agent for such

VASOTONIC: supporting the tone of the blood vessels, or an agent for such

VERMIFUGE: serving to kill parasitical worms, or an agent for such

VERTIGO: a sensation that one is traversing space or that everything is spinning around one; often related to disturbances of the inner ear or of cerebral blood flow

VOLATILE OIL: another term for *essential oil*

VULNERARY: promoting the healing of wounds, or an agent for such

WEED: a small, nonwoody plant growing wild or uncultivated

WHORL: a cluster of three or more leaves radiating from a single *node*

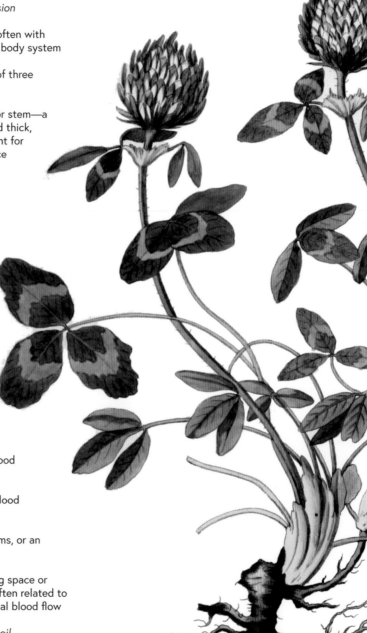

red clover

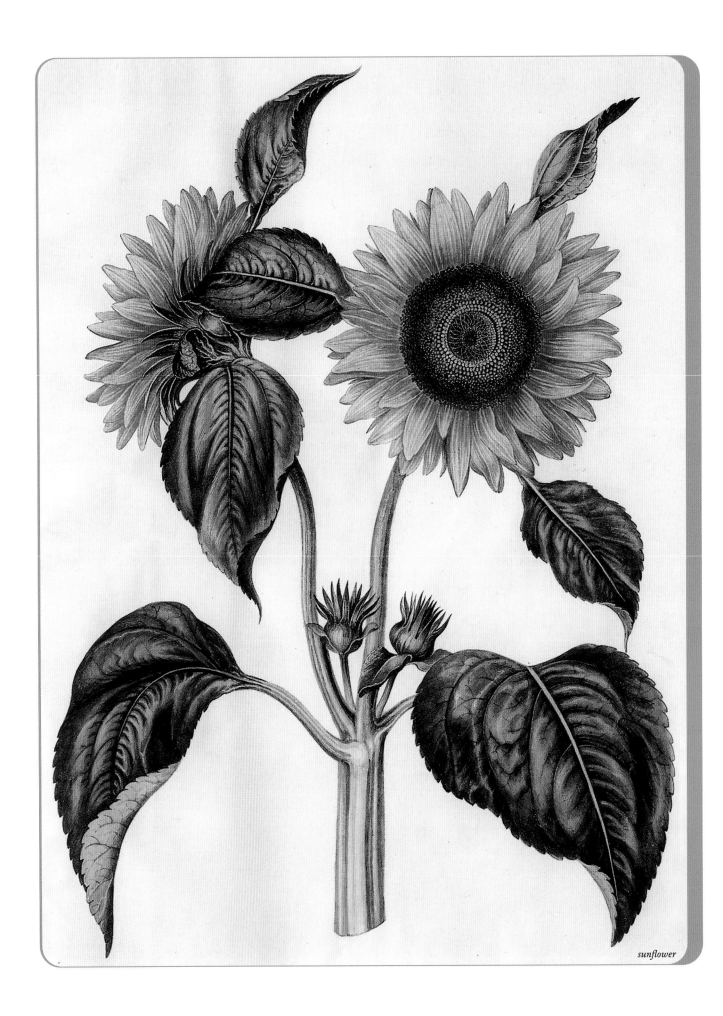

sunflower

Bibliography

Abad, MJ, et al. 1999. "Antiviral Activity of Some South American Plants." *Phytother. Res.* 13(2):142–46.

Abdullin, KK. 1962. *Zap Dazansk, Vet. Inst.* 84:75, through *Chem. Abstr.* 1964. 60:11843b.

Abrams MV, et al. 2012. "The Effectiveness of Jewelweed, *Impatiens capensis*, the Related Cultivar *I. balsamina*, and the Component, Lawsone, in Preventing Post Poison Ivy Exposure Contact Dermatitis." *J. Ethnopharmacol.* 143(1):314–18. Epub 2012 Jul 3.

Abud, MA, et al. 2017. "Hypoglycemic Effect Due to Insulin Stimulation with *Plantago major* in Wistar Rats." *Med. Aromat. Plants.* (Los Angel) 6(3).

Agawane, SB, et al. 2019. "Chemo-biological Evaluation of Antidiabetic Activity of *Mentha arvensis* L. and Its Role in Inhibition of Advanced Glycation End Products." *J. Ayurveda Integr. Med.* 10(3):166–70.

Ageel, AM, et al. 1989. "Experimental Studies on Antirheumatic Crude Drugs Used in Saudi Traditional Medicine." *Drugs Exp. Clin. Res.* 15(8):369–72.

Aggarwal, PK, et al. 1986. "Effect of *Rumex nepalensis* Extracts on Histamine, Acetylcholine, Carbachol, Bradykinin, and PGs-evoked Skin Reactions in Rabbits." *Ann. Allergy.* 56:177–82.

Agha-Hosseini, F, et al. 2010. "Efficacy of Purslane in the Treatment of Oral Lichen Planus." *Phytother. Res.* 24(2):240–44.

Ahsan, SK, et al. 1989. "Studies on Some Herbal Drugs Used in Fracture Healing." *Int. J. Crude Drug Res.* 27(4):235–39.

Airaksinen, MM, et al. 1986. "Toxicity of Plant Material Used as Emergency Food during Famines in Finland." *J. Ethnopharmacol.* 18(3):273–96.

Akanmu, MA, et al. 2002. "Hypnotic Effects of Total Aqueous Extracts of *Vervain hastata* (Verbenaceae) in Rats." *Psychiatry Clin. Neurosci.* 56(3):309–10.

Akhtar, MS, et al. 1985. "Effects of *Portulaca oleracae* (Kulfa) and *Taraxacum officinale* (Dhudhal) in Normoglycaemic and Alloxan-treated Hyperglycaemic Rabbits." *J. Pak. Med. Assn.* 35(7):207–10.

Akihisa, T, et al. 1996. "Triterpene Alcohols from the Flowers of Compositae and Their Anti-inflammatory Effects." *Phytochem.* 43(6):1255–60.

Akkol, EK, et al. 2011. "Evaluation of the Wound Healing Potential of *Achillea biebersteinii* Afan. (Asteraceae), by In Vivo Excision and Incision Models." *Evid.-Based Complement. Altern. Med.* 2011:474026. doi: 10.1093/ecam/nep039. Epub 2011 Jun 16.

Aksornthong, C, et al. 2019. "Cooking Has the Potential to Decrease the Antitumor Effect of Fresh Betong Watercress." *J. Food Biochem.* 43(4):E12783. Epub 2019 Jan 24.

Alothman, EA, et al. 2018. "Evaluation of Anti-ulcer and Ulcerative Colitis of *Sonchus oleraceus* L." *Saud. Pharm. J.* 26(7):956–59.

Aman, MG, et al. 1987. "The Effects of Essential Fatty Acid Supplementation by Efamol in Hyperactive Children." *J. Abnorm. Child Psychol.* 15(1):75–90.

An, HJ, et al. 2006. "*Glechoma hederacea* Inhibits Inflammatory Mediator Release in IFN-gamma and LPS-stimulated Mouse Peritoneal Macrophages." *J. Ethnopharmacol.* 106(3):418–24.

Andros, F. 1883. "The Medicine and Surgery of the Winnebago and Dakota Indians." *Am. Med. Assn. J.* 1:116–18.

Angier, Bradford. 1978. *Field Guide to Medicinal Wild Plants.* Harrisburg, PA: Stackpole Bks. 320pp.

Anisimov, MM, et al. 1972. "The Antimicrobial Activity of the Triterpene Glycosides of *Caulophyllum thalictroides*" [ET]. *Antibiotiki.* 17(9):834–37.

Anonymous. 1977. *A Barefoot Doctor's Manual: The American Translation of the Official Chinese Paramedical Manual.* Philadelphia: Running Press, 942pp.

Anonymous. 1990a. "Debugging Precautions." *Prevention.* 42(6):22.

Anonymous. 1990b. "Vorinformation Pyrrolizidinalkaloid-haltige Humanarzneimittel." *Pharmaceutische Ztg.* 135(1990):2532–33, 2623–24.

Anton, R, et al. 1980. "Therapeutic Use of Natural Anthraquinone for Other than Laxative Actions." *Pharmacol.* 20(1 Suppl):104–12.

Apáti, P, et al. 2003. "Herbal Remedies of *Solidago*—Correlation of Phytochemical Characteristics and Antioxidative Properties." *J. Pharm. Biomed. Anal.* 32(4–5):1045–53.

Arustamova, FA. 1963. "Hypotensive Effect of *Leonurus cardiaca* on Animals in Experimental Chronic Hypertension" [ET]. *Izvestiya Akademii Nauk Armyanski SSR, Biologicheski Nauki.* 16(7):47–52.

Asgary, S, et al. 2000. "Antihypertensive and Antihyperlipidemic Effects of *Achillea wilhlelmsii*." *Drugs Exp. Clin. Res.* 26(3):89–93.

Ashkani-Esfahani, S, et al. 2019. "The Healing Effect of *Plantago Major* and *Aloe Vera* Mixture in Excisional Full Thickness Skin Wounds: Stereological Study." *World J. Plast. Surg.* 8(1):51–57.

Asolkar, LV, et al. 1992. *Second Supplement to Glossary of Indian Medicinal Plants with Active Principles: Part 1 (A–K) (1965–81).* New Delhi, IN: Publications & Information Directorate. 414pp.

Atlee, EA. 1819. "On the Medicinal Properties of *Monarda punctata*." *Am. Med. Rec.* 2:496–501.

Atmaca, H, et al. 2016. "Effects of *Galium aparine* Extract on the Cell Viability, Cell Cycle and Cell Death in Breast Cancer Cell Lines." *J. Ethnopharmacol.* 186:305–10.

Au, TK, et al. 2001. "A Comparison of HIV-1 Integrase Inhibition by Aqueous and Methanol Extracts of Chinese Medicinal Herbs." *Life Sci.* 68(14):1687–94.

Auf'Mkolk, M, et al. 1984. "Inhibition by Certain Plant Extracts of the Binding and Adenylate Cyclase Stimulatory Effect of Bovine Thyrotropin in Human Thyroid Membranes." *Endocrinol.* 115(2):527–34.

Auf'Mkolk, M, et al. 1985. "Extracts and Auto-oxidized Constituents of Certain Plants Inhibit the Receptor-Binding and the Biological Activity of Graves' Immunoglobulins." *Endocrinol.* 116:1687–93.

Austin, S, et al. 1994. "Long-term Follow-up of Cancer Patients Using Contreras, Hoxsey, and Gerson Therapies." *J. Naturopath. Med.* 5(1):74–76.

Awad, R, et al. 2003. "Phytochemical and Biological Analysis of Skullcap (*Scutellaria lateriflora* L.): A Medicinal Plant with Anxiolytic Properties." *Phytomed.* 10(8):640–49.

Awale, S, et al. 2006. "Identification of Arctigenin as an Antitumor Agent Having the Ability to Eliminate the Tolerance of Cancer Cells to Nutrient Starvation." *Cancer Res.* 66(3):1751–57.

Baba, K, et al. 1981. "Antitumor Activity of Hot Water Extract of Dandelion, *Taraxacum officinale*: Correlation between Antitumor Activity and Timing of Administration" [ET]. *Yakugaku Zasshi.* 101(6):538–43.

Bader, G, et al. 1987. "The Antifungal Action of Triterpene Saponins of *Solidago virgaurea* L." [ET]. *Pharmazie.* 42(2):140.

Baillie, N, and Rasmussen, P. 1997. "Black and Blue Cohosh in Labour." *N Z Med. J.* 110(1036):20–21.

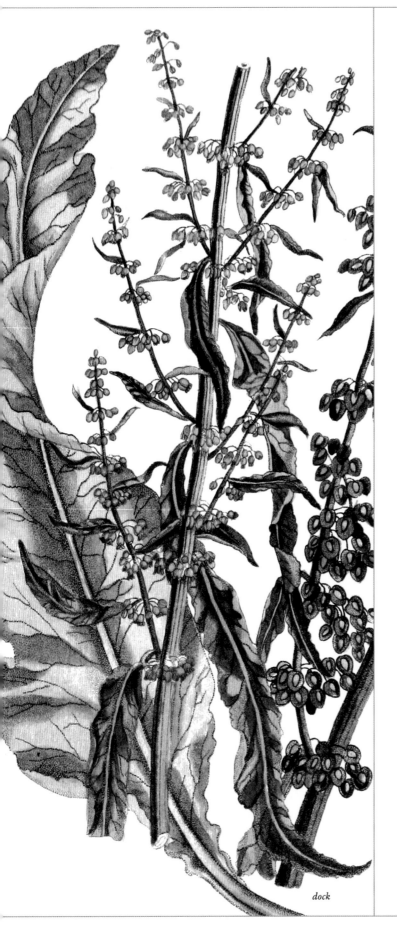

dock

Balbaa, SI, et al. 1973. "Preliminary Phytochemical and Pharmacological Investigation into the Roots of Different Varieties of *Cichorium intybus.*" *Planta Med.* 24(2):133–44.

Bank II, Theodore P. 1953. *Botanical and Ethnobotanical Studies in the Aleutian Islands II. Health and Medical Lore of the Aleuts.* Botanical and Ethnobotanical Studies Papers, Michigan Academy of Science, Arts and Letters.

Banks, WH. 1953. "Ethnobotany of the Cherokee Indians" [master's thesis]. University of Tennessee.

Baradaran, RV, et al. 2019. "Cytotoxicity and Apoptogenic Properties of the Standardized Extract of *Portulaca oleracea* on Glioblastoma Multiforme Cancer Cell Line (U-87): A Mechanistic Study." *EXCLI J.* 18:165–86.

Barrett, SA, and Gifford, EW. 1933. "Miwok Material Culture: Indian Life of the Yosemite Region." *Bull. Public Mus. City of Milwaukee.* 2(4):117–376.

Bartfay, WJ, et al. 2012. "Gram-negative and Gram-positive Antibacterial Properties of the Whole Plant Extract of Willow Herb (*Epilobium angustifolium*)." *Biol. Res. Nurs.* 14(1):85–89.

Barton, Benjamin Smith. 1810. *Collections for an Essay towards a Materia Medica of the United States.* 3rd ed., with additions. Philadelphia: Edward Earle & Co. 106pp.

Barton, Benjamin Smith. 1900. *Collections for an Essay towards a Materia Medica of the United States.* 2nd ed. Philadelphia: A. & G. Way, 1801–1804; reprint, Bulletin of the Lloyd Library, No. 1, Series No. 1, Cincinnati: Lloyd Library. 150pp.

Barton, William PC. 1817–18. *Vegetable Materia Medica of the United States, or Medical Botany.* Philadelphia: M. Carey & Son. 2 vols. 273 + 239pp.

Bartram, William. 1958. *The Travels of William Bartram.* Francis Harper, editor. Naturalist's edition. New Haven: Yale University Press. 727pp.

Bartsch, G, et al. 1998. "Combined *Sabal* and *Urtica* Extract vs. Finasteride in Benign Prostatic Hyperplasia (Alken Stages I to II): Comment on the Contribution by J. Skeland and J. Albrech" [ET]. *Urologe A.* 37(1):83–85.

Battinelli, L, et al. 2001. "Antimicrobial Activity of *Epilobium* spp. Extracts." *Farmaco.* 56(5–7):345–48.

Baumann, IC, et al. 1975. "Studies on the Effects of Wormwood (*Artemisia absinthium* L.) on Bile and Pancreatic Juice Secretion in Man" [ET]. *Z Allgemeinmed.* 51(17):784–91.

Beardsley, G. 1941. "Notes on Cree Medicines, Based on a Collection Made by I. Cowie in 1892." *Mich. Acad. Sci. Arts Let.* 27:483–96.

Becker, H. 2005. "Bioactivity Guided Isolation of Antimicrobial Compounds from *Lythrum salicaria.*" *Fitoterapia.* 76(6):580–84.

Beer, AM, et al. 2008. "*Lycopus europaeus* (Gypsywort): Effects on the Thyroidal Parameters and Symptoms Associated with Thyroid Function." *Phytomed.* 15(1–2):16–22.

Béládi, I, et al. 1977. "Activity of Some Flavonoids against Viruses." *Ann. N Y Acad. Sci.* 284(2):358–64.

Belaiche, P, and Leivoux, O. 1991. "Clinical Studies on the Palliative Treatment of Prostatic Adenoma with Extract of *Urtica* Root." *Phytother. Res.* 5:267–69.

Belanger, Charles. 1997. *The Chinese Herb Selection Guide.* Richmond, CA: Phytotech. 892pp.

Belscak-Cvitanovic, A, et al. 2014. "Phytochemical Attributes of Four Conventionally Extracted Medicinal Plants and Cytotoxic Evaluation of Their Extracts on Human Laryngeal Carcinoma (Hep2) Cells." *J. Med. Food.* 17(2):206–17.

Benedek, B, et al. 2006. "Choleretic Effects of Yarrow (*Achillea millefolium s.l.*) in the Isolated Perfused Rat Liver." *Phytomed.* 13(910):702–6.

Benigni, R, et al. 1964. *Plante medicinali Intervnie Della Betta.* 11:1593.

Benoit, PS, et al. 1976. "Biological and Phytochemical Evaluation of Plants. XIV. Antiinflammatory Evaluation of 163 Species of Plants." *Lloydia.* 39(2–3):160–71.

Bentley, WH. 1884. "Burdock Seed in Epilepsy." *Ther. Gaz.* 8:108–9.

[Bergner, P]. 1994–95. "Essential Oil Research: Mint Gel." *Med. Herbal.* 6(4):12.

[Bergner, P]. 1995–96. "Clinical Correspondence." *Med. Herbal.* 7(4):10–13.

[Bergner, P]. 2001. "Caulophyllum: Cardiotoxic Effects of Blue Cohosh on a Fetus." *Med. Herbal.* 12(1):12–14.

Bernatoniene, J, et al. 2014. "The Effect of *Leonurus cardiaca* Herb Extract and Some of Its Flavonoids on Mitochondrial Oxidative Phosphorylation in the Heart." *Planta Med.* 80(7):525–32.

Best, WP. 1928. "Eupatorium—Boneset." *Eclect. Med. J.* 88(2):93–94.

Bever, BO, and Zahnd, GR. 1979. "Plants with Oral Hypoglycaemic Action." *Q. J. Crude Drug Res.* 17:139–96.

Bhandari, P, et al. 1987. "Triterpenoid Saponins from *Caltha palustris.*" *Planta Med.* 53(1):98–100.

Bigelow, Jacob. 1817–20. *American Medical Botany, Being a Collection of the Native Medicinal Plants of the United States.* Boston: Cummings & Hilliard. 3 vols.

Bishayee, A, et al. 1995. "Hepatoprotective Activity of Carrot *(Daucus carota L.)* against Carbon Tetrachloride Intoxication in Mouse Liver." *J. Ethnopharmacol.* 47:69–74.

Bisset, NG, and Wichtl, Max. 1994. *Herbal Drugs and Phytopharmaceuticals.* Stuttgart: MedPharm GmbH Scientific Publishers. 566pp.

Black, Meredith Jean. 1973. *Algonquin Ethnobotany: An Interpretation of Aboriginal Adaptations in Southwestern Quebec.* Mercury Series, No. 65. Ottawa: National Museums of Canada. 174pp.

Black, Meredith Jean. 1980. *Algonquin Ethnobotany: An Interpretation of Aboriginal Adaptations in Southwestern Quebec.* Rev. ed., Mercury Series, No. 65. Ottawa: National Museums of Canada. 266pp.

Bloyer, WE. 1899. "Epilobium." *Eclect. Med. J.* 59:276.

Bloyer, WE. 1901. "Eupatorium." *Eclect. Med. J.* 61(6):336–37.

Blumenthal, Mark, ed. 1998. *The Complete German Commission E Monographs: Therapeutic Guide to Herbal Medicines.* Austin, TX: American Botanical Council/Boston, MA: Integrative Medicine Communication. 684pp.

Blumenthal, Mark, et al., eds. 2000. *Herbal Medicine: Expanded Commission E Monographs.* Newton, MA: Integrative Medicine Communications. 519pp.

Bocek, Barbara R. 1984. "Ethnobotany of the Costanoan Indians, California, Based on Collections by John P. Harrington." *Econ. Botany.* 38(2):240–55.

Bogoiavlenskii, AP, et al. 1999. "Immunostimulating Activity of a Saponin-containing Extract of *Saponaria officinalis*" [ET]. *Vopr. Virusol.* 44(5):229–32.

Bohm, K. 1959. "Choleretic Action of Some Medicinal Plants." *Arzneimittel-Forschung.* 9:376–78.

Bol'shakova, IV. 1997. "Antioxidant Properties of a Series of Extracts from Medicinal Plants." *Biofizika.* 42(2):480–83.

Bol'shavoka, IV. 1998. "Antioxidant Properties of Plant Extracts" [ET]. *Biofizika.* 43(2):186–88.

Bolyard, Judith L. 1981. *Medicinal Plants and Home Remedies of Appalachia.* Springfield, IL: Chas. C. Thomas. 187pp.

Bombardelli, E, and Morazzoni, P. 1997. "*Urtica dioica* L.: A Review." *Fitoterapia.* 68(5):387–401.

Bora, KS, and Sharma, A. 2010. "Neuroprotective Effect of *Artemisia absinthium* L. on Focal Ischemia and Reperfusion-induced Cerebral Injury." *J. Ethnopharmacol.* 129(3):403–9.

Borawska, MH, et al. 2010. "Enhancement of Antibacterial Effects of Extracts from *Cirsium* Species Using Sodium Picolinate and Estimation of Their Toxicity." *Nat. Prod. Res.* 24(6):554–61.

Bradley, Peter R, et al. 1992. *The British Herbal Compendium.* Kegley, UK: British Herbal Medicine Assn. Vol. 1. 239pp.

Bramwell, W. 1915. "*Scutellaria* in Epilepsy." *Br. Med. J.* 2:880.

Breneman, WR, et al. 1996. "*In vivo* Inhibition of Gonadotropins and Thyrotropin in the Chick by Extracts of *Lithospermum ruderale.*" *Gen. Comp. Endocrinol.* 28(1):24–32.

Brill, Steve, and Dean, Evelyn. 1994. *Identifying and Harvesting Edible and Medicinal Plants in Wild (and Not So Wild) Places.* New York: Hearst Books. 317pp.

Brinker, Francis. 1990. "Inhibition of Endocrine Function by Botanical Agents." *J. Naturopath. Med.* 1:1–14.

Brinker, Francis. 1995. "The Hoxsey Treatment: Cancer Quackery or Effective Physiological Adjuvant?" *J. Naturopath. Med.* 6:9–23.

Brinker, Francis. 2000. *The Toxicology of Botanical Medicines.* 3rd ed. Sandy, OR: Eclectic Medical Pubns. 296pp.

Brock, C, et al. 2014. "American Skullcap (*Scutellaria lateriflora*): A Randomised, Double-blind, Placebo-controlled Crossover Study of Its Effects on Mood in Healthy Volunteers." *Phytother. Res.* 28(5):692–98.

Brooke, Elisabeth. 1992. *Herbal Therapy for Women.* San Francisco: Thorsons. 160pp.

Brown, Tom Jr. 1985. *Tom Brown's Guide to Wild Edible and Medicinal Plants.* New York: Berkeley Bks. 241pp.

Bruneton, Jean. 1995. *Pharmacognosy, Phytochemistry, Medicinal Plants.* Caroline K. Hatton, translator. New York: Lavoissier Publ. Inc. 915pp.

Bruni, A, et al. 1986. "Protoanemonin Detection in *Caltha palustris.*" *J. Nat. Prod.* 49(6):1172–73.

Brush, MG, et al. 1982. "Evening Primrose Oil in the Treatment of Premenstrual Syndrome." In: Horrobin, David F, editor. *Clinical Uses of Essential Fatty Acids: Proceedings of the First Efamol Symposium Held in London, England in November, 1981.* Montreal: Eden Press. 214pp.

Budeiri, D, et al. 1996. "Is Evening Primrose Oil of Value in the Treatment of Premenstrual Syndrome?" *Control. Clin. Trials.* 17(1):60–68.

Buechel, Eugene. 1983. *A Dictionary of Teton Sioux Lakota-English: English-Lakota.* Pine Ridge, SD: Red Cloud Indian School. 853pp.

Burlage, Henry M. 1969. *Index of Plants of Texas with Reputed Medicinal and Poisonous Properties.* Austin: The author. 272pp.

Bussemaker, J. 1936. "On the Choleretic Activity of Dandelion" [ET]. *Naunyn-Shcmiederbergs Archivfuer Experiementelle Pharmakology und Pathologie.* 181:512–13.

Cáceres, A, et al. 1991. "Plants Used in Guatemala for the Treatment of Respiratory Diseases: Screening of 68 Plants against Gram-Positive Bacteria." *J. Ethnopharmacol.* 31(2):193–208.

Cáceres, A, et al. 1995. "Antigonorrhoeal Activity of Plants Used in Guatemala for the Treatment of Sexually Transmitted Diseases." *J. Ethnopharmacol.* 48(2):85–88.

Cai, DG. 1983. "Expectorant Constituents of *Eupatorium fortunei*" [ET]. *Zhong Yao Tung Pao.* 8(6):30–31.

Callegari, Jeff, and Durand, Keith. 1977. *Wild Edible and Medicinal Plants of California.* El Cerrito, CA: The authors. 96pp.

Calzada, F, et al. 2003. "Antiamoebic Activity of Benzyl Glucosinolate from *Lepidium Virginicum.*" *Phytother. Res.* 17(6):618–19.

Calzada, F, et al. 2010. "Effect of Plants Used in Mexico to Treat Gastrointestinal Disorders on Charcoal-Gum Acacia-Induced Hyperperistalsis in Rats." *J Ethnopharmacol.* 128(1):49–51.

Camazine, S, and Bye, RA. 1980. "A Study of the Medical Ethnobotany of the Zuñi Indians of New Mexico." *J. Ethnopharmacol.* 2:365–88.

Campbell, AC, and MacEwan, GC. 1982. *Systematic Treatment of Sjogren's Syndrome and Sicca Syndrome with Efamol (EPO), Vitamin C, and Pyridoxine.* Montreal: Eden Press.

Campbell, TN, and Roberts, FH Jr. 1951. "Medicinal Plants Used by Choctaw, Chickasaw, and Creek Indians in the Early Nineteenth Century." *J. Wash. Acad. Sci.* 41(9):285–90.

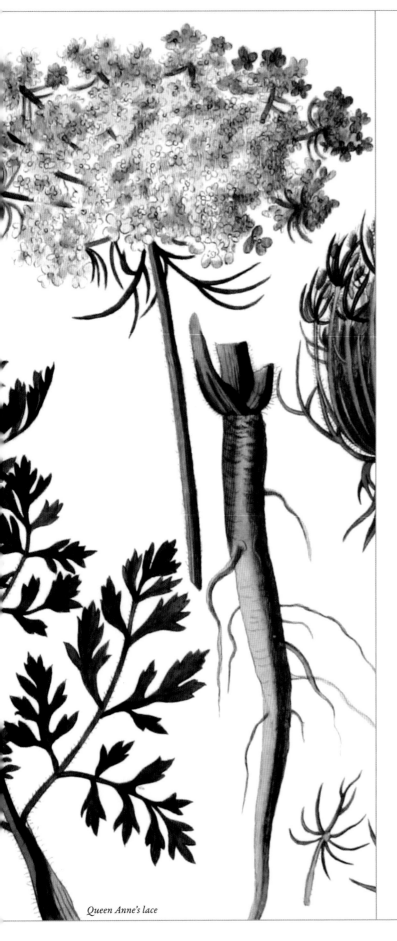

Queen Anne's lace

Canavan, D, and Yarnell, E. 2005. "Successful Treatment of Poison Oak Dermatitis Treated with *Grindelia* spp. (Gumweed)." *J. Altern. Complement. Med.* 11(4):709–10.

Cardoso Vilela, F, et al. 2009. "Anxiolytic-like Effect of *Sonchus oleraceus* L. in Mice." *J. Ethnopharmacol.* 124(2):325–27.

Carr, LG, and Westey, C. 1945. "Surviving Folktales and Herbal Lore among the Shinnecock Indians." *J. Am. Folklore.* 58:113–23.

Carse, Mary. 1989. *Herbs of the Earth: A Self-Teaching Guide to Healing Remedies, Using Common North American Plants and Trees.* Hinesburg, VT: Upper Access Pubns. 238pps.

Carvalho, LH, and Krettli, AU. 1991. "Antimalarial Chemotherapy with Natural Products and Chemically Defined Molecules." *Mem. Inst. Oswaldo Cruz.* 86(2 Suppl):181–84.

Carvalho, LH, et al. 1991. "Antimalarial Activity of Crude Extracts from Brazilian Plants Studied *in vivo* in *Plasmodium-berghei*-infected Mice and *in vitro* against *Plasmodium falciparum* in Culture." *Braz. J. Med. Biol. Res.* 24(11):1113–23.

Cassady, JM, et al. 1969. "Terpene Constituents from *Eupatorium* Species." *Lloydia.* 32:522.

Cassady, JM, et al. 1988. "Use of a Mammalian Cell Culture Benzo(a)pyrene Metabolism Assay for the Detection of Potential Anticarcinogens from Natural Products: Inhibition of Metabolism by Biochanin A, an Isoflavone from *Trifolium pratense* L." *Cancer Res.* 48(22):6257–61.

Castillo, SL, et al. 2011. "Extracts of Edible and Medicinal Plants in Inhibition of Growth, Adherence, and Cytotoxin Production of Campaylobacter jejuni and Campylobacter coli." *J. Food Sci.* 76(6):M421–26.

Castillo-Juárez, I, et al. 2009. "Anti-*Helicobacter pylori* Activity of Plants Used in Mexican Traditional Medicine for Gastrointestinal Disorders." *J. Ethnopharmacol.* 122(2):402–5.

Castleman, Michael. 1991. *The Healing Herbs: The Ultimate Guide to the Curative Power of Nature's Medicines.* Emmaus, NJ: Rodale Press. 436pp.

Catanicin-Hintz, I, et al. 1983. "Action of Some Plant Extracts on the Bacteria Involved in Urinary Infections." *Clujul-Med.* 56:381–84.

Cavalcanti, AM, et al. 2006. "Safety and Antiulcer Efficacy Studies of *Achillea millefolium* L. After Chronic Treatment in Wistar Rats." *J. Ethnopharmacol.* 107(2):277–84.

Celsus. 1938. *De Medicina, with an English Translation by W. G. Spencer.* Reprint ed., Birmingham: Classics of Medicine Library, 1989. 499pp + 649pp.

Chabrol, E, and Charonnat, R. 1935. "Therapeutic Agents in Bile Secretion" [ET]. *Annales de Medecine.* 37:131–42.

Chabrol, E, et al. 1931. "L'action Choleretique des Composees." *C. R. Soc. Biol.* (Paris). 108(12):1100–1102.

Chai, Mary Ann P. 1978. *Herb Walk Medicinal Guide.* Provo, UT: Gluten Co. 127pp.

Chakurski, I [Chakarski, I], et al. 1981. "Treatment of Chronic Colitis with an Herbal Combination of *Taraxacum officinale, Hypericum perforatum, Melissa officinalis, Calendula officinalis,* and *Foeniculum vulgare.*" *Vutr. Boles.* 20(6):51–54.

Chakurski, I [Chakarski, I], et al. 1982. "Clinical Study of a Herb Combination Consisting of *Agrimonia eupatoria, Hypericum perforatum, Plantago major, Mentha piperita, Matricaria chamomilla* for the Treatment of Patients with Gastroduodenitis." *Probl. Vutr. Med.* 10:78–84.

Chamberlain, AF. 1888. "Notes on the History, Customs, and Beliefs of the Mississaugas." *J. Am. Folklore.* 1:150–60.

Chamberlin, RV. 1909. "Some Plant Names of the Ute Indians." *Am. Anthropol.* 11:27–40.

Chamberlin, RV. 1911. "The Ethno-Botany of the Gosiute Indians of Utah." *Memoirs Am. Anthropol. Assoc.* 2(5):329–405.

Chan K, et al. 2000. "The Analgesic and Anti-inflammatory Effects of *Portulaca oleracea* L. subsp. Sativa (Haw.) Celak." *J. Ethnopharmacol.* 73(3):445–51.

Chandler, RF, et al. 1979. "Herbal Remedies of the Maritime Indians." *J. Ethnopharmacol.* 1:49–68.

Chandler, RF, et al. 1982. "Ethnobotany and Phytochemistry of Yarrow, *Achillea millefolium*, Compositae." *Econ. Botany.* 36:203–23.

Chang, CF, and Li, CZ. 1986. "Experimental Studies on the Mechanism of Anti-platelet Aggregation Action of Motherwort" [ET]. *Zhong Xi Yi Jie He Za Zhi.* 6(1):39–40, 5.

Chang, IM, and Choi, HSY. 1985. "Plants with Liver-protective Activities: Pharmacology and Toxicology of Aucubin." In: Chang, Hson-Mou, et al., editors. *Advances in Chinese Medicinal Materials Research.* Singapore: World Scientific. p. 269–85.

Chatterjee, SJ, et al. 2011. "The Efficacy of Dandelion Root Extract in Inducing Apoptosis in Drug-resistant Human Melanoma Cells." *Evid.-Based Complement. Altern. Med.* 2011:129045. Epub 2010 Dec 30.

(ChemAbstr). 1963. *Chem. Abstr.* 59:5535c.

Chen, J, et al. 2003. "Determination of Noradrenaline and Dopamine in Chinese Herbal Extracts from *Portulaca oleracea L.* by High-performance Liquid Chromatography." *J. Chromatog. A.* 1003(1–2):127–32.

Chen, L, et al. 2019. "*Sonchus oleraceus* Linn Extract Enhanced Glucose Homeostasis through the AMPK/Akt/ GSK-3beta Signaling Pathway in Diabetic Liver and HepG2 Cell Culture." *Food Chem. Toxicol.* 136:111072. Epub 2019 Dec 23.

Chenoy, R, et al. 1994. "Effect of Oral Gamolenic Acid from Evening Primrose Oil on Menopausal Flushing." *Br. Med. J.* 308(6927):501–3.

Chestnut, VK. 1902. "Plants Used by the Indians of Mendocino County, California." *Contributions from the U.S. Natl. Herb.* 7:295–408.

Chevallier, Andrew. 1996. *The Encyclopedia of Medicinal Plants.* London: Dorling Kindersley. 336pp.

Chiang, LC, et al. 2002. "Antiviral Activity of *Plantago major* Extracts and Related Compounds *in vitro.*" *Antivir. Res.* 55(1):53–62.

Chiang, LC, et al. 2003. "In vitro Cytotoxic, Antiviral and Immunomodulatory Effects of *Plantago major* and *Plantago asiatica.*" *Am. J. Chin. Med.* 31(2):225–34.

Chidrawar, VR. 2011. "Antiobesity Effect of *Stellaria media* against Drug-induced Obesity in Swiss Albino Mice." *Ayu.* 32(4):576–84.

Chistokhodova, N, et al. 2002. "Antithrombin Activity of Medicinal Plants from Central Florida." *J. Ethnopharmacol.* 81(2):277–80.

Chiu, LC, et al. 2004. "A Polysaccharide Fraction from Medicinal Herb *Prunella vulgaris* Downregulates the Expression of *Herpes simplex* Virus Antigen in Vero Cells." *J. Ethnopharmacol.* 93(1):63–68.

Chodera, A, et al. 1985. "Diuretic Effect of the Glycoside from a Plant of the *Solidago* L. Genus." *Acta Pol. Pharm.* 42(2):199–204.

Chodera, A, et al. 1991. "Effect of Flavonoid Fractions of *Solidago virgaurea* L. on Diuresis and Levels of Electrolytes." *Acta Pol. Pharm.* 48(5–6):35–37.

Choi, ES. 2012. "*Althaea rosea* Cavanil and *Plantago major* L. Suppress Neoplastic Cell Transformation through the Inhibition of Epidermal Growth Factor Receptor Kinase." *Mol. Med. Rep.* 6(4):843–47.

Choi, SB, and Park, S. 2002. "A Steroidal Glycoside from *Polygonatum odoratum* (Mill.) Druce. Improves Insulin Resistance but Does Not Alter Insulin Secretion in 90% Pancreatectomized Rats." *Biosci. Biotechnol. Biochem.* 66(10):2036–43.

Chopra, RN, et al. 1956. *Glossary of Indian Medicinal Plants.* New Delhi, IN: Council of Scientific & Industrial Research. 330pp.

Chou, ST, et al. 2019. "Phytochemical Profile of Hot Water Extract of *Glechoma hederacea* and Its Antioxidant and Anti-inflammatory Activities." *Life Sci.* Aug 15; 231:116519. Epub 2019 May 30.

Christianson, EH. 1987. "The Search for Diagnostic and Therapeutic Authority in the Early American Healer's Encounter with 'The Animals which Inhabit the Human Stomach and Intestines.'" In: Scarborough, John, editor. *Folklore and Folk Medicines.* Madison, WI: American Institute of History of Pharmacy. p. 69–85.

Christopher, John R. 1976. *School of Natural Healing.* Springville, UT: Christopher Pubs. 653pp.

Chrubasik, S, et al. 1997. "Evidence for Antirheumatic Effectiveness of Herba *Urtica dioica* in Acute Arthritis: A Pilot Study." *Phytomed.* 4(2):105–8.

Cicero, AF, et al. 2001. "*Lepidium meyenii* Walp. Improves Sexual Behaviour in Male Rats Independently from its Action on Spontaneous Locomotor Activity." *J. Ethnopharmacol.* 75(2–3):225–29.

Clapp, A. 1852. "A Synopsis, Or Systematic Catalogue of the Indigenous and Naturalized, Flowering, and Filicoid, ... Medicinal Plants of the United States, Being a Report of the Committee on Indigenous Medical Botany and Materia Medica for 1850–51." *Trans. Am. Med. Assoc.* 5:689–906.

Clarke, CB. 1977. *Edible and Useful Plants of California.* Berkeley: University of California Press, 1977. 280pp.

Claus, Edward P. 1961. *Pharmacognosy.* 4th ed. Philadelphia: Lea & Febiger. 565pp.

Clementson, CAB, and Andersen, L. 1966. "Plant Polyphenols as Antioxidants for Ascorbic Acid." *Ann. NY Acad. Sci.* 136:339–78.

Clymer, R. Swinburne. 1973. *Nature's Healing Agents.* Quakertown, PA: Humanitarian Soc. 230pp.

Coffey, Timothy. 1993. *The History and Folklore of North American Wildflowers.* New York: Facts on File. 356pp.

Colegate, SM, et al. 2018. "Potentially Toxic Pyrrolizidine Alkaloids in *Eupatorium perfoliatum* and Three Related Species. Implications for Herbal Use as Boneset." *Phytochem. Anal.* 29(6):613–26. Epub 2018 Jul 2.

Collier, HOJ, and Chesher, GB. 1956. "Identification of 5-Hydroxytryptamine in the Sting of the Nettle (*Urtica dioica*)." *Br. J. Pharmacol. Chemother.* 11(2):186–89.

Colton, HS. 1974. "Hopi History and Ethnobotany." In: Horr, David A, editor. *The Hopi Indians.* New York: Garland. p. 279–386.

Conaway, CC, et al. 2002. "Isothiocyanates as Cancer Chemopreventive Agents: Their Biological Activities and Metabolism in Rodents and Humans." *Curr. Drug Metab.* 3(3):233–55.

Cook, WH. 1985. *The Physio-Medical Dispensatory.* 1869; reprint, Portland, OR: Eclectic Medical Pubns. 832pp. Web version at: www.henriettesherbal.com/eclectic/cook/index.htm.

Coon, JT, et al. 2007. "*Trifolium pratense* Isoflavones in the Treatment of Menopausal Hot Flushes: A Systematic Review and Meta-analysis." *Phytomed.* 14(2–3):153–59.

Cooper, Marion R, and Johnson, Anthony W. 1988. *Poisonous Plants & Fungi: An Illustrated Guide.* London: Her Majesty's Stationery Office. 134pp.

Corbett, R, et al. 1992. "The Effects of Chronic Administration of Ethanol on Synaptosomal Fatty-acid Composition: Modulation by Oil Enriched with Gamma-Linolenic Acid." *Alcohol.* 27(1):11–14.

Couplan, François. 1998. *Encyclopedia of the Edible Plants of North America.* New Canaan, CT: Keats Publ. Co. 584pp.

Court, WE. 1986. "A History of Mustard in Pharmacy and Medicine." *Pharm. Hist.* 6(2):4–11.

Coutinho, HD, et al. 2008. "Enhancement of the Antibiotic Activity against a Multiresistant *Escherichia coli* by *Mentha arvensis* L. and Chlorpromazine." *Chemother.* 54(4):328–30.

Crellin, John K, and Philpott, Jane. 1990a. *Herbal Medicine Past and Present.* Vol. 2: *A Reference Guide to Medicinal Plants.* Durham, NC: Duke University Press. 549pp.

Crellin, John K, and Philpott, Jane. 1990b. *Trying to Give Ease: Tommie Bass and the Story of Herbal Medicine.* Durham, NC: Duke University Press. 335pp.

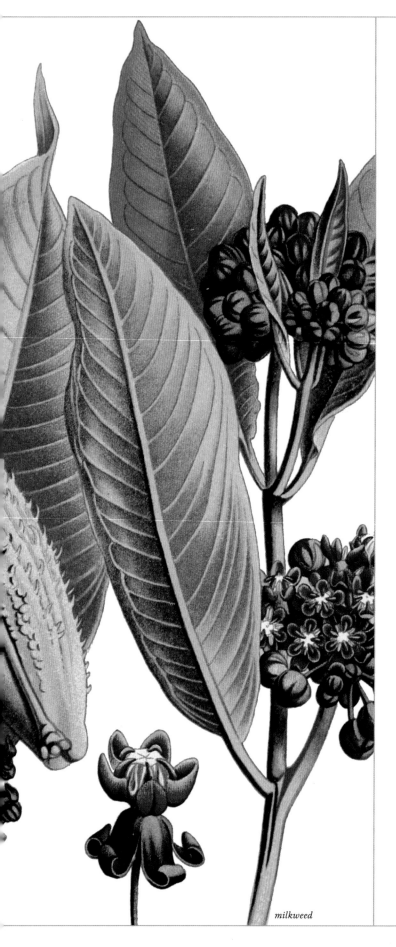

milkweed

Croom, Edward Mortimer. 1983. "Medicinal Plants of the Lumbee Indians" [dissertation]. North Carolina State University, 1982; reprint, Ann Arbor, MI: University Microfilms. 183pp.

Crowhurst, Adrienne. 1972. *The Weed Cookbook*. New York: Lancer Bks. 190pp.

Cui, X, et al. 2018. "A Review: The Bioactivities and Pharmacological Applications of *Polygonatum sibiricum* Polysaccharides." *Molecules*. 23(5):pii: E1170.

Culbreth, David MR. 1927. *A Manual of Materia Medica and Pharmacology*. 7th ed. Philadelphia: Lea & Febiger. 627pp. Web version at: http://swsbm.com/ManualsOther/Culbreth.html.

Culpeper, Nicholas. 1983. *Culpeper's Color Herbal*. London, 1649; reprint, New York: Sterling Publ. Co. 224pp.

Curtis, John T. 1959. *The Vegetation of Wisconsin: An Ordination of Plant Communities*. Madison: University of Wisconsin Press. 657pp.

Cutler, Manasseh. 1903. *An Account of Some of the Vegetable Productions Naturally Growing in this Part of America, Botanically Arranged*. Boston: The author, 1785; reprint, Bulletin of the Lloyd Library, No. 7, Reproduction Series No. 4, Cincinnati, OH: Lloyd Library.

D'Adamo, PJ. 1992. "*Chelidonium* and *Sanguinaria* Alkaloids as Anti-HIV Therapy." *J. Naturopath. Med.* 3(1):31–34.

Dall'Acqua, S, et al. 2011. "Vasoprotective Activity of Standardized *Achillea millefolium* Extract." *Phytomed.* 18(12):1031–16.

D'Amico, L. 1950. "Ricerche Sulla Presenza di Sostanze Ad Azione Antibiotica Nelle Piante Superiori." *Fitoterapia*. 21(1):77–79.

Das, PK, et al. 1976. "Pharmacology of Kutkin and Its Two Organic Constituents, Cinnamic Acid and Vanillic Acid." *Indian J. Exp. Biol.* 14:3456–58.

Daucus, S. 1997. "'A Simple' Cure for Brown Recluse Bites." *Med. Herbal.* 9(4):20.

Davaatseren, M. 2013. "*Taraxacum official* (Dandelion) Leaf Extract Alleviates High-fat Diet-induced Nonalcoholic Fatty Liver." *Food Chem. Toxicol.* 58:30–36.

de Bairacli Levy, Juliette. 1974. *Common Herbs for Natural Health*. New York: Schocken Books. 200pp.

Deepak, M, and Handa, SS. 2000. "Antiinflammatory Activity and Chemical Composition of Extracts of *Verbena officinalis*." *Phytother. Res.* 14(6):463–65.

Deglmann, HE. 1955. "The Effect of *Lycopus europeus* Extracts on the Distribution of Iodine in Human Serum" [ET]. *Arzneim Forsch* 5(8):465–70.

Delas, R, et al. 1947. *Toulouse Medicale* 49:57, cited in Knott and McCutchcon, 1961.

de Laszlo, H, and Henshaw, PS. 1954. "Plant Materials Used by Primitive Peoples to Affect Fertility." *Sci.* 119(3097, May 7):626–31.

Deng, L, et al. 2019. "Evaluation of the Therapeutic Effect against Benign Prostatic Hyperplasia and the Active Constituents from *Epilobium angustifolium* L." *J. Ethnopharmacol.* 232:1–10.

Densmore, Frances. 1918. *Teton Sioux Music*. Washington, DC: Smithsonian Institution, Bureau of American Ethnology Bulletin #61. 561pp.

Densmore, Frances. 1932. *Menominee Music*. Washington, DC: Smithsonian Institution, Bureau of American Ethnology Bulletin #102. 230pp.

Densmore, Frances. 1974. *How Indians Use Wild Plants for Food, Medicine, & Crafts* [*Uses of Plants by the Chippewa Indians*. Forty-fourth Annual Report of the Bureau of American Ethnology, 1926–27]. Washington, DC: Government Printing Office, 1928; reprint, New York: Dover Publications; p. 277–397.

Derksen, A, et al. 2016. "Antiviral Activity of Hydroalcoholic Extract from *Eupatorium perfoliatum* L. against the Attachment of Influenza A Virus." *J. Ethnopharmacol.* 188:144–52.

Didry, N, et al. 1993. "Antibacterial Activity of Thymol, Carvacrol, and Cinnamaldehyde Alone or in Combination" [ET]. *Pharmazie.* 48(4):301–4.

Diehl, JF. 1990. *Safety of Irradiated Foods.* New York and Basel: Marcel Dekker Co. 464pp.

Dioscorides. 1996. *The Greek Herbal of Dioscorides, Illustrated by a Byzantine A.D. 512, Englished by John Goodyear A.D. 1655, Edited and First Printed A.D. 1933.* Robert Gunther, editor. Oxford: John Johnson, 1959; reprint, New York: Classics of Medicine Library. 701pp.

Doan, DD, et al. 1992. "Studies on the Individual and Combined Diuretic Effects of Four Vietnamese Traditional Herbal Remedies (*Zea mays, Imperata cylindrica, Plantago major and Orthosiphon Stamineus*)." *J. Ethnopharmacol.* 36(3):225–31.

Dobelis, Inge N. et al., eds. 1986. *Magic and Medicine of Plants.* Pleasantville, NY: Reader's Digest Association. 464pp.

Dombradi, CA. 1970. "Tumour-Growth Inhibiting Substances of Plant Origin. II. The Experimental Animal Tumour-Pharmacology of Arctigenin-Mustard." *Chemother.* 15:250.

Dombradi, CA and Foldeak, S. 1966. "Screening Report on the Antitumor Activity of Purified *Arctium Lappa* Extracts." *Tumori.* 52(3):173–75.

Donson, Alexandra. 1982. *Healing Herbs for Arthritis and Rheumatism.* New York: Sterling Publishing Co. 143pp.

Dording, CM, et al. 2008. "A Double-blind, Randomized, Pilot Dose-finding Study of Maca Root (L. *meyenii*) for the Management of SSRI-induced Sexual Dysfunction." *CNS Neurosci. Ther.* 14(3):182–91.

Duarte, MC, et al. 2005. "Anti-Candida Activity of Brazilian Medicinal Plants." *J. Ethnopharmacol.* 97(2):305–11.

Duckett, S. 1980. "Plantain Leaf for Poison Ivy." *New Engl. J. Med.* 303(10):583.

Ducrey, B, et al. 1997. "Inhibition of 5a-Reductase and Aromatase by the Ellagitannins Oenothein A and Oenothein B from *Epilobium* Species." *Planta Med.* 63(2):111–14.

Duffy, O, et al. 1992. "Attenuation of the Effects of Chronic Ethanol Administration in the Brain Lipid Content of the Developing Rat by an Oil Enriched in Gamma-Linolenic Acid." *Drug Alcohol Depen.* 31(1):85.

Duke, JA. 1994. "Balm *Monarda punctata*, for the Balmy." *Coltsfoot.* 15(3):12–14.

Duke, James. 1992. *Handbook of Edible Weeds.* Boca Raton, FL: CRC Press. 246pp.

Duke, James. 1997. *The Green Pharmacy.* Emmaus, PA: Rodale Press. 507pp.

Duke, James A. 1985. *CRC Handbook of Medicinal Herbs.* Boca Raton, FL: CRC Press. 704pp.

Duke, James A, and Atchley, Alan A. 1986. *CRC Handbook of Proximate Analysis Tables of Higher Plants.* Boca Raton, FL: CRC Press. 389pp.

Durak, I, et al. 2004. "Aqueous Extract of *Urtica dioica* Makes Significant Inhibition on Adenosine Deaminase Activity in Prostate Tissue from Patients with Prostate Cancer." *Cancer Biol. Ther.* 3(9):855–57.

Dzink, JL, and Socransky, SS. 1985. "Comparative *in vitro* Activity of Sanguinarine against Oral Microbial Isolates." *Antimicrob. Agents Chemother.* 27(4):663–65.

Edmunds, J. 1999. "Blue Cohosh and Newborn Myocardial Infarction?" *Midwifery Today/Int. Midwife.* (Winter)52:34–35.

Eiling, R, et al. 2013. "Improvement of Symptoms in Mild Hyperthyroidism with an Extract of *Lycopus europaeus* (Thyreogutt® Mono)" [ET]. *Wien. Med. Wochenscrh.* 163(3–4):95–101.

Eisner, T. 1965. "Catnip: Its *raison d'etre.*" *Sci.* 146(3649):1318–20.

el-Ghazaly, M, et al. 1992. "Study of the Antiinflammatory Activity of *Populus tremula, Solidago virgaurea,* and *Fraxinus excelsior.*" *Arzneimittelforschung.* 42(3):333–36.

Ellingwood, Finley. 1983. *American Materia Medica, Therapeutics, and Pharmacognosy.* Evanston, IL: Ellingwood's Therapeutist, 1915; reprint, Portland, OR: Eclectic Medical Publications. 564pp.

Elliott, Stephen. 1821–24. *A Sketch of the Botany of South-Carolina and Georgia.* Charleston, SC: Schenk, Hoh. 2 vols. 635pp.

el-Mekkawy, S, et al. 1995. "Inhibitory Effects of Egyptian Folk Medicines on Human Immunodeficiency Virus (HIV) Reverse Transcriptase." *Chem. Pharm. Bull.* (Tokyo). 43:641–48, abstract.

Elmore, Francis H. 1944. *Ethnobotany of the Navajo.* University of New Mexico: Monographs of the School of American Research 8. Albuquerque: University of New Mexico. 136pp.

el-Sayed, MI. 2011. "Effects of *Portulaca oleracea* L. Seeds in Treatment of Type-2 Diabetes Mellitus Patients as Adjunctive and Alternative Therapy." *J. Ethnopharmacol.* 137(1):643–51.

Emmelin, N, and Feldberg, W. 1947. "The Mechanism of the Sting of the Common Nettle (*Urtica urens*)." *J. Physiol.* 106(4):440–55.

Engelmann, U, et al. 2006. "Efficacy and Safety of a Combination of Sabal and Urtica Extract in Lower-urinary-tract Symptoms: A Randomized, Double-blind Study versus Tamsulosin." *Arzneimittelforschung.* 56(3):222–29.

Entezari Heravi, N, et al. 2018. "Doxorubicin-induced Renal Inflammation in Rats: Protective Role of *Plantago major.*" *Avicenna J. Phytomed.* 8(2):179–87.

Erichsen-Brown, Charlotte. 1989. *Medicinal and Other Uses of North American Plants: A Historical Survey with Special Reference to the Eastern Indian Tribes.* Aurora, ON: Breezy Creeks Press, 1979; reprint, New York: Dover Publications. 512pp.

Erickson, DW, and Lindzey, JS. 1983. "Lead and Cadmium in Muskrat and Cattail Tissues." *J. Wildl. Manag.* 47(2):550–55.

(EthnobDB). Ethnobotanical Database. Web resource at: https://phytochem.nal.usda.gov.

Faber, K. 1958. "The Dandelion: *Taraxacum officinale*" [ET]. *Pharmazie.* 13:423–26.

Faddeeva, MD, and Beliaeva, TN. 1997. "Sanguinarine and Ellipticine, Cytotoxic Alkaloids Isolated from Well-known Antitumor Plants: Intracellular Targets of their Action" [ET]. *Tsitologiia.* 39(2–3):181–208.

Fakhrieh-Kashan, Z, et al. 2018. "Induction of Apoptosis by Alcoholic Extract of Combination *Verbascum thapsus* and *Ginger officinale* on Iranian Isolate of *Trichomonas vaginalis.*" *Iran J. Parasitol.* 13(1):72–78.

Falk, AJ, et al. 1975. "Isolation and Identification of Three New Flavones from *Achillea millefolium* L." *J. Pharm. Sci.* 64(11):1838–42.

Fang, X, et al. 2005a. "Immune Modulatory Effects of *Prunella vulgaris* L." *Int. J. Mol. Med.* 15(3):491–96.

Fang, X, et al. 2005b. "Immune Modulatory Effects of *Prunella vulgaris* L. on Monocytes/Macrophages." *Int. J. Mol. Med.* 16(6):1109–16.

Farnsworth, NR. 1966. "Biological and Phytochemical Screening of Plants." *J. Pharm. Sci.* 55(3):225–76.

Farnsworth, NR. 1968. "Biological and Phytochemical Screening of Plants." *Lloydia.* 31:225–76.

Farnsworth, NR. 1985. "Medicinal Plants in Therapy." *Bull. World Health Organ.* 63(6):968–81.

Farnsworth, NR, and Segelman, AB. 1971. "Hypoglycemic Plants." *Tile and Till.* 57:52–56.

Farnsworth, NR, et al. 1975. "Potential Value of Plants as Sources of New Antifertility Agents." *J. Pharm. Sci.* 64:535–98, 717–54.

Farré, M. 1989. "Fatal Oxalic Acid Poisoning from Sorrel Soup." *Lancet.* Dec 23–30, 2(8668–70):1524.

Fearn, J. 1923. "Fearn's Eclectic Therapeutics: Epilobium." *Eclect. Med. J.* 83(12):582–83.

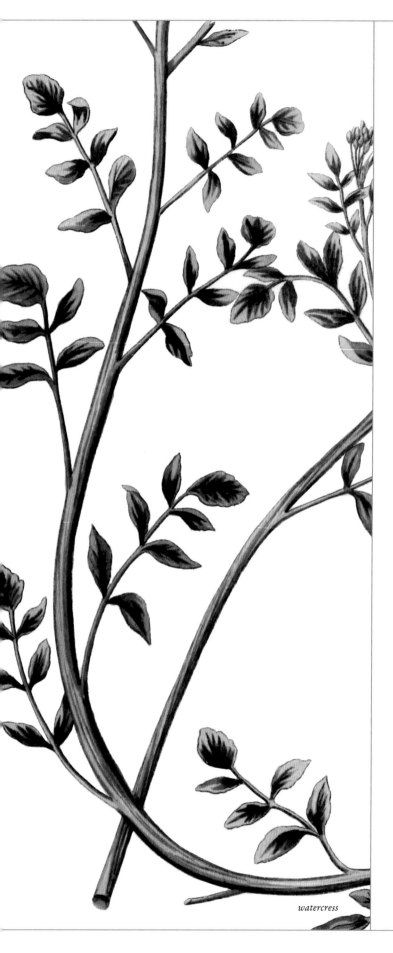

watercress

Feaster, JE, et al. 2009. "Dihydronepetalactones Deter Feeding Activity by Mosquitoes, Stable Flies, and Deer Ticks." *J. Med. Entomol.* 46(4):832–40.

Fell, J. Weldon. 1857. *A Treatise on Cancer, and Its Treatment.* London: J. Churchill. 95pp.

Felter, Harvey Wickes. 1922. *The Eclectic Materia Medica, Pharmacology, and Therapeutics.* Cincinnati, OH: J. K. Scudder. 743pp.

Felter, Harvey Wickes. 1983. *The Eclectic Materia Medica, Pharmacology, and Therapeutics.* Cincinnati: John K. Scudder, 1922; reprint, Portland, OR: Eclectic Medical Publications. 743pp. Web version at: https://www.henriettes-herb.com/eclectic/felter/index.html.

Felter, Harvey Wickes, and Lloyd, John Uri. 1898. *King's American Dispensatory, Entirely Rewritten.* 18th ed., 3rd revision. Cincinnati: Ohio Valley Co. 2 vols. Web version at: https://www.henriettes-herb.com/eclectic/kings/index.html.

Felter, HW. 1924. "Eupatorium (Boneset)." *Eclect. Med. J.* 84(4):200–202.

Feng, L, et al. 2011. "Oleanolic Acid from *Prunella vulgaris* Induces SPC-A-1 Cell Line Apoptosis via Regulation of Bax, Bad, and Bcl-2 Expression." *Asian Pac. J. Cancer Prev.* 12(2):403–8.

Feng, PC, et al. 1961. "High Concentration of (-)-noradrenaline in *Portulaca oleracea* L." *Nat.* 191:1108.

Fernald, Merritt Lyndon, and Kinsey, Alfred Charles. 1958. *Edible Wild Plants of Eastern North America.* Revised by Reed Rollins. New York: Harper and Row. 452pp.

Fetrow, Charles W, and Avila, Juan R. 1999. *Professional's Handbook of Complementary & Alternative Medicines.* Springhouse, PA: Springhouse Publications. 762pp.

Field, EJ. 1978. "Gamma-linolenate in Multiple Sclerosis." *Lancet.* 1:780.

Fischer-Rizzi, Susanne. 1996. *Medicine of the Earth: Legends, Recipes, Remedies, and Cultivation of Healing Plants.* Portland, OR: Rudra Press. 320pp.

Fisher, CN. 1997. "Nettles—An Aid to the Treatment of Allergic Rhinitis." *Eur. J. Herb. Med.* 3(2):34–35.

Fitzpatrick, FK. 1954. "Plant Substances Active against *Mycobacterium tuberculosis.*" *Antibiot. and Chemother.* 4(5):528–36.

Fleming, Thomas, ed. 1998. *PDR for Herbal Medicines.* Montvale, NJ: Medical Economics Co. 1244pp.

Fokina, GI, et al. 1991. "Experimental Phytotherapy of Tick-borne Encephalitis." *Vopr. Virusol.* 36(1):18–21.

Foldeak, S, and Dombradi, GA. 1964. "Tumor-growth Inhibiting Substances of Plant Origin. 1. Isolation of Active Principle of *Arctium lappa.*" *Acta Physiol. Chem. (Szeged).* 10:91–93.

Folsom-Dickerson, W. E. S. 1965. *The White Path: Alabama-Koasati Indians of Texas.* San Antonio, TX: Naylor Co. 148pp.

Foster, Steven. 1993. *Herbal Renaissance: Growing, Using, and Understanding Herbs in the Modern World.* Salt Lake City, UT: Gibbs Smith Publisher. 234pp.

Foster, Steven, and Duke, James A. 1990. *A Field Guide to Medicinal Plants: Eastern and Central North America.* Boston: Houghton Mifflin Co. 366pp.

Frances, D. 2009. "Bloodroot (*Sanguinaria canadensis*)." *Medicines from the Earth: Official Proceedings May 29–June 1, 2009.* p. 58–59.

Freire, RS, et al. 2005. "Synthesis and Antioxidant, Antiinflammatory, and Gastroprotector Activities of Anethole and Related Compounds." *Bioorg. Med. Chem.* 13(13):4353–58.

Fruet, AC, et al. 2012. "Dietary Intervention with Narrow-Leaved Cattail Rhizome Flour Prevents Intestinal Inflammation in the Trinitrobenzenesulphonic Acid Model of Rat Colitis." *BMC Complement. Altern. Med.* 12:62. Published online May 4.

Fukuchi, K, et al. 1989. "Inhibition of *Herpes simplex* Virus Infection by Tannins and Related Compounds." *Antivir. Res.* 11(56):285–98.

Fuller, Thomas C, and McClintock, Elizabeth. 1986. *Poisonous Plants of California*. Berkeley: University of California Press. 433pp.

Fyfe, John William. 1903. *The Essentials of Modern Materia Medica and Therapeutics, with a Complete Formulary*. George W. Boskowitz, compiler. Cincinnati, OH: Scudder Brothers Co., 1903. 344pp. Web version at: http://swsbm.com/ManualsOther/Fyfe.html.

Fyfe, John William. 1909. *Specific Diagnosis and Specific Medication*. Cincinnati, OH: Scudder Brothers Co. 784pp.

Gaertner, EE. 1979. "The History and Use of Milkweed." *Econ. Botany*. 33(2):119–23.

Galecka, H. 1969. "Choleretic and Cholagogic Effects of Certain Hydroxy Acids and Their Derivatives in Guinea Pigs." *Acta Pol. Pharm.* 26:479–84.

Gambhir, SS, et al. 1979. "Antispasmodic Activity of the Tertiary Base of *Daucus carota*, Linn. Seeds." *Indian J. Physiol. Pharmacol.* 23:225–28.

Gansser, D, and Spiteller, G. 1995a. "Aromatase Inhibitors from Urtica dioica Roots." *Planta Med.* 61:138–40.

Gansser, D, and Spiteller, G. 1995b. "Plant Constituents Interfering with Human Sex Hormone-binding Globulin: Evaluation of a Test Method and Its Application to *Urtica dioica* Root Extracts." *Z Naturforsch [C]*. Jan-Feb, 50(1–2):98–104.

Gasperi-Campani, A, et al. 1991. "Inhibition of Growth of Breast Cancer Cells in vitro by the Ribosome-inactivating Protein Saporin 6." *Anticancer Res.* 11:1007–11.

Gassinger, CA, et al. 1981. "Klinische Prüfung zum Nachweis der therapeutischen Wirksamkeit des homöopathischen Arzneimittels Eupatorium perfoliatum D 2 (Wasserhanf composite) bei der Diagnose 'Grippaler Infekt.'" *Arzneim.-Forsch./Drug Res.* 31(1):732–36.

Gateley, CA, et al. 1992. "Drug Treatments for Mastalgia: 17 Years Experience in the Cardiff Mastalgia Clinic." *J. R. Soc. Med.* 85(1):12–15.

Gathercoal, Edmund N, and Wirth, Elmer H. 1936. *Pharmacognosy*. 1st ed. Philadelphia: Lea and Febiger. 852pp.

Gathercoal, Edmund N, and Wirth, Elmer H. 1947. *Pharmacognosy*. 2nd ed. Philadelphia: Lea and Febiger. 756pp.

George, EJ, et al. 1911. "*Lycopus virginicus* as a Remedy for Exophthalmic Goitre: Report of the Cure of a Few Cases." *J. Ophthalmol., Otol. and Laryngol.* 17:94–96.

Gerald, FL. 1878. "Art. XII. Lycopus virginicus." *Eclect. Med. J.* 38:57–59.

Gerard, John. 1975. *The Herball, or Generall Historie of Plantes, the Complete 1633 Edition as Revised & Enlarged by Thomas Johnson*. London; reprint, New York: Dover Publications. 1630pp.

Ghasemi, S, et al. 2016. "Cytotoxic Effects of *Urtica dioica* Radix on Human Colon (HT20) and Gastric (MKN45) Cancer Cells Mediated through Oxidative and Apoptotic Mechanisms." *Cell. Mol. Biol.* (Noisy-le-grand). 62(9):90–96.

Gherase, F, et al. 2002. "The Experimental Evaluation Regarding Analgesic Activity of Some Extracts Isolated from *Achillea collina* J. Becker ex Reichenb." *Rev. Med. Chir. Soc. Nat. Iasi.* 106(4):801–5.

Gibbons, Euell. 1970. *Stalking the Healthful Herbs*. Field Guide ed. New York: David McKay Co. 303pp.

Gibbons, Euell. 1971. *Stalking the Good Life: My Love Affair with Nature*. New York: David McKay Co. 247pp.

Gibbons, Euell. 1973. *Stalking the Faraway Places*. New York: David McKay Co. 279pp.

Gibbons, Euell, and Tucker, Gordon. 1979. *Euell Gibbons' Handbook of Edible Wild Plants*. Virginia Beach, VA: Donning Co. 319pp.

Gibbs, A, et al. 1983. "Isolation and Anticoagulant Properties of Polysaccharides of *Typha angustata* and *Daemonorops* Species." *Thromb. Res.* 32(2):97–108.

Gierlikowska, B, et al. 2019. "*Inula helenium* and *Grindelia squarrosa* as a Source of Compounds with Anti-inflammatory Activity in Human Neutrophils and Cultured Human Respiratory Epithelium." *J. Ethnopharmacol.* 249:112311. Epub 2019 Oct 20.

Gilani, AH, and Janbaz, KH. 1995. "Preventive and Curative Effects of *Artemisia absinthium* on Acetaminophen and CC14-induced Hepatotoxicity." *Gen. Pharmacol.* 26(2):309–15.

Gilani, AH, et al. 1994. "Cardiovascular Actions of *Daucus carota*." *Arch. Pharmacol. Res.* 17:150–53.

Gill, Steven J. 1983. "Ethnobotany of the Makah and Ozette People, Olympic Peninsula, Washington (USA)" [dissertation]. Washington State University.

Gilmore, M. 1913. "A Study in the Ethnobotany of the Omaha Indians." *Collect. Neb. State Historical Soc.* 17:314–57.

Gilmore, M. 1933. "Some Chippewa Uses of Plants." In: *Papers of the Michigan Academy of Science, Arts, & Letters, 17*. Ann Arbor: University of Michigan Press. p. 119–43.

Gilmore, Melvin. 1977. *Uses of Plants by the Indians of the Missouri River Region*. 33rd Annual Report of the Bureau of American Ethnology, 1911–12. Washington, DC: Government Printing Office, 1919, p. 43–154; reprint, Lincoln: University of Nebraska Press. 109pp.

Gilmore, Melvin. 1991. *Uses of Plants by the Indians of the Missouri River Region*. 33rd Annual Report of the Bureau of American Ethnology, 1911–12, Washington, DC: Government Printing Office, 1919:43–154; enlarged ed., Lincoln: University of Nebraska Press. 125pp.

Giuffrida, S, et al. 2000. "Essential Fatty Acids (Linoleic and gamma-Linolenic Acids) on Tear Deficient Dry-eye Treatment." *Investig. Ophthalmol.* 41: Arvo Abstract 1447.

Glen, I, et al. 1987. "The Role of Essential Fatty Acids in Alcohol Dependence and Tissue Damage." *Alcoholism, Clin. and Exp. Res.* 11(1):37–41.

Godowski, KC. 1989. "Antimicrobial Action of Sanguinarine." *J. Clin. Dent.* 1(4):96–101.

Goldberg, AS, and Mueller, EC. 1969. "Isolation of the Antiinflammatory Principles from *Achillea millefolium* (Compositae)." *J. Pharm. Sci.* 58(8):938–41.

Gomez-Flores, R, et al. 2000. "Immunoenhancing Properties of *Plantago major* Leaf Extract." *Phytother. Res.* 14(8):617–22.

Gonzales, GF, et al. 2002. "Effect of *Lepidium Meyenii* (MACA) on Sexual Desire and Its Absent Relationship With Serum Testosterone Levels in Adult Healthy Men." *Andrologia.* 34(6):367–72.

Gonzalez, C, et al. 2002. "Effects of Different Varieties of Maca (*Lepidium meyenii*) on Bone Structure in Ovariectomized Rats." *Forsch. Komplementmed.* 17(3):137–43.

Goodchild, Peter. 1984. *Survival Skills of the North American Indians*. Chicago: Chicago Review Press. 234pp.

Goodrich, Jennie, and Lawson, Claudia. 1980. *Kashaya Pomo Plants*. San Bernardino, CA: Borgo Press. 176pp.

Goranov, K, et al. 1983. "Clinical Results from the Treatment of Hemorrhagic Form of Periodontosis with a Complex Herb Extract and 15% DMSO [ET]. *Stomatologiia* (Sofia). 65(6):25–30.

Gosse, Philip Henry. 1971. *The Canadian Naturalist: A Series of Conversations on the Natural History of Lower Canada*. London: John van Voorst, 1840; facsimile ed., Toronto: Coles. 372pp.

Graber, JD. 1907. "*Sanguinaria* in Eczema." *J. Am. Med. Assoc.* 49:705.

Grases, F, et al. 1994. "Urolithiasis and Phytotherapy." *Int. Urol. Nephrol.* 26:507–11.

Green, James. 1991. *The Male Herbal: Health Care for Men and Boys*. Freedom, CA: Crossing Press. 267pp.

Greenberger, AJ, and Greenberger, ME. 1940. "*Capsella bursa-pastoris* as a Hemostatic After Prostatectomy." *J.-Lancet.* 60:422–23.

Grieve, Maud. 1971. *A Modern Herbal*. Mrs. C. F. Leyel, editor. London: Jonathan Cape, 1931; reprint, New York: Dover Publications. 2 vols. 902pp.

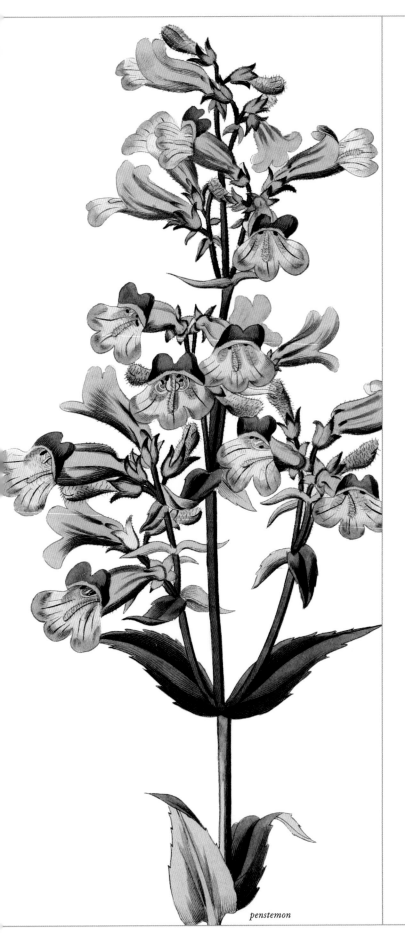

penstemon

Griffith, R. Eglesfeld. 1847. *Medical Botany*. Philadelphia: Lea and Blanchard. 704pp.

Grimé, William, ed. 1979. *Ethno-Botany of the Black Americans*. Algonac, MI: Reference Publications. 237pp.

Grinnell, GB. 1905. "Some Cheyenne Plant Medicines." *Am. Anthropol.* 7:37–43.

Grinnell, George Bird. 1972. *The Cheyenne Indians: Their History and Ways of Life*. Vol. 2. Lincoln: University of Nebraska Press. 402pp.

Gross, SC, et al. 2002. "Antineoplastic Activity of *Solidago virgaurea* on Prostatic Tumor Cells in an SCID Mouse Model." *Nutr. Cancer.* 43(1):76–81.

Grujic-Vasic, J, et al. 2006. "Antimicrobial Activity of Different Extracts from Rhizome and Root of *Potentilla erecta* L. Raeuschel and *Potentilla alba* L. Rosaceae." *Acta Medica Academica.* 35:9–14.

Guérin, JC, and Reveillere, HP. 1985. "Antifungal Activity of Plant Extracts Used Therapeutically. II. Study of 40 Extracts on 9 Fungal Strains" [ET]. *Ann. Pharm. Fr.* 43(1):77–81.

Gui, CH. 1985. "Antitussive Components of *Verbena officinalis*" [ET]. *Zhong Yao Tung Bao.* 10(10):35.

Guillén, MEN, et al. 1997. "Analgesic and Anti-inflammatory Activities of the Aqueous Extract of *Plantago major* L." *Int. J. Pharmacogn.* 35:99–104.

Guin, JD, and Reynolds, R. 1980. "Jewelweed Treatment of Poison Ivy Dermatitis." *Contact Dermat.* 6:287–88.

Gunn, John. 1859–61. *New Domestic Physician, or Home Book of Health.* 2nd rev. ed. Cincinnati, OH: Moore, Wilstach, and Keys. 1046pp.

Gunn, John. 1867. *New Domestic Physician, or Home Book of Health.* Cincinnati, OH: Moore, Wilstach and Baldwin. 1214pp.

Gunn, TR, and Wright, IM. 1996. "The Use of Black and Blue Cohosh in Labour." *N Z Med. J.* (25 Oct) 109(1032):410–11.

Gunther, Erna. 1973. *Ethnobotany of Western Washington.* Rev. ed. Seattle: University of Washington Press. 71pp.

Gupta, MB, et al. 1971. "Pharmacological Studies to Isolate the Active Constituents from *Cyperus rotundus* Possessing Anti-inflammatory, Antipyretic, and Analgesic Activities." *Indian J. Med. Res.* 59(1):76–82.

Habtemariam, S. 1998. "Cistifolin, an Integrin-dependent Cell-adhesion Blocker from the Anti-rheumatic Herbal Drug, Gravel Root (Rhizome of *Eupatorium purpureum*)." *Planta Med.* 64(8):683–85.

Habtemariam, S, and MacPherson, AM. 2000. "Cytotoxicity and Antibacterial Activity of Ethanol Extract from Leaves of a Herbal Drug, Boneset *(Eupatorium perfoliatum*)." *Phytother. Res.* 14(7):575–77.

Hall, TB. 1974. "*Eupatorium perfoliatum*: A Plant with a History." *Mo. Med.* 71(9):527.

Hall, Walter, and Hall, Nancy. 1980. *The Wild Palate: A Serious Wild Foods Cookbook.* Emmaus, PA: Rodale Press. 374pp.

Hamel, Paul B, and Chiltoskey, Mary Ulmer. 1975. *Cherokee Plants and Their Uses: A 400-Year History.* Sylva, NC: Herald Publishing Co. 65pp.

Handa, SS, et al. 1986. "Natural Products and Plants as Liver Protecting Drugs." *Fitoterapia.* 57:307–51.

Harborne, Jeffrey B, and Baxter, Herbert. 1993. *Phytochemical Dictionary: A Handbook of Bioactive Compounds from Plants.* Washington, DC: Taylor and Francis. 791pp.

Harlan, R. 1830. "Experiments Made on the Poison of the Rattle-snake; in which the Powers of the *Hieracium venosum*, as a Specific, Were Tested." *Trans. Am. Philos. Soc.* New Series, 3:300–14.

Harney, JW, et al. 1978. "Behavioral and Toxicological Studies of Cyclopentanoid Monoterpenes from *Nepeta cataria*." *Lloydia.* 41(4):367–74.

Harnyk, TP. 1999. "The Use of Preparations of Plant Origin in Treating and Rehabilitating Elderly Patients with Chronic Hepatitis" [ET]. *Lik. Sprava.* (7–8):168–70.

Harper, DS, et al. 1990a. "Clinical Efficacy of a Dentifrice and Oral Rinse Containing Sanguinaria Extract and Zinc Chloride during 6 Months of Use." *J. Periodontol.* 61(6):352–58.

Harper, DS, et al. 1990b. "Effect of 6 Months Use of a Dentifrice and Oral Rinse Containing Sanguinaria Extract and Zinc Chloride upon the Microflora of the Dental Plaque and Oral Soft Tissues." *J. Periodontol.* 61(6):359–63.

Harper-Shove, Frederick. 1938. *Prescriber and Clinical Repertory of Medicinal Herbs.* London: Homeopathic Publishing Co. 199pp.

Harput, US, et al. 2006. "Effects of Two *Prunella* Species on Lymphocyte Proliferation and Nitric Oxide Production." *Phytother. Res.* 20(2):157–59.

Harrar, Sari, and O'Donnell, Sara Altshul, eds. 1999. *The Woman's Book of Healing Herbs: Healing Teas, Tonics, Supplements, and Formulas.* Emmaus, PA: Rodale Press. 495pp.

Harrington, Harold David. 1967. *Edible Native Plants of the Rocky Mountains.* Albuquerque: University of New Mexico Press. 392pp.

Harris, Ben Charles. 1973. *Eat the Weeds.* New Canaan, CT: Keats Publishing Co. 253pp.

Hart, JA. 1981. "The Ethnobotany of the Northern Cheyenne Indians of Montana." *J. Ethnopharmacol.* 4:1–55.

Hart, Jeff. 1976. *Montana Native Plants and Early Peoples.* Helena. Montana Historical Society Press. 76pp.

Hart, Jeff. 1992. *Montana Native Plants and Early Peoples.* Helena. Montana Historical Society Press. 75pp.

Hartenstein, H, and Mueller, WA. 1961. "Studies on the Effect of *Lycopus europaeus* and *Lithospermum officinale* on Thyroid-gland Metabolism in the Rat" [ET]. *Hippokrates.* 32:284–88.

Hartmann, RW, et al. 1996. "Inhibition of 5 a-reductase and Aromatase by PHL-00801 (Prostatonin), a Combination of PY 102 (*Pygeum africanum*) and UR 102 (*Urtica dioica*) Extracts." *Phytomed.* 3(2):121–28.

Hartwell, JL. 1960. "Plant Remedies for Cancer." *Cancer Chemother. Rep.* 7:19–24.

Hartwell, JL. 1968. "Plants Used Against Cancer: A Survey." *Lloydia.* 31:71–170.

Hartwell, JL. 1970. "Plants Used Against Cancer: A Survey." *Lloydia.* 33:97–124, 288–392.

Hartwell, JL. 1971. "Plants Used Against Cancer: A Survey." *Lloydia.* 34:103–60, 204–55, 310–60, 386–425.

Hartwell, Jonathan L. 1982. *Plants Used Against Cancer: A Survey.* Lawrence, MA: Quarterman Publication. 710pp.

Hausen, BM. 1992. "Sesquiterpene Lactones—General Discussion." In: de Smet, Peter AGM, et al., editors. *Adverse Effects of Herbal Drugs.* Berlin: Springer-Verlag. 2 vols. 1:227–36.

Heatherly, Ana Nez. 1998. *Healing Plants: A Medicinal Guide to Native North American Plants and Herbs.* New York: Lyons Press. 252pp.

Hecht, SS. 1996. "Chemoprevention of Lung Cancer by Isothiacyanates." *Adv. Exp. Med. Biol.* 40(1):1–11.

Hecht, SS, et al. 1995. "Effects of Watercress Consumption on Metabolism of a Tobacco-specific Lung Carcinogen in Smokers." *Cancer Epidemiol. Biomark. Prev.* 4(8):877–84.

Heckewelder, John Gottlieb Ernestus. 1820. *A Narrative of the Mission of the United Brethren among the Delaware and Mohegan Indians.* Philadelphia: McCarty and Davis. 429pp.

Hederos, CA, and Berg, A. 1996. "Epogram Evening Primrose Oil Treatment in Atopic Dermatitis and Asthma." *Arch. Dis. Child.* 75:494–97.

Heinerman, John. 1979. *Science of Herbal Medicine: Pharmacological, Medical, Historical, Anthropological.* Orem, UT: Bi-World Publications. 318pp.

Heinerman, John. 2001. *Folk Medicine in America Today: A Guide for a New Generation of Folk Healers.* New York: Kensington Publishing Corp. 304pp.

Hellson, John C, and Gadd, Morgan. 1974. *Ethnobotany of the Blackfoot Indians.* Canadian Ethnology Service Paper No. 19. Ottawa: National Museums of Canada. 138pp.

Henry, DY, et al. 1987. "Isolation and Characterization of 9-hydroxy-10-trans, 12-cis-octadecadienoic Acid, a Novel Regulator of Platelet adenylate cyclase from *Glechoma hederacea* L., Labiatae." *Eur. J. Biochem.* 170(1–2):389–94.

Hermann, H, and Remy, A. 1922. "Cardiovascular Action of the Aqueous Extract of Stinging Nettle" [ET]. *Comptes Rendus des Seances de la Societe de Biologie et de ses Filiales.* 86:399–400.

Herold, A, et al. 2003. "Hydroalcoholic Plant Extracts with Anti-inflammatory Activity." *Roum. Arch. Microbiol. Immunol.* 62(1–2):117–29.

Herrick, James W. 1995. *Iroquois Medical Botany.* Syracuse, NY: Syracuse University Press. 278pp.

Herrick, James William. 1977. "Iroquois Medical Botany" [dissertation]. Ann Arbor: University Microfilms International. 518pp.

Herz, W, and Sharma, RP. 1976. "Sesquiterpene Lactones of *Eupatorium hyssopifolium*: A Germacranolide with an Unusual Lipid Ester Side Chain." *J. Org. Chem.* 1976:1015–20.

Herz, W, et al. 1977. "Sesquiterpene Lactones of *Eupatorium perfoliatum*." *J. Org. Chem.* 42:2264–71.

Heywood, VH, et al., eds. 1977. *The Biology and Chemistry of the Compositae.* New York: Academic Press. 2 vols. 619 + 567pp.

Hiermann, A, et al. 1986. "Influence of *Epilobium* Extracts on Prostaglandin Biosynthesis and Carrageenin-induced Oedema of the Rat Paw." *J. Ethnopharmacol.* 17(2):161–69.

Hiermann, A, et al. 1991. "Isolation of the Antiphlogistic Principle from *Epilobium angustifolium*" [ET]. *Planta Med.* 57(4):357–60.

Hill, John A. 1751. *A History of the Materia Medica.* London: Longman. 924pp.

Hiller, E, and Deglmann, H. 1955. "The Effect of *Lycopus europeus* Extracts on the Distribution of Iodine in Human Serum." *Arznemittelforschung.* 5:465–70.

Hiller, K. 1987. "New Results on the Structure and Biological Activity of Triterpenoid Saponins." In: Hostettmann, Kurt, and Lea, Peter J, editors. *Biologically Active Natural Products.* Oxford: Clarendon Press. p. 175–84.

Hippocrates. n.d. *The Genuine Works of Hippocrates, Translated from the Greek, with a Preliminary Discourse and Annotations by Francis Adams.* New York: William Wood and Co. 2 vols. in 1. 390 + 366pp.

Hirano, T, et al. 1994. "Effects of Stinging Nettle Root Extracts and Their Steroidal Components on the Na+, K+-ATPase of the Benign Prostatic Hyperplasia." *Planta Med.* 60(1):30–33.

Hirose, M, et al. 2000. "Effects of Arctiin on PhIP-induced Mammary, Colon and Pancreatic Carcinogenesis in Female Sprague-Dawley Rats and MelQx-induced Hepatocarcinogenesis in Male F344 Rats." *Cancer Lett.* 155(1):79–88.

Hocking, George Macdonald. 1997. *A Dictionary of Natural Products.* 2nd ed. Medford, NJ: Plexus Publications. 1024pp.

Hocking, GM. 1956. "Some Plant Materials Used Medicinally and Otherwise by the Navajo Indians in the Chaco Canyon, New Mexico." *El Palacio.* 63:161.

Hoerhammer L. 1961. "Flavone Concentration of Medicinal Plants with Regard to Their Spasmolytic Action." *Congr. Sci. Farm. Conf. Commun.* 21:578–88.

Hoffmann, David. 1986. *The Holistic Herbal: A Herbal Celebrating the Wholeness of Life.* 2nd ed. The Park, Forres, Scotland: Findhorn Press. 281pp.

Hoffman, Walter J. 1891. "The Mide'wiwin or 'Grand Medicine Society' of the Ojibwa." *Seventh Annual Report of the Bureau of American Ethnology, 1885–86, Part 2.* Washington, DC: Government Printing Office. p. 143–300.

Holetz, FB, et al. 2002. "Screening of Some Plants Used in the Brazilian Folk Medicine for the Treatment of Infectious Diseases." *Mem. Inst. Oswaldo Cruz.* 97(7):1027–31.

Holmes, EM. 1884. "Medicinal Plants Used by the Cree Indians, Hudson's Bay Territory." *Pharm. J. Trans.* 15:302–4.

Holmes, Peter. 1989–90. *The Energetics of Western Herbs: Integrating Western and Oriental Herbal Medicine Traditions.* Boulder, CO: Artemis Press. 2 vols. 421pp. + 416pp.

Holmes, Peter. 1997–98. *The Energetics of Western Herbs: Treatment Strategies Integrating Western and Oriental Herbal Medicine.* Rev. 3rd ed. Boulder, CO: Snow Lotus Press. 2 vols. 442 + 442pp.

Honeychurch, Penelope N. 1980. *Caribbean Wild Plants and Their Uses: An Illustrated Guide to Some Medicinal and Wild Ornamental Plants of the West Indies.* Oxford: Caribbean. 166pp.

Hong, L, et al. 2014. "Antibacterial Activity and Mechanism of Action of *Monarda punctata* Essential Oil and Its Main Components against Common Bacterial Pathogens in Respiratory Tract." *Int. J. Clin. Exp. Pathol.* 7(11):7389–98.

Hook, I, et al. 1993. "Evaluation of Dandelion for Diuretic Activity and Variation in Potassium Content." *Int. J. Pharmacogn.* 31:29–34.

Hooper, SN, and Chandler, RF. 1984. "Herbal Remedies of the Maritime Indians: Phytosterols and Triterpenes of 67 Plants." *J. Ethnopharmacol.* 10:181–94.

Horng, CT, et al. 2014. "Antioxidant and Antifatigue Activities of *Polygonatum Alte-lobatum* Hayata Rhizomes in Rats." *Nutr.* 6(11):5327–37.

Horrobin, DF. 1983. "The Role of Essential Fatty Acids and Prostaglandins in the Premenstrual Syndrome." *J. Reprod. Med.* 28(7):465–68.

Horrobin, DF. 1984. "Placebo-controlled Trials of Evening Primrose Oil." *Swed. J. Biol. Med.* 3:13–17.

Horrobin, DF. 1990. "Gamma-linolenic Acid." *Rev. Contemp. Pharmacother.* 1:1–45.

Hostettmann, Kurt, and Lea, Peter J, eds. 1987. *Biologically Active Natural Products.* Oxford: Clarendon Press. 283pp.

Hriscu, A, et al. 1990. "A Pharmacodynamic Investigation of the Effect of Polyholozidic Substances Extracted from *Plantago* sp. on the Digestive Tract" [ET]. *Rev. Med. Chir. Soc. Med. Nat. Iasi.* 94(1):165–70.

Hryb, DJ, et al. 1995. "The Effect of Extracts of the Roots of the Stinging Nettle (*Urtica dioica*) on the Interaction of SHBG with Its Receptor on Human Prostatic Membranes." *Planta Med.* 61(1):31–32.

Huang, YG, et al. 2006. "Novel Selective Cytotoxicity of Wild Sarsaparilla Rhizome Extract." *J. Pharm. Pharmacol.* 58(10):1399–1403.

Hudson, James B. 1990. *Antiviral Compounds from Plants.* Boca Raton, FL: CRC Press. 200pp.

Huseini, HF, et al. 2005. "The Efficacy of Liv-52 on Liver Cirrhotic Patients: A Randomized, Double-blind, Placebo-controlled First Approach." *Phytomed.* 12(9):619–24.

Hussan, F, et al. 2015. "Anti-inflammatory Property of *Plantago major* Leaf Extract Reduces the Inflammatory Reaction in Experimental Acetaminophen-induced Liver Injury." *Evid.-Based Complement. Altern. Med.* 2015:347861, Epub 2015 Aug 2.

Hutchens, Alma. 1991. *Indian Herbalogy of North America.* Boston: Shambala. 382pp.

Hutchens, Alma R. 1973. *Indian Herbalogy of North America: A Study of Anglo-American, Russian and Oriental Literature on Indian Medical Botanics of North America, with Illustrations, Glossary, Index and Annotated Bibliography.* Windsor, ON: Merco. 382pp.

Hyde, Fletcher, et al. 1976–79. *British Herbal Pharmacopoeia.* Keighley: British Medical Association. 3 vols. 229 + 248 + 210pp.

Iauk, L, et al. 2003. "Antibacterial Activity of Medicinal Plant Extracts Against Periodontopathic Bacteria." *Phytother. Res.* 17(6):599–604.

Ibragimov, DI, and Kazanskaia, GB. 1981. ["Antimicrobial Action of Cranberry Bush, Common Yarrow and *Achillea biebersteinii*"] (article in Russian). *Antibiotiki.* 26(2):108–9.

Ikawati, Z, et al. 2001. "Screening of Several Indonesian Medicinal Plants for Their Inhibitory Effect on Histamine Release from RBL-2H3 Cells." *J. Ethnopharmacol.* 75(2–3):249–56.

Ikram, M. 1980. "Medicinal Plants as Hypocholesterolemic Agents." *J. Pak. Med. Assn.* 30(12):278–81.

Inouye, H, et al. 1974. "Purgative Activities of Iridoid Glycosides." *Planta Med.* 25:285–88.

IRCS Med. Sci. 1986. Abstract 14, 212.

Isaev, I, and Boiadzhieva, M. 1960. "Production of Galenic and Neogalenic Preparations and Experience with the Isolation of Active Substances from *Leonurus cardiaca*" [ET]. *Nauchni Tr. Vissh. Med. Inst.* (Sofia). 39(5):145–52.

Ito, Y, et al. 1986. "Suppression of 7, 12-dimethylbenz(a) anthracene-induced Chromosome Aberrations in Rat Bone Marrow Cells by Vegetable Juices." *Mutat. Res.* 182:55–60.

Iurisson, S. 1971. ["Determination of Active Substances of *Capsella bursa-pastoris*"] (article in Russian). *Tartu Riiliku Ulikooli Toim.* 270:71–79.

Iurisson, SM. 1973. ["Flavonoid Substances of *Capsella Bursa Pastoris* (L.) Medic"] (article in Russian). *Farmatsiia.* 22(5):34–35.

Iurisson, SM. 1976. ["Vitamin Content in Shepherd's Purse (*Capsella Bursa Pastoris* [L.] Medic)"] (article in Russian). *Farmatsiia.* 25(4):66–67.

Jabbar, A, et al. 2007. "Anthelmintic Activity of *Chenopodium album* (L) and *Caesalpinia crista* (L) against Trichostrongylid Nematodes of Sheep." *J. Ethnopharmacol.* 114(1):86–91.

Jackson, JR. 1873. "Note on the Reputed Value of *Polygonum aviculare* for Stone." *Pharmaceut. J.* 33:105.

Jackson, JR. 1876. "Notes on Some Medicinal Plants of the Compositae." *Canadian Pharm. J.* 9:231–26.

Jacobs, Marion Lee, and Burlage, Henry M. 1958. *Index of Plants of North Carolina with Reputed Medicinal Uses.* Chapel Hill: Henry M. Burlage. 332pp.

Jang, DS, et al. 2010. "3, 5-Di-O-caffeoyl-epi-quinic Acid from the Leaves and Stems of *Erigeron annuus* Inhibits Protein Glycation, Aldose Reductase, and Cataractogenesis." *Biol. Pharm. Bull.* 33(2):329–32.

Jäntti, J, et al. 1989. "Evening Primrose Oil in Rheumatoid Arthritis: Changes in Serum Lipids and Fatty Acids." *Ann. Rheum. Dis.* 48: 124–27.

Jarred, RA, et al. 2002. "Induction of Apoptosis in Low- to Moderate-grade Human Prostate Carcinoma by Red Clover–derived Dietary Isoflavones." *Cancer Epidemiol. Biomark. Prev.* 11(12):1689–96.

Jashemski, Wilhelmina Feemster. 1999. *A Pompeian Herbal: Ancient and Modern Medicinal Plants.* Austin: University of Texas Press. 107pp.

Jiang, D, et al. 2019. "Potential Anticancer Properties and Mechanisms of Action of Formononetin." *Biomed. Res. Int.* Jul 28:2019:5854315. eCollection 2019.

Jimenez-Arellanes, A, et al. 2003. "Activity against Multidrug-resistant *Mycobacterium tuberculosis* in Mexican Plants Used to Treat Respiratory Diseases." *Phytother. Res.* 17(8):903–8.

Jo, MJ, et al. 2013. "Roots of *Erigeron annuus* Attenuate Acute Inflammation as Mediated with the Inhibition of NF-KB-associated Nitric Oxide and Prostaglandin E2 Production." *Evid. Based Complement. Altern. Med.* 2013:297427. Epub 2013 Feb 24.

John, JF. 1994. "Synergistic Antiretroviral Activities of the Herb, *Prunella vulgaris*, with AZT, ddI and ddC." *Abstr. Gen. Meet. Am. Soc. Microbiol.* 94:481, 484. Abstract S-27.

Johnson, Laurence. 1884. *A Manual of the Medical Botany of North America.* New York: Wood. 292pp.

Johnson, M, et al. 2011. "Antibacterial Activity of Leaves and Inter-nodal Callus Extracts of *Mentha arvensis*." *Asian Pac. J. Trop. Med.* 4(3):196–200.

Johnston, A. 1970. "Blackfoot Indian Utilization of the Flora of the Northwestern Great Plains." *Econ. Botany.* 24:301–24.

Johnston, Alex. 1987. *Plants and the Blackfoot.* Lethbridge, AB: Lethbridge Historical Society. 56pp.

Jones, DE. 1968. "Comanche Plant Medicine." *Papers in Anthropol.* 9:1–13.

Jones, Eli. 1911. *Definite Medication, Containing Therapeutic Facts Gleaned from Forty Years Practice.* Boston: Therapeutic Publishing Co., 1911; reprint, Kila, MT: Kessinger Publishing Co. 312pp.

Jones, NP, et al. 2000. "Antifungal Activity of Extracts from Medicinal Plants Used by First Nations Peoples of Eastern Canada." *J. Ethnopharmacol.* 73(1–2):191–98.

Jones, Pamela. 1991. *Just Weeds: History, Myths, and Uses.* New York: Prentice-Hall Press. 303pp.

Jones, TK, and Larson, BM. 1998. "Profound Neonatal Congestive Heart Failure Caused by Maternal Consumption of Blue Cohosh Herbal Medication." *J. Pediatr.* 132:550–52.

Jones, VH. 1931. "The Ethnobotany of the Isleta Indians" [master's thesis]. University of New Mexico.

Jordan, Michael. 1976. *A Guide to Wild Plants: The Edible and Poisonous Species of the Northern Hemisphere.* London: Millington Books. 240pp.

Juan, H, et al. 1988. "Anti-inflammatory Effects of a Substance Extracted from *Epilobium angustifolium*." *Agents Actions.* 23(1–2):106–7.

Juma, A. 2007. "The Effects of *Lepidium sativum* Seeds on Fracture-induced Healing in Rabbits." *Med. Gen. Med.* 9(2):23.

Jurkstiene, V, et al. 2011. "Investigation of the Antimicrobial Activity of Rhaponticum (*Rhaponticum carthamoides* D. C. Iljin) and Shrubby Cinquefoil (*Potentilla fruticosa* L.)." *Medicina* (Kaunas). 47(3):174–79.

Kageyama, S, et al. 2000. "Extract of *Prunella vulgaris* Spikes Inhibits HIV Replication at Reverse Transcription *in vitro* and Can be Absorbed from Intestine *in vivo*." *Antivir. Chem. Chemother.* 11(2):157–64.

Kakiuchi, N, et al. 1987. "Effect of benzo[c]phenanthridine Alkaloids on Reverse Transcriptase and Their Binding Property to Nucleic Acids." *Planta Med.* 53(1):22–27.

Kalm, Peter. 1937. *Peter Kalm's Travels in North America.* 1770; revised ed., Adolph B. Benson, editor. New York: Wilson-Erickson Inc. 2 vols. 797pp.

Kalm, Peter. 1966. *The America of 1750: Peter Kalm's Travels in North America. The English Version of 1770, Revised from the Original Swedish by Adolph B. Benson.* 2 vols. 1937; reprint, New York: Dover Books. 797pp.

Kamala, A, et al. 2018. "Plants in Traditional Medicine, with Special Reference to *Cyperus rotundus* L.: A Review." *3 Biotech* 8(7):309. Epub 2018 Jul 9.

Kanjanapothi, D, et al. 1981. "Postcoital Antifertility Effect of *Mentha arvensis*." *Contracept.* 24(5):559–67.

Kari, Priscilla Russell. 1977. *Dena'ina K'et'una, Tanaina Plantlore.* Anchorage, AK: Adult Literacy Laboratory. 205pp.

Karlowski, JA. 1991. "Bloodroot: *Sanguinaria canadensis* L." *Canadian Pharm. J.* 124(5):260–67.

Karpilovskaia, ED, et al. 1989. "Inhibiting Effect of the Polyphenolic Complex from *Plantago major* (Plantastine) on the Carcinogenic Effect of Endogenously Synthesized Nitrosodimethylamine." *Farmakol. Toksikol.* 52(4):64–67.

Kartini, SP, et al. 2017. "Effects of *Plantago major* Extracts and Its Chemical Compounds on Proliferation of Cancer Cells and Cytokines Production of Lipopolysaccharide-activated THP-1 Macrophages." *Pharmacogn. Mag.* 13(51):393–99. Epub 2017 Jul 19.

Katoch, R, et al. 2000. "Hepatotoxicity of *Eupatorium adenophorum* to Rats." *Toxicon.* 38(2):309–14.

Kaushal, V, et al. 2001. "Hepatotoxicity in Rat Induced by Partially Purified Toxins from *Eupatorium adenophorum* (*Ageratina adenophora*)." *Toxicon.* 39(5):615–19.

Kavasch, E. Barrie. 1977. *Native Harvests: Botanicals and Recipes of the American Indian.* Washington, CT: American Indian Archaeological Institute. 73pp.

Kay, Margarita. 1996. *Healing with Plants in the American and Mexican West.* Tucson: University of Arizona Press. 315pp.

Kemper, F, et al. 1961. "Antihormonal Effectiveness of *Lycopus* (Wolf's Foot)." *Arzneimittelforschung.* 11:92–94.

Keville, Kathi, and Szolkowski, Roman. 1991. *The Illustrated Herb Encyclopedia: A Complete Culinary, Cosmetic, Medicinal, and Ornamental Guide to Herbs.* New York: Mallard Press. 224pp.

Khan, AU, and Gilani, AH. 2011. "Blood-pressure Lowering, Cardiovascular Inhibiting, and Bronchodilatory Actions of *Achillea millefolium*." *Phytother. Res.* 25(4):577–83.

Khan, AW, et al. 2016. "Anticonvulsant, Anxiolytic, and Sedative Activities of *Verbena officinalis*." *Front. Pharmacol.* Dec 21; 7:499. eCollection 2016.

Khan, MR, et al. 2011. "Prevention of Hepatorenal Toxicity with *Sonchus asper* in Gentamicin-treated Rats." *BMC Complement. Altern. Med.* 11:113.

Khan, RA. 2012. "Evaluation of Flavonoids and Diverse Antioxidant Activities of *Sonchus arvensis*." *Chem. Cent. J.* 6(1):126.

Khan, RA. 2017. "Antidiabetic, Antioxidant, and Hypolipidemic Potential of *Sonchus asper* Hill." *Altern. Ther. Health Med.* 23(7):34–40.

Khan, RA, et al. 2010. "Prevention of CC14-induced Nephrotoxicity with *Sonchus asper* in Rat." *Food Chem. Toxicol.* 48(8–9):2469–76.

Khan, RA, et al. 2012a. "Brain Antioxidant Markers, Cognitive Performance and Acetylcholinesterase Activity of Rats: Efficiency of *Sonchus asper*." *Behav. Brain Funct.* 8:21.

Khan, RA, et al. 2012b. "Evaluation of Phenolic Contents and Antioxidant Activity of Various Solvent Extracts of *Sonchus asper* (L.) Hill." *Chem. Cent. J.* 6(1):12.

Khan, RA, et al. 2012c. "Hepatoprotective Activity of *Sonchus asper* against Carbon Tetrachloride-induced Injuries in Male Rats: A Randomized Controlled Trial." *BMC Complement. Altern. Med.* 12:90.

Khattak, SG, et al. 1985. "Antipyretic Studies on Some Indigenous Pakistani Medicinal Plants." *J. Ethnopharmacol.* 14(1):45–51.

Khazdair, MR, et al. 2019. "Anti-asthmatic Effects of *Portulaca oleracea* and Its Constituents: A Review." *J. Pharmacopuncture.* 22(3):122–30. Epub 2019 Sep 30.

Khuroo, MA, et al. 1988. "Sterones, Iridoids and a Sesquiterpene from *Verbascum thapsus*." *Phytochem.* 27(11):3541–44.

Kim, HI, et al. 2014. "Inhibition of Estrogen Signaling through Depletion of Estrogen Receptor Alpha by Ursolic Acid and Betulinic Acid from *Prunella vulgaris* var. *lilacina*." *Biochem. Biophys Res. Commun.* 451(2):282–87. Epub 2014 Aug 1.

Kim, HK, et al. 1999. "HIV Integrase Inhibitory Activity of *Agastache rugosa*." *Arch. Pharm. Res.* 22(5):520–23.

Kim, HM, et al. 1998. "*Taraxacum officinale* Restores Inhibition of Nitric Oxide Production by Cadmium in Mouse Peritoneal Macrophages." *Immunopharmacol. Immunotoxicol.* 20(2):283–97.

Kim, M, and Shin, HK. 1998. "The Water-soluble Extract of Chicory Influences Serum and Liver Lipid Concentrations, Cecal Short-chain Fatty Acid Concentrations and Fecal Lipid Excretion in Rats." *J. Nutr.* 128(10):1731–36.

Kim, SY, et al. 2007. "Effects of *Prunella vulgaris* on Mast Cell-mediated Allergic Reaction and Inflammatory Cytokine Production." *Exp. Biol. Med.* (Maywood). 232(7):921–26.

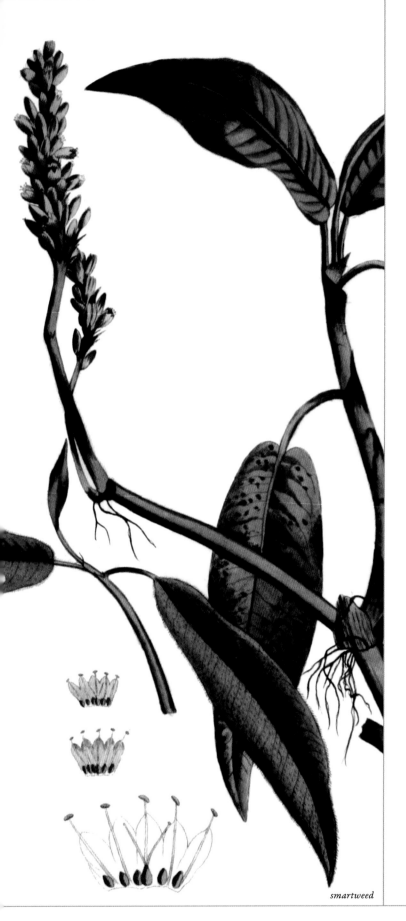

smartweed

Kim, TW, and Yang, KS. 2001. "Antioxidative Effects of *Cichorium intybus* Root Extract on LDL (Low-density Lipoprotein) Oxidation." *Arch. Pharm. Res.* 24(5):431–36.

Kindscher, K, et al. 1998. "Testing Prairie Plants with Ethnobotanical Importance for Anti-cancer and Anti-AIDS Compounds." *J. Ethnobiol.* 18(2):229–45.

Kindscher, Kelly. 1987. *Edible Wild Plants of the Prairie: An Ethnobotanical Guide*. Lawrence: University Press of Kansas. 278pp.

Kindscher, Kelly. 1992. *Medicinal Wild Plants of the Prairie: An Ethnobotanical Guide*. Lawrence: University Press of Kansas. 340pp.

King, John. 1882. *The American Dispensatory*. Cincinnati: Wilstach, Baldwin.

Kirby, ED. 1902. "Violets and Cancer." *Br. Med. J.* 1:55.

Kirchoff, HW. 1983. "Brennesselsaft als Diuretikum." *Z Phytother.* 4:621–26.

Kirk, Donald. R. 1975. *Wild Edible Plants of Western North America*. Happy Camp, CA: Naturegraph Publishers. 307pp.

Kishore, N, et al. 1993. "Fungitoxicity of Essential Oils against Dermatophytes." *Mycoses.* 36(5–6):211–15.

Kiss, A, et al. 2006a. "Effect of *Epilobium angustifolium* L. Extracts and Polyphenols on Cell Proliferation and Neutral Endopeptidase Activity in Selected Cell Lines." *Pharmazie.* 61(1):66–69.

Kiss, A, et al. 2006b. "Induction of Neutral Endopeptidase Activity in PC-3 Cells by an Aqueous Extract of *Epilobium angustifolium* L. and Oenothein B." *Phytomed.* 13(4):284–89.

Kloss, Jethro. 1975. *Back to Eden.* 5th ed. Santa Barbara, CA: Woodbridge Press Publishing Co. 684pp.

Knott, RP, and McCutcheon, RS. 1961. "Phytochemical Investigation of a *Rubiaceae, Galium triflorum*." *J. Pharm. Sci.* 50(11):963–65.

Knutsen, Karl. 1975. *Wild Plants You Can Eat: A Guide to Identification and Preparation*. Garden City, NY: Dolphin Books. 89pp.

Kohrle, J, et al. 1981. "Iodothyronine Deiodinases: Inhibition by Plant Extracts." *Acta Endocrinol.* Suppl 16:188–92.

Koichev, A. 1983. "Complex Evaluation of the Therapeutic Effect of a Preparation from *Plantago major* in Chronic Bronchitis." *Probl. Vutr. Med.* 11:61–69.

Komal, S, et al. 2018. "Antimicrobial Activity of *Prunella vulgaris* Extracts against Multi-drug Resistant *Escherichia coli* from Patients of Urinary Tract Infection." *Pak. J. Med. Sci.* 34(3):616–20.

Kong, YC, et al. 1976. "Isolation of the Uterotonic Principle from *Leonurus cardiaca*, the Chinese Motherwort." *Am. J. Chin. Med.* 4(4):373–82.

Konowalchuk, J, and Speirs, JI. 1976. "Antiviral Activity of Fruit Extracts." *J. Food Sci.* 41(5):1013–17.

Konrad, L, et al. 2000. "Antiproliferative Effect on Human Prostate Cancer Cells by a Stinging Nettle Root (*Urtica dioica*) Extract." *Planta Med.* 66(1):44–47.

Kosalec, I, et al. 2013. "Antimicrobial Activity of Willowherb (*Epilobium angustifolium* L.) Leaves and Flowers." *Curr. Drug Targets.* 14(9):986–91.

Kotobuki, KK. 1979. "*Taraxacum* Extracts as Antitumor Agents." *Chem. Abstr.* 94:14:530.

Kotobuki Seiyaku, KK. 1981. Pat. Jp 81/10117 Japan.

Kraft, Shelly Katheren. 1990. "Recent Changes in the Ethnobotany of Standing Rock Indian Reservation" [master's thesis]. University of North Dakota.

Krenn, L, et al. 2009. "Contribution of Methylated Exudate Flavonoids to the Anti-inflammatory Activity of *Grindelia robusta*." *Fitoterapia.* 80(5):267–69.

Kresanek, Jaroslav, and Krejca, Jindrich. 1989. *Healing Plants: Spotters Guide to Healing Plants*. New York: Dorset Press. 223pp.

Krivenko, VV, et al. 1989. "Experience in Treating Digestive Organ Diseases with Medicinal Plants" [ET]. *Vrach. Delo.* 3:76–78.

Krochmal, Arnold, and Krochmal, Connie. 1973. *A Guide to the Medicinal Plants of the United States*. New York: Quadrangle. 259pp.

Krochmal, Connie, and Krochmal, Arnold. 1974. *A Naturalist's Guide to Cooking with Wild Plants*. New York: Quadrangle/New York Times Book Co. 336pp.

Kroeber, L. 1950. "Pharmacology of Inulin Drugs and Their Therapeutic Use. II. *Cichorium intybus*; *Taraxacum officinale*." *Pharmazie*. 5:122–27.

Krzeski, T, et al. 1993. "Combined Extracts of *Urtica dioica* and *Pygeum africanum* in the Treatment of Benign Prostatic Hyperplasia: Double-blind Comparison of Two Doses." *Clin. Ther.* 15(6):1011–20.

Kuang, PG, et al. 1988. "Motherwort and Cerebral Ischemia." *J. Tradit. Chin. Med.* 8(1):37–40.

Kulze, A, and Greaves, M. 1988. "Contact Urticaria Caused by Stinging Nettles." *Br. J. Dermatol.* 119(2):269–70.

Kumar, S, et al. 2007. "*Chenopodium album* Seed Extract: A Potent Sperm-immobilizing Agent Both *in vitro* and *in vivo*." *Contracept.* 75(1):71–78.

Kumarasamy, Y, et al. 2002. "Biological Activity of *Glechoma hederacea*." *Fitoterapia*. 73:721–23.

Kupchan, SM, et al. 1965. "Tumor Inhibitors VIII. Eupatorin, New CytotoxicFlavone from *Eupatorium semiserratum*." *J. Pharm. Sci.* 54(6):929–30.

Kupchan, SM, et al. 1973. "Structural Elucidation of Novel Tumor-Inhibitory Sesquiterpene Lactones from *Eupatorium cuneifolium*." *J. Org. Chem.* 38(12):2189–96.

Kuroda, K. 1977. "Neoplasm Inhibitor from *Capsella bursa-pastoris*." *Japan Kokai*. 41:207.

Kuroda, K, and Kaku, T. 1969. "Pharmacological and Chemical Studies on the Alcohol Extract of *Capsella bursa-pastoris*." *Life Sci.* 8(3):151–55.

Kuroda, K, and Takagi, K. 1968. "Physiologically Active Substances in *Capsella bursa-pastoris*." *Nat.* 220(5168):707–8.

Kuroda, K, and Takagi, K. 1969a. "Studies on *Capsella bursa pastoris*. I. General Pharmacology of Ethanol Extract of the Herb." *Arch. Int. Pharmacodyn. Ther.* 178(2):382–91.

Kuroda, K, and Takagi, K. 1969b. "Studies on *Capsella bursa pastoris*. II. Diuretic, Anti-inflammatory and Anti-ulcer Action of Ethanol Extracts of the Herb." *Arch. Int. Pharmacodyn. Ther.* 178(2):392–99.

Kuroda, K, et al. 1976. "Inhibitory Effect of *Capsella bursa-pastoris* Extract on Growth of Ehrlich Solid Tumor in Mice." *Cancer Res.* 36(6):1900–1903.

Kuusi, T, et al. 1985. "Bitterness Properties of Dandelion: II. Chemical Investigations." *Lebensm.-Wiss. Technol.* 18:347–49.

Kyi, KK, et al. 1977. "Hypotensive Property of *Plantago major* Linn." *Union Burma J. Life Sci.* 4(1):167–71.

La, VD, et al. 2010. "Active Principles of *Grindelia robusta* Exert Antiinflammatory Properties in a Macrophage Model." *Phytother. Res.* 24(11):1687–92.

Lacey, Laurie. 1993. *Micmac Medicines: Remedies and Recollections*. Halifax: Nimbus Publishing. 125pp.

Lambev, I, et al. 1981. "Study of the Anti-inflammatory and Capillary Restorative Activity of a Dispersed Substance from *Plantago major* L." *Probl. Vutr. Med.* 9:162–69.

Lamela, M, et al. 1985. "Effects of *Lythrum salicaria* in Normoglycemic Rats." *J. Ethnopharmacol.* 14(1):83–91.

Lamela, M, et al. 1986. "Effects of *Lythrum salicaria* Extracts on Hyperglycemic Rats and Mice." *J. Ethnopharmacol.* 15(2):153–60.

Landis, Robyn. 1997. *Herbal Defense: Positioning Yourself to Triumph over Illness and Aging*. New York: Warner Books. 562pp.

Lang, G, et al. 2001. "Non-Toxic Pyrrolizidine Alkaloids from *Eupatorium semialatum*." *Biochem. Syst. Ecol.* 29(2):143–47.

Lans, C, et al. 2007. "Ethnoveterinary Medicines Used to Treat Endoparasites and Stomach Problems in Pigs and Pets in British Columbia, Canada." *Vet. Parasitol.* 148(3–4):325–40.

Lapinina, LO, and Sisoeva, TF. 1964. "Investigation of Some Plants to Determine Their Sugar Lowering Action." *Farmatsevt. Zhurnal*. 19(4):52–58.

Lavoie, S, et al. 2017. "Chemical Composition and Anti-herpes Simplex Virus Type 1 (HSV-1) Activity of Extracts from *Cornus canadensis*." *BMC Complement. Altern. Med.* 17(1):123.

Law, Donald. 1976. *Herbs and Herbal Remedies*. London: Foyles Handbooks. 63pp.

Laws, OS. 1896. "Tincture of Mullein Flowers." *Calif. Med. J.* 17:174.

Lee, AS. 2012. "An Aqueous Extract of *Portulaca oleracea* Ameliorates Diabetic Nephropathy through Suppression of Renal Fibrosis and Inflammation in Diabetic db/db Mice." *Am. J. Chin. Med.* 40(3):495–510.

Lee, AS, et al. 2012a. "Anti-TNF-α Activity of *Portulaca oleracea* in Vascular Endothelial Cells." *Int. J. Mol. Sci.* 13(5):5628–44.

Lee, AS, et al. 2012b. "*Portulaca oleracea* Ameliorates Diabetic Vascular Inflammation and Endothelial Dysfunction in db/db Mice." *Evid. Based Complement. Altern. Med.* Epub 2012 Mar 1.

Lee, H, and Lin, JY. 1988. "Antimutagenic Activity of Extracts from Anticancer Drugs in Chinese Medicine." *Mutat. Res.* 204(2):229–34.

Lee, KH, et al. 1988. "The Cytotoxic Principles of *Prunella vulgaris*, *Psychotrial terpens*, and *Hyptis capitata*: Ursolic Acid and Related Derivatives." *Planta Med.* 54:308–11.

Legssyer, A, et al. 2002. "Cardiovascular Effects of *Urtica dioica* L. in Isolated Rat Heart and Aorta." *Phytother. Res.* 16(6):503–7.

Leighton, Anna. 1985. *Wild Plant Use by the Woods Cree (Nihithawak) of East-Central Saskatchewan*. Mercury Series, Canadian Ethnology Service Paper No. 101. Ottawa: Canadian Museum of Civilization. 128pp.

Lenfeld, J, et al. 1986. "Anti-inflammatory Activity of Extracts from *Conyza canadensis*." *Pharmazie*. 41(4):268–69.

Leonard, SS, et al. 2006. "Essiac Tea: Scavenging of Reactive Oxygen Species and Effects on DNA Damage." *J. Ethnopharmacol.* 103(2):288–96.

Lepore, Donald. 1988. *The Ultimate Healing System: Breakthrough in Nutrition, Kinesiology and Holistic Healing Techniques: Course Manual*. Provo, UT: Woodland Books. 402pp.

Lesuisse, D, et al. 1996. "Determination of Oenothein B as the Active 5-alpha-reductase-inhibiting Principle of the Folk Medicine *Epilobium parviflorum*." *J. Nat. Prod.* 59(5):490–92.

Leung, Albert Y. 1980. *Encyclopedia of Common Natural Ingredients Used in Food, Drugs, and Cosmetics*. New York: John Wiley and Sons. 409pp.

Leung, Albert Y, and Foster, Steven. 1996. *Encyclopedia of Common Natural Ingredients Used in Food, Drugs, and Cosmetics*. 2nd ed. New York: John Wiley and Sons. 688pp.

Leuschner, J. 1995. "Anti-inflammatory, Spasmolytic, and Diuretic Effects of a Commercially Available *Solidago gigantea* Herb Extract." *Arzneimittelforschung*. 45(2):165–68.

Leventhal, LJ, et al. 1993. "Treatment of Rheumatoid Arthritis with gamma-Linolenic Acid." *Ann. Intern. Med.* 119(9):867–73.

Lewis, Walter H, and Elvin-Lewis, Memory PF. 1977. *Medical Botany: Plants Affecting Man's Health*. New York: John Wiley Co. 515pp.

Lexa, A, et al. 1989. "Choleretic and Hepatoprotective Properties of *Eupatorium cannabinum* in the Rat." *Planta Med.* 55(2):127–32.

Li, H, et al. 2012. "Anti-mycobacterial Diynes from the Canadian Medicinal Plant *Aralia nudicaulis*." *J. Ethnopharmacol.* 140(1):141–44.

Li, H, et al. 2015. "Antimycobacterial Natural Products from Endophytes of the Medicinal Plant *Aralia nudicaulis*." *Nat. Prod. Commun.* 10(10):1641–42.

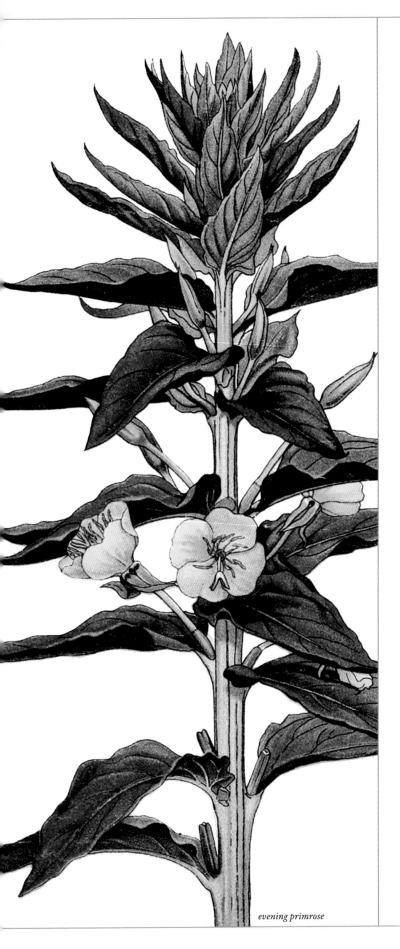

evening primrose

Li, XH, et al. 2017. "*Taraxacum mongolicum* Extract Induced Endoplasmic Reticulum Stress Associated Apoptosis in Triple-negative Breast Cancer Cells." *J. Ethnopharmacol.* 206:55–64. Epub 2017 Apr 28.

Lichius, JJ, and Muth, C. 1997. "The Inhibiting Effects of *Urtica dioica* Root Extracts on Experimentally Induced Prostatic Hyperplasia in the Mouse." *Planta Med.* 63(4):307–10.

Lichius, JJ, et al. 1999. "Antiproliferative Effect of a Polysaccharide Fraction of a 20%-methanolic Extract of Stinging-nettle Roots upon Epithelial Cells of the Human Prostate (LNCaP)." *Pharmazie.* 54(10):768–71.

Lin, CC, et al. 1996. "Anti-inflammatory and Radical-scavenge Effects of *Arctium lappa*." *Am. J. Chin. Med.* 24(2):127–37.

Lin, LT, et al. 2002. "*In vitro* Anti-hepatoma Activity of Fifteen Natural Medicines from Canada." *Phytother. Res.* 16(5):440–44.

Lin, YC, et al. 1972. "Search for Biologically Active Substances in Taiwan Medicinal Plants. I. Screening for Anti-tumor and Anti-microbial Substances." *Chin. J. Microbiol.* 5(1):76–81.

Linnaeus, C. 1829. *Vegetable Materia Medica.* In: Whitlaw, Charles. *Whitlaw's New Medical Discoveries, with a Defence of the Linnaean Doctrine and a Translation of His Vegetable Materia Medica.* London: Privately published. 2 vols in 1. 254pp.

Lipton, RA. 1958. "The Use of *Impatiens biflora* (Jewelweed) in the Treatment of *Rhus* Dermatitis." *Ann. Allergy.* 16(5):526–27.

List, Paul Heinz, and Hörhammer, Ludwig, eds. 1969–79. *Hager's Handbuch der Pharmazeutischen Praxis.* Berlin: Springer-Verlag. 6 vols.

Lithander, A. 1992. "Intracellular Fluid of Waybread (*Plantago major*) as a Prophylactic for Mammary Cancer in Mice." *Tumour Biol.* 13(3):138–41.

Liu, J, et al. 2001. "Evaluation of Estrogenic Activity of Plant Extracts for the Potential Treatment of Menopausal Symptoms." *J. Agric. Food Chem.* 49(5):2472–79.

Liu, K, et al. 2016. "3-beta-Erythrodiol Isolated from *Conyza canadensis* Inhibits MKN-45 Human Gastric Cancer Cell Proliferation by Inducing Apoptosis, Cell Cycle Arrest, DNA Fragmentation, ROS Generation and Reduces Tumor Weight and Volume in Mouse Xenograft Model." *Oncol. Rep.* 35(4):2328–38. Epub 2016 Feb 3.

Lloyd, John Uri. 1929. *Origin and History of All the Pharmacopeial Vegetable Drugs, Chemicals, and Preparations.* 8th & 9th Decennial Revisions. Vol 1. Cincinnati: Caxton Press, 1921; reprint, Cincinnati: Lloyd Library. 449pp.

Lloyd, John Uri, and Lloyd, Curtis Gates. 1930–31. *Drugs and Medicines of North America.* Cincinnati: J.U. and C.G. Lloyd, 1884–85; reprint, Lloyd Library Bulletin #29–31, Reproduction Series 9, Cincinnati: Lloyd Library. 2 vols. 299 + 162pp.

Locock, RA. 1965. "A Phytochemical Investigation of *Eupatorium* Species" [dissertation]. Ohio State University.

Locock, RA. 1990. "Boneset (Eupatorium)." *Canadian Pharm. J.* 123(5):229–33.

Long, D, et al. 1997. "Treatment of Poison Ivy/Oak Allergic Contact Dermatitis with an Extract of Jewelweed." *Am. J. Contact Dermat.* 8(3):150–53.

Long, X, and Tian, J. 1990. "Antifatigue and Anoxia-tolerating Effects of the Root of *Tragopogon porrifolius* L." [ET]. *Chung Kuo Chung Yao Tsa Chih.* 15(12):741–43, 765.

Lust, John. 1974. *The Herb Book.* New York: Bantam Books. 659pp.

Lytle, David. 1992. "Forgotten and Neglected American Medicinal Plants." In: Tierra, Michael, editor. *American Herbalism: Essays on Herbs and Herbalism by Members of the American Herbalists Guild.* Freedom, CA: Crossing. p. 100–107.

Mabey, Richard, et al, eds. 1988. *The New Age Herbalist: How to Use Herbs for Healing, Nutrition, Body Care, and Relaxation.* New York: Collier Books. 288pp.

MacFarlane, WV. 1963. "The Stinging Properties of *Laportea*." *Econ. Botany.* 17(4):303–11.

Mahady, GB, et al. 2003. "*In-vitro* Susceptibility of *Helicobacter pylori* to Isoquinoline Alkaloids from *Sanguinaria canadensis* and *Hydrastis canadensis*." *Phytother. Res.* 17(3):217–21.

Mahady, GB, et al. 2005. "*In-vitro* Susceptibility of *Helicobacter pylori* to Botanical Extracts Used Traditionally for the Treatment of Gastrointestinal Disorders." *Phytother. Res.* 19(11):988–91.

Mahdavi, S, et al. 2019. "The Antioxidant, Anticarcinogenic, and Antimicrobial Properties of *Verbascum thapsus* L." *Med. Chem.* Aug 28. Online ahead of print.

Makkar, MK, et al. 2018. "Evaluation of *Mentha arvensis* Essential Oil and Its Major Constituents for Fungotoxicity." *J. Food Sci. Technol.* 55(9):3840–44. Epub 2018 Jul 11.

Maksyutina, NP. 1971a. "Hydroxycinnamic Acids from *Plantago major* and *P. lanceolata*." *Khim Prir Soedin.* 7:824–25.

Maksyutina, NP. 1971b. "Hydroxycinnamic Acids of *Plantago major* and *Pl. lanceolata*." *Chem. Nat. Compd.* 7(6):795.

Maksyutina, NP, et al. 1978. "Chemical Composition and Hypocholesterolemic Action of Some Drugs from *Plantago major* Leaves. Part 1: Polyphenolic Compounds." *Farm Zh* (Kiev). 33(4):56–61.

Malagón, F, et al. 1997. "Antimalaric Effect of an Alcoholic Extract of *Artemisia ludoviciana mexicana* in a Rodent Malaria Model." *Parassitologia.* 39(1):3–7.

Malek, F, et al. 2004. "Bronchodilatory Effect of *Portulaca oleracea* in Airways of Asthmatic Patients." *J. Ethnopharmacol.* 93(1):57–62.

Malten, KE. 1983. "Chicory Dermatitis from September to April." *Contact Dermat.* 9(3):232.

Manning, David, Jason, Dan, and Jason, Nancy. 1972. *Some Useful Wild Plants for Nourishment and Healing.* Rev. ed. Vancouver, BC: Talonbooks. 174pp.

Manthorpe, R, et al. 1984. "Primary Sjögren's Syndrome Treated with Efamol/Efavit: A Double-blind Cross-over Investigation." *Rheumatol. Int.* 4(4):165–67.

March, Kathryn G, and March, Andrew L. 1986. *The Wild Plant Companion: A Fresh Understanding of Herbal Food and Medicine.* [Bailey, CO]: Meridian Hill Publications. 166pp.

Marker, RE. 1947. "Analysis of Trilliums, *Smilacina* and *Clintonia*." *J. Am. Chem. Soc.* 69:2242.

Marker, RE, et al. 1942. "Sterols. CXLVI. Sapogenins. LX. Some New Sources of Diosgenin." *J. Am. Chem. Soc.* 64:1283–85.

Marková, H, et al. 1997. "*Prunella vulgaris*: A Rediscovered Medicinal Plant." *Ceska Slov. Farm.* 46(2):58–63.

Martinez, G, et al. 1993. "Effect of the Alkaloid Derivative Ukrain in AIDS Patients with Kaposi's Sarcoma." *Int. Conf. AIDS.* 9(1):401.

Martins, WB, et al. 2016. "Neuroprotective Effect of *Portulaca oleracea* Extracts against 6 hydroxydopamine-induced Lesion of Dopaminergic Neurons." *An. Acad. Bras. Cienc.* 88(3):1439–50. Epub 2016 Aug 4.

Masaki, H, et al. 1995. "Active-oxygen Scavenging Activity of Plant Extracts." *Biol. Pharm. Bull.* 18(1):162–66.

Mascolo, N, et al. 1987. "Biological Screening of Italian Medicinal Plants for Anti-inflammatory Activity." *Phytother. Res.* 1(1):28–31.

Matev, M, et al. 1982. "Clinical Trial of *Plantago major* Preparation in the Treatment of Chronic Bronchitis" [ET]. *Vutr. Boles.* 21(2):133–37.

Matsumoto, T, et al. 2006. "Antiproliferative and Apoptotic Effects of Butyrolactone Lignans from *Arctium lappa* on Leukemic Cells." *Planta Med.* 72(3):276–78.

Mattson, Morris. 1841. *The American Vegetable Practice; or, A New and Improved Guide to Health, Designed for the Use of Families.* Boston: Daniel L. Hale. 2 vols. in 1. 592pp.

Mauriello, SM, and Bader, JD. 1988. "Six-month Effects of a Sanguinarine Dentifrice on Plaque and Gingivitis." *J. Periodontol.* 59(4):238–43.

Mayes, Vernon O, and Lacy, Barbara Bayless. 1989. *Nanise', A Navajo Herbal: One Hundred Plants from the Navajo Reservation.* Tsaile, AZ: Navajo Community College Press. 153pp.

McClintock, Walter. 1923. *Old Indian Trails.* Boston: Houghton Mifflin. 336pp.

McCutcheon, AR, et al. 1992. "Antibiotic Screening of Medicinal Plants of the British Columbian Native Peoples." *J. Ethnopharmacol.* 37(3):213–23.

McCutcheon, AR, et al. 1994. "Antifungal Screening of Medicinal Plants of British Columbian Native Peoples." *J. Ethnopharmacol.* 44(3):157–69.

McCutcheon, AR, et al. 1995. "Antiviral Screening of British Columbian Medicinal Plants." *J. Ethnopharmacol.* 49(2):101–10.

McDowell, A, et al. 2011. "Antioxidant Activity of Puha (*Sonchus oleraceus* L.) as Assessed by the Cellular Antioxidant Activity (CAA) Assay." *Phytother. Res.* 25(12):1876–82.

McIntyre, Anne. 1995. *The Complete Woman's Herbal: A Manual of Healing Herbs and Nutrition for Personal Well-Being and Family Care.* New York: Henry Holt and Co. 287pp.

McQuade-Crawford, Amanda. 1996. *The Herbal Menopause Book: Herbs, Nutrition, and Other Natural Therapies.* Freedom, CA: Crossing Press. 218pp.

McQuade-Crawford, Amanda. 1997. *Herbal Remedies for Women: Discover Nature's Wonderful Secrets Just for Women.* Rocklin, CA: Prima Publishing. 291pp.

Mechling, WH. 1959. "The Malecite Indians, with Notes on the Micmacs." *Anthropolog.* 8:239–63.

Medjakovic, S, and Jungbauer, A. 2008. "Red Clover Isoflavones Biochanin A and Formononetin Are Potent Ligands of the Human Artyl Hydrocarbon Receptor." *J. Steroid Biochem. Mol. Biol.* 108(1–2):171–77.

Medsger, Oliver Perry. 1972. *Edible Wild Plants.* New York: Collier Books. 323pp.

Medve, Richard J, and Medve, Mary Lee. 1990. *Edible Wild Plants of Pennsylvania and Neighboring States.* University Park: Pennsylvania State University Press. 242pp.

Mellanby, Alex, et al. 1996. *Evening Primrose Oil for Cyclical Mastalgia.* Development and Evaluation Committee Report 65. Southampton: Wessex Institute for Health Research and Development (WIHRD).

Melo, EA. 2002. "Evaluating the Efficiency of a Combination of *Pygeum africanum* and Stinging Nettle (*Urtica dioica*) Extracts in Treating Benign Prostatic Hyperplasia (BPH): Double-blind, Randomized, Placebo-controlled Trial." *Int. Braz. J. Urol.* 28(5):418–25.

Melzig, MF. 2004. "Goldenrod: A Classical Exponent in the Urological Phytotherapy" [ET]. *Wien. Med. Wochenschr.* 154(21–22):523–27.

Menke, K, et al. 2018. "*Taraxacum officinale* Extract Shows Antitumor Effects on Pediatric Cancer Cells and Enhance Mistletoe Therapy." *Complement. Ther. Med.* 40:158–64. Epub 2018 Mar 13.

Meral, I, and Kanter, M. 2003. "Effects of *Nigella sativa* L. and *Urtica dioica* L. on Selected Mineral Status and Hematological Values in CCl4-treated Rats." *Biol. Trace Elem. Res.* 96(1–3):263–70.

Merriam, C. Hart. 1966. "Ethnographic Notes on California Indian Tribes." Robert F Heizer, compiler and editor. Reports of the University of California Archaeological Survey, No. 68, Pt. 1. Berkeley: University of California Archaeological Research Facility. 175pp.

Messenger, W. 1992. "Common Smartweed: *Polygonum hydropiper*." *Coltsfoot.* 13:2–5.

Metzner, J, et al. 1984. "Antiphlogistic and Analgesic Effects of Leiocarposide, a Phenolic Bisglucoside of *Solidago virgaurea* L." *Pharmazie.* 39(12):869–70.

Micota, B, et al. 2014. "*Leonurus cardiaca* L. Herb: A Derived Extract and an Ursolic Acid as the Factors Affecting the Adhesion Capacity of *Staphylococcus aureus* in the Context of Infective Endocarditis." *Acta Biochim. Pol.* 61(2):385–88.

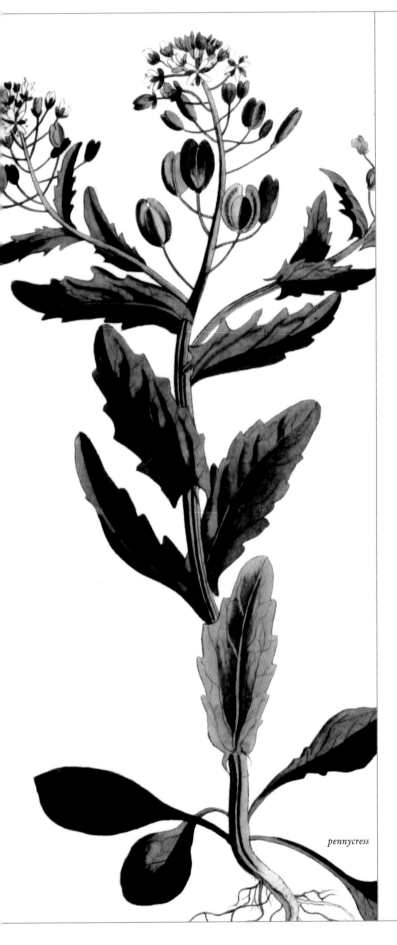

pennycress

Middleton, E Jr. 1988. "Plant Flavonoid Effects on Mammalian Cell Systems." In: Craker, Lyle E, and Simon, James E, editors. *Herbs, Spices, and Medicinal Plants: Recent Advances in Botany, Horticulture, and Pharmacology.* Phoenix: Oryx Press. 4 vols. 3:103–44.

Midge, MD, and Rama-Rao, AV. 1975. "Synthesis of Eupatilin & Eupafolin, the Two Cytotoxic Principles from the *Eupatorium* Species." *Indian J. Chem.* 13(6):541–42.

Miller, FM, and Chow, LM. 1954. "Alkaloids of *Achillea millefolium* L. I. Isolation and Characterization of Achilleine." *J. Am. Chem. Soc.* 76:1353–54.

Mills, Simon, and Bone, Kerry. 2000. *Principles and Practice of Phytotherapy: Modern Herbal Medicine.* Edinburgh: Churchill Livingstone. 643pp.

Millspaugh, Charles. 1974. *American Medicinal Plants.* Philadelphia: John C. Yorston, 1892; reprint, New York: Dover Publications. 806pp.

Min, BS, et al. 1999. "Inhibitory Constituents against HIV-1 Protease from *Agastache rugosa.*" *Arch. Pharm. Res.* 22(1):75–77.

Mitchell, WA Jr. 1998. "The Eclectic Therapeutic Categories: The Two Best Remedies in Each Category." In: *Medicines from the Earth: Phytomedicines, Their Expanding Role, 1998 Official Proceedings.* Brevard, NC: Gaia Herbal Research Institute. p. 90–92.

Mitchell, William A. Jr. 2003. *Plant Medicine in Practice: Using the Teachings of John Bastyr.* St. Louis, MO: Churchill Livingstone, 272pp.

Mittman, P. 1990. "Randomized, Double-blind Study of Freeze-dried *Urtica dioica* in the Treatment of Allergic Rhinitis." *Planta Med.* 56(1):44–47.

Miura, T, and Kato, A. 1995. "The Difference in Hypoglycemic Action between Polygonati Rhizoma and Polygonati officinalis Rhizoma." *Biol. Pharm. Bull.* 18(11):1605–6.

Miyazawa, M, and Kameoka, H. 1983. "Constituents of the Essential Oil from *Rumex crispus.*" *Yakagaku.* 32:45–47.

Mockle, JA. 1955. "Contributions a l'etude des plantes medicinales du Canada" [dissertation]. University of Paris.

Moerman, Daniel. 1986. *Medicinal Plants of Native America.* Technical Reports, No. 19. Ann Arbor: University of Michigan Museum of Anthropology. 2 vols. 912pp.

Moerman, Daniel E. 1977. *American Medical Ethnobotany: A Reference Dictionary.* New York: Garland Publishing. 527pp.

Moerman, DE. 1996. "An Analysis of the Food Plants and Drug Plants of Native North America." *J. Ethnopharmacol.* 52(1):1–22.

Moga, MM. 2003. "Alternative Treatment of Gallbladder Disease." *Med. Hypotheses.* 60(1):143–47.

Mohammadi, A, et al. 2016. "The Herbal Medicine *Utrica dioica* Inhibits Proliferation of Colorectal Cancer Cell Line by Inducing Apoptosis and Arrest at the G2/M Phase." *J. Gastrointest. Cancer.* 47(2):187–95.

Mooney, J. 1890. "Cherokee Theory and Practice of Medicine." *J. Am. Folklore.* 3:44–50.

Moore, Michael. 1979. *Medicinal Plants of the Mountain West.* Santa Fe: Museum of New Mexico Press. 200pp.

Moore, Michael. 1989. *Medicinal Plants of the Desert and Canyon West: A Guide to Identifying, Preparing, and Using Traditional Medicinal Plants Found in the Deserts and Canyons of the West and Southwest.* Santa Fe: Museum of New Mexico Press. 216pp.

Moore, Michael. 1993. *Medicinal Plants of the Pacific West.* Santa Fe, NM: Red Crane Books. 359pp.

Moore, Michael. 1994a. *Herbal Materia Medica.* 4th ed. Albuquerque, NM: Southwest School of Botanical Medicine. Unpaginated.

Moore, Michael. 1994b. *Herbal Repertory in Clinical Practice: A Manual of Differential Therapeutics for the Health Care Professional.* 3rd ed. Albuquerque, NM: Southwest School of Botanical Medicine. 36pp.

Morita, K, et al. 1984. "A Desmutagenic Factor Isolated from Burdock (*Arctium lappa* Linne.)." *Mutat. Res.* 129(1):25–31.

Morita, K, et al. 1985. "Chemical Nature of a Desmutagenic Factor from Burdock (*A. lappa* L.)." *Agric. Biol. Chem.* 49:925–32.

Morse, PF, et al. 1989. "Meta-analysis of Placebo-controlled Studies of the Efficacy of Epogram in Treatment of Atopic Eczema: Relationship between Plasma Essential-fatty-acid Changes and Response." *Br. J. Dermatol.* 121(1):75–90.

Morton, Julia. 1974. *Folk Remedies of the Low Country.* Miami: E. A. Seemann Publishing. 176pp.

Moskalenko, SA. 1986. "Preliminary Screening of Far-Eastern Ethnomedicinal Plants for Antibacterial Activity." *J. Ethnopharmacol.* 15(3):231–59.

Moss, Ralph. 1998. *Herbs against Cancer: History and Controversy.* Brooklyn, NY: Equinox Press. 300pp.

Motz, VA, et al. 2015. "Efficacy of the Saponin Component of *Impatiens capensis* Meerb. in Preventing Urushiol-induced Contact Dermatitis." *J. Ethnopharmacol.* 162:163–67. Epub 2014 Dec 24.

Mowrey, Daniel B. 1986. *The Scientific Validation of Herbal Medicine.* New Canaan, CT: Keats Publishing Co. 316pp.

Munson, PJ. 1981. "Contributions to Osage and Lakota Ethnobotany." *Plains Anthropol.* 26(93):229–40.

Murai, M, et al. 1995. "Phenylethanoids in the Herb of *Plantago lanceolata* and Inhibitory Effect on Arachidonic Acid-induced Mouse Ear Edema." *Planta Med.* 61(5):479–80.

Murray, Michael, and Pizzorno, Joseph. 1998. *The Encyclopedia of Natural Medicine.* Rocklin, CA: Prima Publishing. 946pp.

Naegele, Thomas A. 1980. *Edible and Medicinal Plants of the Great Lakes.* Calumet, MI: Thomas A. Naegele Survival Seminars. 427pp.

Naiman, Ingrid. 1999. *Cancer Salves: A Botanical Approach to Treatment.* Berkeley, CA: North Atlantic Books. 272pp.

Naji Ebrahimi Yazd, Z, et al. 2018. "Protection against Doxorubicin-induced Nephropathy by *Plantago major* in Rat." *Iran J. Kidney Dis.* 12(2):99–106.

Nalbantsoy, A, et al. 2013. "Viper Venom-induced Inflammation with *Montivipera xanthina* (Gray, 1849) and the Anti Snake-venom Activities of *Artemisia absinthium* L. in Rat." *Toxicon.* 65:34–40.

Namgung, S, et al. 2017. "*Prunella vulgaris* Attenuates Diabetic Renal Injury by Suppressing Glomerular Fibrosis and Inflammation." *Am. J. Chin. Med.* 45(3):475–95. Epub 2017 Mar 30.

Navarro, E, et al. 1994. "Diuretic Action of an Aqueous Extract of *Lepidium latifolium* L." *J. Ethnopharmacol.* 41(1–2):65–69.

Nazaruk, J, et al. 2008. "Polyphenolic Compounds and *in vitro* Antimicrobial and Antioxidant Activity of Aqueous Extracts from Leaves of Some *Cirsium* Species." *Nat. Prod. Res.* 22(18):1583–88. Epub 2008 Dec 15.

Neef, H, et al. 1996. "Platelet Anti-aggregating Activity of *Taraxacum officinale* Weber." *Phytother. Res.* 10:S138–40.

Nene, YL, and Kumar, K. 1966. "Antifungal Properties of *Erigeron linifolius* Willd. Extracts." *Naturwissenschaften.* 53(14):363.

Newall, Carol, et al. 1996. *Herbal Medicines: A Guide for Health-Care Professionals.* London: Pharmaceutical Press. 296pp.

Nguyen, C, et al. 2019. "Dandelion Root and Lemongrass Extracts Induce Apoptosis, Enhance Chemotherapeutic Efficacy, and Reduce Tumor Xenograft Growth *In Vivo* in Prostate Cancer." *Evid. Based Complement. Altern. Med.* 2019:2951428. eCollection 2019.

Nile, SH, et al. 2017. "Total Phenolics, Antioxidant, Antitumor, and Enzyme Inhibitory Activity of Indian Medicinal and Aromatic Plants Extracted with Different Extraction Methods." *3 Biotech.* 7(1):76. Epub 2017 Apr 27.

Noreen, S, et al. 2015. "*Portulaca oleracea* L. as a Prospective Candidate Inhibitor of Hepatitis C Virus NS3 Serine Protease." *Viral Immunol.* 28(5):282–89. Epub 2015 Apr 14.

North, Pamela. 1967. *Poisonous Plants and Fungi in Colour.* London: Pharmaceutical Society of Great Britain. 161pp.

Nuttall, Thomas. 1905. *A Journal of Travels into the Arkansas Territory during the Year 1819.* In: Thwaites, Reuben Gold, editor. *Early Western Travels.* Cleveland: Arthur H. Clark Co. p. 12.

Ockerman, PA, et al. 1986. "Evening Primrose Oil as a Treatment of Premenstrual Syndrome." *Rec. Adv. Clin. Nutr.* 2:404–5.

Ody, Penelope. 1993. *The Complete Medicinal Herbal.* New York: Dorling Kindersley. 192pp.

Oerter Klein, K, et al. 2003. "Estrogen Bioactivity in Fo-ti and Other Herbs Used for Their Estrogen-like Effects as Determined by a Recombinant Cell Bioassay." *J. Clin. Endocrinol. Metab.* 88:4077–79.

Oh, KB, et al. 2000. "Detection of Antifungal Activity in *Portulaca oleracea* by a Single-cell Bioassay System." *Phytother. Res.* 14(5):329–32.

Oh, SM, et al. 2015. "Ethanolic Extract of Dandelion (*Taraxacum Mongolicum*) Induces Estrogenic Activity in MCF-7 Cells and Immature Rats." *Chin. J. Nat. Med.* 13(11):808–14.

Ohigashi, H, et al. 1986. "Search for Possible Antitumor Promoters by Inhibition of 12-O-tetradecanoylphorbol-13-acetate-induced Epstein-Barr Virus Activation; Ursolic Acid, and Oleanolic Acid from an Anti-inflammatory Chinese Medicinal Plant, *Glechoma hederacea* L." *Cancer Lett.* 30(2):143–51.

Okpanyi, SN, et al. 1989. "Anti-inflammatory, Analgesic, and Antipyretic Effect of Various Plant Extracts and their Combinations in an Animal Model." *Arzneimittelforschung.* 39(6):698–703.

Okuda, T, et al. 1989. "Ellagitannins as Active Constituents of Medicinal Plants." *Planta Med.* 55(2):117–22.

Okuyama, E, et al. 1983. "Isolation and Identification of Ursolic Acid-Related Compounds as the Principles of *Glechoma hederacea* having an Anti-ulcerogenic Activity." *Shoyakugaku Zasshi.* 37(1):52–55.

Okwuasaba, F, et al. 1987a. "Comparison of the Skeletal Muscle Relaxant Properties of *Portulaca oleracea* Extracts with Dantholene Sodium and Methoxyverampil." *J. Ethnopharmacol.* 20(2):85–106.

Okwuasaba, F, et al. 1987b. "Investigations into the Mechanism of Action of Extracts of *Portulaca oleracea*." *J. Ethnopharmacol.* 21:91–97.

Oliver, F, et al. 1991. "Contact Urticaria Due to the Common Stinging Nettle *(Urtica dioica)*—Histological, Ultrastructural and Pharmacological Studies." *Clin. Exp. Dermatol.* 16(1):1–7.

Oliver-Bever, B, and Zahnd, GR. 1979–80. "Plants with Oral Hypoglycaemic Action." *Q. J. Crude Drug Res.* 17:139–96.

Oliver-Bever, Bep. 1986. *Medicinal Plants in Tropical West Africa.* Cambridge: Cambridge University Press. 366pp.

Olsen, Cynthia. 1996. *Essiac: A Native Herbal Cancer Remedy.* Pagosa Springs, CO: Kali Press. 129pp.

Omarbasha, B, et al. 1989. "Effect of Coumarin on the Normal Rat Prostate and on the R-3372H Prostatic Adenocarcinoma." *Cancer Res.* 49(11):3045–49.

Omer, B, et al. 2007. "Steroid-sparing Effect of Wormwood (*Artemisia absinthium*) in Crohn's Disease: A Double-blind, Placebo-controlled Study." *Phytomed.* 14(2–3):87–95.

Onuoha, NO, et al. 2017. "Tigernut (*Cyperus esculentus* L.) 'Milk' as a Potent 'Nutri-drink' for the Prevention of Acetaminophen-induced Hepatotoxicity in a Murine Model." *J. Intercult. Ethnopharmacol.* 6(3):290–95. eCollection 2017 Jul-Sep.

Orne, J. 1791. "Experiments Made with the Common Cow Parsnip in the Relief of Epilepsy." *Massachusetts Magazine.* 3:157.

Oswalt, WH. 1957. "A Western Eskimo Ethnobotany." *Anthropol. Pap. Univ. Alsk.* 6(1):17–36.

Ou, ZQ, et al. 2013. "Application of an Online Post-column Derivatization HPLC-DPPH Assay to Detect Compounds

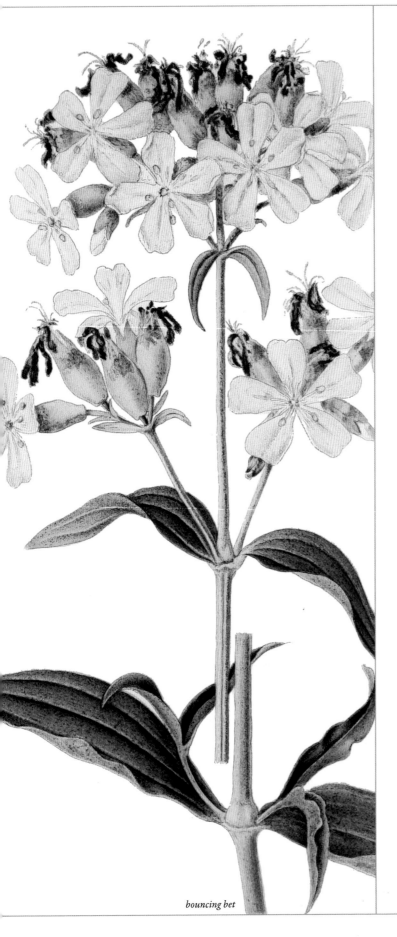

bouncing bet

Responsible for Antioxidant Activity in *Sonchus oleraceus* L. Leaf Extracts." *J. Pharm. Pharmacol.* 65(2):271–79.

Ovadje, P, et al. 2011. "Selective Induction of Apoptosis through Activation of Caspase-8 in Human Leukemia Cells (Jurkat) by Dandelion Root Extract." *J. Ethnopharmacol.* 133(1):86–91. Epub 2010 Sep 16.

Ovadje, P, et al. 2012. "Selective Induction of Apoptosis and Autophagy through Treatment with Dandelion Root Extract in Human Pancreatic Cancer Cells." *Pancreas.* 41(7):1039–47.

Ovadje, P, et al. 2016. "Dandelion Root Extract Affects Colorectal Cancer Proliferation and Survival through the Activation of Multiple Death Signalling Pathways." *Oncotarget.* 7(45):73080–100.

Overk, CR, et al. 2005. "Comparison of the *in-vitro* Estrogenic Activities of Compounds from Hops (*Humulus lupulus*) and Red Cover (*Trifolium pratense*)." *J. Agric. Food Chem.* 53(16):6246–53.

Ownbey, Gerald B, and Morley, Thomas. 1991. *Vascular Plants of Minnesota: A Checklist and Atlas.* Minneapolis: University of Minnesota. 307pp.

Ozaslan, M, et al. 2007. "*In-vivo* antitumoral Effect of *Plantago major* L. Extract on Balb/C Mouse with Ehrlich Ascites Tumor." *Am. J. Chin. Med.* 35(5):841–51.

Pahlow, Mannfried. 1993. *Healing Plants.* Hauppauge, NY: Barron's Educational Series. 224pp.

Palmer, E. 1878. "Plants Used by the Indians of the United States." *Am. Naturalist.* 12(10):593–606, 646–55.

Palmer, G. 1975. "Shuswap Indian Ethnobotany." *Syesis.* 8:29–81.

Palopoli, J, and Waxman, J. 1990. "Recurrent Aphthous Stomatitis and Vitamin B12 Deficiency." *South. Med. J.* 83:475–77.

Panicera, RJ, et al. 1990. "Acute Oxalate Poisoning Attributable to Ingestion of Curly Dock (*Rumex crispus*) in Sheep." *J. Am. Vet. Med. Assoc.* 196(12):1981–84.

Parhizgar, S, et al. 2016. "Renoprotective Effect of *Plantago major* against Nephrotoxicity and Oxidative Stress Induced by Cisplatin." *Iran J. Kidney Dis.* 10(4):182–88.

Park, SY, et al. 2007. "Induction of Apoptosis by Isothiocyanate Sulforaphane in Human Cervical Carcinoma HeLa and Hepatocarcinoma HepG2 Cells through Activation of Caspase-3." *Oncol. Rep.* 18(1):181–87.

Parke, Davis and Co. 1890. *Organic Materia Medica.* Detroit: Parke, Davis and Co. 301pp.

Parks, GF. 1909. "Capsella bursa-pastoris." *Ellingwood's Therapeutist.* 3(12):12.

Parry, O, et al. 1987a. "Preliminary Clinical Investigation into the Muscle-relaxant Actions of an Aqueous Extract of *Portulaca oleracea* Applied Topically." *J. Ethnopharmacol.* 21(1):99–106.

Parry, O. et al. 1987b. "Skeletal Muscle Relaxant Action of an Aqueous Extract of *Portulaca oleracea* in the Rat." *J. Ethnopharmacol.* 19(3):247–53.

Parry, O, et al. 1993. "The Skeletal-muscle-relaxant Action of *Portulaca oleracea*: Role of Potassium Ions." *J. Ethnopharmacol.* 40(3):187–94.

Pashby, NL, et al. 1981. "A Clinical Trial of Evening Primrose Oil in Mastalgia." *Br. J. Surg.* 68:801.

Patnaik, GK, et al. 1987. "Spasmolytic Activity of Angelicin: A Coumarin from *Heracleum thomsoni*." *Planta Med.* 53(6):517–20.

Pedersen, Mark. 1998. *Nutritional Herbology: A Reference Guide to Herbs.* Rev. ed. Warsaw, IN: Wendell W. Whitman Co. 336pp.

Peng, Y, et al. 1983. "65 Cases of Urinary-tract Infection Treated by Total Acid of *Achillea alpine*." *J. Tradit. Chin. Med.* 3(3):217–18.

Peredery, O, and Persinger, MA. 2004. "Herbal Treatment Following Post-seizure Induction in Rat by Lithium Pilocarpine: *Scutellaria lateriflora* (Skullcap), *Gelsemium sempervirens* (Gelsemium) and *Datura stramonium* (Jimson Weed) May Prevent Development of Spontaneous Seizures." *Phytother. Res.* 18(9):700–705.

Perkins, AE. 1929. "Colloquial Names of Maine Plants." *Torreya.* 29(6):149–51.

Perry, F. 1952. "Ethnobotany of the Indians in the Interior of British Columbia." *Mus. and Art Notes.* 2(2):36–43.

Peterson, CJ, and Coats, JR. 2011. "Catnip Essential Oil and Its Nepetalactone Isomers as Repellents for Mosquitoes." In: Paluch, Gretchen E, and Coats, Joel R, editors. *Recent Developments in Invertebrate Repellents.* Washington, DC: American Chemical Society. p. 59–65.

Peterson, W. 1851. "On *Eupatorium perfoliatum*." *Am. J. Pharm.* 17:206–10.

Phelan, JT, and Juardo, J. 1963a. "Chemosurgical Management of Carcinoma of the External Ear." *Surg. Gynecol. Obstet.* 117:244–46.

Phelan, JT, and Juardo, J. 1963b. "Chemosurgical Management of Carcinoma of the Nose." *Surg.* 53(3):310–14.

Phelan, JT, et al. 1962. "The Use of Mohs' Chemosurgery Technique in the Management of Superficial Cancers." *Surg. Gynecol. Obstet.* 114:25–30.

Phillips, Roger, and Foy, Nicky. 1990. *Herbs.* London: Pan Books. 192pp.

(Phytochem DB.) US Department of Agriculture, Agricultural Research Service. 1992–2020. Dr. Duke's Phytochemical and Ethnobotanical Databases. Web resource at: http://phytochem.nal.usda.gov/.

Pitkin, J. 2004. "Red-clover Isoflavones in Practice: A Clinician's View." *J. Br. Menopause Soc.* 10 Suppl 1:7–12.

Pledgie-Tracy, A, et al. 2007. "Sulforaphane Induces Cell Type-specific Apoptosis in Human Breast-cancer Cell Lines." *Mol. Cancer Ther.* 6(3):1013–21.

Pliny the Elder. 1938. *Natural History.* WHS Jones, translator. Cambridge, MA: Harvard University Press. 10 vols.

Ponce-Macotela, M, et al. 1994. "*In-vitro* Effect against Giardia of 14 Plant Extracts." *Rev. Invest. Clin.* 46(5):343–47.

Popowska, E, et al. 1975. "Cholekinetic and Choleretic Action of Radix Inulae, Radix Taraxaci and Herba Hyperici." *Acta Pol. Pharm.* 32(4):491–97.

Porcher, FP. 1849. "Report on the Indigenous Medicinal Plants of South Carolina." *Trans. Am. Med. Assoc.* 2:677–862.

Porcher, Francis Peyre. 1863. *Resources of the Southern Fields and Forests, Medical, Economical, and Agricultural, Being Also a Medical Botany of the Confederate States.* Charleston, NC: Evans and Cogswell. 601pp.

Porcher, Francis Peyre. 1869. *Resources of the Southern Fields and Forests, Medical, Economical, and Agricultural, Being Also a Medical Botany of the Southern States.* Rev. ed. Charleston, NC: Walker, Evans, and Cogswell. 733pp.

Porter, SR, et al. 1988. "Hematologic Status in Recurrent Aphthous Stomatitis Compared to Other Oral Disease." *Oral Surg. Oral Med. Oral Pathol.* 66:41–44.

Potterton, David, ed. 1983. *Culpeper's Color Herbal.* New York: Sterling Publishing Co. 224pp.

Prakash, AO. 1984. "Biological Evaluation of Some Medicinal Plant Extracts for Contraceptive Efficacy in Females." *Contracept. Deliv. Syst.* 5:9.

Puolakka J, et al. 1985. "Biochemical and Clinical Effects of Treating the Premenstrual Syndrome with Prostaglandin Synthesis Precursors." *J. Reprod. Med.* 30(3):149–53.

Puri, BK, and Martins, JG. 2014. "Which Polyunsaturated Fatty Acids Are Active in Children with Attention-deficit Hyperactivity Disorder Receiving PUFA Supplementation? A Fatty Acid Validated Meta-Regression Analysis of Randomized Controlled Trials." *Prostaglandins Leukot. Essent. Fatty Acids.* 90(5):179–89.

Pye, JK, et al. 1985. "Clinical Experience of Drug Treatment for Mastalgia." *Lancet.* 2:373–77.

Qayyum, R, et al. 2016. "Mechanisms Underlying the Antihypertensive Properties of *Urtica dioica*." *J. Transl. Med.* 14(1):254.

Qiao, Z, et al. 2012. "Anti-melanogenesis Effect of *Glechoma hederacea* L. Extract on B16 Murine Melanoma Cells." *Biosci. Biotechnol. Biochem.* 76(10):1877–83. Epub 2012 Oct 7.

Quinlan, MB, et al. 2002. "Ethnophysiology and Herbal Treatments of Intestinal Worms in Dominica, West Indies." *J. Ethnopharmacol.* 80(1):75–83.

Qu, Z, et al. 2017. "*Prunella vulgaris* L., an Edible and Medicinal Plant, Attenuates Scopolamine-induced Memory Impairment in Rats." *J. Agric. Food Chem.* 65(2):291–300. Epub 2017 Jan 3.

Rácz-Kotilla, E, et al. 1974. "The Action of *Taraxacum officinale* Extracts on the Body Weight and Diuresis of Laboratory Animals." *Planta Med.* 26(3):212–17.

Rafinesque, Constantine S. 1828–30. *Medical Flora, or Manual of the Medical Botany of the United States.* Philadelphia: Samuel C. Atkinson. 2 vols. 268 + 276pp.

Rahmat, LT, and Damon LE. 2018. "The Use of Natural Health Products Especially Papaya Leaf Extract and Dandelion Root Extract in Previously Untreated Chronic Myelomonocytic Leukemia." *Case Rep. Hematol.* 2018:7267920. eCollection 2018.

Ramm, S, and Hansen, C. 1995. "Brennessel-Extrakt bei Rheumatischen Beschwerden." *Dtsch. Apoth. Ztg.* 135(Suppl.):3–8.

Ramm, S, and Hansen, C. 1996. "Brennesselblatter-extrakt bei Arthrose und Rheumatoider Arthritis." *Therapiewoche.* 28:3–6.

Randall, C, et al. 1999. "Nettle Sting of *Urtica dioica* for Joint Pain—An Exploratory Study of This Complementary Therapy." *Complement. Ther. Med.* 7(3):126–31.

Randall, C, et al. 2000. "Randomized, Controlled Trial of Nettle Sting for Treatment of Base-of-thumb Pain." *J. R. Soc. Med.* 93(6):305–9.

Rani, N, et al. 2012. "Quality Assessment and Anti-obesity Activity of *Stellaria media*." *BMC Complement. Altern. Med.* 12:145.

Rao, KV, and Alvarez, FM. 1981. "Antibiotic Principle of *Eupatorium capillifolium*." *J. Nat. Prod.* 44(3):252–56.

Rashed, AN, et al. 2003. "Simple Evaluation of the Wound-healing Activity of a Crude Extract of *Portulaca oleracea* L. (Growing in Jordan) in Mus Musculus JVI-1." *J. Ethnopharmacol.* 88(2–3):131–36.

Rashidian, A, et al. 2017. "Anticonvulsant Effects of Aerial Parts of *Verbena officinalis* Extract in Mice: Involvement of Benzodiazepine and Opioid Receptors." *J. Evid. Based Complement. Altern. Med.* 22(4):632–36. Epub 2017 Jun 6.

Rashrash M, et al. 2017. "Prevalence and Predictors of Herbal Medicine Use Among Adults in the United States." *J. Patient Exp.* 4(3):108–13. doi: 10.1177/2374373517706612. Epub 2017 Jun 5.

Rauha, JP, et al. 2000. "Antimicrobial Effects of Finnish Plant Extracts Containing Flavonoids and Other Phenolic Compounds." *Int. J. Food Microbiol.* 56(1):3–12.

Ray, Verne F. 1933. *The Sanpoil and Nespelem: Salishan Peoples of Northeastern Washington.* University of Washington Publications in Anthropology, Vol. 5. Seattle: University of Washington Press. 237pp.

Raymond, M. 1945. "Notes ethnobotaniques sur les Tête-de-Boule de Manouan." *Études Ethnobotaniques Québécoises, Contributions de l'Institut Botanique l'Université de Montréal.* 55:113–35.

Reagan, AB. 1928. "Plants Used by the Bois Forte Chippewa (Ojibwa) Indians of Minnesota." *Wis. Archaeologist.* 7(4):230–48.

Regnier, FE, et al. 1967. "Studies on the Composition of the Essential Oils of Three *Nepeta* Species." *Phytochem.* 6(9):1281–89.

Rehman, G, et al. 2017. "Effect of Methanolic Extract of Dandelion Roots on Cancer Cell Lines and AMP-activated Protein Kinase Pathway." *Front. Pharmacol.* 8:875. eCollection 2017.

Reid, Daniel P. 1993. *Chinese Herbal Medicine.* Boston: Shambhala. 174pp.

Reig, R, et al. 1990. "Fatal Poisoning by *Rumex crispus*: (Curled Dock): Pathological Findings and Application of Scanning Electron Microscopy." *Vet. Hum. Toxicol.* 32(5):468–70.

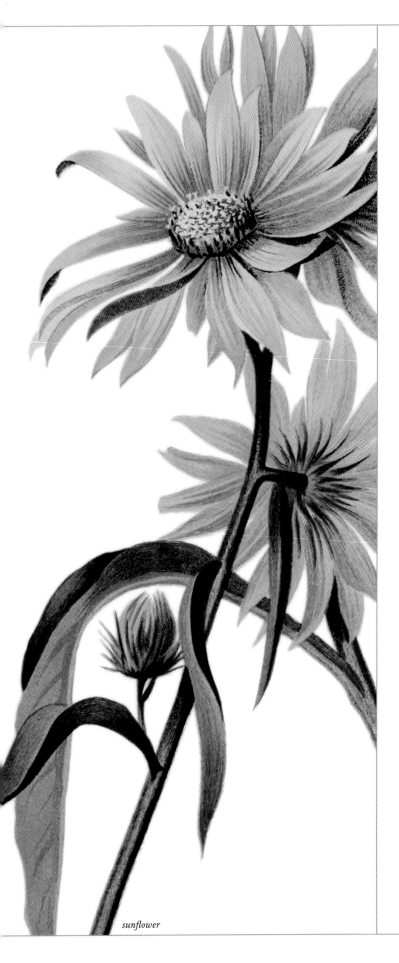

sunflower

Réthy, B, et al. 2007. "Antiproliferative Activity of Hungarian Asteraceae Species against Human Cancer Cell Lines. Part 1." *Phytother. Res.* 21(12):1200–1208.

Reynolds, James EF, ed. 1982. *Martindale: The Extra Pharmacopoeia.* 28th ed. London: Pharmaceutical Press. 2025pp.

Rice, KC, and Wilson, RS. 1976. "(-)-3-Isothujone, a Small Nonnitrogenous Molecule With Antinociceptive Activity in Mice." *J. Med. Chem.* 19(8):1054–57.

Richardson, Joan. 1981. *Wild Edible Plants of New England: A Field Guide, Including Poisonous Plants Often Encountered.* Jane Crosen, editor. Yarmouth, ME: DeLorme Publishing Co. 217pp.

Richardson, MA. 2001. "Assessment of Outcomes at Alternative Medicine Cancer Clinics: A Feasibility Study." *J. Altern. Complement. Med.* 7(1):19–32.

Richardson, MA, et al. 2000. "Flor-Essence Herbal Tonic Use in North America: A Profile of General Consumers and Cancer Patients." *HerbalGram.* 50:40–46.

Riehemann, B, et al. 1999. "Plant Extracts from *Urtica dioica*, an Antirheumatic Remedy, Inhibit Proinflammatory Transcription Factor NF-kappa." *FEBS Lett.* 442(1):89–94.

Ringbom, T, et al. 1998. "Ursolic Acid from *Plantago major*, a Selective Inhibitor of Cyclooxygenase-2 Catalyzed Prostaglandin Biosynthesis." *J. Nat. Prod. (Lloydia).* 61(10):1212–15.

Rinzler, Carol Ann. 1991. *The Complete Book of Herbs, Spices and Condiments: From Garden to Kitchen to Medicine Chest.* New York: Henry Holt and Co. 199pp.

Ritter, M, et al. 2010. "Cardiac and Electrophysiological Effects of Primary and Refined Extracts from *Leonurus cardiaca* L. (Ph. Eur.)." *Planta Med.* 76(6):572–82.

Rodriguez, P, et al. 1995. "Allergic Contact Dermatitis Due to Burdock (*Arctium lappa*)." *Contact Dermat.* 33(2):134–35.

Rogers, Carol. 1995. *The Women's Guide to Herbal Medicine.* London: Hamish Hamilton. 217pp.

Rogers, Dilwyn J. 1980. *Lakota Names and Traditional Uses of Native Plants by Sicangu (Brule) People in the Rosebud Area, South Dakota.* St. Francis, SD: Rosebud Educational Society. 112pp.

Rojas, G, et al. 2001. "Antimicrobial Evaluation of Certain Plants Used in Mexican Traditional Medicine for the Treatment of Respiratory Diseases." *J. Ethnopharmacol.* 74(1):97–101.

Romero, John Bruno. 1954. *The Botanical Lore of the California Indians.* New York: Vantage Press. 82pp.

Rousseau, J. 1945a. "Le folklore botanique de Caughnawaga: Etudes Ethnobotaniques quebecoises." *Contributions de l'Institut Botanique de l'Universite Montreal.* 55:7–74.

Rousseau, J. 1945b. "Le folklore botanique de l'Ile aux Coudres." *Contributions de l'Institut Botanique de l'Universite Montreal.* 55:75–111.

Rousseau, J. 1947. "Ethnobotanique Abenkaise." *Arch. Folklore.* 11:145–82.

Rücker, G, et al. 1991. "Antimalarial Activity of Some Natural Peroxides." *Planta Med.* 57(3):295–96.

Rumessen, JJ, et al. 1990. "Fructans of Jerusalem Artichokes: Intestinal Transport, Absorption, Fermentation, and Influence on Blood Glucose, Insulin, and C-peptide Responses in Healthy Subjects." *Am. J. Clin. Nutr.* 52(4):675–81.

Ryu, SY, et al. 2000. "Anti-allergic and Anti-inflammatory Triterpenes from the Herb of *Prunella vulgaris*." *Planta Med.* 66(4):358–60.

Sabudak, T, et al. 2017. "Investigation of Some Antibacterial and Antioxidant Properties of Wild *Cirsium vulgare* from Turkey." *Indian J. Pharm. Educ. and Res.* 51(3):S363–67.

Sadeghi, H, et al. 2014. "In vivo Anti-inflammatory Properties of Aerial Parts of *Nasturtium officinale*." *Pharm. Biol.* 52(2): 169–74. Epub 2013 Oct 25.

Sadowska, B, et al. 2019. "Molecular Mechanisms of *Leonurus cardiaca* L. Extract Activity in Prevention of Staphylococcal

Endocarditis: Study on in Vitro and ex Vivo Models." *Molecules.* 24(18): E3318.

Safarinejad, MR. 2005. "*Urtica dioica* for Treatment of Benign Prostatic Hyperplasia: A Prospective, Randomized, Double-blind, Placebo-controlled, Crossover Study." *J. Herb. Pharmacother.* 5(4):1–11.

Said-Fernández, S, et al. 2005. "In-vitro Antiprotozoal Activity of the Leaves of *Artemisia ludoviciana.*" Fitoterapia. 76(5):466–68.

Sakai, Saburo. 1963. "Pharmacological Actions of *Verbena officinalis* L." *Gifu Daigaku Igakubu Kiyo.* 11(1):6–17.

Salvucci, ME, et al. 1987. "Purification and Species Distribution of Rubisco Activase." *Plant Physiol.* 84(3):930–36.

Samec, V. 1961. ["Effect of *Lycopus* Extracts on Thyroid Metabolism and Autonomic Disorders"] (article in German). *Wien. Med. Wochenschr.* 111:513–16.

Samuelsen, AB. 2000. "The Traditional Uses, Chemical Constituents and Biological Activities of *Plantago major* L. A review." *J. Ethnopharmacol.* 71(1–2):1–21.

Sánchez, E, et al. 2010. "Extracts of Edible and Medicinal Plants Damage Membranes of *Vibrio cholerae.*" *Appl Environ Microbiol.* 76(20):6888–94.

Sankaran, J. 1977. "Livr-Doks in Viral Hepatitis." *The Antiseptic.* 74:621–26.

Santillo, Humbart. 1984. *Natural Healing with Herbs.* Subhuti Dharmananda, editor. Prescott Valley, AZ: Hohm Press. 370pp.

Sanyal, A, and Varma, KC. 1969. "*In-Vitro* Antibacterial and Antifungal Activity of *Mentha Arvensis* var. *Piperascens* Oil Obtained from Different Sources." *Indian J. Microbiol.* 9(1):23–24.

Saratale, RG, et al. 2018. "Bio-fabrication of Silver Nanoparticles Using the Leaf Extract of an Ancient Herbal Medicine, Dandelion (*Taraxacum officinale*), Evaluation of Their Antioxidant, Anticancer Potential, and Antimicrobial Activity Against Phytopathogens." *Environ. Sci. Pollut. Res. Int.* 25(11):10392–406.

Sarbhoy, AK, et al. 1978. "Efficacy of Some Essential Oils and Their Constituents on a Few Ubiquitous Molds." *Zentralbl. Bakteriol.* [Naturwiss]. 133(7–8):723–25.

Sarrell, EM, et al. 2001. "Efficacy of Naturopathic Extracts in the Management of Ear Pain Associated with Acute Otitis Media." *Arch. Pediatr. Adolesc. Med.* 155(7):796–99.

Sarrell, EM, et al. 2003. "Naturopathic Treatment of Ear Pain in Children." *Pediatr.* 111(5.1):e574–79.

Saxena, PR, et al. 1965. "Identification of Pharmacologically Active Substances in the Indian Stinging Nettle, *Urtica Parviflora* (Roxb.)." *Canadian J. Physiol. Pharmacol.* 43(6):869–76.

Sayyah, M, et al. 2005. "Anticonvulsant Activity of *Heracleum persicum* Seed." *J. Ethnopharmacol.* 98(1–2):209–11.

Schenck, SM, and Gifford, EW. 1952. "Karok Ethnobotany." *Anthropol. Records.* 13(6):389.

Schepetkin, IA, et al. 2009. "Immunomodulatory Activity of Oenothein B Isolated from *Epilobium angustifolium.*" *J. Immunol.* 183(10):6754–66.

Schneider, HJ, et al. 1995. "Treatment of Benign Prostatic Hyperplasia: Results of a Treatment Study with the Phytogenic Combination of Sabal Extract WS 1473 and Urtica Extract WS 1031 in Urologic Specialty Practices" [ET]. *Fortschr. Med.* 113(3):37–40.

Schofield Eaton, Janice J. 1989. *Discovering Wild Plants: Alaska, Western Canada, the Northwest.* Anchorage: Alaska Northwest Books. 354pp.

Schöttner, M, et al. 1997. "Lignans from the Roots of *Urtica dioica* and Their Metabolites Bind to Human Sex Hormone Binding Globulin (SHBG)." *Planta Med.* 63(6):529–32.

Schulte, KE, et al. 1967. "Polyacetylenes in Burdock Root." *Arzneimittel-Forschung.* 17(7):829–33.

Scott, Julian. 1990. *Natural Medicine for Children.* New York: Avon Books. 191pp.

Scudder, John Milton. 1870. *Specific Medication & Specific Medicines.* Cincinnati, OH: Wilstach, Baldwin, and Co. 253pp.

Scully, Virginia. 1970. *A Treasury of American Indian Herbs: Their Lore and Their Use for Food, Drugs, and Medicine.* New York: Crown Books. 306pp.

Selway, JWT. 1986. "Antiviral Activity of Flavones and Flavanes." In: Cody, Vivian, et al., editors. *Plant Flavonoids in Biology and Medicine: Biochemical, Pharmacological, and Structure-Activity Relationships.* New York: Alan R. Liss. p. 521–36.

Serkedjieva, J. 2000. "Combined Antiinfluenza Virus Activity of Flos Verbasci Infusion and Amantadine Derivatives." *Phytother. Res.* 14(7):571–74.

Serkedjieva, J, et al. 1990. "Antiviral Activity of the Infusion (SHS-174) from Flowers of *Sambucus nigra* L., Aerial Parts of *Hypericum perforatum* L., and Roots of *Saponaria officinalis* L. against Influenza and Herpes simplex Viruses." *Phytother. Res.* 4(3):97–100.

Serkedzhieva, I, et al. 1986. ["Antiviral Action of a Polyphenol Complex Isolated from the Medicinal Plant *Geranium sanguineum* L. II. Its Inactivating Action on the Influenza Virus"] (article in Bulgarian). *Acta Microbiol. Bulg.* 18:73–82.

Serkedzhieva, I, et al. 1987. ["Antiviral Action of a Polyphenol Complex Isolated from the Medicinal Plant *Geranium sanguineum* L. V. Mechanism of the Anti-influenza Effect *in vitro*"] (article in Bulgarian). *Acta Microbiol. Bulg.* 21:66–71.

Serkedzhieva, I, et al. 1988. ["Antiviral Action of a Polyphenol Complex Isolated from the Medicinal Plant *Geranium sanguineum* L. VI. Reproduction of the Influenza Virus Pretreated with the Polyphenol Complex"] (article in Bulgarian). *Acta Microbiol. Bulg.* 22:16–21.

Setzer, WN. 2018. "The Phytochemistry of Cherokee Aromatic Medicinal Plants." *Medicines* (Basel). 5(4):121.

Sévenet, T. 1991. "Looking for New Drugs: What Criteria?" *J. Ethnopharmacol.* 32(1–3):83–90.

Shafi, G, et al. 2012. "*Artemisia absinthium* (AA): A Novel Potential Complementary and Alternative Medicine for Breast Cancer." *Mol. Biol. Rep.* 39(7):7373–79.

Sharifi-Rad, M, et al. 2016. "Anti-methicillin-resistant Staphylococcus aureus (MRSA) Activity of Rubiaceae, Fabaceae, and Poaceae Plants: A Search for New Sources of Useful Alternative Antibacterials against MRSA Infections." *Cell. Mol. Biol.* (Noisy-le-grand). 62(9):39–45.

Sharma, H, et al. 2016. "Antifungal Efficacy of Three Medicinal Plants: *Glycyrrhiza glabra, Ficus religiosa,* and *Plantago major* against Oral *Candida albicans*: A Comparative Analysis." *Indian J. Dent. Res.* 27(4):433–36.

Sharma, N, and Jacob, D. 2001. "Antifertility Investigation and Toxicological Screening of the Petroleum Ether Extract of *Mentha arvensis* L. in Male Albino Mice." *J. Ethnopharmacol.* 75(1):5–12.

Sharma, N, and Jacob, D. 2002. "Assessment of Reversible Contraceptive Efficacy of Methanol Extract of *Mentha arvensis* L. Leaves in Male Albino Mice." *J. Ethnopharmacol.* 80(1):9–13.

Sharma, OP, et al. 1998. "A Review of the Toxicosis and Biological Properties of the Genus *Eupatorium.*" *Nat. Toxins.* 6(1):1–14.

Shemluck, M. 1982. "Medicinal and Other Uses of the *Compositae* by Indians in the United States and Canada." *J. Ethnopharmacol.* 5(13):303–58.

Shen, L, and Lu, FE. 2003. "Effects of Portulaca oleracea on Insulin Resistance in Rats with Type 2 Diabetes mellitus." *Chin. J. Integr. Med.* 9(4):289–92.

Sherry, CJ, and Hunter, PS. 1979. "The Effect of an Ethanolic Extract of Catnip (*Nepeta cataria*) on the Behavior of the Young Chick." *Experientia.* 35(2):237–38.

Sherry, CJ, and Koontz, JA. 1979. "Pharmacologic Studies of 'Catnip Tea': The Hot Water Extract of *Nepeta cataria.*" *Q. J. Crude Drug Res.* 17(2):68–72.

Sherry, CJ, and Mitchell, JP. 1983. "The Behavioral Effects of the 'Lactone-free' Hot Water Extract of Catnip (*Nepeta cataria*) on the Young Chick." *Int. J. Crude Drug Res.* 21(2):89–92.

Shi, G, et al. 2016. "Separation and Purification and in vitro Anti-proliferative Activity of Leukemia Cell K562 of *Galium aparine* L. Petroleum Ether Phase." *Saudi Pharm. J.* 24(3):241–44.

Shikov, AN, et al. 2011. "Effect of *Leonurus cardiaca* Oil Extract in Patients with Arterial Hypertension Accompanied by Anxiety and Sleep Disorders." *Phytother. Res.* 25(4):540–43.

Shim, KS, et al. 2017. "Water Extract of *Rumex crispus* Prevents Bone Loss by Inhibiting Osteoclastogenesis and Inducing Osteoblast Mineralization." *BMC Complement. Altern. Med.* 17(1):483.

Shin, S. 2004. "Essential Oil Compounds from *Agastache rugosa* as Antifungal Agents against *Trichophyton* Species." *Arch. Pharm. Res.* 27(3):295–99.

Shin, S, and Kang, CA. 2003. "Antifungal Activity of the Essential Oil of *Agastache rugosa* Kuntze and Its Synergism with Ketoconazole." *Lett. Appl. Microbiol.* 36(2):111–15.

Shin, TY, et al. 2001. "Inhibition of Immediate-type Allergic Reactions by *Prunella vulgaris* in a Murine Model." *Immunopharmacol. Immunotoxicol.* 23(3):423–35.

Shin, TY, et al. 2005. "Anti-allergic Effects of *Lycopus lucidus* on Mast Cell-mediated Allergy Model." *Toxicol. Appl. Pharmacol.* 209(3):255–62.

Shipochliev, T. 1981. "Uterotonic Action of Extracts from a Group of Medicinal Plants." *Vet. Med. Nauki.* 18(4):94–98.

Shipochliev, T, and Fournadjiev, G. 1984. "Spectrum of the Anti-inflammatory Effect of *Arctostaphylos uva-ursi* and *Achillea millefolium* L." *Prob. Vutr. Med.* 12:99–107.

Shipochliev, T, et al. 1981. "Anti-inflammatory Action of a Group of Plant Extracts" [ET]. *Vet. Med. Nauki.* 18(6):87–94.

Shirley, KP, et al. 2017. "In vitro Effects of *Plantago major* Extract, Aucubin, and Baicalein on *Candida albicans* Biofilm Formation, Metabolic Activity, and Cell Surface Hydrophobicity." *J. Prosthodont.* 26(6):508–15. Epub 2015 Nov 30.

Shook, Dr. Edward E. 1978. *Advanced Treatise in Herbology.* Beaumont, CA: Trinity Center Press. 360pp.

Siena, S, et al. 1989. "Activity of Monoclonal Antibody-Saporin-6 Conjugate against B-Lymphoma Cells." *Cancer Res.* 49:3328–32.

Sigstedt, SC, et al. 2008. "Evaluation of Aqueous Extracts of *Taraxacum officinale* on Growth and Invasion of Breast and Prostate Cancer Cells." *Int. J. Oncol.* 32(5):1085–90.

Silló, S, et al. 2014. ["Phytochemical and Antimicrobial Investigation of *Epilobium angustifolium* L."] (article in Hungarian). *Acta Pharm. Hung.* 84(3):105–10.

Silver, AA, and Krantz, JC. 1931. "The Effect of the Ingestion of Burdock Root on Normal and Diabetic Individuals: A Preliminary Report." *Ann. Intern. Med.* 5(3):274–84.

Silverman, Maida. 1990. *A City Herbal: A Guide to the Lore, Legend & Usefulness of 34 Plants that Grow Wild in the Cities, Suburbs & Country Places.* Boston: David R. Godine. 181pps.

Silverstein, Alvin, et al. 1990. *Lyme Disease, The Great Imitator: How to Prevent and Cure It.* Lebanon, NJ: Avstar Publishing. 104pp.

Sim, Stephen K. 1967. *Medicinal Plant Glycosides: An Introduction for Pharmacy Students.* Toronto: University of Toronto Press. 76pp.

Simon, JA, and Hudes, ES. 1999. "Relationship of Ascorbic Acid to Blood Lead Levels." *JAMA.* 281(24):2289–93.

Slagowska, A, et al. 1987. "Inhibition of Herpes Simplex Virus Replication by *Flos verbasci* Infusion." *Pol. J. Pharmacol. Pharm.* 39(1):55–61.

Smith, Ed. 1999. *Therapeutic Herb Manual.* Williams, OR: The author. 131pp.

Smith, GW. 1973. "Arctic Pharmacognosia." *Arct.* 26(4) (Dec):324–33.

Smith, HI. 1929. "Materia Medica of the Bella Coola and Neighboring Tribes of British Columbia." *Bulletin of the National Museum of Canada: Annual Report 1927.* 56:47–68.

Smith, HH. 1923. "Ethnobotany of the Menomini Indians." *Bull. Public Mus. City Milwaukee.* 4(1):1–174.

Smith, HH. 1928. "Ethnobotany of the Meskwaki Indians." *Bull. Public Mus. City Milwaukee.* 4(2):175–326.

Smith, HH. 1932. "Ethnobotany of the Ojibwe Indians." *Bull. Public Mus. City Milwaukee.* 4(3):327–525.

Smith, HH. 1933. "Ethnobotany of the Forest Potawatomi Indians." *Bull. Public Mus. City Milwaukee.* 7(1):1–230.

Smyk, GK, and Krivenko, VV. 1975. "*Potentilla alba* L: An Effective Agent for Treatment of Thyroid Disease" [ET]. *Farm. Zh.* 30(2):58–62.

Smythe, BB. 1903. "Preliminary List of Medicinal and Economic Kansas Plants." *Kansas Acad. Sci. Trans.* 18:191–209.

Sökeland, J, and Albrecht, J. 1997. "Combination of *Sabal* and *Urtica* Extract vs. Finasteride in Benign Prostatic Hyperplasia (Aiken Stages I to II). Comparison of Therapeutic Effectiveness in a One-year, Double-blind Study" [ET]. *Urologe A.* 36(4):327–33.

Soliman, SSM, et al. 2017. "Assessment of Herbal Drugs for Promising Anti-Candida Activity." *BMC Complement. Altern. Med.* 17(1):257.

Sonneland, J. 1972. "The 'Inoperable' Breast Carcinoma: A Successful Result Using Zinc Chloride Fixative." *Am. J. Surg.* 124(3):391–93.

Soranus. 1991. *Soranus' Gynecology.* Owsei Temkin, translator. Baltimore, MD: Johns Hopkins University Press. 258pp.

Spalding, Lyman. 1819. *History of the Introduction and Use of Scutellaria lateriflora, Scullcap, as a Remedy for Preventing and Curing Hydrophobia Occasioned by the Bite of Rabid Animals.* New York: Treadwell. 30pp.

Speck, FG. 1917. "Medicine Practices of the Northeastern Algonquians." In: *Proceedings of the 19ᵗʰ International Congress of Americanists, 1915.* Washington, DC: The congress. p. 303–21.

Speck, FG. 1937. "Catawba Medicines and Curative Practices." *Publications of the Phila. Anthropol. Soc.* 1:179–98.

Speck, FG. 1941. "A List of Plant Curatives Obtained from the Houma Indians of Louisiana." *Primitive Man.* 14(4):49–73.

Speck, FG, et al. 1942. "Rappahannock Herbals, Folk-lore and Science of Cures." *Proceedings Del. Cty. Inst. Sci.* 10:7–55.

Speck, Frank G. 1915. *The Nanticoke Community of Delaware.* New York: Museum of the American Indian, Heye Foundation. 88pp.

Spoerke, David G. 1990. *Herbal Medications.* Santa Barbara, CA: Woodbridge Press. 192pp.

Stanford, EE. 1927. "*Polygonum hydropiper* in Europe and North America." *Rhodora.* 29(341):77–87.

Stansbury, J. 1997. "Botanical Therapies for Fibrocystic Breast Disease." *Med. Herbal.* 9(2):1, 8–13.

Starý, František, and Jirásek, Václav. 1983. *Herbs: A Concise Guide in Color.* O Kuthanova, translator. London: Hamlyn. 238pp.

Steedman, Elsie V. 1928. "Ethnobotany of the Thompson Indians of British Columbia, Based on Field Notes by James A. Teit." *Bureau of American Ethnology Annual Report.* 45:441–522.

Steinmetz, EF. 1957. *Codex Vegetabilis.* Amsterdam: The author. Unpaginated.

Stevenson, Matilda C. 1915. "Ethnobotany of the Zuñi Indians." *Thirtieth Annual Report of the Bureau of American Ethnology, 1908–09.* Washington, DC: Government Printing Office. p. 31–102.

Stewart, Anne Marie, and Kronoff, Leon. 1975. *Eating from the Wild.* New York: Ballantine Books. 387pp.

Stewart, JCM, et al. 1991. "Treatment of Severe and Moderately Severe Atopic Dermatitis with Evening Primrose Oil (Epogram): A Multi-centre Study." *J. Nutr. Med.* 2:9–15.

Stickl, O. 1929. "Chemotherapeutische Versuche gegen das Ubertraghore Mausecarcinom." *Virchows Arch. Pathol. Anat.* 270:801–67.

Stolarczyk, M, et al. 2013a. "Extracts from *Epilobium* sp. Herbs Induce Apoptosis in Human Hormone-dependent Prostate Cancer Cells by Activating the Mitochondrial Pathway." *J. Pharm. Pharmacol.* 65(7):1044–54. Epub 2013 Apr 21.

Stolarczyk, M, et al. 2013b. "Extracts from *Epilobium* sp. Herbs, their Components and Gut Microbiota Metabolites of *Epilobium* Ellagitannins, Urolithins, Inhibit Hormone-dependent Prostate Cancer cells-(LNCaP) Proliferation and PSA Secretion." *Phytother. Res.* 27(12):1842–48. Epub 2013 Feb 25.

Stone, M, et al. 2009. "A Pilot Investigation into the Effect of Maca Supplementation on Physical Activity and Sexual Desire in Sportsmen." *J. Ethnopharmacol.* 126(3):574–76.

Strike, Sandra S, and Roeder, Emily D. 1994. *Ethnobotany of the California Indians. Vol. 2: Aboriginal Uses of California's Indigenous Plants.* Champaign, IL: Koeltz Scientific Books. 250pp.

Stripe, F, et al. 1987. "Hepatoxicity of Immunotoxins Made with Saporin, a Ribosome-inactivating Protein from *Saponaria officinalis.*" *Virchows Arch. B Cell Pathol.* 53(5):259–71.

Stuart, Malcolm, ed. 1982. *VNR Color Dictionary of Herbs and Herbalism.* New York: Van Nostrand Reinhold Co. 160pp.

Sultana, S, et al. 1995. "Crude Extracts of Hepatoprotective Plants, *Solanum nigra and Cichorium intybus,* Inhibit Free Radical-Mediated DNA Damage." *J. Ethnopharmacol.* 45(3):189–92.

Sun, HX, et al. 2005. "In-vitro and in-vivo Immunosuppressive Activity of Spica Prunellae Ethanol Extract on the Immune Responses in Mice." *J. Ethnopharmacol.* 101(1–3):31–36.

Sun, J, et al. 2005. "Anti-oxidative Stress Effects of Herba Leonuri on Ischemic Rat Hearts." *Life Sci.* 76(26):3043–56.

Susnik, F. 1982. "Present State of Knowledge of the Medicinal Plant *Taraxacum officinale* Weber." *Med. Razgledi.* 21:323–28.

Suter, Chester Merle., ed. 1951. *Medicinal Chemistry.* New York: John Wiley & Sons, Inc. 3 vols. 1200pp.

Swank, George R. 1932. "The Ethnobotany of the Acoma and Laguna Indians" [master's thesis]. University of New Mexico. 86pp.

Swanton, John Reed. 1928. "Religious Beliefs and Medical Practices of [the Kindscher] Creek Indians." *Forty-second Annual Report of the Bureau of American Ethnology, 1924–25.* Washington, DC: Government Printing Office. p. 473–900.

Szczawinski, Adam F, and Turner, Nancy J. 1980. *Edible Wild Plants of Canada.* Edible Wild Plants of Canada 4. Ottawa: National Museum of Natural Sciences, National Museums of Canada. 179pp.

Tabba, HD, et al. 1989. "Isolation, Purification, and Partial Characterization of Prunellin, an Anti-HIV Component, from Aqueous Extracts of *Prunella vulgaris.*" *Antivir. Res.* 11(5–6):263–73.

Tahri, A, et al. 2000. "Acute Diuretic, Natriuretic and Hypotensive Effects of a Continuous Perfusion of Aqueous Extract of *Urtica dioica* in the Rat." *J. Ethnopharmacol.* 73(1–2):95–100.

Tai, J, and Cheung, S. 2005. "In-vitro Culture Studies of FlorEssence on Human Tumor Cell Lines." *Phytother. Res.* 19(2):107–12.

Tai, J, et al. 2004. "In-vitro Comparison of Essiac and Flor-Essence on Human Tumor Cell Lines." *Oncol. Rep.* 11(2):471–76.

Takasaki, M, et al. 1999. "Anti-carcinogenic Activity of *Taraxacum* Plant." *Biol. Pharm. Bull.* 22(6):602–10.

Tantaquidgeon, Gladys. 1928. "Mohegan Medicinal Practices, Weather-lore, and Superstition." *Forty-third Annual Report of the Bureau of American Ethnology, 1925–1926.* Washington, DC: Government Printing Office. p. 264–79.

Tantaquidgeon, Gladys. 1942. *A Study of Delaware Indian Medicine Practice and Folk Beliefs.* Harrisburg: Pennsylvania Historical Commission. 91pp.

Tantaquidgeon, Gladys. 1972. *Folk Medicine of the Delaware and Related Algonkian Indians.* Harrisburg: Pennsylvania Historical and Museum Commission. 145pp.

Tarle, D. 1981. "Antibiotic Effect of Aucubin, Saponins and Extract of Plantain Leaf—Herba or Folium *Plantaginis lanceolata.*" *Farm. Glas.* 37:351–54.

Taylor, Lyda Averhill. 1940. *Plants Used as Curatives by Certain Southeastern Tribes.* Cambridge, MA: Botanical Museum of Harvard University. 88pp.

Tecce, R, et al. 1991. "Saporin 6 Conjugated to Monoclonal Antibody Selectively Kills Human Melanoma Cells." *Melanoma Res.* 1(2):115–23.

Teit, James A. 1928. "The Salishan Tribes of the Western Plateau." In: Boas, Franz, editor. *Forty-fifth Annual Report of the Bureau of American Ethnology.* Washington, DC: Government Printing Office. p. 23–396.

Testai, L, et al. 2002. "Cardiovascular Effects of *Urtica dioica* L. (Urticaceae) Roots Extracts: *In vitro* and *in vivo* Phamarcological Studies." *J. Ethnopharmacol.* 81(1):105–9.

Teugwa, CM, et al. 2013. "Antioxidant and Antidiabetic Profiles of Two African Medicinal Plants: *Picralima nitida* (Apocynaeceae) and *Sonchus oleraceus* (Asteraceae)." *BMC Complement. Altern. Med.* 13:175. Epub 2013 Jul 13.

Thayer, S. 2001. "The Milkweed Phenomenon: You Most Certainly Cannot Believe Everything You Read." *The Forager* 1(2):2–4.

Thomas, Richard. 1993. *The Essiac Report: The True Story of a Canadian Herbal Cancer Remedy and of the Thousands of Lives it Continues to Save.* Los Angeles: Alternative Treatment Information Network. 95pp.

Thomas, Rolla. 1907. *The Eclectic Practice of Medicine.* 2nd ed. Cincinnati, OH: Scudder Bros. 1033pp.

Thomé, RG, et al. 2012. "Evaluation of Healing Wound and Genotoxicity Potentials from Extracts Hydroalcoholic of *Plantago major* and *Siparuna guianensis.*" *Exp. Biol. Med.* (Maywood). 237(12):1379–86.

Thurston, EL. 1974. "Morphology, Fine Structure, and Ontogeny of the Stinging Emergence of *Urtica Dioica.*" *Am. J. Botany.* 61(8):809–17.

Thurston, EL, and Lursten, Nels R. 1969. "The Morphology and Toxicology of Plant Stinging Hairs." *Bot. Rev.* 35(4):393–412.

Tierra, Michael. 1988. *Planetary Herbology: An Integration of Western Herbs into the Traditional Chinese and Ayurvedic Systems.* Twin Lakes, WI: Lotus Press. 485pp.

Tierra, Michael. 1998. *The Way of Herbs.* New York: Pocket Books. 378pp.

Tierra, Michael, ed. 1992. *American Herbalism: Essays on Herbs & Herbalism by Members of the American Herbalists Guild.* Freedom, CA: Crossing Press. 321pp.

Tilgner, S. 1998. "Kidney Support." *Med. Herbal.* 10(3):1–16.

Tilgner, S. 2000. "Urinary Tract Health." *Herb. Transitions.* 5(2):1–12.

Tilgner, Sharol. 1999. *Herbal Medicine: From the Heart of the Earth.* Creswell, OR: Wise Acres Press. 384pp.

Tintera, J. 1959. "What You Should Know About Your Glands and Allergies." *Woman's Day.* February: 28–29, 92.

Tintera, JW. 1955. "The Hypoadrenocortical State and Its Management." *New York State J. Med.* 55(13):1869–76.

Tintera, JW. 1966. "Stabilizing Homeostasis in the Recovered Alcoholic through Endocrine Therapy: Evaluation of the Hypoglycemic Factor." *J. Am. Geriatr. Soc.* 14(7):126–50.

Tokuda, H, et al. 1986. "Inhibitory Effects of Ursolic Acid and Oleanolic Acid on Skin Tumor Promotion by 12-O-tetradecanolyphorbol-13-acetate." *Cancer Lett.* 33(3):279–85.

Torres, IC, and Suarez, JC. 1980. "A Preliminary Study of Hypoglycemic Activity of *Lythrum salicaria.*" *J. Nat. Prod.* 43(5):559–63.

Tozyo, T, et al. 1994. "Novel Antitumor Sesquiterpenoids in *Achillea millefolium.*" *Chem. Pharm. Bull.* 42(5):1096–1100.

Train, Percy, et al. 1988. *Medicinal Uses of Plants by Indian Tribes of Nevada.* Beltsville, MD: USDA, 1957. Rev. ed., Lawrence, MA: Quarterman Publications. 139pp.

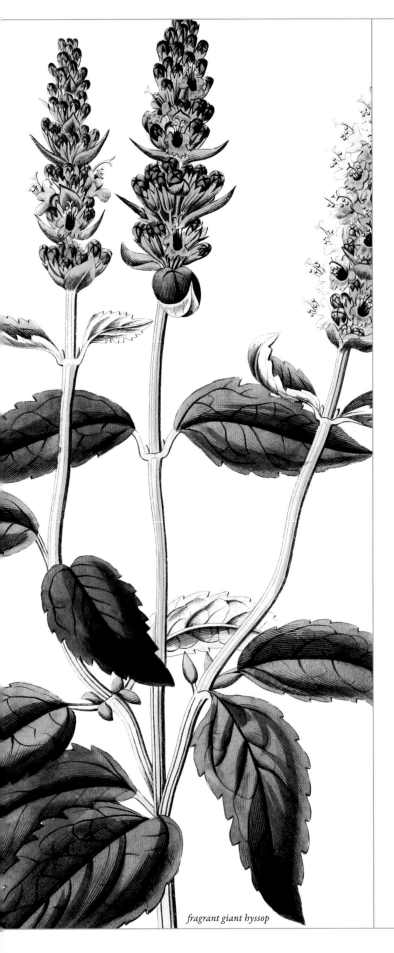

fragrant giant hyssop

Trease, George Edward, and William Charles Evans. 1957. *Pharmacognosy.* London: Baillière Tindall. 795pp.

Trease, George Edward, and William Charles Evans. 1973. *Pharmacognosy.* 10th ed. London: Baillière Tindall. 795pp.

Treasure, J. 2003. "Urtica Semen Reduces Serum Creatinine Levels." *J. Am. Herbal. Guild.* 4(2):22–25.

Truong, HKT, et al. 2019. "Evaluating the Potential of *Portulaca oleracea* L. for Parkinson's Disease Treatment Using a Drosophila Model with dUCH-Knockdown." *Parkinsons Dis.* Apr 18; 2019:1818259. eCollection 2019.

Tsuda, Y, and Marion, L. 1963. "The Alkaloids of *Eupatorium maculatum.*" *Canadian J. Chem.* 41(8):1919–23.

Tull, Delena. 1987. *Edible and Useful Plants of Texas and the Southwest, Including Recipes, Harmful Plants, Natural Dyes and Textile Fibers: A Practical Guide.* Austin: Texas Monthly Press. 400pp.

Tunón, H, et al. 1995. "Evaluation of Anti-inflammatory Activity of Some Swedish Medicinal Plants: Inhibition of Prostaglandin Synthesis and PAF-induced Exocytosis." *J. Ethnopharmacol.* 48(2):61–76.

Turner, Nancy J. 1975. *Food Plants of British Columbia Indians, Part I: Coastal Peoples.* British Columbia Provincial Handbooks 34. Victoria: British Columbia Provincial Museum. 264pp.

Turner, Nancy J, and Efrat, Barbara S. 1982. *Ethnobotany of the Hesquiat Indians of Vancouver Island.* Victoria: British Columbia Provincial Museum. 101pp.

Turner, Nancy J, and Szczawinski, Adam F. 1978. *Wild Coffee and Tea Substitutes of Canada.* Edible Wild Plants of Canada 2. Ottawa: National Museum of Natural Sciences, National Museums of Canada. 111pp.

Turner, Nancy J, et al. 1980. *Ethnobotany of the Okanagan-Colville Indians of British Columbia and Washington.* Victoria: British Columbia Provincial Museum. 110pp.

Turner, Nancy J, et al. 1983. *Ethnobotany of the Nitinaht Indians of Vancouver Island.* Victoria: British Columbia Provincial Museum. 165pp.

Turner, Nancy J, et al. 1990. *Thompson Ethnobotany: Knowledge and Usage of Plants by the Thompson Indians of British Columbia.* Victoria: Royal British Columbia Museum. 335pp.

Turner, NJ. 1973. "The Ethnobotany of the Bella Coola Indians of British Columbia." *Syesis.* 6:193–220.

Turner, NJ. 1981. "A Gift for the Taking: The Untapped Potential of Some Food Plants of North American Native Peoples." *Canadian J. Botany.* 59(11):2331–57.

Turner, NJ, and Bell, MAM. 1971. "The Ethnobotany of the Coast Salish Indians of Vancouver Island, I and II." *Econ. Botany.* 25(1):63–104, 335–39.

Turner, NJ, and Bell, MAM. 1973. "The Ethnobotany of the Southern Kwakiutl Indians of British Columbia." *Econ. Botany.* 27:257–310.

Tyler, Varro E. 1985. *Hoosier Home Remedies.* West Lafayette, IN: Purdue University Press. 212pp.

Tyler, Varro E. 1993. *The Honest Herbal: A Sensible Guide to the Use of Herbs and Related Remedies.* 3rd ed. New York: Pharmaceutical Products Press. 375pp.

Veres, K, et al. 2012. "Antifungal Activity and Composition of Essential Oils of *Conyza canadensis* Herbs and Roots." *ScientificWorldJournal.* 2012: 489646. Epub 2012 May 1.

Vermathen, M, and Glasl, H. 1993. "Effect of the Herb Extract of *Capsella bursa-pastoris* on Blood Coagulation." *Planta Med.* 59(Suppl.):A670.

Verzan-Petri, G, and Banh-Nhu. 1977. *Scienta Pharm.* 45, c. 24 [cited in Mabey, Richard, et al., eds. 1988].

Vestal, PA. 1952. "The Ethnobotany of the Ramah Navaho." *Pap. Peabody Mus. American Archaeol. Ethnol.* 40(4):1–94.

Vestal, Paul A, and Schultes, Richard Evans. 1939. *The Economic Botany of the Kiowa Indians.* Cambridge, MA: Botanical Museum of Harvard University. 110pp.

Viereck, Eleanor G. 1987. *Alaska's Wilderness Medicines: Healthful Plants of the Far North*. Edmonds, WA: Alaska Northwest Publishing Co. 108pp.

Vilela, FC, et al. 2009. "Evaluation of the Antinociceptive Activity of Extracts of *Sonchus oleraceus* L. in Mice." *J. Ethnopharmacol.* 124(2):306–10. Epub 2009 May 3.

Vilela, FC, et al. 2010a. "Antidepressant-like Activity of *Sonchus oleraceus* in Mouse Models of Immobility Tests." *J. Med. Food.* 13(1):219–22.

Vilela, FC, et al. 2010b. "Anti-inflammatory and Antipyretic Effects of *Sonchus oleraceus* in Rats." *J. Ethnopharmacol.* 127(3):737–41. Epub 2009 Dec 3.

Vincent, E, and Segonzac, G. 1948. "Higher Plants Having Antibiotic Properties." *Toulouse Medicale.* 49:669.

Vitalone, A, et al. 2001. "Anti-proliferative Effect on a Prostatic Epipthelial Cell Line (PZ-HPV-7) by *Epilobium angustifolium* L." *Farmaco.* 56(5–7):483–89.

Vitalone, A, et al. 2003. "Characterization of the Effect of Epilobium Extracts on Human Cell Proliferation." *Pharmacol.* 69(2):79–87.

Vogel, Virgil J. 1970. *American Indian Medicine*. Norman: University of Oklahoma Press. 585pp.

Vollmar, A, et al. 1986. "Immunologically Active Polysaccharides *Eupatorium cannabinum* and *Eupatorium perfoliatum*." *Phytochem.* 25(2):377–81.

Vonhoff, C. 2006. "Extract of *Lycopus europaeus* L. Reduces Cardiac Signs of Hyperthyroidism in Rats." *Life Sci.* 78(10):1063–70.

Vontobel, HP, et al. 1985. "Results of a Double-blind Study on the Effectiveness of ERU (Extractum Radicis Urticae) Capsules in Conservative Treatment of Benign Prostatic Hyperplasia" [ET]. *Urologe A.* 24(1):49–51.

Vuilleumier, BS. 1973. "The Genera of *Lactucaea* (*Compositae*) in the Southeastern United States." *J. Arnold Arboreum.* 54:42–93.

Wagner, H. 1988. "Non-Steroid, Cardioactive Plant Constituents." In: Wagner, Hildebert, et al., editors. *Economic and Medicinal Plant Research*. San Diego, CA: Academic Press. 5 vols. 2:17–38.

Wagner, H, and Jurcik, K. 1991. "Immunologic Studies of Plant Combination Preparations: *In Vitro* and *in Vivo* Studies on the Stimulation of Phagocytosis" [ET]. *Arzneimittelforschung.* 41(10):1072–76.

Wagner, H, and Proksch, A. 1985. "Immunostimulatory Drugs of Fungi & Higher Plants." In: Wagner, Hildebert, et al., editors. *Economic and Medicinal Plant Research*. New York: Academic Press. 6 vols. 1:113–53.

Wagner, H, et al. 1972. "Flavonol-3-Glycosides in Eight Eupatorium Species." *Phytochem.* 11:1504–5.

Wagner, H, et al. 1984. "Immunostimulant Action of Polysaccharides (heteroglycans) from Higher Plants. Preliminary Communication" [ET]. *Arzneimittelforschung.* 34(6):659–61.

Wagner, H, et al. 1985a. "Immunostimulating Action of Polysaccharides (Heteroglycans) from Higher Plants" [ET]. *Arzneimittelforschung.* 35(7):1069–75.

Wagner, H, et al. 1985b. "Immunstimulierend wirkende Polysaccharide (Heteroglykane) aus hoheren Pflanzen." *Arzneim.-Forsch./Drug Res.* 34(6):659–61.

Wagner, H, et al. 1985c. "*In-vitro* Phagozytose-Stimulierung durch isolierte Pflanzenstoffe gemessen im Phagozytose-Chemolumineszenz(CL)-Modell." *Planta Med.* 51(2):139–44.

Wagner, H, et al. 1989. "Biologically Active Compounds from the Aqueous Extract of *Urtica Dioica*." *Planta Med.* 55(5):452–54.

Wagner, H, et al. 1994. "Search for the Antiprostatic Principle of Stinging Nettle (*Urtica dioica*) Roots." *Phytomed.* 1(3):213–24.

Walters, Richard. 1993. *Options: The Alternative Cancer Therapy Book*. Garden City Park, NY: Avery Publishing Group, Inc. 396pp.

Wang, HK, et al. 1998. "Recent Advances in the Discovery and Development of Flavonoids and Their Analogous Antitumor and Anti-HIV Agents." *Adv. Exp. Med. Biol.* 439:191–225.

Wang, J, et al. 2006. "Anticancer Effect of Extracts from a North-American Medicinal Plant—Wild Sarsaparilla." *Anticancer Res.* 26(3A):2157–64.

Wang, Y, et al. 2008. "The Red Clover (*Trifolium pratense*) Isoflavone Biochanin A Inhibits Aromatase Activity and Expression." *Br. J. Nutr.* 99(2):303–10.

Ward-Harris, Joan. 1983. *More than Meets the Eye: The Life and Lore of Western Wildflowers*. Toronto: Oxford University Press. 242pp.

Webster, D, et al. 2008. "Antifungal Activity of Medicinal Plant Extracts: Preliminary Screening Studies." *J. Ethnopharmacol.* 115(1):140–46.

Weed, Susun S. 1986. *Wise Woman Herbal for the Childbearing Year*. Woodstock, NY: Ash Tree Publishing. 171pp.

Weiner, Michael. 1980. *Earth Medicine—Earth Food: Plant Remedies, Drugs, and Natural Foods of the North American Indians*. Rev. and expanded ed. New York: Collier Books. 230pp.

Weiner, Michael A. 1994. *Herbs that Heal: Prescription for Herbal Healing*. Mill Valley, CA: Quantum Books. 436pp.

Weiss, Rudolf Fritz. 1960. *Lehrbuch der Phytotherapie*. Stuttgart, Germany: Hippokrates-Verlag. 408pp.

Weiss, Rudolf Fritz. 1988. *Herbal Medicine*. AR Meuss, translator. Beaconsfield, UK: Beaconsfield Publishers. 362pp.

Weiss, Rudolf Fritz, and Fitnelmann, Volker. 2000. *Herbal Medicine*. 2nd ed., rev. and expanded. Stuttgart, Germany: Thieme. 438pp.

Westrich, LoLo. 1989. *California Herbal Remedies*. Houston, TX: Gulf Publishing Co. 180pp.

White, LA. 1945. "Notes on the Ethnobotany of the Keres." *Pap. Mich. Acad. Sci. Arts Lett.* 30:557–68.

Wigmore, Ann. 1985. *The Wheatgrass Book: How to Grow and Use Wheatgrass to Maximize Your Health and Vitality*. Wayne, NJ: Avery Publishing Group. 144pp.

Wilasrusmee, C, et al. 2002. "*In-vitro* Immunomodulatory Effects of Herbal Products." *Am. Surg.* 68(10):860–64.

Willard, Terry. 1991. *The Wild Rose Scientific Herbal*. Calgary, AB: Wild Rose College of Natural Healing. 416pp.

Willard, Terry. 1992a. *Edible and Medicinal Plants of the Rocky Mountains and Neighbouring Territories*. Calgary, AB: Wild Rose College of Natural Healing. 278pp.

Willard, Terry. 1992b. *Textbook of Advanced Herbology*. Calgary, AB: Wild Rose College of Natural Healing. 436pp.

Willard, Terry. 1993. *Textbook of Modern Herbology*. 2nd rev. ed. Calgary, AB: Wild Rose College of Natural Healing. 389pp.

Willard, Terry. 1994. *Herbology 101: Course Workbook*. Calgary, AB: Wild Rose College of Natural Healing.

Willer, F, and Wagner, H. 1990. "Immunologically Active Polysaccharides and Lectins from the Aqueous Extract of Urtica dioica" [ET]. *Planta Med.* 56(6):669.

Williams, CA, et al. 1996. "Flavonoids, Cinnamic Acids, and Coumarins from the Different Tissues and Medicinal Preparations of *Taraxacum officinale*." *Phytochem.* 42(1):121–27.

Willigmann, I, et al. 1991. "Occurrence of Omega-3 Fatty Acids in *Portulaca oleracea*." *Planta Med.* 57(Suppl. 2):A91.

Winder, W. 1846. "On Indian Diseases and Remedies." *Boston Med. Surg. J.* 34(1):10–13.

Winston, David. 1992. "Nvwote: Cherokee Medicine and Ethnobotany." In: Tierra, Michael, editor. *American Herbalism: Essays on Herbs & Herbalism by Members of the American Herbalists Guild*. Freedom, CA: Crossing Press. p. 86–89.

Winston, David. 1998. "Little-known, but Important, Herbal Medicines for the Pharmacy." Discourse given at: "Medicines from the Earth" herbal medicine convention, Black Mountain, NC.

Winston, David. 1999. *Herbal Therapeutics: Specific Indications for Herbs & Herbal Formulas*. 6th ed. Broadway, NJ: Herbal Therapeutics Research Library. 55pp.

Winterhoff, H, et al. 1988. "On the Antigonadotropic Activity of *Lithospermum* and *Lycopus* species and Some of Their Phenolic Constituents." *Planta Med.* 54(2):101–6.

Winterhoff, H, et al. 1994. "Endocrine Effects of *Lycopus europaeus* L. Following Oral Application." *Arzneimittelforschung.* 44(1):41–45.

Woerdenbag, HJ. 1986. "*Eupatorium cannabinum* L.: A Review Emphasizing the Sesquiterpene Lactones and Their Biological Activity." *Pharm. Weekbl. Sci.* 8(5):245–51.

Woerdenbag, HJ. 1993. "*Eupatorium* Species." In: de Smet, Peter AGM, et al., editors. *Adverse Effects of Herbal Drugs.* Berlin: Springer Verlag. 2 vols. 2:171–94.

Wojcikowski, K, et al. 2004. "Medicinal Herbal Extracts—Renal Friend or Foe? Part Two: Herbal Extracts with Potential Renal Benefits." *Nephrol.* (Carlton). 9(6):400–405.

Wojtyniak, K, et al. 2013. "*Leonurus cardiaca* L. (Motherwort): A Review of Its Phytochemistry and Pharmacology." *Phytother. Res.* 27(8):1115–20. Epub 2012 Oct 8.

Wolfson, P, and Hoffmann, DL. 2003. "An Investigation into the Efficacy of *Scutellaria lateriflora* in Healthy Volunteers." *Altern. Ther. Health Med.* 9(2):74–78.

Wood, George P, and Ruddock, EH. 1925. *Vitalogy, or Encyclopedia of Health and Home, Adapted for Family Use.* Chicago: Vitalogy Assn. 971pp.

Wood, Horatio, et al. 1926. *The Dispensatory of the United States of America.* 21ˢᵗ ed. Philadelphia: J. B. Lippincott Co. 1792pp.

Wood, Matthew. 1997. *The Book of Herbal Wisdom.* Berkeley, CA: North Atlantic Books. 580pp.

Woodward, Lucia. 1985. *Poisonous Plants: A Color Field Guide.* New York: Hippocrene Books. 192pp.

Wray, D, et al. 1978. "Nutritional Deficiencies in Recurrent Aphthae." *J. Oral Pathol.* 7(6):418–23.

Wren, RC. 1972. *Potter's New Cyclopaedia of Medicinal Herbs and Preparations.* Edited and enlarged, R. W. Wren. New York: Harper/Colophon Books. 400pp.

Wren, RC. 1988. *Potter's New Cyclopaedia of Botanical Drugs and Preparations.* Rewritten Elizabeth M. Williamson and Fred J. Evans. London: Saffron Walden; New York: C. W. Daniel Co. 400pp.

Wright, IM. 1999. "Neonatal Effects of Maternal Consumption of Blue Cohosh." *J. Pediatr.* 134(3):384–85.

Wright, S, and Burton, JL. 1982. "Oral Evening-Primrose-Seed Oil Improves Atopic Eczema." *Lancet.* 320(8308):1120–22.

Wunderlin, RP, and Lockey, RF. 1988. "Questions and Answers." *JAMA* 260: 3064–65.

Wyman, Leland C, and Harris, Stuart K. 1951. *The Ethnobotany of the Kayenta Navaho: An Analysis of the John and Louisa Wetherill Ethnobotanical Collection.* University of New Mexico Publications in Biology 5. Albuquerque: University of New Mexico Press. 66pp.

Xia, DZ, et al. 2011. "Antioxidant and Antibacterial Activity of Six Edible Wild Plants (*Sonchus* spp.) in China." *Nat. Prod. Res.* 25(20):1893–1901.

Xia, YX. 1983. "The Inhibitory Effect of Motherwort Extract on Pulsating Myocardial Cells *in vitro.*" *J. Trad. Chin. Med.* 3(3):185–88.

Xia, Z, et al. 2010. "Sesquiterpene Lactones from *Sonchus arvensis* L. and Their Antibacterial Activity against *Streptococcus mutans* ATCC 25175." *Fitoterapia.* 81(5):424–28.

Xu, HX, et al. 1999. "Isolation and Characterization of an Anti-HSV Polysaccharide from *Prunella vulgaris.*" *Antivir. Res.* 44(1):43–54.

Yaeesh S, et al. 2006. "Studies on Hepatoprotective, Antispasmodic and Calcium-antagonist Activities of the Aqueous-methanol Extract of *Achillea millefolium.*" *Phytother. Res.* 20(7):546–51.

Yaginuma, T, et al. 1982. ["Effect of Traditional Herbal Medicine on Serum Testosterone Levels and Its Induction of Regular Ovulation in Hyperandrogenic and Oligomenorrheic Women"] (article in Japanese). *Nihon Sanka Fujinka Gakkai Zasshi.* 34(7):939–44.

Yamasaki, K, et al. 1993. "Screening Test of Crude Drug Extract on Anti-HIV Activity" [ET]. *Yakugaku Zasshi.* 113(11):818–24.

Yamasaki, K, et al. 1996. "Anti-HIV-1 Activity of *Labiatae* Plants, Especially Aromatic Plants." *Int. Conf. AIDS.* 11(1):65, Abstract Mo.A.1062.

Yamasaki, K, et al. 1998. "Anti-HIV-1 Activity of Herbs in Labiatae." *Biol. Pharm. Bull.* 21(8):829–33.

Yamashita, K, et al. 1984. "Effects of Fructooligosaccharides on Blood Glucose and Serum Lipids in Diabetic Subjects." *Nutr. Res.* 4:961–66.

Yanchi, Liu. 1995. *The Essential Book of Traditional Chinese Medicine. Volume 2: Clinical Practice.* New York: Columbia University Press. 479pp.

Yang, Y, et al. 2012. "In vitro and in vivo Anti-Inflammatory Activities of *Polygonum hydropiper* Methanol Extract." *J. Ethnopharmacol.* 139(2):616–25.

Yang, Y, et al. 2017. "A Cell-based High-throughput Protocol to Screen Entry Inhibitors of Highly Pathogenic Viruses with Traditional Chinese Medicines." *J. Med. Virol.* 89(5):908–16. Epub 2016 Oct 14.

Yanovsky, Elias. 1936. *Food Plants of the North American Indians.* USDA Miscellaneous Publication 237. Washington, DC: Government Printing Office; reprint, New York: Gordon Press. 84pp.

Yao, XJ, et al. 1992. "Mechanism of Inhibition of HIV-1 Infection *in vitro* by Purified Extract of *Prunella vulgaris.*" *Virology.* 187(1):56–62.

Yearsley, C. 2020. "American Herbal Pharmacopoeia Publishes Boneset Monograph and Therapeutic Compendium." *HerbalGram.* 125:26–28.

Yeung, HW, et al. 1977. "The Structure and Biological Effect of Leonurine, a Uterotonic Principle from the Chinese Drug, I-mu Ts'ao." *Planta Med.* 31(1):51–56.

Yin, MH, et al. 2005. "Screening of Vasorelaxant Activity of Some Medicinal Plants Used in Oriental Medicines." *J. Ethnopharmacol.* 99(1):113–17.

Yoshikawa, M, et al. 1996. "Medicinal Foodstuffs. II. On the Bioactive Constituents of the Tuber of *Sagittaria trifolia* L. (Kuwai, Alismataceae): Absolute Stereostructures of Trifoliones A, B, C, and D, Sagittariosides A and B, and Arabinothalictroside." *Chem. Pharm. Bull.* (Tokyo). 44(3):492–99.

Young, Kay. 1993. *Wild Seasons: Gathering and Cooking Wild Plants of the Great Plains.* Lincoln: University of Nebraska Press. 318pp.

Youngken, Heber W. 1948. *A Text Book of Pharmacognosy.* 6ᵗʰ ed. Philadelphia: Blakiston Publishing Co. 1063pp.

Youngken, HW. 1924. "The Drugs of the North American Indian." *Am. J. Pharm.* 96:485–502.

Youngken, HW. 1925. "The Drugs of the North American Indian II." *Am. J. Pharm.* 97:158–85, 257–71.

Zafar, MM, et al. 1990. "Screening of *Artemisia absinthium* for Antimalarial Effects on *Plasmodium berghei* in Mice: A Preliminary Report." *J. Ethnopharmacol.* 30(2):223–26.

Zafar, R, and Ali, SM. 1998. "Anti-hepatoxic Effects of Root and Root Callus Extracts of *Cichorium intybus.*" *J. Ethnopharmacol.* 63(3):227–31.

Zenico, T, et al. 2009. "Subjective Effects of *Lepidium meyenii* (Maca) Extract on Well-being and Sexual Performances in Patients with Mild Erectile Dysfunction: A Randomised, Double-blind Clinical Trial." *Andrologia.* 41(2):95–99.

Zennie, TM, and Ogzewalla, CD. 1977. "Ascorbic Acid and Vitamin A Content of Edible Wild Plants of Ohio and Kentucky." *Econ. Botany.* 31(1):76–79.

Zevin, Igor Vilevich. 1997. *A Russian Herbal: Traditional Remedies for Health and Healing.* Rochester, VT. Healing Arts Press 250pp.

Zgórniak-Nowosielska, I, et al. 1991. "Antiviral Activity of *Flos verbasci* Infusion against Influenza and Herpes simplex Viruses." *Arch. Immunol. Ther. Exp.* 39(1–2):103–8.

Zhang, CF, et al. 1982. "Studies on Actions of Extract of Motherwort." *J. Tradit. Chin. Med.* 2(4):267–70.

Zhang, RH, et al. 2018. "Phytochemistry and Pharmacology of the Genus Leonurus: The Herb to Benefit the Mothers and More." *Phytochem.* 147:167-83. Epub 2018 Jan 12.

Zhang, Y, et al. 2007. "Chemical Properties, Mode of Action, and in-vivo Anti-herpes Activities of a Lignin Carbohydrate Complex from *Prunella vulgaris.*" *Antivir. Res.* 75(3):242–49.

Zhang, Z, et al. 2009. "Characterization of Chemical Ingredients and Anticonvulsant Activity of American Skullcap (*Scutellaria lateriflora*)." *Phytomed.* 16(5):485–93.

Zhao, P, et al. 2018. "The Genus *Polygonatum*: A Review of Ethnopharmacology, Phytochemistry, and Pharmacology." *J. Ethnopharmacol.* 214:274–91. Epub 2017 Dec 12.

Zhao, XL, et al. 1987. "A Comparative Study on the Pyrrolizidine Alkaloid Content and Pattern of Hepatic Pyrrolic Metabolite Accumulation in Mice Given Extracts of *Eupatorium* Plant Species, *Crotalaria assamica*, and Indian Herbal Mixture." *Am. J. Chin. Med.* 15(1–2):59–67.

Zheng, BL. 2000. "Effect of a Lipid Extract from *Lepidium meyenii* on Sexual Behavior in Mice and Rats." *Urol.* 55(4):598–602.

Zheng, M. 1990. "Experimental Study of 472 Herbs with Antiviral Action against the Herpes Simplex Virus" [ET]. *Zhong Xi Yi Jie He Za Zhi.* 10(1):39–41.

Zheng, Y, et al. 2019. "Synergistic Action of *Erigeron annuus* L. Pers and *Borago officinalis* L. Enhances Anti-obesity Activity in a Mouse Model of Diet-induced Obesity." *Nutr. Res.* 69:58–66. Epub 2019 Jul 30.

Zhu, H, et al. 2017. "Dandelion Root Extract Suppressed Gastric Cancer Cells Proliferation and Migration through Targeting lncRNA-CCAT1." *Biomed. Pharmacother.* 93:1010–17. Epub 2017 Jul 14.

Zigmond, Maurice. 1981. *Kawaiisu Ethnobotany.* Salt Lake City: University of Utah Press. 293pp.

Ziyin, Shen, and Zelin, Chen. 1996. *The Basis of Traditional Chinese Medicine.* Boston: Shambala. 244pp.

Zomorodian, K, et al. 2013. "Chemical Composition and Antimicrobial Activities of Essential Oil of *Nepeta cataria* L. against Common Causes of Oral Infections." *J. Dent* (Tehran). 10(4):329–37. Epub 2013 May 31.

Zou, QZ, et al. 1989. "Effect of Motherwort on Blood Hyperviscosity." *Am. J. Chin. Med.* 17(1–2):65–70.

Zubair, M, et al. 2012. "Effects of *Plantago major* L. Leaf Extracts on Oral Epithelial Cells in a Scratch Assay." *J. Ethnopharmacol.* 141(3):825–30.

Zubair, M, et al. 2016. "Promotion of Wound Healing by *Plantago major* L. Leaf Extracts: Ex Vivo Experiments Confirm Experiences from Traditional Medicines." *Nat. Prod. Res.* 30(5):622–24.

Zubair, M, et al. 2018. "Water and Ethanol Extracts of *Plantago major* Leaves Show Anti-inflammatory Activity on Oral Epithelial Cells." *J. Tradit. Complement. Med.* 9(3):169–71.

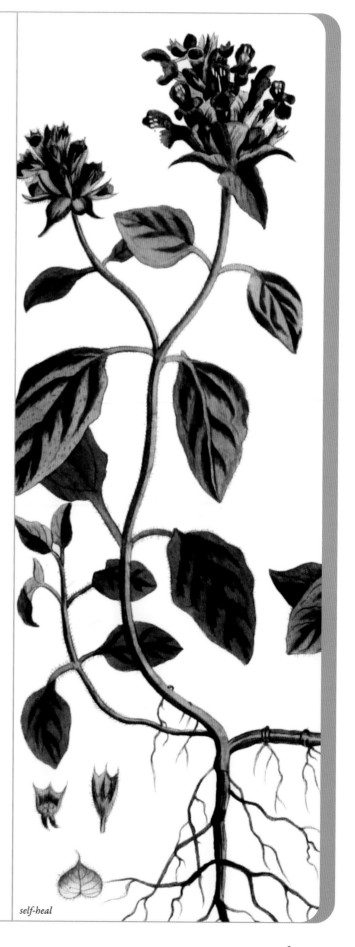

self-heal

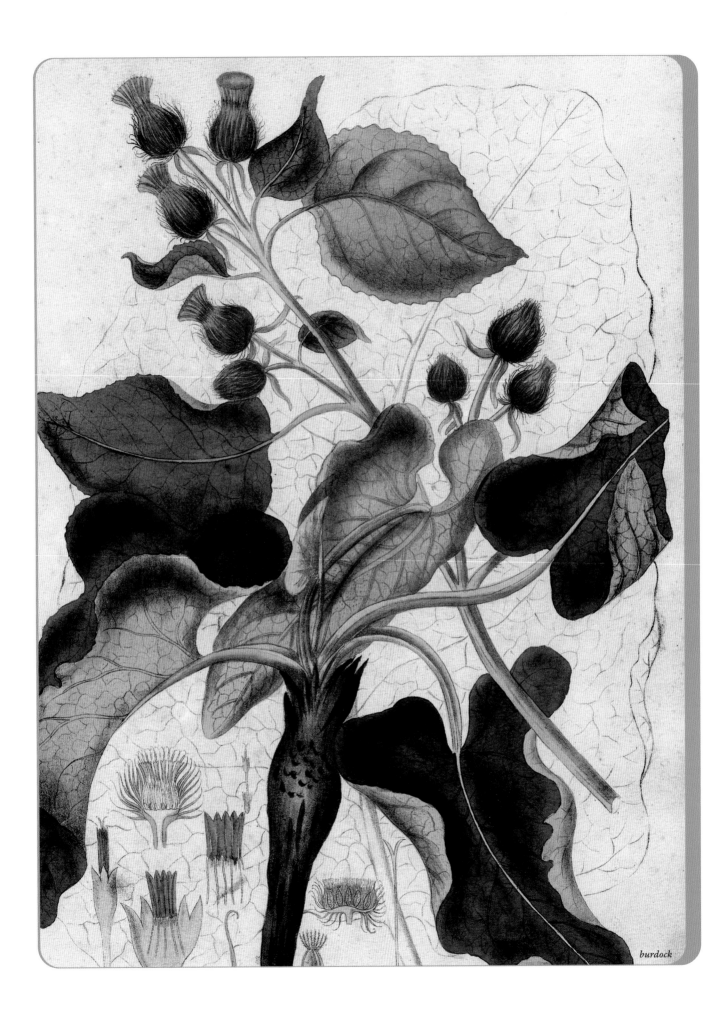

burdock

Index

Aaron's rod. *See Verbascum thapsus* (mullein)
abdomen: bloating, 166; cramps, 29; pain, 89, 272, 285
Abenaki people, 244, 284, 294
abortive effects, 147, 197, 265
abrasions, 190
abscesses, 56, 163, 169, 183, 291
absinthe, 281
acetaminophen poisoning, 280
acetic acid, 31, 60, 215
acetylcholine, 133, 203, 208, 226, 231
Achillea millefolium (yarrow), 5, 11, 12, 14, 119, 181, 209, 210, 264, 282–87, 298, 299, 300, 301, 302, 303
Achilles, 11, 283
acne, 38, 40, 62, 63, 102
Acorus calamus (calamus), 294
Actaea spp. (baneberry), 239
adaptogenic effects, 174
adaptogens, 238
addictions, 213, 222
ADHD (attention-deficit/hyperactivity disorder), 110
Aethusa cynapium (fool's parsley), 197
African violet, 251
afterbirth, expelling, 276
Agastache spp. (fragrant giant hyssop), 120–21, 281, 298, 300, 301, 303, *342*
agitation, 70
Agrimonia eupatoria (agrimony), 209
ague, 82, 262
AIDS, 29, 106, 263
albumin, 158, 232, 235
alcoholism, 110
ale hoof. *See Glechoma hederacea* (creeping Charlie)
Aleut people, 179
Algonquin people, 25, 31, 74, 182, 183, 294
alimentary canal: bleeding in, 283; inflammation, 116, 296
alkaloids, 11–12, 89, 156, 165, 195, 218, 282, 284, 286, 292
alkanes, 242, 266, 282
allantoin, 112, 180
allergic rhinitis. *See* hay fever
allergies, 5, 6, 12, 74, 185, 203, 229, 275. *See also* antiallergics
Allium stellatum (wild onion), 6, 269–70, 298, 302, 303
aloe vera, 183
alteratives. *See* depuratives
aluminum, 161

alum root. *See Geranium maculatum* (wild geranium)
Alzheimer's disease, 133
amaranth, 13
Amaranthus retroflexus (pigweed), 176–77, 300, 301, 302
amenorrhea, 26, 29, 118, 125, 139, 156, 158, 212, 216, 217, 272, 281, 286. *See also* emmenagogues
American cowslip. *See Caltha palustris* (marsh marigold); *Dodecatheon* spp. (shooting star)
American cranesbill. *See Geranium maculatum* (wild geranium)
American sarsaparilla. *See Aralia nudicaulis* (wild sarsaparilla)
American vervain. *See Verbena hastata* (blue vervain)
amino acids, 66, 145, 180, 193, 232, 254, 282
analgesics, 12, 14, 42, 58, 163, 166, 171, 172, 194, 265, 280, 284, 293, 294. *See also* pain
anal inflammation or irritation, 65, 115, 199
Anaphalis margaritacea (pearly everlasting), 167–68, 298, 300
anaphrodisiacs, 294
anemia, 76, 77, 254, 274
anesthetics, 74
angelicin, 91, 92, 93
angina pectoris, 287. *See also* chest
anise hyssop. *See Agastache* spp. (fragrant giant hyssop)
Anishinabe people. *See* Ojibwe people
anodynes, 26, 143, 152, 163, 241, 250. *See also* pain
anorexia, 42
anthelmintics, 12, 14, 15, 48, 133, 144, 147, 166, 197, 210, 235, 247, 280. *See also* vermifuges
anthocyanins, 14, 191, 275
anthraquinones, 12, 75, 86, 104, 105, 107, 204, 218, 220
antiabortives, 34–35
antiallergics, 54, 124, 166, 202, 284
anti-arrhythmics, 29
antibacterials, 12, 14, 47, 95, 105, 115, 183, 192, 220, 222, 256
antibiotics (herbal), 76, 183, 194, 245
antibradykinin, 105
anticancer effects, 14, 125, 200, 250, 256. *See also* cancer
anticariogenics, 166
anticatarrhals, 12, 48, 96, 141, 152, 185, 241
anticholinergics, 105
anticoagulants, 12, 74
anticonstipationals, 77
anticonvulsives, 42, 43, 92, 149–50, 166, 213
antidementia activity, 203
antidepressants, 222

℔

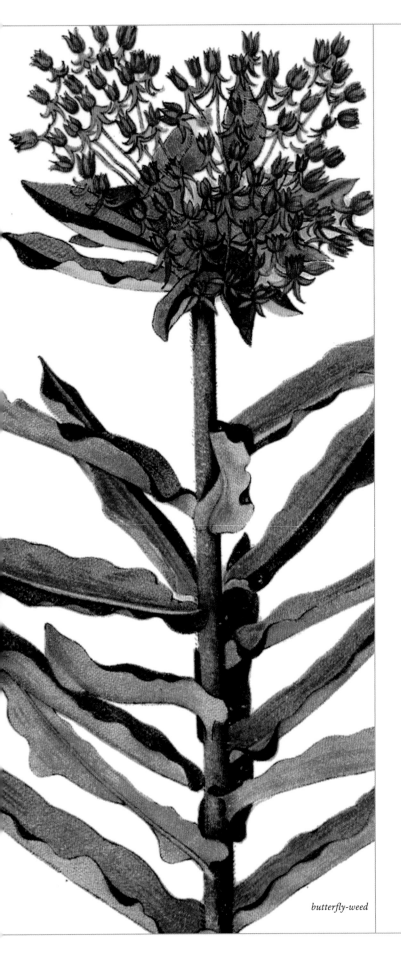

butterfly-weed

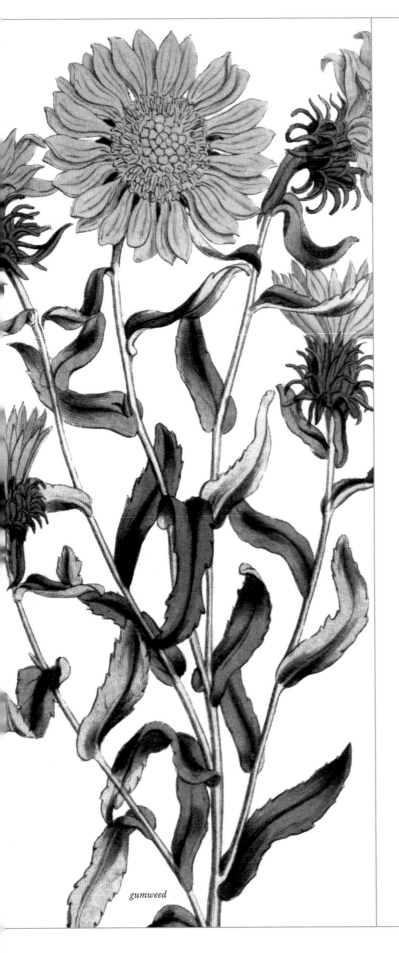

gumweed

freezing plants, 8
fructose, 100, 104
fuller's herb. *See Saponaria officinalis* (bouncing bet)
fungicides, 265
fungistatics, 132
furanocoumarins, 12, 91, 92, 282
furunculosis, 62

galactagogues, 41, 153, 178–79, 230
Galium aparine (cleavers), 40, 65, 77, 86–88,
    163, 298, 299, 300, 301, 302, 303
gallbladder, 39, 42, 48, 97, 101, 203, 280, 291, 296
gallic acid, 44, 52, 66, 86, 108, 114, 117, 215, 243, 260
gallstones, 95, 152
gamma-linolenic acid (GLA), 108, 109, 110
garlic, 5, 6
gastric catarrh, 125, 236
gastric discomfort, 109, 143, 257, 297
gastric hemorrhage, 207
gastric inflammation, 141, 181
gastric secretion stimulants, 62
gastric ulcers, 261, 285
gastritis, 14, 59, 95, 101, 115
gastroenteritis, 115
gastrointestinal cramps, 179
gastrointestinal inflammation, 142
gastrointestinal pain, 257
gastrointestinal tract atony, 280
gastroprotectives, 166
gein, 186
genitourinary afflictions, 128, 139, 149, 194
George, Edgar J., 52–53
geraniol, 41, 159, 257, 259
Geranium maculatum (wild geranium),
    260–63, 298, 300, 301, 302
German Commission E, 90, 124, 141,
    157, 182, 229, 285, 286
German rampion. *See Oenothera bien-
    nis* (evening primrose)
Geum triflorum (prairie smoke), 186–88, 300
giant hogweed. *See Heracleum* spp. (cow-parsnip)
Giardia, 181, 279
Gibbons, Euell, 3, 4, 10, 11, 60, 69, 84,
    109, 180, 228, 274, 293
gill-over-the ground. *See Glechoma hed-
    eracea* (creeping Charlie)
Gilmore, Melvin, 7
gingivitis, 29–30
Gitksan people, 92, 112
glaucoma cautions, 30
Glechoma hederacea (creeping Charlie),
    94–96, 298, 300, 301, 303
gleet, 293

glycosides, 12, 52, 65, 76, 78, 143, 148, 151, 153,
    165, 169, 178, 192, 195, 271, 273
goiter, 83
goldenrod. *See Solidago* spp. (goldenrod)
golden seal, 67
gonorrhea, 47, 87, 209, 262, 275, 294
goosefoot. *See Chenopodium album* (lamb's quarters)
goosegrass. *See Galium aparine* (cleavers)
Gosiute people, 55, 89, 129, 265, 286
gout, 12, 42, 76, 95, 102, 118, 125, 139, 163, 185, 196, 203,
    210, 217, 219, 229, 231, 234, 250, 255, 275, 280
gravel root. *See Eutrochium* spp. (joe-pye weed)
Graves' disease, 52–53, 54, 83
great willow herb. *See Epilobium angustifolium* (fireweed)
Green People movement, 16–17
Grindelia squarrosa (gumweed), 126–28,
    298, 299, 300, 301, 302, 303, *354*
gromwell. *See Lithospermum* spp. (puccoon)
Gros Ventre people, 279
ground ivy. *See Glechoma hederacea* (creeping Charlie)
guggul, 40
gum, 38, 44, 50, 260
gumplant. *See Grindelia squarrosa* (gumweed)
gums: discomfort of, 92; infection, 261, 264;
    inflammation, 182, 249; sore, 82, 182,
    275; spongy, 82, 106; tonic for, 255
gumweed. *See Grindelia squarrosa* (gumweed)
Gunn, John C., 17, 41, 138, 153, 216, 220, 247, 272

hair: dry, 110; lice infestation, 90, 119,
    128; loss, 174, 230, 231
halitosis, 268
hands, chapped, 172
hangovers, 249, 296
Hartwell, Jonathan, 63, 206, 250
harvesting guidelines, 6–7
hawk's beard, 129
hawkweed. *See Hieracium* spp. (hawkweed)
hawthorn. *See Crataegus* spp. (hawthorn)
hay fever, 12, 37, 229, 231, 284
headache, 25, 42, 58–59, 69, 95, 97, 113, 118, 127,
    146, 156, 159, 168, 175, 203, 213, 217, 240, 249,
    257, 258, 265, 267, 279, 280, 284, 294, 296
heal-all. *See Prunella vulgaris* (self-heal)
heart: attack, 109, 158; disease, 194; disorders, 213; dispir-
    ited, 121; palpitations, 222; problems, 32, 141, 144,
    157, 160, 234, 250, 255, 265, 294; *qi* constraint, 128;
    rapid heartbeat, 53; relaxant, 128; weak, 202, 265
heartburn, 101, 289, 296
heart-leaved aster. *See Aster* spp. (aster)
heart's-ease. *See Polygonum persicaria* (lady's thumb)
heartweed. *See Polygonum persicaria* (lady's thumb)
heat exhaustion, 77
heating energies, 27, 217

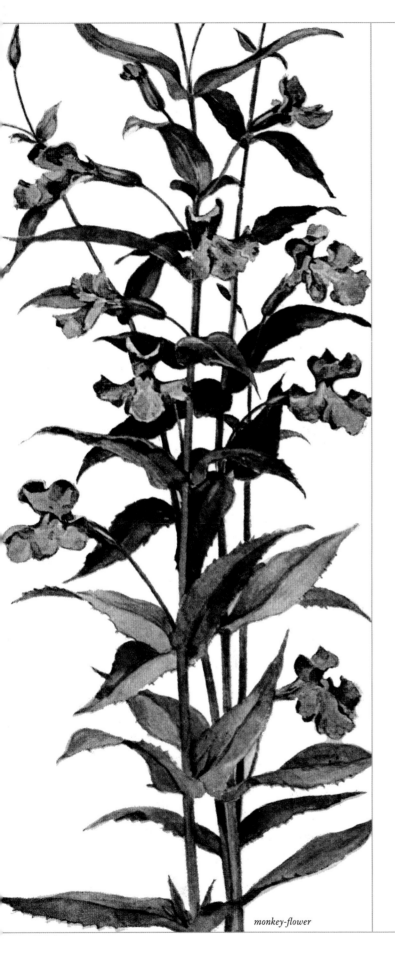

monkey-flower

lung(s): fluid in, 255; hemorrhage, 34, 190, 262; infection, 113, 152; inflammation, 29; problems, 34

Lust, Benedict, 17

Lust, John, 17, 65, 109, 144, 177, 289

luteal tonics, 43

lutein, 254, 273

luteinizing actions, 42

luteinizing hormone (LH), 54

luteolin, 52, 86, 94, 99, 100, 117, 126, 161, 178, 180, 193, 195, 212, 242, 243, 264, 282

Lycopus americanus (cut-leaved water horehound), *53*

Lycopus spp. (bugleweed), 52–54, 80, 83, 157, 158, 298, 300, 302

Lyme disease, 5, 244

lymphadenitis, 87

lymphangitis, 39

lymphatics, 198

lymphedema, 87

lymph nodes: congestion, 251; swollen, 38–39, 87, 163, 170, 198, 203, 250, 259

lymphoma, 50

Lysimachia spp. (yellow loosestrife), 290–91, 299, 300

Lythrum salicaria (purple loosestrife), 114, 191–92, 298, 300, 302, 303, *370*

maca, 174

magnesium, 10, 41, 60, 76, 78, 100, 108, 161, 193, 198, 201, 212, 264, 273, 282

Mahuna people, 37, 42, 174, 183

Maidu people, 118, 154, 174, 179

Makah people, 270

malaria, 15, 29, 45, 70, 166, 234, 281

Malecite people, 29, 56, 74, 163, 217, 275, 284

malic acid, 27, 161, 204, 208, 215

manganese, 10, 69, 76, 100, 104, 161, 201, 226, 254

marsh marigold. *See Caltha palustris* (marsh marigold)

marsh milkweed. *See Asclepias incarnata* (swamp milkweed)

mastalgia, 109, 110

masterwort. *See Heracleum* spp. (cow-parsnip)

mastitis, 102, 169, 263

Matricaria discoidea (pineapple-weed), 14, 178–79, 298, 300, 301, 302, 303

Matricaria recutita (chamomile), 5, 178

Mausert, Otto, 17

Mazatec people, 88

McIntosh, John, 48, 236

McQuade-Crawford, Amanda, 34, 102

meadow salsify. *See Tragopogon* spp. (yellow goatsbeard)

measles, 70, 188, 257

Medical Flora (Rafinesque), 17

melancholy, 121

melanoma, 50, 103

melatonin, 193

Melissa officinalis (lemon balm), 52, 54, 83, 121, 157

Mendocino people, 146

Menomini people, xi, 34, 41, 45, 68, 70, 98, 113, 174, 189, 210, 216, 220, 237, 253, 264, 284

menopause, 42, 199, 220, 294

menorrhagia, 54, 115, 118, 119, 176, 205, 209, 210, 262, 283, 287, 290

menstruation: backache, 118; bloating, 229; cramps, 12, 34, 42, 118, 166, 179, 286; excitant of, 195; irregular, 275; painful, 113, 156, 216, 220; problems, 118; profuse, 34; promotion of, 70, 125

Mentha arvensis (wild mint), 109, 168, 264–65, 298, 299, 300, 301, 303

menthol, 15, 264, 265

Meskwaki people, xi, 34, 37, 43, 48, 89, 91, 98, 102, 129, 132, 137, 146, 160, 216, 220, 224, 235, 241, 257, 258, 260, 261, 263, 267, 272, 276, 277, 279

methyl salicylate, 198, 249, 250

metrorrhagia, 209

Mexican Americans, 106

Mexican people, 217, 241

Meyer, Joseph, 43

Micmac people, 29, 32, 56, 58, 59, 74, 87, 88, 162, 217, 275, 284, 294

migraines, 42, 109, 240, 284

mild arssmart. *See Polygonum persicaria* (lady's thumb)

milfoil. *See Achillea millefolium* (yarrow)

milk sickness, 49

milkweed. *See Asclepias syriaca* (milkweed)

Mimulus spp. (monkey-flower), 154–55, 300, 303, *358*

minerals: boron, 100, 108; calcium, 41, 76, 78, 100, 104, 108, 136, 161, 165, 191, 193, 198, 201, 204, 212, 226, 254, 260, 264, 266, 273, 282, 288; iron, 60, 68, 76, 78, 94, 100, 104, 108, 134, 149, 161, 176, 193, 201, 204, 208, 226, 229, 254, 264, 266, 273, 282; lithium, 193; magnesium, 41, 60, 76, 78, 100, 108, 161, 193, 198, 201, 212, 264, 273, 282; manganese, 69, 76, 100, 104, 161, 201, 226, 254; phosphorus, 22, 72, 76, 78, 94, 100, 104, 198, 221, 226, 228, 254, 266, 282, 288, 295; potassium, 22, 69, 72, 76, 78, 94, 100, 102, 104, 108, 180, 193, 195, 198, 201, 204, 208, 212, 226, 232, 264, 266, 273, 282, 288, 295; selenium, 68, 100, 104, 136, 161, 270; silica, 161, 180, 226, 230, 278, 282; silicon, 60, 76, 94, 100; sodium, 100, 104, 108, 161, 193, 201, 226; sulfur, 76, 94, 160, 226, 254, 269, 273; zinc, 76, 94, 100, 104, 180, 201, 254, 264

mint, 15. *See also Mentha arvensis* (wild mint)

Mitchella repens (partridgeberry), 156

Miwok people, 117, 118, 119, 179, 279

Mohawk people, 153, 168, 264

Mohegan people, 34, 45, 70, 105, 133, 153, 162, 183, 197, 210, 244, 272, 280

moistening effects, 76, 126, 249

molluscicides, 150

molybdenum, 94

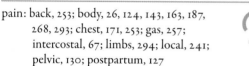

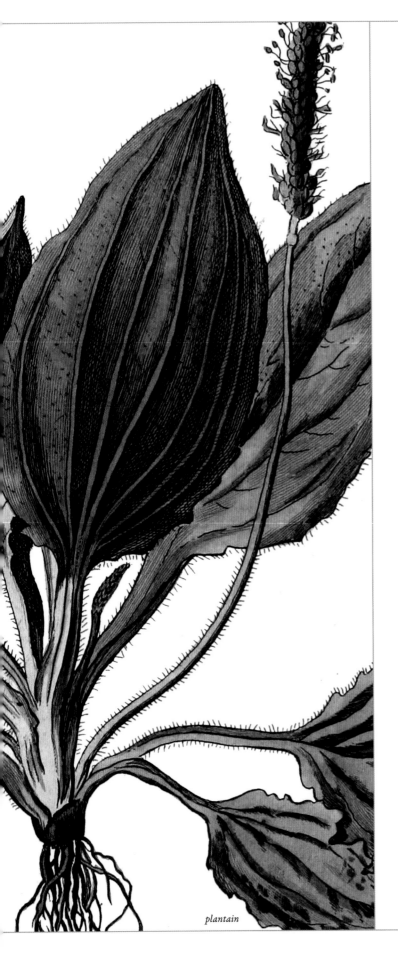

plantain

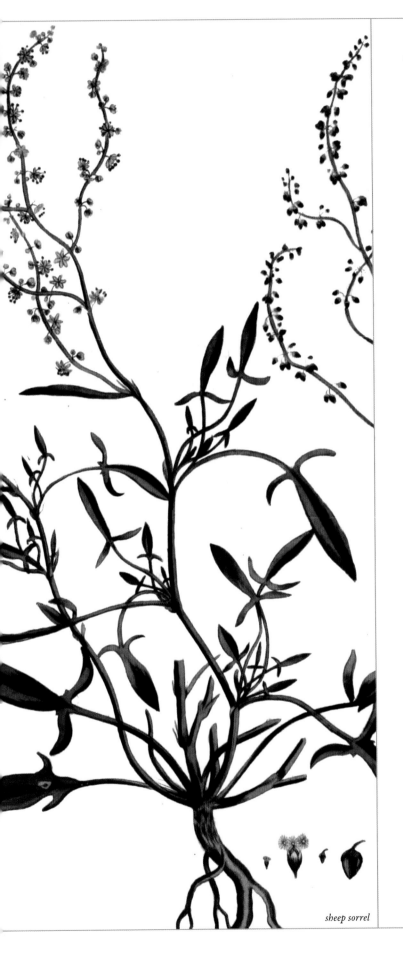

sheep sorrel

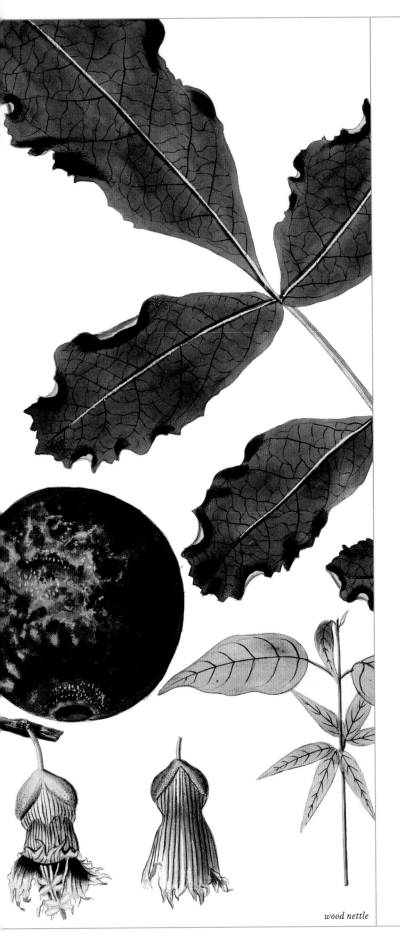

wood nettle

wounds, 11, 12, 25, 31, 39, 56, 58, 68, 74, 76, 82,
  92, 106, 109, 112, 118, 123, 124, 127, 146, 166,
  171, 182, 183, 187, 189, 192, 194, 202, 205,
  209, 228, 239, 262, 271–72, 276, 283, 290
woundwort. *See Prunella vulgaris* (self-heal)

X

Xanthoxylum americanum (prickly ash), 197

Y

yarrow. *See Achillea millefolium* (yarrow)
yeast infections, 102, 121
yellow fever, 45
yellow goatsbeard. *See Tragopogon*
  spp. (yellow goatsbeard)

yellowjacket stings, 123, 183
yellow loosestrife. *See Lysimachia* spp. (yellow loosestrife)
yellow oxalis. *See Oxalis* spp. (yellow wood-sorrel)
yellow pond-lily. *See Nuphar* spp. (yellow pond-lily)
yellow salsify. *See Tragopogon* spp. (yellow goatsbeard)
yellow snapdragon. *See Linaria vul-
  garis* (butter-and-eggs)
yellow wood-sorrel. *See Oxalis* spp. (yellow wood-sorrel)
Yuki people, 211

Z

Zigadenus venenosus (death camas), 270
zinc, 10, 76, 94, 100, 104, 108, 180, 201, 254, 264
Zulu people, 147
Zuni people, 25, 123, 124, 234, 244

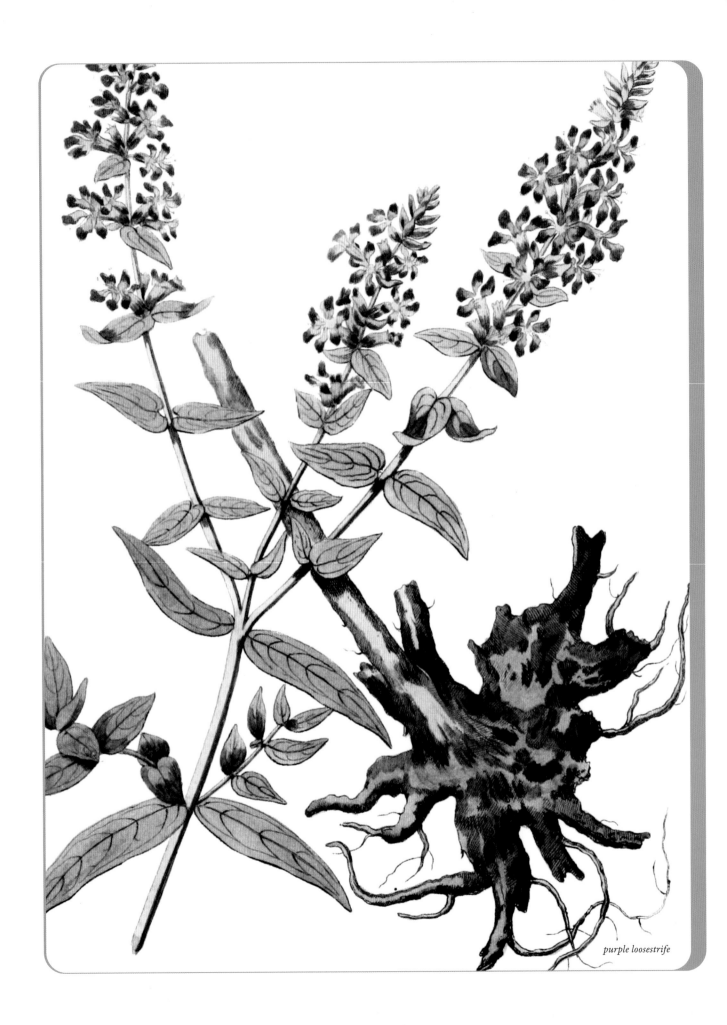

purple loosestrife

Image Credits

Images not listed below are in the public domain. Many come from the journal *Flora Batava*, vols. 1–28 (Amsterdam, 1800–1934) or Otto Wilhelm Thomé, *Flora von Deutschland, Österreich und der Schweiz* (Gera, Germany, 1885).

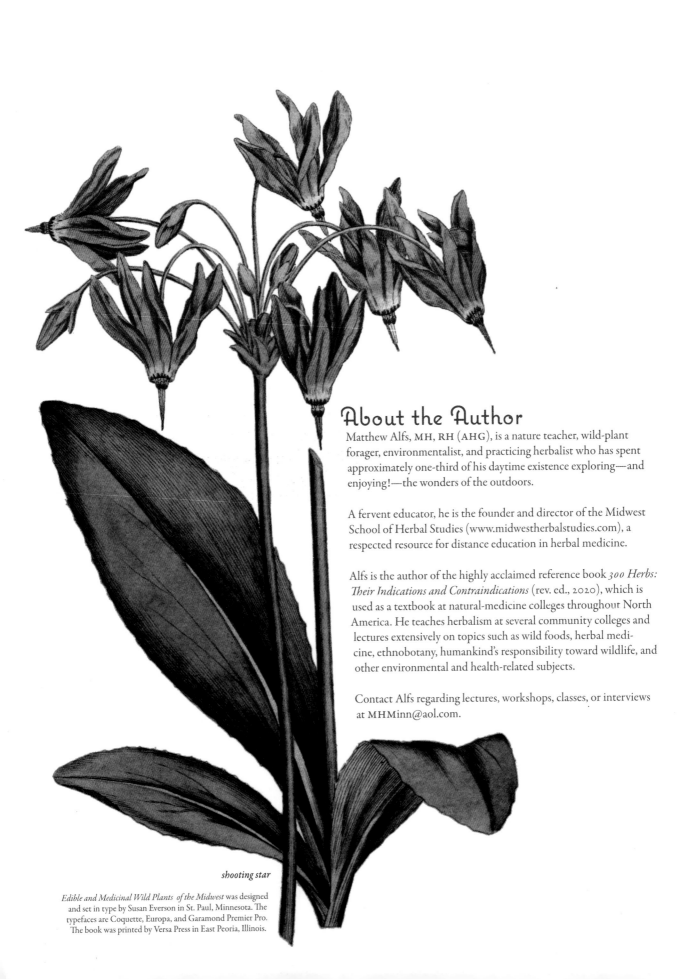

About the Author

Matthew Alfs, MH, RH (AHG), is a nature teacher, wild-plant forager, environmentalist, and practicing herbalist who has spent approximately one-third of his daytime existence exploring—and enjoying!—the wonders of the outdoors.

A fervent educator, he is the founder and director of the Midwest School of Herbal Studies (www.midwestherbalstudies.com), a respected resource for distance education in herbal medicine.

Alfs is the author of the highly acclaimed reference book *300 Herbs: Their Indications and Contraindications* (rev. ed., 2020), which is used as a textbook at natural-medicine colleges throughout North America. He teaches herbalism at several community colleges and lectures extensively on topics such as wild foods, herbal medicine, ethnobotany, humankind's responsibility toward wildlife, and other environmental and health-related subjects.

Contact Alfs regarding lectures, workshops, classes, or interviews at MHMinn@aol.com.

shooting star

Edible and Medicinal Wild Plants of the Midwest was designed and set in type by Susan Everson in St. Paul, Minnesota. The typefaces are Coquette, Europa, and Garamond Premier Pro. The book was printed by Versa Press in East Peoria, Illinois.